Cancer Pain

Nearly one in three people will be diagnosed with cancer. Although pain continues to be widely feared by cancer patients, knowledge about the causes and management of cancer pain has increased dramatically in recent years and many new treatment options are available. This comprehensive book discusses the unique characteristics of cancer pain, including its pathophysiology, clinical assessment, diagnosis, pharmacological management, and nonpharmacological treatment. Internationally recognized leaders in cancer pain research apply their first-hand knowledge in summarizing the principal issues in the clinical management of cancer pain. This state-of-the-art book cohesively addresses the full range of disciplines regularly involved in cancer pain management including pharmacology, communication studies, and psychology. *Cancer Pain* is a scholarly but accessible text that will be an essential resource for physicians, nurses, and medical students who treat suffering from cancer pain.

Eduardo D. Bruera, MD, is Professor of Medicine, F. T. McGraw Chair in the Treatment of Cancer, and Chairman of the Department of Palliative Care and Rehabilitation Medicine at The University of Texas M. D. Anderson Cancer Center in Houston. Formerly the Director of the University of Alberta's Division of Palliative Care Medicine, Dr. Bruera researches amphetamine derivatives, patient-controlled analgesia, and methadone for cancer pain, as well as delirium, dementia, and dyspnea in terminal cancer.

Russell K. Portenoy, MD, is Chairman of the Department of Pain Medicine and Palliative Care at Beth Israel Medical Center and Professor of Neurology at the Albert Einstein College of Medicine in New York. Formerly the Co-Chief of the Pain and Palliative Care Service at Memorial Sloan-Kettering Cancer Center, Dr. Portenoy is a past president of the American Pain Society and recent recipient of the American Academy of Pain Medicine's Founder's Award. His research is devoted to pain and analgesics, symptom assessment, and quality of life.

Cancer Pain

Assessment and Management

EDITED BY

Eduardo D. Bruera, MD

The University of Texas
M. D. Anderson Cancer Center
Houston, Texas

Russell K. Portenoy, MD

Beth Israel Medical Center and
Albert Einstein College of Medicine
New York, New York

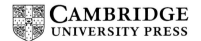

CAMBRIDGE
UNIVERSITY PRESS

PUBLISHED BY THE PRESS SYNDICATE OF THE UNIVERSITY OF CAMBRIDGE
The Pitt Building, Trumpington Street, Cambridge, United Kingdom

CAMBRIDGE UNIVERSITY PRESS
The Edinburgh Building, Cambridge CB2 2RU, UK
40 West 20th Street, New York, NY 10011-4211, USA
477 Williamstown Road, Port Melbourne, VIC 3207, Australia
Ruiz de Alarcón 13, 28014 Madrid, Spain
Dock House, The Waterfront, Cape Town 8001, South Africa

http://www.cambridge.org

First published 2003

Printed in the United States of America

Typeface Times Roman 10.25/13pt   *System* QuarkXPress™   [HT]

A catalog record for this book is available from the British Library.

Library of Congress Cataloging in Publication Data

Cancer pain / edited by Eduardo D. Bruera, Russell K. Portenoy.
    p. cm.
  Includes bibliographical references and index.
  ISBN 0 521 77332 6
  1. Cancer pain. I. Bruera, Eduardo. II. Portenoy, Russell K.
RC262 .C291184 2003
616.99′4 – dc21   2002035072

ISBN 0 521 77332 6   hardback

To Susan Portenoy and Ed, Sofia, and Sebastian Bruera;
their love and support make our work possible.

Contents

Contributors

Anderson, Karen O., PhD
Assistant Professor
Department of Symptom Research
Division of Anesthesiology & Critical Care
The University of Texas M. D. Anderson Cancer Center
Houston, Texas

Ballo, Matthew, MD
Assistant Professor
Department of Radiation Oncology
The University of Texas M. D. Anderson Cancer Center
Houston, Texas

Berde, Charles B., MD, PhD
Director
Pain Treatment Service
Children's Hospital
Professor
Department of Anesthesia
Harvard University Medical School
Boston, Massachusetts

Breitbart, William S., MD
Chief, Psychiatry Service and Attending Psychiatrist
Department of Psychiatry and Behavioral Sciences
Memorial Sloan-Kettering Cancer Center
Professor of Clinical Psychiatry
Weill Medical College of Cornell University
New York, New York

Bruera, Eduardo D., MD
Chairman
Department of Palliative Care & Rehabilitation Medicine
Professor of Medicine
The University of Texas M. D. Anderson Cancer Center
Houston, Texas

Brune, Kay, MD
Professor
Department of Experimental and Clinical Pharmacology
    and Toxicology
Friedrich Alexander University Erlangen-Nuremberg
Erlangen, Germany

Cleeland, Charles S., PhD
McCullough Professor of Cancer Research
Chairman
Department of Symptom Research
Division of Anesthesiology & Critical Care
The University of Texas M. D. Anderson Cancer Center
Houston, Texas

Collins, John J., MB BS, PhD, FRACP
Head
Pain and Palliative Care Service
The Children's Hospital at Westmead
Sydney, New South Wales, Australia

Conn, Maria, MD, MBA
Assistant Attending and Clinical Instructor
Harlem Hospital Center, an affiliate of Columbia
    University School of Medicine
New York, New York

Cousins, Michael J., MB BS, MD, FANZCA, FRCA, FFPMANZCA, FAChPM(RACP)
Professor and Head
University of Sydney Pain Management and Research
    Center
Department of Anesthesia and Pain Management
Royal North Shore Hospital
St. Leonards, New South Wales, Australia

Crane, Christopher, MD
Assistant Professor
Department of Radiation Oncology
The University of Texas M. D. Anderson Cancer Center
Houston, Texas

Dahl, June L., PhD
Professor
Department of Pharmacology
University of Wisconsin-Madison School of Medicine
Madison, Wisconsin

Delclos, Marc, MD
Assistant Professor
Department of Radiation Oncology
The University of Texas M. D. Anderson Cancer Center
Houston, Texas

Dickenson, Anthony H., PhD
Professor
Department of Pharmacology
University College London
London, United Kingdom

Farrar, John T., MD
Senior Scholar
Center for Clinical Epidemiology and Biostatistics
Adjunct Assistant Professor
Department of Biostatistics and Epidemiology
Adjunct Assistant Professor
Department of Anesthesia
University of Pennsylvania School of Medicine
Philadelphia, Pennsylvania

Fine, Perry G., MD
The Pain Management Center
University of Utah Health Sciences Center
Professor
Department of Anesthesiology
University of Utah School of Medicine
Salt Lake City, Utah

Fisch, Michael J., MD, MPH
Assistant Professor
Center Medical Director
Department of Palliative Care and Rehabilition
Division of Cancer Medicine
The University of Texas M. D. Anderson Cancer Center
Houston, Texas

Gillis, Theresa A., MD
Attending Physician
Christiana Care Health System and the Helen F. Graham
    Cancer Center
Newark, Delaware

Glajchen, Myra, DSW
Director
Institute for Education and Research in Pain and
    Palliative Care
Department of Pain Medicine and Palliative Care
Beth Israel Medical Center
Instructor
Department of Neurology
Albert Einstein College of Medicine
New York, New York

Halpern, Scott D., MD, PhD
Fellow
Center for Clinical Epidemiology and Biostatistics
University of Pennsylvania School of Medicine
Philadelphia, Pennsylvania

Hassenbusch, Samuel J., MD, PhD
Professor
Department of Neurosurgery
The University of Texas M. D. Anderson Cancer Center
Houston, Texas

Hearn, Julie, PhD
Research Officer
Department of Palliative Care and Policy
Guy's, King's and St. Thomas' School of Medicine and
    St. Christopher's Hospice
London, United Kingdom

Higginson, Irene J., BMBS, PhD
Head
Department of Palliative Care and Policy
Guy's, King's & St. Thomas' School of Medicine and
    St. Christopher's Hospice
London, United Kingdom

Hinz, Burkhard, PhD
Department of Experimental and Clinical Pharmacology
    and Toxicology
Friedrich Alexander University Erlangen-Nuremberg
Erlangen, Germany

Inturrisi, Charles E., PhD
Professor
Department of Pharmacology
Weill Medical College of Cornell University
New York, New York

Janjan, Nora A., MD
Professor
Department of Radiation Oncology
The University of Texas M. D. Anderson Cancer Center
Houston, Texas

Johns, Lauren
Department of Neurosurgery
The University of Texas M. D. Anderson Cancer Center
Houston, Texas

Kirsh, Kenneth L., PhD
Research Associate
Symptom Management and Palliative Care Program
Markey Cancer Center
University of Kentucky
Lexington, Kentucky

Lawlor, Peter G., MB
Consultant
Palliative Medicine
St. Francis Hospice, Mater Misericordiae Hospital, and
    James Connolly Memorial Hospital
Dublin, Ireland
Assistant Professor (Adjunct)
Division of Palliative Care Medicine
Department of Oncology
University of Alberta
Edmonton, Alberta, Canada

Lesage, Pauline, MD
Attending Physician
Department of Pain Medicine and Palliative Care
Beth Israel Medical Center
New York, New York

Moulin, Dwight E., MD, FRCP
Associate Professor
Departments of Clinical Neurological Sciences and
    Oncology
University of Western Ontario
London, Ontario, Canada

Mullen, Vincent, MD
Assistant Professor
Department of Psychiatry
University of Kentucky College of Medicine
Lexington, Kentucky

Novy, Diane M., PhD
Associate Professor
Departments of Anesthesiology and Psychiatry and
    Behavioral Sciences
The University of Texas M. D. Anderson Cancer Center
Houston, Texas

O'Mahony, Sean, MB, BCH, BAO
Medical Director
Palliative Care Service
Montefiore Medical Center
Albert Einstein College of Medicine
Bronx, New York

Passik, Steven D., PhD
Director
Symptom Management and Palliative Care Program
Markey Cancer Center
Associate Professor
Departments of Internal Medicine and Behavioral
    Sciences
University of Kentucky
Lexington, Kentucky

Portenoy, Russell K., MD
Chairman
Department of Pain Medicine and Palliative Care
Beth Israel Medical Center
Professor of Neurology
Albert Einstein College of Medicine
New York, New York

Ripamonti, Carla, MD
Vice-Director of Pain Therapy & Palliative Care
Rehabilitation & Palliative Care Division
National Cancer Institute of Milan
Milan, Italy

Rouhani, Marjaneh, MD
Counselor
Behavioral Health Care
Battle Creek, Michigan

Rowe, Germaine, MD, CAc, FAAPMR
Attending Physician
Pain Management, Healthcare Associates in Medicine, PC
Medical Director of Physical Therapy
Neuroscience Associates of New York, a Division of
    Healthcare Associates in Medicine, PC
Attending Physician
Department of Rehabilitation Medicine
Staten Island University Hospital
Staten Island, New York

Saifollahi, Jahandar, MD
Resident
Michigan State University School of Medicine
Kalamazoo, Michigan

Suzuki, Rie, BSc, PhD
Senior Research Fellow
Department of Pharmacology
University College
London, United Kingdom

Sweeney, Catherine, MD, MB, MICGP
Research Fellow
Department of Palliative Care & Rehabilitation
    Medicine
The University of Texas M. D. Anderson Cancer Center
Houston, Texas

**Walker, Suellen M., MB BS, MMed(PM), MSc,
    FANZCA, FFPMANZCA**
Clinical Senior Lecturer
University of Sydney Pain Management and Research
    Centre
Department of Anesthesia and Pain Management
Royal North Shore Hospital
St. Leonards, New South Wales, Australia

Watling, Christopher J., MD, FRCP
Assistant Professor
Departments of Clinical Neurological Sciences and
    Oncology
University of Western Ontario
London, Ontario, Canada

Wollner, David I., MD, FACP, AGSF
Director
Palliative Care Services
Veterans Administration New York Harbor Healthcare
    System
Brooklyn, New York

Zeilhofer, Hanns Ulrich, MD
Professor
Department of Experimental and Clinical Pharmacology
    and Toxicology
Friedrich Alexander University Erlangen-Nuremberg
Erlangen, Germany

Preface

Approximately one in three individuals in the developed world will be diagnosed with cancer. The incidence of cancer is also increasing rapidly in developing countries. Approximately 50% of patients in developed countries and 70% of patients in developing countries will die as a result of their cancer. More than 80% of those who die of cancer will develop severe pain. The increased frequency of cancer around the world suggests that the burden of cancer pain is likely to increase dramatically over the next decade.

A large number of studies have documented that cancer pain is poorly assessed and managed in many patients. The main reason for these problems is inadequate health care professional education.

The purpose of this book is to provide a comprehensive, clinically oriented, and scholarly review of all aspects of this complex and multidimensional problem. It is our hope that this comprehensive text will lead to improved understanding in treating this devastating disease and will contribute to improvement in care.

Eduardo D. Bruera
Russell K. Portenoy

SECTION I MECHANISMS AND EPIDEMIOLOGY

1 Nociception: basic principles

RIE SUZUKI AND ANTHONY H. DICKENSON
University College London

Introduction

Pain has been a major concern in the clinic for many decades. In recent years, considerable progress has been made with respect to our understanding of both acute and chronic pain mechanisms. This has largely been attributed to advancements in molecular biology and genomic techniques, as well as the use of animal models, which has allowed us to explore potential targets for pain. This has fundamentally altered our understanding of the pathophysiology of pain mechanisms and has led to the hope of development of novel analgesics.

The study of the receptor systems involved in the transmission of pain and its modulation involves investigation of processes occurring at the peripheral endings of sensory neurons, as well as central events. The mechanisms of inflammatory and neuropathic pain are different from those of acute pain, and there is considerable plasticity in both the transmission and modulating systems in these prolonged pain states. The search for new treatments for these pain states requires the development of valid animal models. For such models to be valid, a number of criteria must be fulfilled. First, the model must provide reproducible and quantifiable behavioral data. Second, the model must produce behaviors in the animal that resemble some of the pain syndromes observed in humans (e.g. allodynia, hyperalgesia). Third, the behavioral data must correlate with pain responses in humans. Through the use of these animal models, we can broaden our understanding of pain mechanisms and possibly identify or develop potential agents for treatment.

Mechanisms of pain and analgesia

The anatomy and physiology of pain

The somatosensory primary afferent fiber, which conveys sensory information to the spinal cord, can be grouped into several classes, according to the transduction properties of the individual nerve fiber. The properties of each afferent fiber are summarized in Table 1.1.

The afferent fibers differ in their conduction velocities and degrees of myelination, and can be distinguished by their diameter. The large diameter $A\beta$-fibers are myelinated by Schwann cells and hence have a fast conduction velocity. This group of nerve fibers innervates receptors in the dermis and is involved in the transmission of low-threshold, non-noxious information, such as touch. The $A\delta$-fiber is less densely myelinated and conveys both non-noxious and noxious sensory information. The unmyelinated C-fiber conveys high-threshold noxious inputs and has the slowest conduction velocity of all three fiber types.

On entry into the spinal cord, each primary afferent fiber ($A\beta$-, $A\delta$- or C-fiber) exhibits a specific termination pattern in the dorsal horn (Fig. 1.1). This has been studied extensively through the use of use of specific markers. Dorsal root afferents send most of their collaterals into the segment of entry. However, there is also a degree of rostrocaudal distribution, and some collaterals may spread to several segments above or below the target segment. Thus, there is an anatomical substrate for the spreading of pain beyond the segment in which it originates.

The large diameter $A\beta$-fiber enters the spinal dorsal horn through the medial division of the dorsal root and

Table 1.1. *Classification of somatosensory primary afferent fibers innervating the skin*

Primary afferent fiber type	Mean diameter (μm)	Myelination	Mean conduction velocity (m/s)
$A\beta$	6–12	Myelinated	25–70
$A\delta$	1–5	Thin myelination	10–30
C	0.2–1.5	None	<2.5

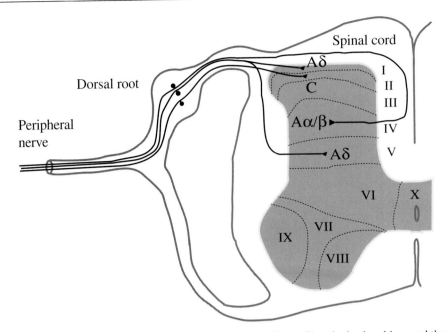

Fig. 1.1. Cross-section of the lumbar spinal cord illustrating the termination sites of afferent fibers in the dorsal horn and the organization of the gray matter into laminae I to X.

terminates in laminae III and IV, where it forms a characteristic termination pattern (1). The densest arborization appears to occur in lamina III. Some also extend to laminae VIII and IX of the ventral horn, where they synapse directly onto motor neurons and form the basis of monosynaptic reflexes (2). The terminals of Aδ-fibers, on the other hand, form a plexus at the surface of the spinal cord in laminae I and IIo. Unmyelinated C-fibers enter the spinal cord through the lateral part of the dorsal white matter and terminate in the superficial dorsal horn. Current evidence suggests that lamina II is the main termination area for cutaneous primary afferent C-fibers, whereas that for Aδ-fibers is in lamina I (1).

Pharmacology of pain transmission

Peripheral events

The transmission of acute pain involves activation of sensory receptors on peripheral C-fibers, the nociceptors. However, once tissue damage and inflammation occur, the actions of prostanoids, bradykinin and 5-hydroxytryptamine (5HT), on their excitatory receptors play a major role in sensitization and activation of C-fibers (Fig. 1.2). Other factors, such as nerve growth factor (NGF) and cytokines are also important at the peripheral level, and resultant changes in the phenotype of the sensory neurons may be another important process. C-fibers have unique sodium channels with very low tetrodotoxin

(TTX) sensitivity and some C-fibers are "sleeping"; that is, they do not respond to natural stimuli until after inflammation. The former channels may become important targets for drugs.

These polymodal C-fiber receptors can be selectively activated by noxious thermal and mechanical stimuli. In the case of activation by noxious heat, we now suspect that a recently characterized channel that also responds to the extract of hot peppers, capsaicin, may be responsi-

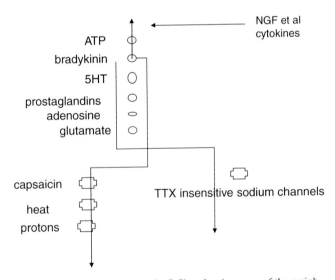

Fig. 1.2. A schematic diagram of a C-fiber showing some of the peripheral mediators of pain and inflammation in the periphery.

ble for the generation of action potentials after application of heat. Other channels have been identified that respond to protons, namely, acid sensing ion channels (ASICs). In inflammation, the pH of the tissue is known to be low.

Thus, the peripheral terminals of small diameter neurons may be excited by a number of endogenous chemical mediators, especially in conditions of tissue damage. These can be released from local non-neuronal cells, the afferent fibers themselves, and from products from immune cells triggered by activation of the body's defense mechanisms. These chemical mediators then interact to cause a sensitization of nociceptors so that afferent activity induced by a given stimulus is increased. This produces primary hyperalgesia, a zone of increased sensitivity to painful stimuli in the center of the damaged tissue (3,4).

One of the most important components in inflammation is the production of arachidonic acid metabolites. Arachidonic acid, a component of cell membranes, is liberated by phospholipase A2 and is subsequently metabolized by two main pathways controlled by two enzymes, cyclooxygenase (COX) and lipoxygenase. This metabolism gives rise to a large number of eicosanoids, (leukotrienes, thromboxanes, prostacyclins, and prostaglandins). These chemicals are still poorly understood, but it is clear that they do not normally activate nociceptors directly but, by contrast, reduce the C-fiber threshold and so sensitize them to other mediators and stimuli. The use of both steroids and the nonsteroidal anti-inflammatory (NSAIDs) drugs is based on their ability to block the conversion of arachidonic acid to these mediators. However, these drugs can only prevent further conversion and will not change the effects of eicosanoids that have already been produced. The main action of most NSAIDs is to inhibit COX-1, but as this form is the constitutive enzyme, COX-1 inhibition results in the gastric and renal side effects of NSAIDs. The new generation of selective COX-2 inhibitors has improved therapeutic profiles, as this form of the enzyme is induced at the site of tissue damage. Interestingly, COX-2 is normally present in the brain and spinal cord and so may be responsible for some of the central analgesic effects of NSAIDs.

Bradykinin is another chemical with important peripheral actions, but as yet cannot be manipulated in any direct way by drugs. It is a product of plasma kininogens that find their way to C-fiber endings following plasma extravasation in response to tissue injury. Bradykinin receptors have been characterized and here again, there are two forms. The B_1-receptor is constitutively expressed less than the B_2-receptor, but in chronic inflammation, it is upregulated. Pain may arise via the activation of the B_2-receptor, which is abundant in most tissues; this can activate C-polymodal receptors. The response to bradykinin can be enhanced by prostaglandins, heat, and serotonin, indicating the extent of interactions between these peripheral pain mediators.

After tissue damage, there is an accumulation of hydrogen ions; the pH is lowered in inflammation and ischemia. These protons may activate nociceptors directly via their own family of ion channels and sensitize them to mechanical stimulation. ASICs are a family of sodium channels that are activated by protons. Of special interest is one type found only in small dorsal root ganglion neurons that are responsible for activation of nociceptors.

Mast cells can release histamine, which causes vasodilation, edema, and itch. Adenosine is also involved in inflammatory conditions. Substance P (SP) and calcitonin gene-related peptide (CGRP) released from the peripheral terminals of primary afferents (via axon reflex) cause neurogenic inflammation. These peptides produce vasodilation, plasma extravasation, and mast cell degranulation. Adenosine 5'-triphosphate (ATP) can cause direct nociceptor activation. The vascular changes produced by SP, CGRP, prostaglandins, and bradykinins lead to vasodilation, and plasma extravasation that underlie the swelling that accompanies tissue damage (3).

Serotonin is released from a number of non-neuronal cells, such as platelets and mast cells, and can produce an excitation of nociceptive afferents via the activation of a large number of receptors ($5HT_{1A}$, $5HT_2$ and $5HT_3$), as well as sensitizing nociceptors, especially to bradykinin. The key role, but not the mechanism of action, of 5HT in the pain associated with migraine and other headaches is well established, but little is known about the actions of this mediator in other non-cranial pains. The aura of neurological symptoms and/or signs is thought to be caused by a vascular or a neuronal mechanism, or a combination of the two. One theory suggests that changes in the vasculature are responsible for causing migraine. A related idea is that peripheral nerves are the source of the problem and then cause the associated vascular changes via release of 5HT and other inflammatory mediators. A third theory suggests that the primary abnormality is neuronal but originates within the brain itself (5).

Sumatriptan, which is commercially available for the treatment of migraine, is an agonist at $5HT_{1B}$ and $5HT_{1D}$ receptors. It has three distinct pharmacological actions. Stimulation of the presynaptic $5HT_{1D}$ receptors on trigeminal Aδ-fibers inhibits the release of CGRP, which inhibits dural vasodilation. $5HT_{1D}$ receptors on trigeminal C-fibers are also stimulated, inhibiting the release of SP and, therefore, blocking neurogenic inflammation and dural plasma extravasation. A further possible action is a direct attenuation of excitability of trigeminal nuclei, as $5HT_{1B/1D}$ receptors in the brainstem are stimulated. Stimulation of these receptors is caused by second-generation triptans that cross the blood-brain barrier, such as zolmitriptan. They all bind to neurons in the trigeminal nucleus caudalis and in the upper cervical cord.

Direct vasoconstriction is mediated by the stimulation of vascular $5HT_{1B}$ receptors. These receptors are also found systemically, and coronary arteries also undergo vasoconstriction. Sumatriptan constricts cerebral arteries, but if the vasculature is normal, this does not affect cerebral blood flow.

Other factors such as NGF and cytokines are also important at the peripheral level. The changes in the phenotype of sensory neurons are produced by these mediators. This contributes to the complex changes in the transduction of painful stimuli.

Central events

Nociceptive sensory information arriving from primary afferent fibers enters the spinal cord via the dorsal horn. On entering the spinal cord, nociceptive signals undergo considerable convergence and modulation. The pharmacology of the spinal cord is extremely rich and contains a diverse range of neurotransmitters and receptors, which may be excitatory or inhibitory depending on the consequence of their activation and their location on neuronal circuitry. The transmission of pain can therefore be seen as a complex process involving the interplay between excitatory and inhibitory systems acting at different levels of the central nervous system. All these systems are subject to plasticity, and alterations in pharmacological systems may occur during pathological conditions (6).

In the spinal cord, nociceptive signaling systems undergo convergence and modulation through interactions that involve peripheral inputs, interneurons, and descending controls. One consequence of this modulation is that the relationship between stimulus and response to pain is not straightforward. The response of output cells could be greatly altered via the interaction of various pharmacological systems in the spinal cord.

Excitatory transmission. The excitatory amino acids, glutamate and aspartate, have been implicated in the transmission of nociceptive information in acute and chronic pain states (7). Several receptors for glutamate have been identified in the brain and spinal cord including the ionotropic glutamate receptors (*N*-methyl-D-aspartate [NMDA], alpha-amino-3-hydroxy-5-methyl-4-isoxazole-propionic acid [AMPA], kainate) and the metabotropic glutamate receptors. The three ionotropic receptor types have a prominent localization in the superficial dorsal horn (laminae I-III) and in deeper layers (laminae IV-VI). The parallel neuroanatomical distribution of these receptors in laminae I-III of the spinal cord provides support for functional interactions between NMDA and non-NMDA receptors in modulating nociceptive transmission.

The excitatory amino acids are found in most sensory fibers, including both large- and small-diameter fibers. In the latter case, they are co-localized with peptides, such as SP. The coexistence of these two transmitters suggests that they are released together in response to a noxious stimulus and thereby contribute to the transmission of pain. Whereas AMPA receptors are activated in response to brief acute stimuli and are involved in the fast events of pain transmission, NMDA receptors are activated only after repetitive noxious inputs, under conditions where the stimulus is maintained (7). NMDA receptors have been implicated in the spinal events underlying "wind-up," whereby the responses of dorsal horn neurons are significantly increased after repetitive C-fiber stimulation despite the constant input (8) (Fig. 1.3). This increased responsivity of dorsal horn neurons is probably the basis for central hyperexcitability and is responsible for the amplification and prolongation of neuronal responses in the spinal cord (6,9).

The NMDA receptor has a heteromeric structure composed of two subunit types: the NR1 subunit and one of four subunits (NR2A-NR2D). It is an ionotropic receptor coupled to a cation channel, which is blocked by physiological levels of Mg^{2+} at the resting membrane potential. The channel is blocked in a voltage-dependent manner. The receptor can operate only after sufficient repeated depolarization. The removal of the Mg^{2+} block is mediated by tachykinins, which are co-released with glutamate. After a brief acute stimulus, pain transmission from C-fibers is largely mediated by the action of glutamate on AMPA receptors. When the stimulus is sustained or its intensity is increased, however, the action of SP on NK-1 receptors produces sufficient membrane depolarization so that the Mg^{2+} block can now be removed and the NMDA receptor activated (6). SP (and also other peptides in the spinal cord), therefore, plays an important role in recruiting NMDA receptors and contributes to the

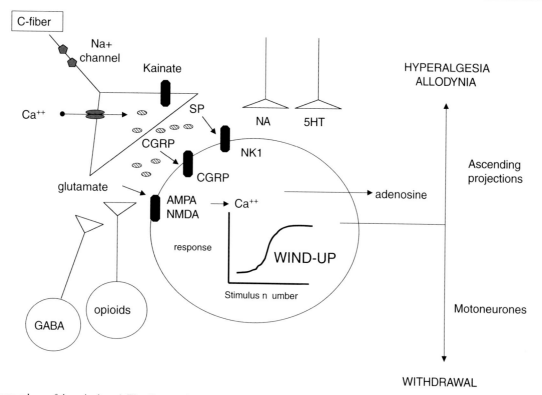

Fig. 1.3. Pharmacology of the spinal cord. The diagram depicts many of the transmitters and receptors involved. Action potentials in a peripheral C-fiber, propagated by sodium channels, arrive in the central terminals and open calcium channels. The influx of calcium causes the release of glutamate, SP, and CGRP, which activate their respective receptors on spinal neurons. NMDA receptor activation produces the wind-up depicted in the figure. Plasticity in these systems can result in hyperalgesia and allodynia. The excitatory events can be controlled by activity or drugs acting on opioid, GABA, and adenosine systems.

cascade of events leading to the enhancement and prolongation of the neuronal response. Indeed, the administration of SP receptor antagonists has been shown to produce antinociception and decrease spinal excitability.

Functional modulation of the NMDA receptor can be achieved through actions at various recognition sites including the primary transmitter site (competitive), the phencyclidine site (uncompetitive), polyamine modulatory site, and the strychnine-insensitive glycine site. Potentially, there are several ways in which the effect of released glutamate can be antagonized through NMDA receptor blockade. Numerous studies have investigated the potential use of antagonists acting through the different recognition sites; however, because of the ubiquitous nature of the receptor, it has often been difficult to achieve therapeutic effects at the target site in the absence of adverse side effects. Evidence suggests that drugs acting at the glycine site in particular appear to lack some of the typical NMDA receptor antagonist side effects. In addition, the fact that there are four subtypes of the receptor (NR1/NR2A-NR2D) might allow the pro-

duction of drugs with selective actions. If these receptors had different distributions, it may be possible to target pain while avoiding forebrain receptors that may mediate problematic side effects.

Substantial evidence exists for the involvement of NMDA receptors in various pathological pain states. Studies have demonstrated the effectiveness of NMDA receptor antagonists in animal models of inflammation (10–12), neuropathic pain (13), allodynia (14), and ischemia (15). Both presurgical and postsurgical administration of antagonists was shown to be effective, suggesting that the induction and maintenance of these ongoing pain states are dependent on NMDA receptor-mediated events. Antagonists at multiple sites on the NMDA receptor complex, including the licensed drugs, ketamine, dextromethorphan, and memantine, have been shown to be effective not only in a number of animal models, but also in humans.

It is now clear that neuropathic pain states are, at least in part, mediated by NMDA receptor-mediated events based on earlier findings from animal studies (16). After nerve injury, there appears to be a greater contribution of the NMDA receptor system to neuronal activity, and this may play a role in the spinal hyperexcitability that underlies this condition. Neuropathy may produce a prolonged activation of NMDA receptors as a result of a sustained afferent input to the spinal cord, and this may result in a relatively small, but continuous increase in the extracellular level of glutamate. Increased glutamate levels have been reported in the ipsilateral dorsal horn of nerve-injured rats. Furthermore, there is evidence for an upregulation of glutamate receptors after nerve injury. Hence, a greater proportion of channels are likely to be in their open state during neuropathy, and this could enable NMDA channel blockers to exert greater effects as a result of their use-dependency.

Central inhibitory systems

The discovery and use of opium date back for many centuries. The roles of the μ, δ, and κ opioid receptors have been established. Most clinically used drugs act on the μ receptor, and the δ receptor may provide a target for opioids with fewer side effects as compared with morphine. The endogenous opioid peptides, the enkephalins, have clear controlling influences on the spinal transmission of pain, whereas the dynorphins have complex actions. Inhibitors of the degradation of the enkephalins have been produced.

To date, four opioid receptor subtypes have been cloned and isolated, which include the μ, δ, and κ receptors (17), and the recently identified ORL-1 (opioid receptor-like) receptor (18) (Table 1.2). The endogenous opioid peptides for these receptors are endorphin, enkephalin, dynorphin, and nociceptin, respectively. The recently discovered ORL-1 receptor, which exhibits considerable sequence homology with the other three classical opioid receptors, shows unique pharmacological properties because it exhibits only a low affinity for

naloxone, a universal opioid receptor antagonist. The endogenous peptide for the receptor has been termed nociceptin, or orphanin FQ, and although its functional role is still somewhat unclear, extensive studies are currently being conducted to elucidate its role in pain modulation (19,20). Overall, this peptide produces spinal analgesia but may well function as an "anti-opioid" at supraspinal sites.

The cloning and isolation of opioid receptors were a major breakthrough in understanding the molecular basis of opioid actions, as well as their localization on nerve fibers. Autoradiographic and immunohistochemical studies have shown opioid receptors to be localized primarily in the superficial dorsal horn (laminae I-II); a smaller population has been demonstrated in deeper layers (21,22). The relative proportion of opioid receptor subtypes in the rat spinal cord has been reported to be approximately 70%, 20–30%, and 5–10% for mu, delta, and κ receptors, respectively (21,22). The majority of these receptors appear to be located on presynaptic terminals of fine afferent fibers. Hence, the predominant presynaptic localization suggests a main presynaptic action of opioids through the inhibition of transmitter release. Indeed, more than 70% of the total mu receptor sites in the spinal cord are localized presynaptically on primary afferent terminals, and only 25% of the receptor population is found on postsynaptic sites, on interneurons, or on dendrites of deep cells in the C-fiber terminal zone (22).

Morphine acts on the mu receptor, as do most of the clinically used opioid drugs. The mu receptor is remarkably similar in structure and function in all species studied so that basic studies will be good predictors for human applications. The best-described central sites of action of morphine are at spinal and brainstem (midbrain) loci.

The spinal actions of opioids and their mechanisms of analgesia involve 1) reduced transmitter release from

Table 1.2. *Opioid receptors and their ligands*

	Mu	Delta	Kappa	ORL-1
Endogenous agonist	Beta-endorphin Endomorphin	Met-enkephalin Leu-enkephalin	Dynorphin A$_{(1-8)}$ Dynorphin A$_{(1-13)}$ Dynorphin B	Nociceptin/OFQ
Other Agonists	Morphine DAMGO	DPDPE DSTBULET	U50488H	–
Antagonists	Naloxone	Naltrindole Naloxone	Naloxone Nor-BNI	[Phe^{1}Ψ(CH$_2$NH) Gly^2]NC$_{(1-13)}$NH$_2$

Abbreviations: [D-Ala2, N-Me-Phe4, Gly5-ol] enkephalin (DAMGO); [D-Pen2, D-Pen5]- enkephalin (DPDPE); Tyr-D-Ser(OtBu)-Gly-Phe-Leu-Thr (DSTBULET); orphanin FQ (OFQ).

nociceptive C-fibers and 2) postsynaptic inhibitions of neurons conveying information from the spinal cord to the brain (Fig. 1.4). The presynaptic action of opioids is the predominant one, and here activation of inhibitory opioid receptors on C-fiber terminals blocks the release of glutamate, SP, and other afferent transmitters. This reduction of transmitter release markedly reduces the activation of spinal pain transmitting neurons by C-fiber activity. Any activation of these neurons by peripheral activity would be countered by the postsynaptic opioid receptors that inhibit firing of the neuron. Furthermore, opioids can also exert indirect postsynaptic actions through a disinhibitory effect on the inhibitory interneuronal system (enkephalin and gamma-aminobutyric acid [GABA] neurons) in the substantia gelatinosa. In a system where an inhibitory interneuron is held under inhibitory control by another interneuron, activation of opioid receptors on the first neuron would result in hyperpolarization, thereby disinhibiting the second neuron and producing a net inhibition (23). Hence, through the combined effect of these mechanisms, opioids can produce powerful antinociceptive effects, and this has been demonstrated in a large number of studies in various pain states (24–26). Some opioids, such as methadone and ketobemidone, may have additional NMDA blocking actions and so may be valuable in cases where morphine effectiveness is reduced, such as in neuropathic pain.

It is known that the opioid system is subject to a considerable degree of plasticity after various pain states (17,27). Hence, whereas inflammation results in an overall increase in the analgesic effect of opioids, neuropathic pain states after nerve injury often display decreased opioid sensitivities, leading to difficulties in achieving good opioid analgesia. The issue of opioid responsiveness in neuropathic pain states has been somewhat controversial and a subject of much debate over the past decade. Reports on the efficacy of opioids have been conflicting and various effects have been reported, ranging from no analgesia (28) to adequate pain relief after sufficient dose escalation (29). It is now generally acknowledged, however, that neuropathic pain states are not completely refractory to opioid treatments, and clinical reports have demonstrated beneficial effects in some patients (30). Various factors are responsible for bringing about these changes in opioid actions after nerve injury, including a loss of opioid receptors. This is seen after nerve section and may account for the poor opioid sensitivity of postamputation pains. Less severe nerve damage can increase the levels of the non-opioid peptides, FLFQPQRFamide or cholecystokinin (CCK), either spinally or supraspinally, which act as negative influences on opioid actions. There is now evidence that this has physiological relevance and the levels of CCK in the cord can determine the potency of morphine. Antagonists at the CCK_B receptor have predicted actions in enhancing or restoring morphine analgesia (17).

Changes after nerve damage can result in hyperexcitability of spinal neurons, against which opioid controls

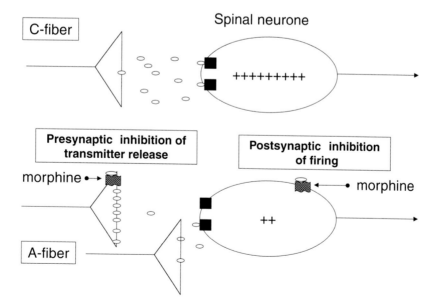

Fig. 1.4. Spinal analgesic actions of opioids. Transmitter release from the terminals of peripheral sensory C-fibers are controlled by opioids, but not that from A-fibers. Postsynaptic inhibitory controls act to modulate firing of spinal neurones.

are insufficiently efficacious. The NMDA receptor is a strong candidate for generation of hyperalgesic states in neuropathic and ischemic pain models. An associated reduction in opioid effects has frequently been observed. Transmission of painful messages via the normally innocuous A-fiber population (allodynia) can occur as a result of pathological changes in peripheral and/or central processes. There are no opioid receptors on the central terminals of these fibers so that any inhibition of A-fiber-mediated allodynia could arise only from activation of the smaller population of postsynaptic opioid receptors. This may be the reason for the difficulties of controlling allodynia by opioids.

Together with the opioid receptor system, GABA forms another important inhibitory transmitter system within the spinal cord. GABA is found extensively within the central nervous system (CNS) and appears to be localized in the superficial dorsal horn (laminae I-III), where it is found mainly within interneurons (6). GABAergic terminals contact Aδ- and nonglomerular C-fiber terminals (31) and exert tonic inhibitory controls on excitatory transmission.

During inflammation, there appears to be an increase in the GABAergic inhibitory control, as demonstrated by an increase in GABA immunoreactivity after carageenan-induced inflammation (32). The increase in inhibitory control after inflammation may possibly reflect a mechanism by which the enhanced neuronal excitability is counteracted. In direct contrast, there appears to be a significant decrease in spinal GABA levels, GABA receptor binding, and the number of GABA immunoreactive neurons after nerve injury (33–35). However, an alternative explanation may be that the reduced levels of GABA may reflect an increased use of the transmitter. Whatever the case, GABA appears to be part of a compensatory mechanism to counteract increased afferent input via the activation of endogenous inhibitory systems. This has important implications because the loss of endogenous inhibitory controls may disturb the physiological equilibrium between excitatory and inhibitory transmitter systems and contribute to the induction of central hyperexcitability.

Another inhibitory system includes the adenosine receptor system. The purines, adenosine and ATP, have been implicated in the modulation of nociceptive transmission, both in the periphery and in the central nervous system (CNS) (36,37).

Receptor sites for adenosine in the spinal cord have been identified in the substantia gelatinosa, where they are localized primarily on intrinsic neurons. Two main subclasses of adenosine receptors (A$_1$/A$_{2A/B}$) have so far been described and it appears to be predominantly the A$_1$ receptor subtype that plays a major role in inhibiting the nociceptive input in the dorsal spinal cord (38). The predominant localization of adenosine A$_1$ receptors in the spinal cord appears to be on postsynaptic sites, and only a minor population has been observed presynaptically on afferent terminals. The mechanism by which adenosine produces antinociception involves an interaction with the excitatory amino acids and the neurokinins. Hyperpolarization of transmission neurons through the activation of postsynaptic A$_1$ receptors reduces the excitatory actions of glutamate or SP, which also acts on postsynaptic sites and consequently inhibits synaptic transmission. In support of this, A$_1$ receptor agonists have been shown to inhibit wind-up, an NMDA receptor-mediated event (39).

There is now a growing interest in the development of therapeutic agents that interact with adenosine systems for the treatment of neuropathic pain. Patients with neuropathic pain have been reported to have a deficiency in the plasma and cerebrospinal fluid adenosine level. Neuropathic pain states are associated with neuronal hyperexcitability, and adenosine administration may be beneficial in attenuating excessive neuronal activity through interactions with the NMDA receptor system. The direct and indirect manipulation of the adenosine system may prove to be a useful approach in producing spinally mediated antinociception during neuropathy (37).

Monoamine systems, originating in the midbrain and brainstem act on the spinal transmission of pain. There are other important sites of opioid actions located in these 5HT and noradrenergic nuclei of the brainstem (e.g. midbrain), including the raphe nuclei, the periaqueductal gray matter, and the locus coeruleus. Opioid receptors in these zones (μ, δ, and κ), when activated, alter the level of activity in descending pathways from these zones to the spinal cord. The mechanisms of action of opioids at supraspinal levels are still poorly understood. One idea is that descending controls filter sensory messages at the spinal level, allowing a pain message to be extracted from the incoming barrage. Supraspinal morphine is thought to reduce these controls, thereby blurring the perception of pain. The second theory is that morphine turns on descending controls that simply inhibit spinal pain transmission. The relative roles of the 5HT receptors in the spinal cord are yet unknown, but the spinal target for the noradrenaline released from descending pathways are α-2 receptors that have similar actions and distribution to the opioid receptors. Sedation and hypotension with α-2 agonists presently limit their use as analgesics.

Opioid mechanisms at a number of other supraspinal sites (thalamic levels, the amyglada, and the sensory cortex) are likely to be of relevance to analgesia (23). Sites in the monoamine nuclei, such as the well-demonstrated actions of opioids on noradrenergic transmission in the locus coeruleus and enhancing dopamine release in the ventral tegmental area, are likely to be associated with reward processes and so relate to dependence. Because pain produces aversive psychological effects, it may be that the sensory stimulus "switches off" the neural circuitry that leads to reward and reinforcement. Thus, opioids in the presence of pain may not produce reward, whereas street use of the same drugs in the absence of pain may result in psychological dependence.

The relative extent of the unwanted effects caused by selective agonists at the different opioid receptors is of great importance in determining if non-μ opioids will have more favorable actions than morphine. There are good indications that the κ and δ receptor agonists cause less respiratory depression than μ agonists, and that prolonged protection of the enkephalins by the peptidase inhibitors has no dependence liability. This lack of dependence is also seen with κ agonists but is accompanied by aversive or non-rewarding effects that limit the usefulness of these agents in man.

Mechanisms of neuropathic pain

After nerve injury, there is considerable plasticity in the peripheral and central nervous system, which may be related to the pathogenesis of neuropathic pain states. The mechanisms underlying these chronic pain states are heterogeneous. The complex nature of these syndromes is largely responsible for the limited number of therapeutic strategies.

The sequence of events that follow peripheral nerve injury, and consequently contribute to the development of neuropathic pain, can be seen at various levels of the nervous system. Nerve injury is associated with anatomical, neurochemical, pharmacological, and electrophysiological changes (40). After a nerve lesion develops, there are alterations in the anatomy of the peripheral nerves; demyelination occurs through phagocytosis by macrophages. A number of neurochemical changes also take place. Studies have reported a complex change in the expression of neuropeptides in the dorsal root ganglia (DRG), including a reduction in the levels of SP and CGRP. In contrast, there is evidence for an upregulation of galanin, as well as for a novel induction of vasoactive intestinal polypeptide (VIP) and neuropeptide Y (NPY). These changes may be related to the degenerative and regenerative processes that take place in the central and peripheral branches of the sensory neuron.

One prominent feature of nerve injury is a marked increase in neuronal excitability, which is manifested as abnormal ectopic activities. Ectopic impulses appear to originate from the DRG as well as from the neuroma of the injured peripheral nerve (41). The incidence and level of spontaneous activity depend on several factors, including animal species, time elapsed from injury onset, type of nerve injury, and the nerve studied. One factor contributing to the electrogenesis of ectopic discharges is thought to be the alteration in the expression of voltage-gated sodium channels on peripheral afferents after nerve injury. Immunohistochemical studies have demonstrated that nerve injury induces remodeling of axolemmal sodium channels, and channels have been shown to accumulate in neuromas, especially in regions of demyelination (42).

DRG neurons express multiple distinct sodium channels encoded by different genes, and there is considerable plasticity in its expression during development and various pain states. Two types of sodium currents have so far been identified in the DRG, the TTX-resistant (NaN, SNS) and TTX-sensitive (types I, IIA, III, PN1, NaCh6) currents, which differ in their kinetics and sensitivity to TTX (43). Changes in the expression and function of these sodium channels may make an important contribution to the establishment of certain chronic pain states. There is evidence for a loss of immunolabeling for the TTX-resistant sodium channels, NaN and SNS, in small-diameter DRG neurons after peripheral nerve injury. This appears to be correlated with its redistribution and accumulation in the peripheral nerve, proximal to the site of injury. Furthermore, there is a switch in the expression of certain sodium channels, and a previously silent type III sodium channel gene has been reported to emerge after nerve injury (44). The type III sodium channel mRNA is normally expressed in embryonic neurons and is subsequently downregulated during development. Activation of these previously quiescent channels may therefore induce abnormal repetitive firing in injured neurons and potentially act as ectopic impulse generators. The change in expression of both TTX-S and TTX-R channels implies that the kinetics and voltage-dependent characteristics of sodium currents may be considerably altered in neuropathic pain states. This, together with the pathological accumulation of sodium channels at the neuroma, may promote inappropriate action potential initiation and may form the basis of the therapeutic use of local anaesthetics and excitability blockers, such as carbamazepine, for neuropathic pain states (45).

Another feature of nerve injury is axonal sprouting, whereby injured axons undergo regeneration and reinnervation of target peripheral tissues including the deafferentated territory. In addition, nerve injury can induce adjacent undamaged sensory axons to sprout collateral fibers into an area that has been denervated owing to the nerve lesion over a limited distance (collateral sprouting).

Similarly, studies have reported a structural reorganization of the spinal cord after nerve injury, such that the central terminals of axotomized Aβ-fibers sprout into lamina II, an area of the cord that normally only processes C-fiber input (46). As a result of this sprouting, low-threshold mechanoreceptive afferent terminals have been proposed to establish functional contacts with cells that normally would have a C-nociceptor input, leading to inappropriate responses to innocuous peripheral stimuli. The mechanism by which Aβ-fibers sprout into lamina II is unclear, although several mechanisms have been proposed. These include a creation of a vacant synaptic space in lamina II resulting from the transganglionic degeneration of C-fiber terminals, and the release of a chemoattractant for A-fibers. Such structural reorganization of primary afferent central terminals has been proposed to underlie the development of some of the sensory abnormalities associated with peripheral nerve injuries (46).

Despite the substantial evidence that exists for the phenomenon of Aβ-fiber sprouting, these findings have been questioned in a recent study, where it was demonstrated that the increased CB-HRP labeling may represent an enhanced uptake and transganglionic transport of the tracer in small DRG neurons, rather than sprouting of large diameter neurons from deeper laminae (47). Although under normal conditions, only large neuronal profiles are labeled with CB-HRP, axotomy induces labeling in both small and large neuronal profiles, suggesting that there is a novel uptake of the marker by small neuronal profiles after nerve injury. Although its significance remains unclear, this finding suggests that CTB-HRP may not be an appropriate marker to study the events underlying Aβ-fiber sprouting, as the tracer may not be strictly selective for large-diameter fibers after nerve injury.

A number of studies suggest that there is a complex change in the pattern of the evoked neuronal responses, as well as in the receptive field size of dorsal horn neurons after nerve injury. Thus, there are important changes in the spinal processing of neuropathic pain. Alterations in the response profile of spinal neurons appear to be modality dependent and are characterized by both increases and decreases to selected peripheral stimuli. It is not clear what underlies this differential plasticity of spinal neurons, although it is likely that the changes result from both de novo acquired neuronal responses, as well as from alterations in the existing response profiles of spinal neurons.

Behavioral studies have shown that NMDA receptor activation is required for both the induction and maintenance of pain-related behaviors (48). Thus, it is likely that aberrant peripheral activity is amplified and enhanced by NMDA receptor-mediated spinal mechanisms in neuropathic pain. The degree of hyperexcitability after peripheral nerve damage is hard to gauge, as peripheral fibers, central neurons, and pharmacological systems may all change their properties after injury. As the operation of the NMDA receptor/channel depends critically on the underlying level of excitability, spinal neurons are probably hyperactive and compensate for much of the peripheral nerve damage. Although there is human evidence for effectiveness of agents acting at the NMDA receptor complex, especially ketamine (16,49), it would appear that although some patients get good pain relief, the majority cannot achieve complete pain control because dose escalation is compromised by the narrow therapeutic window. The same would apply to the potential use of glutamate receptor/channel antagonists in the treatment of epilepsy. Success of new therapies for pain and epilepsy, based on blocking the actions of glutamate on NMDA or other receptors such as AMPA/kainate receptors, will depend on strategies that increase their therapeutic window over existing drugs.

Recent studies with agents that block neuronal voltage-sensitive calcium channels would also suggest that there is an increase in central neuronal excitability. N-type channels, blocked by omega-conotoxin, appear to be important in behavioral allodynia and play a major role in the neuronal responses to low- and high-threshold natural stimuli and in the C-fiber evoked central hyperexcitability. Blockers of this channel are considerably more effective after nerve injury. Because the channel is voltage operated, these results again suggest increased excitability of the spinal cord neurons after injury. SNX-111 is an example of a drug that works to block calcium channels. Its use is restricted to the spinal route. Interestingly, although the exact mechanism of action of gabapentin remains unknown, there is a body of evidence to suggest that it may act as a calcium channel blocker.

Although the extent of the loss of myelinated and unmyelinated fibers after nerve injury is unknown, a large proportion of input is expected to be lost as a result of neuropathy. Despite this marked loss of afferent input, however, the overall changes in the responses of spinal neurons appear to be comparatively small. Hence, this may represent an increase in spinal cord excitability, which could compensate for the loss of afferent drive. The high level and incidence of spontaneous activity seen after nerve injury may be one contributing factor to the global spinal hyperexcitability. This activity may well produce an ongoing level of transmitter release in the spinal cord, which may, in turn, favor hyperexcitability of responses to subsequent evoked stimuli. Furthermore, there may be a drop in the mechanical threshold of spinal neurons after nerve injury, which could facilitate neuronal activation with a low-intensity stimulus. This, together with an enlargement of neuronal receptive fields, could form the electrophysiological basis for the mechanism underlying the behavioral manifestation of allodynia, hyperalgesia, and spontaneous pain after neuropathy (Fig. 1.5).

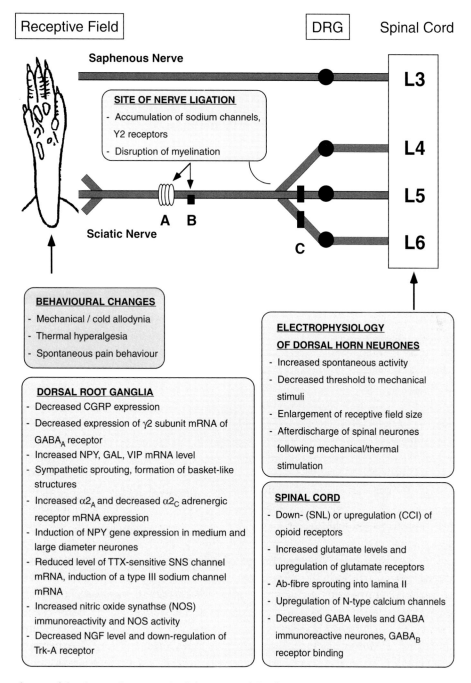

Fig. 1.5. An overview of some of the changes that occur after injury to a peripheral nerve together with the types of animal models used to study the mechanisms of neuropathy. A: CCI model, B: PSTL model, C: selective SNL model.

Animal models of persistent pain

Formalin-induced inflammation

Subcutaneous injection of formalin is widely used to study tonic tissue-injury induced changes and has become an established model of inflammatory pain (50). The introduction of formalin into the peripheral receptive field is believed to activate the afferents directly through the activation of peripheral chemoreceptors (50) and gives rise to an acute/phasic response. Electrophysiologically, the formalin test is characterized by a typical biphasic response—an early acute phase followed by a prolonged tonic phase. The initial acute phase can last up to 10 minutes after formalin injection, after which activity subsides into a silent interphase (51). This phase is followed by a second tonic phase, which begins approximately 25 minutes after injection. The firing of dorsal horn neurons subsides within an hour. These findings are comparable to those seen behaviorally, where a similar two-phased paw-licking/flinching response has been observed (50). It has been proposed that the first phase activity is mediated by the activation of AMPA receptors resulting from an acute afferent barrage in response to formalin. The tonic second phase, by contrast, is a consequence of the sustained afferent input and is produced by a series of biochemical and cellular events (central and peripheral sensitization) (12,50). This latter phase is driven centrally by activation of the spinal NMDA receptor (51).

Carrageenan-induced inflammation

Carrageenan-induced inflammation represents a model of inflammatory cutaneous hyperalgesia. The injection of carrageenan produces rapid development of edema and inflammatory changes, which reach their maximum 3 to 5 hours after administration. The time course of this model is much longer than that seen with formalin inflammation and is maintained up to 72 hours (52). Animals display hyperalgesia to mechanical and thermal stimuli on the injected paw, which is manifested as a decrease in paw withdrawal latency and vocalization threshold. The inflammatory changes that occur in the periphery can have consequences for events at the spinal level. For example, the levels of opioid peptides and transcription markers are elevated after carrageenan inflammation (53). Similarly, the effects of exogenous opioids are enhanced when given spinally (54), and opioids acquire a novel peripheral effect after inflammation (55).

Animal models of neuropathic pain

Neuropathic pain is defined as *pain initiated or caused by a primary lesion, dysfunction in the nervous system.*

Neuropathy can be divided broadly into peripheral and central neuropathic pain, depending on whether the primary lesion or dysfunction is situated in the peripheral or central nervous system. In the periphery, neuropathic pain can result from disease or inflammatory states that affect peripheral nerves (e.g., diabetes mellitus, herpes zoster) or alternatively as a result of neuroma formation (amputation, nerve transection), nerve compression (e.g., tumors, entrapment), or other injuries (e.g., nerve crush, trauma) (56). Central pain syndromes, by contrast, result from alterations in different regions of the brain or the spinal cord. Examples include tumor or trauma affecting particular CNS structures (e.g., brainstem and thalamus) or spinal cord injury. Both the symptoms and origins of neuropathic pain are extremely diverse, and this makes the clinical conditions difficult to treat. Current treatment is still inadequate (16); hence, the availability of good animal models is clearly needed.

Several models of nerve injury have so far been described, which include models of total denervation (dorsal rhizotomy, total nerve section/crush, cryolysis), partial denervation (chronic constriction injury, partial sciatic nerve ligation, selective spinal nerve ligation), and spinal cord injury. Additionally, neuropathy models that involve systemic treatments have also been described (streptozocin-induced diabetic neuropathy).

Models of partial denervation of the hindpaw

Since the introduction of the first animal model of neuropathy involving complete nerve transection (57), models of partial hindpaw denervation based on restricted sciatic nerve injury have been used more frequently. Unlike models of total denervation, such as complete spinal transection or dorsal root rhizotomy, models of partial nerve injury preserve at least some of the sensory information passing into the spinal cord (58–60). Three models that are widely used are the chronic constriction injury (CCI) model (58), partial sciatic tight ligation (PSTL) model (59), and the selective spinal nerve ligation (SNL) model (60). These animal models produce sensory abnormalities in rats, some of which resemble those observed in human neuropathic pain states.

CCI model of neuropathy. The CCI model introduced by Bennett and Xie (58) involves the unilateral ligation of the sciatic nerve using chromic gut sutures. Four loose ligatures are placed around the common sciatic nerve, proximal to the trifurcation. The tightness of the ligatures is such that the nerve is barely constricted but not tight enough to obliterate the superficial epineurial vasculature supply. When placed around the nerve, the chromic gut suture may cause chemical irritation and produce an inflammatory reaction, which may contribute to the development of behavioral abnormalities (61). Hence, CCI may represent a model of inflammatory neuropathy. After surgery, rats show spontaneous pain-like behavior, consistent with the presence of ongoing neuropathic pain; they exhibit signs of allodynia and hyperalgesia (58). These abnormal behaviors are maintained up to 90 days after nerve injury. Some rats also appear to display autotomy on the ipsilateral hindpaw, where animals show signs of self-mutilation, possibly in an attempt to rid themselves of the unpleasant sensory experience coming from the partially denervated limb. Although the extent to which autotomy reflects a sensation of pain has been questioned, it appears to be a response to pain or dysesthesia. The clinical relevance of this behavior in human neuropathic pain states remains debatable. One of the problems associated with this model is the considerable variation in the amount of nerve damage that occurs after the application of the loose ligatures. The variation arises mainly because of the difficulty in placing ligatures with a consistent degree of compression, which could affect the number and type of injured afferent fibers (62). This fact may account for the considerable variability in the incidence of autotomy and mechanical allodynia observed among studies.

PSTL model of neuropathy. Partial denervation of the hindpaw is produced by tightly ligating one third to one half of the common sciatic nerve (59). Similar to the CCI model, the PSTL results in an immediate onset of allodynia and hyperalgesia, as well as behavioral signs of spontaneous pain, which persist for several months. Rats exhibit a change in foot posture of the ipsilateral hindpaw and also display signs of guarding behavior. Autotomy has not been observed in this model. One of the problems associated with this model is that the number and type of sciatic nerve axons that are ligated differ among animals, as it is not possible to damage exactly the same proportion of the nerve in each animal. Hence, there may be a considerable degree of variability associated with this model.

Selective SNL model of neuropathy. Peripheral nerve injury is produced by the unilateral tight ligation of two (L5 and L6) of the three spinal nerves (L4-L6), which make up the sciatic nerve (60). Selective SNL (L5/L6) produces allodynia and hyperalgesia on the ipsilateral hindpaw, which persist for several weeks (5–10 weeks) (60). Rats often exhibit signs of spontaneous pain and

also display guarding behavior of the ipsilateral hindpaw. Autotomy is not observed in this model.

As compared with the other two models of sciatic nerve injury (58,59), this model produces less variability among experiments because the same spinal nerves (L5/L6) are ligated in each animal. The only potential variability may arise from differences among individual rats in the proportion of the sciatic nerve contributed by its three spinal segments.

One key feature of this model is that the location of the injured fibers is in completely separate spinal segments from the uninjured fibers (60). Hence the DRG, which contains the injured nerves, is separated from the neighboring DRG, which contains intact neurons. This allows us to selectively manipulate inputs from injured and intact fibers to spinal segments in an independent manner. This ability is unique to this model of nerve injury because in the CCI and PSTL models, the injured and intact primary afferent neurons are mixed within all the DRGs innervating the sciatic nerve territory.

Models of central pain
A model of central pain has been developed by Xu and colleagues that involves ischemic spinal cord injury induced photochemically by laser irradiation (63). The model produces allodynia-like behaviors whose severity can be titrated by changing the duration of the light exposure.

Models of diabetic neuropathy
Various models have been recently developed to study the complications associated with the clinical condition of diabetes mellitus. The most widely used is the streptozocin-induced diabetes produced by a single injection of streptozocin, which results in an insulin-dependent diabetic neuropathy (64). Studies have shown that the pharmacological characteristics of this model correspond well to the clinical experience from patients with painful diabetic neuropathy, thus making it a useful model to study the mechanisms underlying this condition (65).

Models of bone cancer pain
A murine model of bone cancer pain has been reported in a recent study, which shares many similarities with human cancer-induced bone pain (66). Tumor cells that form lytic lesions in the bone are implanted into the quadriceps muscle and mice develop nociceptive behaviors 3 weeks after injection. Mice displayed signs of guarding behavior, and these nocifensive behaviors were significantly correlated with the extent of bone destruction. In parallel

with these behavioral changes, neurochemical alterations have also been reported in the ipsilateral spinal cord, including an increased expression of GFAP, dynorphin, and c-Fos protein (66).

Use of present animal models of pain: benefits and problems

The development of animal models has contributed to the understanding of the mechanisms underlying clinical pain states. Animal models may enable the replication of some of the symptoms associated with human disease and have been invaluable in providing information about the pathophysiological processes occurring after inflammation or nerve injury. Furthermore, animal models have contributed to the clinical management of various pain states by providing information about the therapeutic value of existing drugs, as well as revealing potential novel targets.

Despite the apparent benefits of these animal models, it is important to be aware of some of the limitations and problems associated with their use. One must be cautious when extrapolating data from animal studies for clinical application. Although animal models produce behavioral responses that resemble those of various human pain states, it is not clear how these behavioral features correspond to the human perception of pain. We can only assume that the behavioral manifestation of the animal represents a similar clinical presentation of the pain in a patient.

Another limitation of an animal model is that it is not possible to distinguish or discriminate the different types of pain sensations of the animal. Whereas clinicians can rely on descriptions given by patients to determine the clinical characteristic of the pain (e.g., "burning" pain or "shooting" pain), information from animal studies is confined to observations made on physical features and behavioral responses that are suggestive of pain.

A question one needs to bear in mind when using animal models is: Which model relates to which clinical condition? Although some animal models represent specific clinical conditions (trigeminal CCI-induced neuropathy and diabetic neuropathy model), others are not as specific. Furthermore, even when the model appears to have a close resemblance to a specific condition, it is difficult to determine whether it represents the same pathological entity as that seen in patients and whether it would respond to the same pharmacological interventions. Hence the direct clinical application of animal findings may not necessarily be straightforward.

Acknowledgements

The authors thank Dr. Vesa Kartiren for his contribution to the figures in this article.

References

1. Sorkin L, Carlton S. Spinal anatomy and pharmacology of afferent processing. In: Yaksh T, Lynch C, Zapol W, et al, eds. Anesthesia. Biologic foundations. Philadelphia: Lippincott-Raven, 1997, pp 577–610.
2. Bonica J. Anatomic and physiologic basis of nociception and pain. In: Bonica J, ed. The management of pain. Philadelphia: Lea & Febiger, 1990, pp. 28–94.
3. Besson J. The neurobiology of pain. Lancet 353:1610–15, 1999.
4. LaMotte RH, Shain CN, Simone DA, et al. Neurogenic hyperalgesia: psychophysical studies of underlying mechanisms. J Neurophysiol 66:190–211, 1991.
5. Goadsby P. New aspects of the pathophysiology of migraine and cluster headaches. In: Max M, ed. Pain 1999—an updated review. Refresher Course Syllabus. Seattle: IASP Press, 1999, pp 181–92.
6. Dickenson AH, Chapman V, Green GM. The pharmacology of excitatory and inhibitory amino acid-mediated events in the transmission and modulation of pain in the spinal cord. Gen Pharmacol 28:633–8, 1997.
7. Dickenson AH. Pharmacology of pain transmission and control. In: Campbell J, ed. Pain 1996—an updated review. Refresher Course Syllabus. Seattle: IASP Press, 1996, pp 113–22.
8. Dickenson AH. Spinal cord pharmacology of pain. Br J Anaesth 75:193–200, 1995.
9. Dickenson A, Stanfa L, Chapman V, et al. Response properties of dorsal horn neurones: pharmacology of the dorsal horn. In: Yaksh T, Lynch C, Zapol W, et al., eds. Anesthesia. Biologic foundations. Philadelphia: Lippincott-Raven, 1997, pp 611–24.
10. Eisenberg E, LaCross S, Strassman AM. The effects of the clinically tested NMDA receptor antagonist memantine on carrageenan-induced thermal hyperalgesia in rats. Eur J Pharmacol 255:123–9, 1994.
11. Ren K, Hylden JL, Williams GM, et al. The effects of a noncompetitive NMDA receptor antagonist, MK-801, on behavioral hyperalgesia and dorsal horn neuronal activity in rats with unilateral inflammation. Pain 50:331–44, 1992.
12. Coderre TJ, Melzack R. The contribution of excitatory amino acids to central sensitization and persistent nociception after formalin-induced tissue injury. J Neurosci 12:3665–70, 1992.
13. Mao J, Price DD, Hayes RL, et al. Intrathecal treatment with dextrorphan or ketamine potently reduces pain-related behaviors in a rat model of peripheral mononeuropathy. Brain Res 605:164–8, 1993.
14. Yaksh TL. Behavioral and autonomic correlates of the tactile evoked allodynia produced by spinal glycine inhibition:

effects of modulatory receptor systems and excitatory amino acid antagonists. Pain 37:111–23, 1989.

15. Sher GD, Cartmell SM, Gelgor L, et al. Role of N-methyl-D-aspartate and opiate receptors in nociception during and after ischaemia in rats. Pain 49:241–8, 1992.

16. Rabben T, Skjelbred P, Oye I. Prolonged analgesic effect of ketamine, an N-methyl-D-aspartate receptor inhibitor, in patients with chronic pain. J Pharmacol Exp Ther 289:1060–6, 1999.

17. Dickenson A, Suzuki R. Function and dysfunction of opioid receptors in the spinal cord. In: Kalso E, McQuay H, Wiesenfeld-Hallin Z, eds. Opioid sensitivity of chronic Noncancer pain. Progress in pain research and management. Seattle: IASP Press, 1999, pp 17–44.

18. Wick MJ, Minnerath SR, Lin X, et al. Isolation of a novel cDNA encoding a putative membrane receptor with high homology to the cloned mu, delta, and kappa opioid receptors. Brain Res Mol Brain Res 27:37–44, 1994.

19. Darland T, Heinricher MM, Grandy DK. Orphanin FQ/nociceptin: a role in pain and analgesia, but so much more. Trends Neurosci 21:215–21, 1998.

20. Taylor F, Dickenson A. Nociceptin/orphanin FQ. A new opioid, a new analgesic? Neuroreport 9:R65–70, 1998.

21. Rahman W, Dashwood MR, Fitzgerald M, et al. Postnatal development of multiple opioid receptors in the spinal cord and development of spinal morphine analgesia. Brain Res Dev Brain Res 108:239–54, 1998.

22. Besse D, Lombard MC, Zajac JM, et al. Pre- and postsynaptic distribution of mu, delta and kappa opioid receptors in the superficial layers of the cervical dorsal horn of the rat spinal cord. Brain Res 521:15–22, 1990.

23. Dickenson AH. Where and how do opioids act? In: Gebhart G, Hammond D, Jensen T, eds. Proceedings of the 7th world congress on pain. Progress in pain research and management. Seattle: IASP Press, 1994: pp 525–52.

24. Attal N, Chen YL, Kayser V, et al. Behavioural evidence that systemic morphine may modulate a phasic pain related behaviour in a rat model of peripheral mononeuropathy. Pain 47:65–70, 1991.

25. Kayser V, Chen YL, Guilbaud G. Behavioural evidence for a peripheral component in the enhanced antinociceptive effect of a low dose of systemic morphine in carrageenin induced hyperalgesic rats. Brain Res 560:237–44, 1991.

26. Ossipov MH, Lopez Y, Nichols ML, et al. Inhibition by spinal morphine of the tail-flick response is attenuated in rats with nerve ligation injury. Neurosci Lett 199:83–6, 1995.

27. Ossipov M, Malan Jr T, Lai J, et al. Opioid pharmacology of acute and chronic pain. In: Dickenson A, Besson J, eds., The pharmacology of pain. Handbook of experimental pharmacology. Berlin: Springer, 1997, pp 305–33.

28. Arner S, Meyerson BA. Lack of analgesic effect of opioids on neuropathic and idiopathic forms of pain. Pain 33:11–23, 1988.

29. Portenoy RK, Foley KM, Inturrisi CE. The nature of opioid responsiveness and its implications for neuropathic pain: new hypotheses derived from studies of opioid infusions. Pain 43:273–86, 1990.

30. Rowbotham MC, Reisner-Keller LA, Fields HL. Both intravenous lidocaine and morphine reduce the pain of postherpetic neuralgia. Neurology 41:1024–8, 1991.

31. Bernardi PS, Valtschanoff JG, Weinberg RJ, et al. Synaptic interactions between primary afferent terminals and GABA and nitric oxide-synthesizing neurons in superficial laminae of the rat spinal cord. J Neurosci 15:1363–71, 1995.

32. Castro-Lopes JM, Tavares I, Tolle TR, et al. Carrageenan-induced inflammation of the hind foot provokes a rise of GABA-immunoreactive cells in the rat spinal cord that is prevented by peripheral neurectomy or neonatal capsaicin treatment. Pain 56:193–201, 1994.

33. Castro-Lopes JM, Tavares I, Coimbra A. GABA decreases in the spinal cord dorsal horn after peripheral neurectomy. Brain Res 620:287–91, 1993.

34. Ibuki T, Hama AT, Wang XT, et al. Loss of GABA-immunoreactivity in the spinal dorsal horn of rats with peripheral nerve injury and promotion of recovery by adrenal medullary grafts. Neuroscience 76:845–58, 1997.

35. Castro-Lopes JM, Malcangio M, Pan BH, et al. Complex changes of GABAA and GABAB receptor binding in the spinal cord dorsal horn following peripheral inflammation or neurectomy. Brain Res 679:289–97, 1995.

36. Sawynok J. Adenosine receptor activation and nociception. Eur J Pharmacol 347:1–11, 1998.

37. Dickenson A, Suzuki R, Reeve AJ. Adenosine as a potential analgesic target in inflammatory and neuropathic pains. CNS Drugs 13:77–85, 2000.

38. Sawynok J, Sweeney MI, White TD. Classification of adenosine receptors mediating antinociception in the rat spinal cord. Br J Pharmacol 88:923–30, 1986.

39. Reeve AJ, Dickenson AH. The roles of spinal adenosine receptors in the control of acute and more persistent nociceptive responses of dorsal horn neurones in the anaesthetized rat. Br J Pharmacol 116:2221–8, 1995.

40. Garry M, Tanelian D. Afferent activity in injured afferent nerves. In: Yaksh T, Lynch C, Zapol W, et al., eds. Anesthesia. Biologic foundations. Philadelphia: Lippincott-Raven, 1997, pp 531–42.

41. Wall PD, Devor M. Sensory afferent impulses originate from dorsal root ganglia as well as from the periphery in normal and nerve injured rats. Pain 17:321–39, 1983.

42. Devor M, Govrin-Lippmann R, Angelides K. Na+ channel immunolocalization in peripheral mammalian axons and changes following nerve injury and neuroma formation. J Neurosci 13:1976–92, 1993.

43. Waxman SG, Dib Hajj S, Cummins TR, et al. Sodium channels and pain. Proc Natl Acad Sci USA 96:7635–9, 1999.

44. Black J, Cummins T, Plumpton C, et al. Upregulation of a silent sodium channel after peripheral, but not central, nerve injury in DRG neurons. J Neurophysiol 82:2776–85, 1999.

45. Sindrup S, Jensen T. Efficacy of pharmacological treatments of neuropathic pain: an update and effect related to mechanism of drug action. Pain 83:389–400, 1999.

46. Woolf C, Mannion R. Neuropathic pain: aetiology, symptoms, mechanisms, and management. Lancet 353:1959–64, 1999.

47. Tong YG, Wang HF, Ju G, et al. Increased uptake and transport of cholera toxin B subunit in dorsal root ganglion neurons after peripheral axotomy: possible implications for sensory sprouting. J Comp Neurol 404:143–58, 1999.

48. Bennett G. Neuropathic pain. In: Wall P, Melzack R, eds. Textbook of pain. London: Churchill Livingstone, 1994, pp 201–24.

49. Eide K, Stubhaug A, Oye I, et al. Continuous subcutaneous administration of the N-methyl-D-aspartic acid (NMDA) receptor antagonist ketamine in the treatment of post-herpetic neuralgia. Pain 61:221–8, 1995.

50. Dubuisson D, Dennis S. The formalin test: a quantitative study of the analgesic effects of morphine, meperidine, and brain stem stimulation in rats and cats. Pain 4:161–74, 1977.

51. Haley JE, Sullivan AF, Dickenson AH. Evidence for spinal N-methyl-D-aspartate receptor involvement in prolonged chemical nociception in the rat. Brain Res 518:218–26, 1990.

52. Winter C, Risley E, Nuss G. Carrageenan-induced edema in hindpaw of the rat as an assay for anti-inflammatory drugs. Proc Soc Exp Biol Med 111:544–7, 1962.

53. Iadarola M, Brady L, Draisci G, et al. Enhancement of dynorphin gene expression in spinal cord following experimental inflammation: stimulus specificity, behavioural parameters and opioid receptor binding. Pain 35:313–26, 1988.

54. Stanfa LC, Sullivan AF, Dickenson AH. Alterations in neuronal excitability and the potency of spinal mu, delta and kappa opioids after carrageenan-induced inflammation. Pain 50:345–54, 1992.

55. Stein C, Millan M, Shippenberg T, et al. Peripheral effect of fentanyl upon nociception in inflamed tissue of the rat. Neurosci Lett 84:225–8, 1988.

56. Ralston D. Present models of neuropathic pain. Pain Rev 5:83–100, 1998.

57. Wall PD, Devor M, Inbal R, et al. Autotomy following peripheral nerve lesions: experimental anaesthesia dolorosa. Pain 7:103–113, 1979.

58. Bennett GJ, Xie YK. A peripheral mononeuropathy in rat that produces disorders of pain sensation like those seen in man. Pain 33:87–107, 1988.

59. Seltzer Z, Dubner R, Shir Y. A novel behavioral model of neuropathic pain disorders produced in rats by partial sciatic nerve injury. Pain 43:205–18, 1990.

60. Kim SH, Chung JM. An experimental model for peripheral neuropathy produced by segmental spinal nerve ligation in the rat. Pain 50:355–63, 1992.

61. Kawakami M, Weinstein JN, Spratt KF, et al. Experimental lumbar radiculopathy. Immunohistochemical and quantitative demonstrations of pain induced by lumbar nerve root irritation of the rat. Spine 19:1780–94, 1994.

62. Carlton SM, Dougherty PM, Pover CM, et al. Neuroma formation and numbers of axons in a rat model of experimental peripheral neuropathy. Neurosci Lett 131:88–92, 1991.

63. Xu X, Hao J, Aldskogius H, et al. Chronic pain related syndrome in rats after ischemic spinal cord lesion: a possible animal model for pain in patients with spinal cord injury. Pain 48:279–90, 1992.

64. Ahlgren SC, Levine JD. Mechanical hyperalgesia in streptozotocin-diabetic rats. Neuroscience 52:1049–55, 1993.

65. Courteix C, Eschalier A, Lavarenne J. Streptozocin-induced diabetic rats: behavioural evidence for a model of chronic pain. Pain 53:81–8, 1993.

66. Schwei M, Honore P, Rogers S, et al. Neurochemical and cellular reorganization of the spinal cord in a murine model of bone cancer pain. J Neurosci 19:10886–97, 1999.

2 Cancer pain epidemiology: a systematic review

JULIE HEARN AND IRENE J. HIGGINSON

Guy's, King's & St. Thomas' School of Medicine and St. Christopher's Hospice

Introduction

Cancer pain afflicts millions of people worldwide every year, yet it can be well or completely controlled in 80%–90% of patients (1–3). Exactly how many of the estimated 6.6 million people worldwide who died from cancer last year (4) experienced pain at any one time is difficult to ascertain. The reasons for this are discussed below. Nevertheless, in spite of the major advances in pain control over the last 15 years, cancer-related pain continues to be a major international public health problem (5–21).

Although pain is recognized as an extremely common symptom in patients with cancer, studies to date show a wide variation in the reported prevalence (22–24). Three main factors influence this:

1. Difficulty in making generalizations to different health care settings or different patient groups because of variation in the design of prevalence studies (25,26)
2. Inherent difficulties in assessing the presence or absence of pain, particularly because no one "gold standard" assessment system exists, exacerbated by attempts to grade the severity of cancer pain in a variety of ways
3. Difficulty in defining the type of pain (27), because pain associated with cancer has features of both chronic and acute pain and can be either the direct or indirect result of the cancer (28,29)

Pain and cancer are not synonymous (30). Evaluation of pain in advanced cancer is primarily clinical and is based on pattern recognition. Attention to detail is necessary to prevent inappropriate treatment (31). Comprehensive pain assessment is important, but initial treatment with analgesics should not be withheld until these have been carried out (30). There are many reasons that pain remains unrelieved, associated with both the patient or family, and the doctor or nurse.

Definition and diagnosis

The definition of pain

Pain is defined as "an unpleasant sensory and emotional experience associated with actual or potential tissue damage, or described in terms of such damage" (32). There is no definitive way to distinguish pain occurring in the absence of tissue damage and pain resulting from damaged tissue (33). By definition, pain is subjective and each person's interpretation is dependent on experiences in earlier life. Not only is it a sensation in a part or parts of the body, but it is also "always unpleasant and therefore an emotional experience" (32). Pain is a complex and unique experience. In addition to its physiological basis, it can be affected by situational factors and by psychological processes including emotion, cognition, and motivation. The perception of pain is therefore modulated by the patient's mood, the patient's morale, and the meaning of pain for the patient (30). Moreover, the situational and psychological factors are all susceptible to cultural, ethnic, and linguistic influences (30,34).

Difficulties in cancer pain assessment

There are several problems associated with cancer pain classification in epidemiology. Study designs are often limited and not generalizable for the reasons given next. Variation among studies makes it difficult to combine data effectively.

First, pain is usually studied in health care settings rather than in communities of people. Therefore the prevalence estimates relate to a group of patients referred to a specific service (e.g., a pain clinic). For example, the study carried out by Coyle (35) reviewed later in this chapter was carried out on patients referred to the Supportive Care

Program of the Pain Service at the Memorial Sloan-Kettering Cancer Center. The patients studied were a subgroup of 90 problematic patients whose management "taxes the clinical skills and compassion of practitioners, as well as the psychologic and financial resources of the patient and family." Hence, although this study provided detailed insight into the management and symptomatology of this particular population, there are obvious limitations in making generalizations from a population who are all experiencing intractable pain. Some studies include only those patients who have pain. Although these give valuable information on pain syndromes, mechanisms, and treatment, they do not give prevalence estimates (see for example Lin [36], who examined relationships between disclosure and pain management, or Uki et al. [37], who examined utility of a pain assessment tool).

Second, measures of pain are not constant among studies. Although severity and its impact on patient function are both critical to assessment, severity is the main factor that determines the impact of pain (38,39). Failure to assess the severity of pain and the variety of methods used for its categorization compound the difficulties in assessment. Further work is needed to develop systematic assessments of pain, which can be used in routine care and for epidemiological monitoring.

Third, pain in cancer is not a well-defined entity (27). A patient may have several pains, which in turn can have features of both acute and chronic pain. Although the site of the tumor influences the characteristics of the pain and the type of intervention (40), the situation is complicated because the definition of cancer pain also incorporates the pathology of pain (e.g., nociceptive or neuropathic (28), pain related to the cancer (bedsores), pain related to the cancer treatment (postoperative scar pain), or pain caused by a concurrent disorder (spondylosis) (41).

In addition to these problems in assessment, in some instances the incidence of pain is determined from records of analgesic use. These estimates are likely to be lower than would have been obtained if pain had been systematically assessed.

Aspects of assessment

First of all, the physician must believe the patient's report of pain and *initiate* discussions about pain. The assessment should define the nature and extent of the underlying disease, evaluate concomitant problems (physical, psychological, and social) that may contribute to patient distress, and clarify the goals of care (42). The assessment should thereby clarify the pain characteristics and

syndrome, infer the putative mechanisms that may underlie the pain, and determine the impact of the pain on function and psychological well-being (42). If necessary additional investigations should be carried out to clarify uncertainties in the assessment (43).

When selecting a mode of measuring pain severity, the response mode must be (39) 1. sufficiently graded to identify changes, 2. clear to both subjects and investigators, and, 3. easy to score.

Visual analo scales, verbal descriptor scales, and numeric rating scales have been used in clinical setting to assess pain severity and shown to approach equivalency in their results (44). Numeric rating scales have been endorsed for use in cancer clinical trial instruments because they are easier to understand and easier to score (45). These have also been shown to be unaffected by language or cultural interpretation of pain severity. A study comparing the rating of pain's interference in four countries using multidimensional scaling consistently revealed two dimensions to the reporting of pain, irrespective of pain severity or cultural or linguistic background (34). The two dimensions used by patients in the study to report how they react to pain were activity and affect. Activity was defined in terms of walking, work, general activity, and sleep. Affect related to functions such as relationships with others, mood, and enjoyment of life (34). Both these dimensions should be included in any assessment measure.

Some general assessment tools include pain alongside other symptoms and problems and thus can be valuable in monitoring pain. As more and more standardized assessment tools become available (46) comparisons between settings may become feasible. Such measures include the Edmonton Symptom Assessment System (ESAS) (47), the Palliative Care Outcome Scale (48), and the Support Team Assessment Schedule (STAS) (49).

Assessment can also be carried out by interview, with either the patient or in certain situations with the assistance of the family. Whether an assessment is carried out by the physician, the nurse, or the patient will obviously affect the data collected. In a study validating a staff-rated outcome measure for use in palliative care, staff were found to underrate the level of pain and family or caregivers overrated the level of pain as compared to the patient's self-report of pain (49). The limitations of each method of measurement need to be understood and noted when reporting cancer pain prevalence data because the methods used will affect the outcomes of the study.

The classification of cancer pain is a controversial issue. Ventafridda and Caraceni (50) suggest:

1. Every study involving patients with cancer pain and analgesic treatments should provide a precise description of the symptoms, including details of all clinical and instrumental diagnostic criteria.
2. A classification of pain according to the definition of somatic, visceral, and nerve pains should separate differentiation, neuropathic, or dysesthetic pain from nerve trunk pains.
3. Temporary patterns of pain and their precipitating factors should always be specified.

This classification reflects an ideal situation and would overcome many of the problems encountered when reviewing the prevalence estimates in this area. Unfortunately, logistic and resource limitations prevent the classification of pain in this way for all studies of cancer pain, and we are therefore restricted to making generalizations from studies with caveats attached.

Prevalence of cancer pain

To determine the prevalence of cancer pain, a systematic literature review involving four stages was undertaken: literature searching and study retrieval, the assessment of studies for inclusion on the basis of relevance and design, data extraction, and data synthesis (51).

Literature identification

The following databases were searched:

- Medline (1980– August 2000);
- BIDS (Bath Information and Data Services), EMBASE, SOCIAL SCISEARCH (Social Sciences Citation Index), and IBSS (International Bibliography of the Social Sciences), (1994 to August 2000).

The databases were searched using the words *cancer pain* as the main search term in the title, abstract, or key words of an article. Searches were carried out using either *cancer pain* alone, or in combination with the following words: *epidemiology, epidemiological, epidemiologic, incidence, prevalence, survey, cross-sectional, cohort, follow-up, prospective, longitudinal, case-control, case-referent, retrospective study, determinant(s), predictor, etiology, causative, risk factor, prevention.*

The following journals were searched by hand to identify articles that may have been missed in the database searches: *Pain, The Journal of Pain Symptom Management, The Clinical Journal of Pain, and Palliative Medicine.*

Cancer sites on the Internet were also investigated for more up to date information on the most recent cancer publications. CancerWEB (www.graylab.ac.uk) compiled by the National Cancer Institute and OncoLink (www. oncolink.upenn.edu/, The Trustees of the University of Pennsylvania) were searched. Both sites provided useful overview information, but neither provided any articles of relevance to the review that had not been identified by the other search mechanisms. The American Pain Society (www.ampainsoc.org/) and Roxane Pain Institute (www.Roxane.com) sites were used for additional reference.

Inclusion/exclusion and data extraction

The inclusion criteria of studies into the review were defined based on the work of Portenoy (24), who proposed using two related sets of survey data to provide epidemiological estimates of cancer pain prevalence. Hence, a study was included in the review if the article reported the prevalence of cancer pain in a clearly defined cancer population, which was derived from:

1. A survey on the natural history of the neoplasm that included information on pain
2. The preliminary stage of a broader study on pain management or cancer service evaluation

In addition, a seminal review article by Bonica (52) was also included. This inclusion was thought to be appropriate, as the original studies mentioned in the review were especially difficult to locate (due to the age and location mainly of the unpublished gray literature), and the data from some would not have been included otherwise. Studies were excluded if they selected only those patients who had pain, or were historical accounts, personal opinion, or case studies.

Data were extracted directly into tables of a predefined format under the headings study type, disease definition and tumor type, source of sample, sample size, pain severity, duration of symptoms, type of prevalence estimate, prevalence, and reference.

Comprehensive patient assessment and thorough patient ascertainment are prerequisites for meaningful data, but the absence of laboratory or radiographic correlates of pain make data gathering a challenge (53). Because of the problems of varied measurement, a meta-analysis of the data could not be carried out. Data extracted from the published studies were reviewed as a whole (Tables 2.1 and 2.2) and are synthesized next.

Table 2.1. *The prevalence of cancer pain in general cancer populations*

Study type	Disease definition and tumor type	Source of sample	Sample size	Pain severity	Duration of symptoms	Type of prevalence estimate	Prevalence[a]	Reference
Prospective survey	General cancer population	Two studies of inpatients of a cancer center, United States	1.540 2.397	• Pain requiring analgesic drugs • Any pain			• 29% (specified by site) • 38% (60% of the terminal patients)	Foley, 1979 (22)
Prospective survey	General cancer population	Outpatients of an oncology unit, UK	237	• Any pain	Not stated—recorded at referral	Period (?)	• 72%	Trotter et al., 1981 (106)
Prospective survey	Breast, prostate, colon or rectum and three gynecological tumors	Inpatient and outpatient services of the oncology, urology, and gynecology departments of a university hospital, United States	667	• Any pain • Type of pain • Intensity	At diagnosis and in the past month	Point and period	• 18% to 49% had had pain as an early symptom (specified by site) • 48% had pain in the past month • Due to the cancer in 56% and 17% with metastatic or non-metastatic disease, respectively • Mean scores for worst pain: 4.0 (SD 3.6) to 6.7 (SD 7.1)[b] • Mean scores for average pain: 2.5 (SD 3.5) to 5.7 (SD 2.1)[b]	Daut and Cleeland, 1982 (38)
Prospective survey	Lung, pancreas, prostate, and uterine cervix	Identified from Cancer Surveillance System (CSS)—a register of cancer cases in northwest Washington, United States	536	• Any pain • Intensity • Severity of worst pain	Last 7 days	Period	• 64% with typical pain (specified by site) • 30% slight pain, 30% moderate pain, 4% very bad pain • 19% had very bad worst pain	Greenwald et al., 1987 (107)
Prospective survey	General cancer population	Inpatients of a Cancer Institute, Netherlands	240	• Any pain • Severity • Interference with daily activities	At admission or over past several days	Point and period together	• 45% • Mean score for present intensity 2.9 (SD 2.5)[b] • Mean score for most severe pain in past week 7.2 (SD 2.4) • 28% maximal interference, 55% extensive interference	Dorrepall et al., 1988 (84)
Quasi-meta-analysis	General cancer population	All studies to 1990, separated into "all stages" and "advanced or terminal"	14,417	• Any pain	Not given	Not known	• 51% patients at all stages • 74% advanced/terminal patients	Bonica, 1990 (52)
Prospective study	Pediatric cancer patients with current or past malignancy	Inpatients and outpatients at the Mayo Clinic and 8 community-based and tertiary cancer institutions, United States	160	• Any pain • Type of pain • Patient setting • Severity	Not stated	Point	• 18% • 21% of which cancer-related, 58% treatment-related, 21% unrelated • 39% of those with pain were inpatients, 13% outpatients • 7% severe (staff reported)	Elliott et al., 1991 (55)

22

Study type	Population	Setting	N	Measure	Time frame	Point/Period	Results	Reference
Retrospective patient record survey	General cancer population	Cancer centers, cancer clinics, University hospitals, and general hospitals chosen at random, Japan	35,683	• Any, indicated by use of analgesics	During care	Point	• 32.6% overall • in 11.4% before treatment, 24.9% in curative stage, 48.7% in conservative stage, 71.3% in terminal stage	Hiraga et al., 1991 (54)
Prospective survey	Newly diagnosed general cancer population	Patients diagnosed or primarily treated at a tertiary care referral hospital, Finland	240	• Any pain • Type of pain	Past 2 weeks/now	Period and point	• 35%, a total of 28% still had pain • 46% pain related to the cancer, 67% had pain secondary to cancer or its treatment, 18% had unrelated pain	Vuorinen, 1993 (56)
Prospective survey	General cancer population with intractable pain	Pain clinic of the anesthesiology department in a university hospital, Germany	1635	• Frequency • Intensity	Assessed at admission	Point	• 99% with continuous pain, 1% with incident or breakthrough pain • 3% mild, 11% moderate, 33% severe, 49% very severe/maximal	Grond et al., 1994 (25)
Prospective study	Prostate, colon, breast or ovarian cancer patients	Four inpatient units and three outpatient clinics of a cancer center, United States	243	• Any pain	Not stated	Point	• 64% (specified by site)	Portenoy et al., 1994 (67)
Prospective survey	Ovarian cancer patients	Inpatient unit and outpatient clinics of the gynecology service of a cancer center, United States	151	• Persistent or frequent pain • Severity • Frequency • Duration	During past 2 weeks	Period	• 42% • 62% had had pain preceding diagnosis or recurrence • Mean severity of pain in general was moderate, mean severity for worst pain was severe • 40% experienced any pain almost constantly, 21% experienced worst pain almost constantly • Median duration of worst or only pain 2 weeks (range <1–756)	Portenoy et al., 1994 (65)
Prospective survey	Advanced general cancer population	Adult outpatients in 16 ambulatory care settings, United States	369	• Any pain • Intensity • Duration	Past month	Period	• 54% with cancer-related pain • Mean score for average daily pain 3.6 (SD 2.2) (between mild and moderate) • Mean number of hours per day in pain 9.2 (SD 9.1) • Mean number of days per week in pain 4.2 (SD 2.8)	Glover et al., 1995 (108)

(continues)

Table 2.1 (Continued)

Study type	Disease definition and tumor type	Source of sample	Sample size	Pain severity	Duration of symptoms	Type of prevalence estimate	Prevalence[a]	Reference
Prospective cross-sectional multicenter survey	General cancer population	Cancer treatment centers, university hospitals, state hospitals, private clinics, home care, France	605	• Any pain • Severity	During past week	Period	• 57% (specified by site), 65% of whom had metastatic disease • 69% rated pain as significant (score of 5 or more)[b] • 54% rated average pain significant	Larue et al., 1995 (70)
Descriptive survey (unclear if it was cross-sectional or prospective)	Ambulatory patients with breast cancer	Adult outpatients in 16 ambulatory care settings—4 affiliated to university medical centers, 12 community-based, United States	97	• Any pain • Type of pain • Intensity • Duration	In the past month	Period	• 64% • 73% of which was cancer-related • Mean score for average daily pain 3.4 (SD 2.3) (mild to moderate) • Mean number of hours per day in pain 8.9 (SD 10.1) • Mean number of days per week in significant pain 3.8 (SD 3.0)	Miaskowski and Dibble, 1995 (109)
Prospective survey	Pain clinic cancer population	Anesthesiology-based pain service of a university hospital, Germany	2266	• Type of pain • Intensity • Number of pains	Previous day	Point	• 85% caused by cancer, 17% treatment-related, 9% associated with cancer disease, 9% unrelated • 77% had an average pain intensity of severe or worse on previous day • 30% had one pain, 39% had two pains, 31% had 3 or more	Grond et al., 1996 (110)
Prospective study	General cancer population all with pain	Patients with pain for at least 1 month treated in hospital and about to be discharged home	383	• Number • Duration • Intensity	At time of discharge from hospital	Point and period	Patients had a mean of 1.8 pain locations, and mean pain duration of 14.2 months (SD 33.4) • Mean present pain intensity on a numeric rating scale (maximum score 10) was 3.3 (SD 2.3), mean average pain intensity over previous week was 4.9 (SD 2.1)	De Wit et al., 1997 (111)

Study design	Population	Description	N	Measures	Timeframe	Point/Period	Results	Reference
Randomized controlled trial	General cancer population	Cancer patients 18 years and older were identified from lists of patients with a cancer diagnosis who had seen a physician during the previous 6 months in a community health care institution	438	• Pain intensity • Brief pain inventory • Pain prevalence in the 3 months before interview	1. Pain now, worst pain in last 7 days, least pain in last 7 days, and average pain in last 7 days 2. Pain in prior 3 months	Point and period	• Pain score—mean 9.9 in treatment group and 111 in control group (range 0–40) • Prevalence—42% in treatment group and 36% in control group at pretest and 39% in both groups at posttest	Elliott et al., 1997 (112)
Retrospective cross-sectional study	General cancer population	Patients aged 65 years and older with cancer admitted from hospital to US nursing homes between 1992 and 1995	13,625	• Any pain	Assessed at admission and for next 7 days	Period	• 29% reported daily pain	Bernabei et al., 1998 (113)
Prospective survey	Patients with recurrent breast or gynecological cancers	Outpatients already in a larger study of the psychosocial needs of patients with cancer who had had a period of stability and recurred	114	• Frequency of pain • Amount of pain • Interference in the patient's life	Pain over the past 4 weeks	Period	• 70% of patients with breast cancer and 63% of patients with gynecological cancer had had at least a little pain over the past 4 weeks • 51% had mild to moderate pain • 62% stated their pain interfered with their ability to function	Rummans et al., 1998 (114)
Prospective study	Newly diagnosed general cancer population	Patients admitted to one hospital during an 18-month period	296	• Presence • Intensity	During week before interview	Period	• 38% had cancer-related pain • Of these, 65% had significant worst pain (i.e. worst pain level scores ≥5 on a 10-point scale), and 31% has significant average pain (i.e. average pain level scores ≥5 on a 10-point scale)	Ger et al., 1998 (57)
Cross-sectional study	General cancer population	Outpatient clinic in a cancer center (50% of patients attending center)	217	• Presence or absence of pain	At any time in the last 2 weeks	Period	• 64% had pain at some time in the last 2 weeks	Wells et al., 1998 (115)
Prospective cross-sectional international survey	General cancer population all with pain requiring opioid medication	10–50 patients from each of 58 cancer practitioners in 24 countries treating patients with severe cancer pain	1095	• Duration • Intensity • Number of pains • Type of pains	Current pain and pain during the past day	Point	• Mean duration of pain 5.9 months (SD 105) • 67% reported worst pain intensity over past day was ≥7 on a 10 point numeric scale • 25% experienced 2 or more pains • 80% had pain due to the cancer, 18% had treatment-related pain	Caraceni and Portenoy, 1999 (116)
Prospective longitudinal study	Patients with cancers of the head and neck	Treated patients disease free at 2 years	93	• Any pain • Pain intensity • Shoulder pain	1. At admission 2. 12 months 3. 24 months	Point	1. 48% had pain at admission, 8% severe, 14% in the shoulder 2. 25% had pain at 12 months, 3% severe, 37% in the shoulder 3. 26% had pain at 24 months, 3% severe, 26% in the shoulder	Chaplin and Morton, 1999 (117)

(continues)

25

Table 2.1 (*Continued*)

Study type	Disease definition and tumor type	Source of sample	Sample size	Pain severity	Duration of symptoms	Type of prevalence estimate	Prevalence[a]	Reference
Prospective study	General cancer population all with pain	Patients with pain being treated by a pain service according to WHO guidelines	593	• Type • Intensity	At admission, after 3 days, and at last follow-up visit	Point	• 64% nociceptive pain, 5% neuropathic pain, 31% mixed • Mean intensity on a numeric rating scale (maximum score 100) at admission was 66 (nociceptive), 70 (neuropathic) and 65 (mixed), reducing to 26, 28 and 30 after 3 days, and 18, 21 and 17 at the end of the survey	Grond et al., 1999 (118)
Secondary analysis of prospective data from 4 studies including a clinical trial	Patients with primary lung cancer or cancer metastatic to bone	Three western states at three medical school affiliated teaching hospitals and several community hospitals. Patients were over 18 years old	125	• McGill pain questionnaire	At interview	Point	• 72% had pain • McGill pain questionnaire total score—mean 19.7 (SD 12.5) range 0–53	Berry et al., 1999 (119)
Prospective study	Patients with pancreas cancer all with pain	Consecutive patients scheduled for neurolytic celiac plexus block separated into patients with cancer (1) of the head of the gland, or (2) of the corpus and tail	50	• Pain intensity	At admission	Point	• The 36 patients in group 1 scored 5.4 (SD 0.54) on a pain visual analog scale (VAS) (maximum score possible 10) • The 14 patients in group 2 scored 7.6 on VAS (SD 0.88)	Rykowski and Hilger, 2000 (120)

Studies are listed in date order of publication.

[a] Percentages for severity breakdowns may not equal overall percentages quoted due to missing values.

[b] 0 = no pain, 10 = worst pain as assessed by a pain rating scale.

[c] Period of terminal care period of care from end of active treatment to the patient's death (median time 9 weeks).

[d] Scores relate to hours of pain multiplied by a severity coefficient values can range from 0 to 240.

Prevalence estimates

Point: measured at the time of the survey for each person, although not necessarily the same point in time for all people in the defined population.

Period: cases that were present at any time during a specified period of time (e.g., any in the last three months)

Lifetime: as read.

Study types

Survey: the main purpose of the study was to survey pain or symptom prevalence.

Study: there may have been other reasons for the study (e.g., as a service evaluation or evaluation of management/control).

Table 2.2. *The prevalence of cancer pain in patients with advanced or terminal disease, or at the end of life*[a]

Study type	Disease definition and tumor type	Source of sample	Sample size	Pain severity	Duration of symptoms	Type of prevalence estimate	Prevalence[a]	Reference
Retrospective record review, and interviews with general practitioners and caregivers	Patients who had died from cancer of the pharynx, breast, bronchus, stomach, colon, rectum	Patients who died in a 4-month period at home or in a hospital in the city of Sheffield, UK	279	• Any pain	During the terminal illness	Period	• 62%	Ward, 1974 (58)
Retrospective interview study	Bereaved caregivers of advanced general cancer population	Caregivers under 65 whose spouse had died during a 4-year period in 2 London boroughs, UK	165	• Severity	During the period of terminal care[b]	Period	• 36% had none to mild pain, 31% moderate, 33% had severe to very severe pain	Parkes, 1978 (59)
Prospective survey	Far-advanced general cancer population; all in pain	Referrals to a special care hospice unit, UK	100	• Type • Intensity • Duration • Number of sites	Several categories used	Point and period	• Only 41% had all their pain caused directly by the cancer • 90% had had pain for > 4 weeks, 57% of these for > 16 weeks • For those who had pain for > 8 weeks, 77% severe to excruciating • 80% had more than one pain, 34% of these had four or more	Twycross and Fairfield, 1982 (66)
Prospective study	Terminal general cancer population or their primary care persons	40 hospital- and home-based hospices and 14 conventional care settings, United States	1754	• Any pain • Severity	Assessed at study entry	Point	• 69% • 19% mild, 21% discomfort, 16% distressing, 7% horrible, 5% excruciating	Morris et al. 1986 (121)
Prospective evaluation study	Advanced general cancer population	Hospice inpatients, UK	256	• Any pain	Assessed at admission	Point	• 53%	McIllmurray and Warren, 1989 (122)
Prospective study	Terminal general cancer population	Patients in the care of a home care service and an inpatient hospital pain therapy and palliative care service, Italy	60	• Daily pain score	Assessed at study entry	Point	• Mean scores 53.5 (SD 37.5) and 41.9 (SD 29.1) for home care and hospital care patients, respectively[c]	Ventafridda et al., 1989 (123)
Retrospective record review but with prospective data collection	Advanced clinically challenging cancer patients	In care for more than 4-weeks before death of a supportive care program of a cancer center, United States	90	• Any pain • Intensity • Degree of activity interference	Reported at 4-weeks before death	Point	• 100% • 27% mild, 19% mild to moderate, 34% moderate, 20% moderate to severe • Major limitation for 94% of those rating pain as moderate to severe	Coyle et al., 1990 (35)

(continues)

Table 2.2. (Continued)

Study type	Disease definition and tumor type	Source of sample	Sample size	Pain severity	Duration of symptoms	Type of prevalence estimate	Prevalence[a]	Reference
Prospective study	Advanced general cancer population	Two community-based support teams, UK	65	• Any pain	Past week	Period	• 68% pain rated as a problem	Higginson et al., 1990 (124)
Prospective study	Terminal general cancer population	Patients assisted by a home care team, Italy	120	• Treatment for pain	During care	Period	• 100%	Ventafridda et al., 1990 (125)
Prospective survey	Advanced general cancer population	Hospital inpatients, UK	78	• Any • Severity • Number of sites	During care	Point	• 71% (specified by site) • 24% mild, 40% moderate, 36% severe • 60% had one main site of pain, 35% two, 5% three or more	Simpson, 1991 (64)
Retrospective record review	Advanced cancer population	Referrals to a general teaching hospital, Australia	110	• Any pain • Type	Present at admission	Point	• 69% • 34% related to the primary cancer, 43% related to metastatic disease	Chan and Woodruff, 1991 (89)
Retrospective record review	Advanced general cancer population who died on the unit	Inpatients of a hospital palliative care unit, Canada	100	• Pain requiring treatment	Assessed at admission	Point	• 99%	Fainsinger et al., 1991 (93)
Retrospective interview study	Bereaved caregivers or informants of people who had died from cancer	Random sample of deaths in 1969 and 1987 from death registration data in areas of England/Wales	383	• Any pain	In the last year of life	Period	• 87% in 1969 • 84% in 1987	Cartwright, 1991 (60)
Retrospective record review	Advanced general cancer population over 65 years old	Community-based hospice organization, United States	239	• Any pain • Severity	Assessed at admission	Point	• 58% with discomfort/pain • 12% mild, 18% discomfort, 17% distress, 7% horrible, 6% excruciating	Stein and Miech, 1993 (126)
Prospective study	Lung cancer patients	New referrals to a palliative care service, treated at home or as an outpatient, Italy	52	• Any pain	Assessed at admission	Point	• 88%	Mercadante et al., 1994 (127)
Prospective study	General advanced cancer population	Inpatients and outpatients of a palliative care service, United States	1000	• Any pain • Severity	Assessed at admission	Point	• 83% with pain • ranked as most severe symptom out of 30 common symptoms	Donnelly et al., 1995 (63)
Prospective survey	Advanced general cancer population	Hospital palliative care team, UK	125	• Any pain • Pain dominating daily life	Assessed at admission	Point	• 74% • > 25%	Ellershaw, 1995 (68)
Retrospective interview study	Bereaved caregivers of general cancer population	Random sample of deaths in 1990 from 20 selected areas, UK	2018	• Any pain	In the last year of life	Period	• 88%	Addington-Hall and McCarthy, 1995 (61)

Study design	Population	Setting/sample	N	Measure	Time frame	Point/Period	Findings	Reference
Prospective study	Far-advanced general cancer population	Hospital inpatients, United States	98	• Any pain	Assessed at 3 days after admission	Point	• 64%	Shannon et al., 1995 (128)
Prospective survey	Advanced general cancer population; all in pain	Inpatients and new outpatients attending a specialist palliative care unit associated with a University medical school, UK	111	• Type • Intensity • Number of sites	Past week	Period and point	• 46% had all pain caused by the cancer, 29% had associated pains, 5% had pain related to the treatment • Median score 4 for average pain, median score 6 for worst pain[c] • 85% had > 1 pain, > 40% of these had 4 or more	Twycross et al., 1997 (30)
Prospective study	Advanced cancer population	Referrals to 7 palliative care units including hospital ward, hospice care or home care, United States, UK, Finland, Australia, Switzerland	1640	• Any pain • Severity	Assessed at admission	Point	• 72% (specified by site) • 24% mild, 30% moderate, 21% severe	Vainio et al., 1996 (129)
Prospective study	Advanced general cancer population	11 multidisciplinary palliative care teams, England and Ireland	695	• Any pain • Severity	Past week	Period	• 70% (specified by site) • 54% mild or moderate, 16% severe or overwhelming	Higginson Hearn, 1997 (26)
Retrospective study	Caregivers of general cancer population	46% from a randomized stratified sample of family caregivers of patients who died in one US state in 1994	170	• Pain intensity • Pain relief	Last 4 weeks of life	Period	• 86% stated pain was a problem; 61% reported a great deal or quite a bit of pain; 25% some or little • 82% reported data on pain relief intervention; 46% of which made pain stop/get better, 56% of which made pain a little better or had no effect or made it worse.	Bucher et al., 1999 (62)
Retrospective cross-sectional survey	Advanced general cancer population	Convenience sample of Chinese patients recruited from hospices and oncology units in Hong Kong	100	• Any pain • Intensity • Analgesic use	Current pain	Point	• 77% had current pain • Majority had mild pain • 76% had regular analgesics for their pain	Chung et al., 1999 (130)
Prospective study	Advanced general cancer population	Patients referred to a home palliative care program over a 9-year period (1988–1997)	3577	• Any pain • Intensity	At referral, after 1 week, and in last week of life	Point	• 70.3% had pain at referral • Mean intensity on a visual analog scale (maximum score 10) was 4.4 at referral, 2.5 at 1 week, 2.3 in the last week of life	Mercadante, 1999 (131)

(continues)

29

Table 2.2 (*Continued*)

Study type	Disease definition and tumor type	Source of sample	Sample size	Pain severity	Duration of symptoms	Type of prevalence estimate	Prevalence[a]	Reference
Retrospective cohort study	Advanced cancer patients who subsequently died	Patients cared for in one of three Colorado home-based hospice programs	223	• 0–10 pain rating scale • Patient reports of change • Hospice nurse	At visit—each patient usually had 3–5 visits	Point	• Pain reported in 66% of all abstracted patient visits • 13.2% of patients never had a documented pain complaint • 19% had pain complaints documented at each visit • Presence of metastases not significantly associated with presence of pain • Hospice programs differed in the proportion of visits for which pain was reported (75%, 64%, and 48%)	Nowels and Lee, 1999 (132)

[a]Studies are listed in date order of publication.
Prevalence estimates
Point: measured at the time of the survey for each person, although not necessarily the same point in time for all people in the defined population.
Period: cases that were present at any time during a specified period of time (e.g. any in the last 3 months).
Lifetime: as read
Study types
Survey: the main purpose of the study was to survey pain or symptom prevalence.
Study: there may have been other reasons for the study (e.g., as a service evaluation or evaluation of management/control).

Prevalence of pain

A total of 54 studies met the criteria for inclusion into the review (Tables 2.1 and 2.2). It became apparent that although cancer pain is prevalent at all stages of the disease and may often be the first symptom of cancer, it is more common in advanced and terminal cancer. For this reason those studies focusing on people with cancer at all stages or who are newly diagnosed (Table 2.1) are considered separately from those concentrating on patients with advanced or terminal disease (Table 2.2).

The prevalence of pain at all stages and in early disease

Twenty-seven studies reported on the prevalence of pain in the *general* adult cancer population (i.e., studies usually at a varying stage of presentation) (Table 2.1). These gave a combined weighted mean prevalence of pain 40%, range 18%–100%.

Note, this estimate includes three low estimates determined from the use of analgesics alone as a measure of pain prevalence (Foley [22]: 29% and 38%; Hiraga et al. [54]: 33%). In addition, Elliott et al. (55) reported a prevalence of 18% among pediatric patients with current or past malignancy. Excluding these studies would provide a weighted mean prevalence of pain of 48%, range 38%–100%.

There is little evidence on the prevalence of pain at or around the time of diagnosis. One study by Vuorinen (56)

reported 35% of newly diagnosed patients had experienced pain in the past 2 weeks; Daut and Cleeland (38) reported that 18%–49% of patients had had pain as an early symptom of the disease. Ger et al. (57) found that 38% of newly diagnosed cancer patients had pain.

Prevalence of pain in advanced cancer

Twenty-seven studies reported data on pain prevalence in the advanced or terminal cancer population (Table 2.2). In the majority of cases the data are for point prevalence estimates, obtained at referral to a particular service. Period prevalence estimates mainly related to pain over the past week, and occasionally the past 2 weeks or month. As a result of the variation in methods of measuring and reporting the data, the values were simply combined to provide a crude overall mean prevalence based on the number of patients in each study and the number reported to be experiencing pain (i.e., a weighted estimate). The combined weighted mean prevalence of pain was 74%, range 53%–100%. There was no relationship between prevalence and study sample size (Fig. 2.1).

Five studies had used retrospective data collected from bereaved caregivers of patients with cancer or from other informants who could provide information on particular patients (58–62). Obviously there are limitations to this data in that the interviews with the bereaved caregivers or

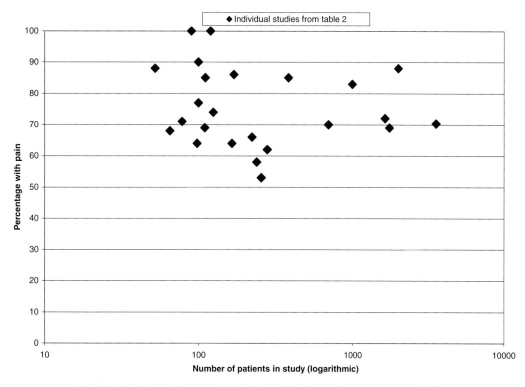

Fig. 2.1. Prevalence of cancer pain in patients with advanced cancer versus sample size.

informants took place at least 6 months after the death of the patient. The data are therefore subject to some recall bias, as well as being subjective assessments. Overall, the estimates were slightly higher than for patient reports. Reports from the Regional Studies for the Care of the Dying (60,61) provided period prevalence estimates of pain in "the last year of life" at three time points: 87% in 1969, 84% in 1987, and 88% in 1995. The studies by Ward (58) and Parkes (59) considered pain in "the period of terminal illness" and gave a pain prevalence of 62%–64%. Bucher et al. (62) reported that 86% of patients had a problem with pain in the last 4 weeks of life.

The prevalence of pain by primary tumor site

Nine studies were identified that provided prevalence data on pain in more than one cancer type in the general adult cancer population. These show a wide range in reported prevalence by tumor site, but those cancers with more than 70% of patients with pain reported in more than one study are:

- Head and neck (mean 80%, range 67%–91%)
- Genitourinary (mean 77%, range 58%–90%)
- Esophagus (mean 74%, range 71%–77%)
- Prostate (mean 74%, range 56%–94%)

One hundred percent of patients with advanced multiple myeloma (65) and with advanced sarcoma (64) were experiencing pain. Portenoy et al. (65) found that 42% of ovarian cancer patients had pain. This evidence must be viewed with caution, as the data are from only one study for each cancer type; however, it does illustrate the extent of the problem.

Cancers of the blood are said to have little pain associated with the disease, particularly in the early stages. This opinion could be substantiated by the evidence from the study by Foley (22), which reported only 5% of patients with leukemia experiencing pain. Nevertheless, the range of pain prevalence values for lymphoma was from 20% to 87%; hence pain in cancers of the blood should not be underestimated.

The severity and effect of pain

The various stages of disease considered and the methods of measurement make it difficult to summarize the data in the tables to provide valid estimates of the prevalence of severe pain, or the proportion of pain affecting or dominating the daily life of patients. However, it is obvious by looking qualitatively at the data that there is a great deal of unrelieved pain at referral to all the services carrying out these studies.

In the study by Grond et al. (25) of patients referred to a pain clinic, patients experiencing very severe or maximal pain complained more frequently of insomnia, sweating, vomiting, and paresis. In this study the use of strong opioids was associated with a higher prevalence of anorexia, constipation, nausea, neuropsychiatric symptoms, vomiting, urinary symptoms, and paresis.

Those studies assessing the number of pains a patient is experiencing have shown that a large proportion of patients have two or more distinct kinds or causes of pain, reflecting the complexity of disease associated with malignancy (30,64,66,67).

High-risk groups

When considering risk factors for cancer pain, it is important to be clear which "type" of cancer pain is under investigation. In this section pain associated with direct tumor involvement is discussed. Pain associated with either the cancer therapy, such as postoperative pain syndromes, or pain syndromes related or unrelated to the cancer itself, such as myofascial pains or constipation, are not considered.

The evidence shows that the prevalence of pain varies according to the site of the cancer and the stage of the disease. Although there are limitations to the data, as discussed earlier, it is possible to draw several conclusions as to who is more likely to be at risk.

Patients reported as more likely to experience pain may be those with primary tumors of the head and neck, the genitourinary system, the esophagus, and the prostate (mean prevalence values for these tumors from more than one study were more than 70%). In addition, the higher prevalence estimates found for patients with far-advanced cancer would indicate that these patients are more likely to be experiencing pain at referral to a service than those at earlier stages of the disease.

Daut and Cleeland (38) found that more pain is usually associated with metastatic than nonmetastatic disease. For example, 64% of those patients with metastatic breast cancer had pain as compared to 40% of patients with nonmetastatic disease, a pattern that is consistent throughout cancer types. This may be related to stage of disease.

Age is not necessarily associated with a greater number of symptoms in cancer (25), and there is no evidence as to whether age is a predictor of pain in cancer patients. There is some suggestion that pain is actually lower among the elderly, but it is not clear whether this is due to physiological changes, different cultural systems, or ageism.

There is no evidence on whether specific psychological factors predispose to the initial onset of pain. However, the effect of pain on increasing psychological distress has been well documented, and it is likely that patients with unresolved psychosocial problems will experience more frequent or more intense pain compared to those patients who are not experiencing psychological distress, according to the models of "suffering" and "total pain."

The severity of pain is determined by the previously mentioned factors combined with the method of pain control therapy administered, and whether it has been appropriate to the needs of the individual patient.

The continued reports of high levels of pain prevalence on referral to cancer services suggests that pain is not being managed as well as it should be (26,68–70). Health professionals should not assume that those patients previously receiving care elsewhere have adequate pain control.

Challenges for the future in the epidemiology of cancer pain

The reality of addressing cancer pain control, coupled with the increasing number of people living to older ages and living longer with cancer, makes reducing the prevalence of pain at any stage of the disease process of paramount importance. Collaboration is needed with the nonmedical sectors of society to ensure that palliative care becomes an integral part of patient care (71). Just as important as research in the purely medical aspects of pain and palliative care are the social, economic, and cultural attitudes toward pain, suffering, and the terminally ill (100–107). This is especially true as the proportion of caregivers declines relative to the growing number of patients who need care (3). Much more work is needed to study the epidemiology of pain in general and community populations, rather than in specialist centers, but using standardized assessments. Work is also needed on pain in different cultural populations and among older people. As cancer treatments change, so the nature and prevalence of pain in cancer may change and this will require careful assessment (80–82).

The gap between what is possible in pain control and what is achieved is due to reasons such as the following (1,83–96):

1. A lack of awareness that established methods already exist for cancer pain management
2. A lack of systematic teaching of medical students, doctors, nurses, and other health care workers about cancer pain management

3. Fears about addiction in both cancer patients and the wider public if strong opioids are more readily available for medical purpose
4. Nonavailability of necessary pain relief drugs in many parts of the world
5. Use of special "triplicate prescription" forms for controlled drugs, which discourages the use of strong opioids
6. A lack of concern by governments

Quality improvement guidelines for the treatment of acute pain and cancer pain were published by the American Pain Society Quality of Care Committee in 1995 (97), building on guidelines published by others (98–103). There are five key elements to the guidelines for improving quality of care for people with acute or cancer pain:

1. Ensuring that a report of unrelieved pain raises a "red flag" that attracts clinicians' attention
2. Making information about analgesics convenient where orders are written
3. Promising patients responsive analgesic care and urging them to communicate pain
4. Implementing policies and safeguards for the use of modern analgesic technologies
5. Coordinating and assessing implementation of these measures

Clinicians often do not recognize how frequently pain remains untreated or inadequately managed (23). It should not be assumed that if a person has been receiving cancer care or treatment in a health care setting that the pain is being adequately controlled (26,104). Continual assessment of the response of the patient's pain complaint is essential to ensure continual pain control and to prevent breakthrough pain (81,105). There is also a need for training and education, a key function of the specialist in palliative care. Health care professionals in all health care settings need to monitor pain and know how to treat cancer pain effectively.

References

1. Grond S, Zech D, Schug SA, et al. Validation for the World Health Organization guidelines for cancer pain relief in the last days and hours of life. J Pain Symptom Manage 6:411–22, 1991.
2. Zech DFJ, Grond S, Lynch J, et al. Validation of the World Health Organization Guidelines for cancer pain relief: a 10-year prospective study. Pain 63:65–76, 1995.
3. Stjernsward J, Colleau SM, Ventafridda V. The World Health Organisation Cancer Pain and Palliative Care

Program: past, present, and future. J Pain Symptom Manage 12(2):65–72, 1996.

4. World Health Organization (WHO). The World Health Report 1996, fighting disease, fostering development executive summary. Geneva: The World Health Organisation, 1996.

5. Allende S, Carvell HC. Mexico: status of cancer pain and palliative care. J Pain Symptom Manage 12(2):121–3, 1996.

6. Cherny NI. Israel: status of cancer pain and palliative care. J Pain Symptom Manage 12(2):116–7, 1996.

7. Erdine S. Turkey: status of cancer pain and palliative care. J Pain Symptom Manage 12(2):139–40, 1996.

8. Fernandez A, Acuna G. Chile: status of cancer pain and palliative care. J Pain Symptom Manage 12(2):102–3, 1996.

9. Goh CR. Singapore: status of cancer pain and palliative care. J Pain Symptom Manage 12(2):130–2, 1996.

10. Larue F, Fontaine A, Brasseur L, Neuwirth L. France: status of cancer pain and palliative care. J Pain Symptom Manage 12(2):106–8, 1996.

11. Laudico AV. The Phillipines: status of cancer pain and palliative care. J Pain Symptom Manage 12(2):133–5, 1996.

12. Lickiss JN. Australia: status of cancer pain and palliative care. J Pain Symptom Manage 12(2):99–101, 1996.

13. Merriman A. Uganda: status of cancer pain and palliative care. J Pain Symptom Manage 12(2):141–3, 1996.

14. Moyano J. Colombia: status of cancer pain and palliative care. J Pain Symptom Manage 12(2):102–3, 1996.

15. Soebadi RD, Tejawinata S. Indonesia: status of cancer pain and palliative care. J Pain Symptom Manage 12(2):112–5, 1996.

16. Strumpf M, Zenz M, Donner B. Germany: status of cancer pain and palliative care. J Pain Symptom Manage 12(2):109–11, 1996.

17. Sun WZ, Hou WY, Li JH. Republic of China: status of cancer pain and palliative care. J Pain Symptom Manage 12(2):127–9, 1996.

18. Takeda F. Results of field-testing in Japan of the WHO draft interim guideline on relief of cancer pain. Pain Clinic 1:83–9, 1986.

19. Wenk R, Ochoa J. Argentina: status of cancer pain and palliative care. J Pain Symptom Manage 12(2):97–9, 1996.

20. Zylicz Z. The Netherlands: status of cancer pain and palliative care. J Pain Symptom Manage 12(2):136–8, 1996.

21. Zhang H, Gu WP, Joranson DE, Cleeland C. People's Republic of China: status of cancer pain and palliative care. J Pain Symptom Manage 12(2):124–6, 1996.

22. Foley KM. Pain syndromes in patients with cancer. In: Bonica JJ, Ventafridda V, eds. Advances in pain research and therapy. New York: Raven Press, 1979:59–75.

23. Bonica JJ. Treatment of cancer pain: current status and future needs. In: Fields HL, ed. Advances in pain research and therapy, Vol 9. New York: Raven, 1985:589–616.

24. Portenoy RK. Epidemiology and syndromes of cancer pain. Cancer 63:2298–307, 1989.

25. Grond S, Zech D, Diefenbach C, Bischoff A. Prevalence and pattern of symptoms in patients with cancer pain: a prospectice evaluation of 1635 cancer patients referred to a pain clinic. J Pain Symptom Manage 9:372–82, 1994.

26. Higginson IJ, Hearn J. A multicentre evaluation of cancer pain control by palliative care teams. J Pain Symptom Manage 13:1–7, 1997.

27. Banning A, Sjorgen P, Henriksen H. Pain causes in 200 patients referred to a multidisciplinary cancer pain clinic. Pain 45:45–8, 1991.

28. Portenoy RK. Cancer pain: pathophysiology and syndromes. Lancet 39:1026–31, 1992.

29. Welsh Office NHS Directorate. Pain, discomfort and palliative care. Welsh Health Planning Forum: Welsh Office, 1992.

30. Twycross R. Cancer pain classification. Acta Anaesthesiol Scand 41:141–5, 1997.

31. Twycross RG. Attention to detail. Progress Palliative Care 2:222–7, 1994.

32. International Association for the study of pain. Subcommittee on taxonomy of pain terms: a list with definitions and notes on usage. Pain 6:249–52, 1979.

33. Foley KM. Pain assessment and cancer pain. In: Doyle D, Hanks G, Macdonald N, eds. The Oxford textbook of palliative medicine. Oxford: Oxford University Press, 1993, pp 140–8.

34. Cleeland CS, Nakamura Y, Mendoza TR, et al. Dimensions of the impact of cancer pain in a four country sample: new information from multidimensional scaling. Pain 67:267–73, 1996.

35. Coyle N. The last four weeks of life. Am J Nurs 90(12):75–8, 1990.

36. Lin CC. Disclosure of the cancer diagnosis as it relates to the quality of pain management among patients with cancer pain in Taiwan. J Pain Symptom Manage 18(5):331–7, 1999.

37. Uki J, Mendoza T, Cleeland CS, et al. A brief cancer pain assessment tool in Japanese: the utility of the Japanese Brief Pain Inventory—BPI-J. J Pain Symptom Manage 16(6):364–73, 1998.

38. Daut RL, Cleeland CS. The prevalence and severity of pain in cancer. Cancer 50:1913–8, 1982.

39. Serlin RC, Mendoza TR, Nakamura Y, et al. When is cancer pain mld, moderate or severe? Grading pain severity by its interference with function. Pain 61:277–84, 1995.

40. Spross JA, McGuire DB, Schmitt RM. Oncology nursing forum position paper on cancer pain; part I. Oncol Nurs Forum 17:595–614, 1991.

41. World Health Organization (WHO). Cancer pain relief and palliative care, 2nd ed. Geneva: WHO, 1996.

42. Cherny N, Portenoy RK. Cancer pain management: current strategy. Cancer Supplement 72(11):3393–415, 1993.

43. Baines M, Kirkham SR. Cancer pain. In: Wall PD, Melzack R, eds. Textbook of pain, 2nd ed. Edinburgh: Churchill Livingstone, 1993.

44. Jensen MP, Karoly P, Braver S. The measurement of clinical pain intensity: a comparison of six methods. Pain 27:117–26, 1986.

45. Moinpour CM, Feigl P, Metch B, et al. Quality of life end points in cancer clinical trials: review and recommendations. J Natl Cancer Inst 81:485–95, 1989.

46. Hearn J, Higginson IJ. Outcome measures in palliative care for advanced cancer patients: a review. J Public Health Med 19:193–9, 1997.

47. Bruera E, Kuehn N, Miller MJ, et al. The Edmonton Symptom Assessment System (ESAS): a simple method for the assessment of palliative care patients. J Palliative Care 7(2):6–9, 1991.

48. Hearn J, Higginson IJ, on behalf of the Palliative Care Audit Project Advisory Group. Development and validation of a core outcome measure for palliative care: the palliative care outcome scale. Qual Healthcare 8:219–27, 1999.

49. Higginson IJ, McCarthy M. Validity of the support team assessment schedule: do staffs' ratings reflect those made by patients or their families? Palliative Med 7:219–28, 1993.

50. Ventafridda V, Caraceni A. Cancer pain classification: a controversial issue. Pain 46:1–2, 1991.

51. Higginson IJ, Finlay I, Goodwin DM, et al. Do hospital-based palliative care teams improve care for patients or families at the end of life? Journal Pain and Symptom Management 23:96–106, 2002.

52. Bonica JJ. Cancer pain. In: Bonica JJ, ed. The management of cancer pain. Philadelphia: Lea and Febiger, 1990:400–60.

53. Walley BA, Hagen NA. The epidemiology of cancer pain. Pain Digest 5:237–44, 1995.

54. Hiraga K, Mizuguchi T, Takeda F. The incidence of cancer pain and improvement of pain management in Japan. Postgrad Med J 67:S14–S25, 1991.

55. Elliott SC, Miser AM, Dose AM, et al. Epidemiologic features of pain in pediatric cancer patients: a co-operative community based study. North Central Cancer Treatment Group and Mayo Clinic. Clin J Pain 7(4):263–8, 1991.

56. Vuorinen E. Pain as an early symptom in cancer. Clin J Pain 9(4):272–8, 1993.

57. Ger LP, Ho ST, Wang JJ, Cherng CH. The prevalence and severity of cancer pain: a study of newly-diagnosed cancer patients in Taiwan. J Pain Symptom Manage 15(5):285–93, 1998.

58. Ward AWM. Terminal care in malignant disease. Soc Sci Med 8:413–20, 1974.

59. Parkes CM. Home or hospital? Terminal care as seen by the surviving spouse. J R Coll Gen Pract 28:19–23, 1978.

60. Cartwright A. Changes in life and care in the year before death 1969–1987. J Public Health Med 13(2):81–7, 1991.

61. Addington-Hall J, McCarthy M. Dying from cancer: results of a national population based investigation. Palliative Med 9:295–305, 1995.

62. Bucher JA, Trostle GB, Moore M. Family reports of cancer pain, pain relief, and prescription access. Cancer Practice 7(2):71–7, 1999.

63. Donnelly S, Walsh D, Rybicki L. The symptoms of advanced cancer: identification of clinical and research priorities by assessment of prevalence and severity. J Palliative Care 11(1):27–32, 1995.

64. Simpson M. The use of research to facilitate the creation of a hospital palliative care team. Palliative Med 5:122–9, 1991.

65. Portenoy RK, Kornblith AB, Wong G, et al. Pain in ovarian cancer patients-prevalence, characteristics and associated symptoms. Cancer 74(3):907–15, 1994.

66. Twycross R. Pain in far-advanced cancer. Pain 14:303–10, 1982.

67. Portenoy RK, Thaler HT, Kornblith AB, et al. Symptom prevalence, characteristics and distress in a cancer population. Qual Life Res 3:183–9, 1994.

68. Ellershaw JE, Peat SJ, Boys LC. Assessing the effectiveness of a hospital palliative care team. Palliative Med 9:145–52, 1995.

69. Larue F, Colleau SM, Fontaine A, Brasseur L. Oncologists and primary care physicians' attitudes towards pain control and morphine prescribing in France. Cancer 76(11):2375–82, 1995.

70. Larue F, Colleau SM, Brasseur L, Cleeland CS. Multicentre study of cancer pain and its treatment in France. BMJ 310:1034–7, 1995.

71. Stjernsward J, Koroltchouk V, Teoh N. National policies for cancer pain relief and palliative care. Palliative Med 6:273–6, 1992.

72. Ahles TA, Blanchard EB, Ruckdeschel JC. The multidimensional nature of cancer-related pain. Pain 17(3):277–88, 1983.

73. Baile WF, Di Maggio JR, Schapira DV, Janofsky JS. The requests for assistance in dying: the need for psychiatric consultation. Cancer 72:2786–91, 1993.

74. Barkwell DP. Ascribed meaning: a critical factor in coping and pain attenuation in patients with cancer-related pain. J Palliative Care 7(3):5–14, 1991.

75. Bolund C. Medical and care factors in suicides by cancer patients in Sweden. J Psychosom Oncol 3:31–52, 1985.

76. Bond MR, Pearson IB. Psychosocial aspects of pain in women with advanced cancer of the cervix. J Pyschosom Res 13:13–21, 1969.

77. Bond MR. Psychologic and emotional aspects of cancer pain. In: Bonica JJ, Ventafridda V, eds. Advances in pain research and therapy. New York: Raven Press, 1979:81–8.

78. Breitbart W. Cancer pain management guidelines: implications for psychooncology. Psychooncology 3:103–18, 1994.

79. Breitbart W. Suicide in the cancer patient. Oncology 1:49–54, 1987.

80. Bruera E, Macmillan K, Hanson J, MacDonald RN. The Edmonton staging system for cancer pain. Pain 37(2):203–9, 1989.

81. Bruera E. A prospective multicentre assessment of the Edmonton staging system for cancer pain. J Pain Symptom Manage 10(5):348–55, 1995.

82. Portenoy RK, Foley KM, Inturisi CE. The nature of opioid responsiveness and its implications for neuropathic pain: new hypotheses derived from studies of opioid infusions. Pain 43:273–86, 1990.

83. Cleeland CS. The impact of pain on the patient with cancer. Cancer 54:2635–41, 1984.

84. Dorrepaal KL, Aaronson NK, van Dam FS. Pain experience and pain management among hospitalised cancer patients. A clinical study. Cancer 63(3):593–8, 1989.

85. World Health Organisation (WHO). Cancer pain relief. Geneva: World Health Organization, 1986.

86. Zenz M, Willweber-Strumpf A. Opiophobia and cancer pain in Europe. Lancet 341:1075–6, 1993.

87. Vainio A. Treatment of terminal cancer pain in France: a questionnaire study. Pain 62:155–62, 1995.

88. Takeda F. Japan: status of cancer pain and palliative care. J Pain Symptom Manage 12(2):118–20, 1996.

89. Chan A, Woodruff RK. Palliative care in a general teaching hospital. Med J Aust 155:597–9, 1991.

90. Cherny NI, Catane R. Professional negligence in the management of cancer pain. Cancer 76(11):2181–5, 1995.

91. Cherny NI, Coyle N, Foley KM. Suffering in the advanced cancer patient: a definition and taxonomy. J Palliative Care 10:57–70, 1994.

92. Au E, Loprinzi CL, Dhodapkar M, et al. Regular use of a verbal pain scale improves the understanding of oncology inpatient pain intensity. J Clin Oncol 12:2751–5, 1994.

93. Fainsinger R, Miller MJ, Bruera E, et al. Symptom control in the last week of life on a palliative care unit. J Palliat Care 7(1):5–11, 1991.

94. Foley KM. The treatment of cancer pain. N Engl J Med 313:84–95, 1985.

95. Goldberg R, Guadagnoli E, Silliman RA, Glicksman A. Cancer patients' concerns: congruence between patients and primary care physicians. J Cancer Educ 5(3):193–9, 1990.

96. Kelsen DP, Portenoy RK, Thaler HT, et al. Pain and depression in patients with newly diagnosed pancreas cancer. J Clin Oncol 13:748–55, 1995.

97. American Pain Society Quality of Care Committee. Quality improvement guidelines for the treatment of acute pain and cancer pain. JAMA 274(23):1874–80, 1995.

98. Stjernsward J, Teoh N. Current status of the global cancer control program of the World Health Organisation. J Pain Symptom Manage 8:340–7, 1993.

99. Stjernsward J, Stanley K, Koroltchouk V. WHO guidelines for cancer pain relief. Cancer Nur 10(Suppl 1):135–7, 1987.

100. Portenoy RK. Report form the International Association for the Study of Pain Task Force on cancer pain. J Pain Symptom Manage 12(2):93–6, 1996.

101. Max M. American Pain Society quality assurance standards for relief of acute pain and cancer pain. In: Bond MR, Charlton JE, Woolf CJ, eds. Proceedings of the VI World Congress on Pain. Amsterdam, The Netherlands: Elsevier, 1990.

102. Jacox A, Carr DB, Payne R. The new clinical practice guidelines for the management of pain in patients with cancer. N Engl J Med 330:651–5, 1994.

103. Foley KM, Portenoy RK. World Health Organisation-International Association for the study of pain: joint initiatives in cancer pain relief. J Pain Symptom Manage 8(6):335–9, 1993.

104. Kaasa S, Malt U, Hagen S, et al. Psychological distress in cancer patients with advanced cancer. Radiother Oncol 27:93–197, 1993.

105. Cassell EJ. The relief of suffering. Arch Intern Med 143:552–3, 1983.

106. Trotter JM, Scott R, Macbeth FR, et al. Problems of oncology outpatients: role of the liaison health visitor. Br Med J Clin Res Ed 282:122–4, 1981.

107. Greenwald HP, Bonica JJ, Bergner M. The prevalence of pain in four cancers. Cancer 60:2563–9, 1987.

108. Glover J, Dibble SL, Dodd MJ, Miaskowski C. Mood states of oncology outpatients: does pain make a difference. J Pain Symptom Manage 10(2):120–8, 1995.

109. Miaskowski C, Dibble SL. The problem of pain in outpatients with breast cancer. Oncol Nurs Forum 22(5):791–7, 1995.

110. Grond S, Zech D, Diefenbach C, et al. Assessment of cancer pain: a prospective evaluation in 2266 cancer patients referred to a pain service. Pain 64:107–14, 1996.

111. De Wit R, van Dam F, Zandbelt L, et al. A pain education program for chronic cancer pain patients: follow-up results from a randomised controlled. Pain 79:55–69, 1999.

112. Elliott TE, Murray DM, Oken MM, et al. Improving cancer pain management in communities: main results from a randomized controlled trial. J Pain Symptom Manage 13(4):191–203, 1997.

113. Bernabei R, Gambassi G, Lapane K, et al, for the SAGE Study Group. Management of pain in elderly patients with cancer. JAMA 279(23):1877–82, 1998.

114. Rummans TA, Frost M, Suman VJ, et al. Quality of life and pain in patients with recurrent breast and gynecologic cancer. Psychosomatics 39:437–45, 1998.

115. Wells N, Johnson RL, Wujick D. Development of a short version of the Barriers Questionnaire. J Pain Symptom Manage 15(5):285–93, 1998.

116. Caraceni A, Portenoy RK, a working group of the IASP Task Force on Cancer Pain. An international survey of cancer pain characteristics and syndromes. Pain 82:263–74, 1999.

117. Chaplin JM, Morton RP. A prospective, longitudinal study of pain in head and neck cancer patients. Head Neck 21(6):531–7, 1999.

118. Grond S, Radbruch L, Meuser T, et al. Assessment and treatment of neuropathic cancer pain following WHO guidelines. Pain 79:15–20, 1999.

119. Berry DL, Wilkie DJ, Huang HY, Blumenstein BA. Cancer pain and common pain: a comparison of patient-reported intensities, Oncol Nurs Forum 26(4):721–6, 1999.

120. Rykowski JJ, Hilger M. Efficacy of neurolytic celiac plexus block in varying locations of pancreatic cancer. Anesthesiology 92:347–54, 2000.

121. Morris JN, Mor V, Goldberg RJ, et al. The effect of treatment setting and patient characteristics on pain in terminal cancer patients: a report from the national hospice study. J Chronic Dis 39(1):27–35, 1986.

122. McMurray MB, Warren MR. Evaluation of a new hospice: the relief of symptoms in cancer patients in the first year. Palliative Med 3:135–40, 1989.

123. Ventafridda V, De Conno F, Vigano A, et al. Tumori 75:619–625, 1989.

124. Higginson I, Wade A, McCarthy M. Palliative care: view of patients and their families. BMJ 301:277–81, 1990.

125. Ventafridda V, Ripamonti C, De Conno F, et al. Symptom prevalence and control during cancer patients' last days of life. J Palliative Care 6(3):7–11, 1990.
126. Stein WM, Miech RP: Cancer pain in the elderly hospice patient. J Pain Symptom Manage 8(7):474–82, 1993.
127. Mercadante S, Armata M, Salvaggio L. Pain characteristics of advanced lung cancer patients referred to a palliative care service. Pain 59:141–5, 1994.
128. Shannon MM, Ryan MA, D'Agostino N, Brescia FJ. Assessment of pain in advanced cancer patients. J Pain Symptom Manage 10(4):274–8, 1995.
129. Vainio A, Auvinen A. Prevalence of symptoms among patients with advanced cancer: an international collaborative study. Symptom Prevalence Group. J Pain Symptom Manage 12(1):3–10, 1996.
130. Chung JW, Yang JC, Wong TK. The significance of pain among Chinese patients with cancer in Hong Kong. Acta Anaesthesiol Sin 37(1):9–14, 1999.
131. Mercadante S. Pain treatment and outcomes for patients with advanced cancer who receive follow-up care at home. Cancer 85:1849–58, 1999.
132. Nowels D, Lee JT. Cancer pain management in home hospice settings: a comparison of primary care and oncologic physicians. J Palliative Care 15(3):5–9, 1999.

3 Cancer pain: prevalence and undertreatment

SEAN O'MAHONY
Albert Einstein College of Medicine

Introduction

Today, for every death caused by cancer there are two caused by infection and parasitic infestation. It is projected that this number will reach parity by 2015. Most of this increase will occur in the developing world, where 55%–60% of the world's cancer patients reside, and the majority of patients will present for palliation until primary prevention programs are in place. Palliative care is not available to eight out of nine cancer patients in the developing world (1).

Cancer pain affects 17 million people worldwide. Its prevalence increases with extent of disease. Its type, location, and intensity vary with tumor type, spread of disease, and disease treatments (2–6). Prevalence rates of 30%–40% are reported for patients receiving active treatment; these increase to 70% to 90% for patients with advanced cancer (7). The National Hospice Report of 1754 patients with advanced cancer demonstrated that only 25% of patients reported persistent pain within 48 hours of death because only 26% of the patients studied could use the assessment tool included in the study (8). This statistic may exemplify a tendency to underestimate pain prevalence in this group. The unexpectedly low estimates of pain prevalence in this population may relate to the high prevalence of cognitive impairment. Other studies observe pain prevalence rates ranging from 12%–99% in the last week of life, with greater than 30% prevalence in seven of nine studies assessed. This variability may relate to the wide variety of scales used to report pain (9).

Chronic cancer pain may occur in relation to disease progression, a complication of the illness or its treatment, or conditions unrelated to the patient's cancer. Cancer pain may also be acute and occur as a consequence of diagnostic or therapeutic interventions or as a result of an acute complication of the disease (10,11).

Cancer pain often occurs at multiple sites. A prospective survey of 2266 cancer patients referred to a pain service demonstrated that 30% of patients presented with one pain syndrome, 39% with two pain syndromes, and 31% with three or more pain syndromes (12). The duration of cancer pain varies, but it can extend to several months or years (13). Transient flares of pain, or breakthrough pains, occur in approximately half the patients with cancer pain and are often associated with patient dissatisfaction with pain control. Breakthrough pain may be associated with the presence of baseline neuropathic pain (14,15).

Persistent pain interferes with multiple domains of function, including social relations and activity level. In the United States, an Eastern Cooperative Oncology Group survey of 1308 ambulatory cancer patients found that 67% reported recent pain, and 36% reported their pain severity as sufficient to interfere with their function (16). In a French study, 69% of patients similarly rated their pain as sufficient to interfere with their function (17). Pain is also associated with an increased prevalence of depression, anxiety, suicidality, hopelessness, and desire for hastened death (18–21). A study at Memorial Sloan-Kettering Cancer Center demonstrated a 17% prevalence of suicidality in patients receiving cancer pain management (18). More than 50% of ambulatory patients receiving treatment for metastatic colon and lung cancer reported moderate or greater pain interference with sleep, mood, and enjoyment of life (22).

Undertreatment of cancer pain

Although reviews of the literature confirm that cancer pain may be relieved in 70%–90% of patients (23), an increasing body of evidence suggests that cancer pain remains undertreated internationally. In 1993, Solomon et al. (24) reported that eight out of ten physicians stated that the most serious form of opioid abuse was undertreatment of pain.

A chart review study of 311 patients treated in a community hospital setting revealed that fewer than one third of patients, including patients with cancer pain, were receiving opioid medications more often than every 6 hours; there was a tendency to use a limited range of opioids (25). A French national questionnaire study of general practitioners and specialists indicated that only 10% of patients treated by general practitioners and 21% of patients treated by specialists were receiving treatment regimens appropriate to their pain severity (26).

An analysis of the computerized medical records of more than 1 million German patients revealed that only 1.9% of patients with cancer were receiving prescriptions for strong opioid medications, and many patients were receiving medications at inappropriate intervals and often on an "as required" basis (27). A random sample of 10% and 5% of Finnish physicians in 1985 and 1990, respectively, demonstrated improvements in pain control. During this period there was increased activity by patient organizations and the development of specialized pain clinics; however, up to 39% of physicians regularly treating patients with cancer pain did not have the requisite prescription sheets for opioid medications (28). A Swedish nationwide questionnaire survey of practitioners treating 10% of the country's cancer patients suggested that many patients were still receiving opioids by intermittent subcutaneous and intramuscular administration rather than continuously (29). Fear of addiction and respiratory depression appears to limit physicians' use of strong opioids (30).

In a study of 13,625 U.S. nursing home residents with daily pain, factors predictive of undertreatment of cancer pain included poor cognitive status, polypharmacy, and advanced age (> 85 years) (31). A study of 1308 ambulatory cancer patients suggested that up to 42% of patients with cancer pain were not receiving adequate analgesic regimens. Predictors of inadequate pain management included minority status, discrepancy between patient and physician rating of pain severity, age, female sex, and poor performance status. Minority patients in the United States are more likely to have undertreated cancer pain (16,31,32). Low income and minority status were also predictive of undertreatment of pain in the Study to Understand Prognoses and Preferences For Outcomes and Risks of Treatments (SUPPORT) (33).

Prevalence of cancer pain and undertreatment in special populations

Cancer pain in the elderly

Life expectancy is increasing in both the industrialized and developing world. In the developing world, the total population is predicted to increase by 95%, and the elderly population is expected to increase by 240% between 1980 and 2020 (34). In absolute numbers, the total number of elderly patients in the developing world is expected to increase from the current 286 million (6.9%) to just over 1 billion in 2030 (15.2%). In the industrialized world, the proportion of elderly is expected to increase from 18% to 28% (203 million to 358 million) (35). The incidence of most cancers is higher in the elderly population.

Although the epidemiology of cancer pain in the elderly has not been widely studied, it has been suggested that as many as 80% will have substantial pain (36). The prevalence of the complications of pain in the elderly also has not been adequately studied; these complications include gait disturbances, falls, delayed rehabilitation, malnutrition, and cognitive dysfunction. Data suggest an association between increased mortality and chest, head, abdominal, and rectal pain, but not shoulder back, or hip pain, in the elderly (37).

The SAGE study group report of 4003 elderly nursing home residents with cancer demonstrated a correlation between undermedication of pain and advanced age. A total of 38% had evidence of daily pain, and 26% of these patients received no analgesics (31). In all 13% of patients with cancer pain older than 85 received opioid medications in comparison with 38% of patients aged 65 to 74. Patients older than 85 were also more likely to receive no analgesia (31).

The undertreatment of cancer pain in the elderly is also found in studies of pain in the ambulatory and hospitalized elderly. In a survey of 1308 patients treated at 54 treatment locations affiliated with the Eastern Cooperative Oncology Group, age greater than 70 years was predictive of poorly controlled pain as well as greater functional impairment secondary to pain (16). In the SUPPORT study, which included 903 hospitalized patients with cancer, increased age was predictive of pain level (33). A total of 44% of 239 consecutive patients over the age of 65 reported pain on admission to a hospice, and of those not initially reporting pain, 55% later required analgesic medication. Nearly one third of elderly patients dying at home were found to have pain in the last 24 hours of life according to interviews with next of kin (38,39).

Cancer pain in children

Children may be undertreated for pain because of the misconception that pain is not experienced by the very young or because of the difficulty of pain assessment. The problem of pain assessment is particularly significant in children younger than age 3 years. The use of visual analog scales has been validated in children as young as 8 years and the use of happy/sad faces has been used in patients as young as 3 years (40). Nevertheless, the use of validated measures in clinical practice is uncommon. In a national Swedish survey of pediatric oncology clinicians, 63% followed the World Health Organization (WHO) analgesic "ladder principle," 72% of clinicians felt that pain could be more effectively managed, and use of validated assessment instruments was rare. Only 31% of clinicians used visual analog scales, 23% used faces, 16% used systematic behavioral observation, and 4% used pain diaries (41).

Miser et al. (42) demonstrated that pain is a common presenting complaint of cancer in a pediatric population. In their study, 57 of 92 cancer patients had pain as an initial presenting complaint, and in 42 patients, this pain was sufficient to interfere with sleep patterns.

The prevalence of pain in children with cancer who are hospitalized reaches 50% in some surveys; this contrasts with a prevalence rate of 25% in outpatients (43). Therapy-related pain predominates in pediatric oncology. In epidemiological surveys, fewer than 30% of patients had tumor-related pain. In another survey, even with the exclusion of procedure-related pain, 58% of pain was related to the complications of cancer treatment, 21% of patients had pain unrelated to their cancer, and 21% of patients had pain directly related to their cancer (44). Recent evidence suggests that although procedural pain becomes less severe later in treatment protocols for childhood cancers, there does not appear to be a decrease in treatment-related pain (45). These data contrast with adult surveys, which indicated that up to 85% of patients have pain related to their cancer and only 17% have pain related to their cancer treatment (7).

Miser et al. (42) demonstrated that 68% of tumor-related pain in pediatric cancer patients was caused by bone lesions, 16% by soft tissue lesions, 5% by cord compression, and 11% by other causes. This survey, however, was characterized by a greater prevalence of sarcoma patients and relative underrepresentation of leukemia and lymphoma. Cornaglia et al. (46) demonstrated a higher prevalence of pain in children with solid malignancies than in patients with hematological malignancies.

Several studies confirm undermedication of pain in children (47,48), and population studies suggest that reports of pain in children may be predictive of pain at later ages. Future research may highlight the relationship between pediatric pain reports and parental and sibling experience of pain and whether patterns of disproportion-ate health care utilization and self-medication can be predicted in children presenting with pain (49).

Cancer pain in minorities

In a study of outpatients with metastatic cancer treated at centers that predominantly treat minorities, patients were three times more likely than patients treated elsewhere to receive inadequate pain management (16). Much of this was attributed to language differences.

In the SAGE study, minority patients were less likely to have pain recorded (even after adjustment for language differences (31). In a more recent report of 281 outpatients with cancer, minority patients were less likely than white patients to be medicated for pain; 65% of minority patients received inadequate analgesia as compared with 50% of non-minority patients (50). This tendency to undermedicate and underassess pain is more marked for minority women (51).

Part of this tendency toward the undertreatment of cancer pain in minorities may relate to both patient and family reluctance to report pain or take analgesics. Clinician concerns about patient resources also may affect prescription practices and lead to difficulty assessing pain because of differences in language and cultural differences. Hispanic patients reported less adequate pain relief than black patients and tended to receive less adequate analgesic treatment and to raise more concerns about analgesic side effects. This suggests a role for culturally targeted education programs.

Little research has been done on the reliability of conventional assessment tools and their translations for different ethnic groups. Health care providers may misinterpret less verbal expression of pain as being indicative of a need for less aggressive pain management.

Some clinicians suggest that targeted interviews for some ethnic groups rather than printed, translated assessment tools including Hispanics may prove more effective in data collection, independent of literacy level (52). Several assessment instruments have been validated cross-culturally, including non-verbal rating scales (53,54).

Pharmacies in minority neighborhoods are frequently reported to have a lower availability of opioids (55). This lack of opioid availability in minority neighborhoods is matched by a tendency to undermedicate pain in minority patients. Non-cancer pain has been shown to be medicated with different morphine equivalent doses for different ethnic groups, suggesting a role for clinician adherence to racial stereotypes with regard to the medication of pain, its assessment, and concerns about substance abuse (56).

Cancer pain in the developing world

In the year 2015, it is predicted that 10 of the 15 million new cases of cancer worldwide will occur in the developing world; as many as 80% to 90% of these will continue to present with advanced disease (57). The WHO uses national morphine consumption for medical purposes as a marker for progress by a country in the treatment of cancer pain; 50% of countries use little or no morphine (58,59). Although codeine is more widely used worldwide than morphine, its use for non-analgesic purposes limits its utility as a marker of cancer pain management resources.

Almost all morphine is consumed in the developed world. The WHO cancer pain relief initiative was implemented in 1984. Between 1984 and 1991, the global consumption of morphine for medical purposes increased by 272%. The 20 countries with the highest per capita consumption of morphine were all developed countries. Together the top 20 countries account for 86% of the morphine consumed globally. The 10 countries consuming 57% of all morphine in 1991 have ranked highest in morphine consumption for many years. They include Australia, Canada, Denmark, Iceland, Ireland, New Zealand, Norway, Sweden, the United Kingdom, and the United States. The remaining 14% of morphine was consumed by approximately 100 other countries, the majority of the world's population (57). Changes in opioid consumption have been mixed during this time. Although many developing countries have demonstrated some increase in morphine usage during this time, many have reported decreases, including Malaysia, Mexico, Cuba, Bulgaria, India, Nicaragua, Kenya, Albania, Zambia, and Bangladesh. The 1995 report of the International Narcotics Control Board demonstrated an 80.19 mg per capita consumption of morphine for Denmark in comparison with a consumption of less than 0.1 mg for many developing nations (59).

Many countries lack economic resources and medical infrastructure to produce and distribute oral opioid medications. Treatment is directed at disease rather than pain. Oral morphine has only recently been recognized as a potentially useful opioid in many countries.

Barriers include a lack of clinician knowledge of opioid pharmacology, and insufficient education of patients and family of their diagnosis and prognosis. Many countries adhere to restrictive regulations requiring triplicate prescriptions and limiting the period during which a patient may receive oral morphine; some even limit the locations where opioids can be dispensed (60). Between 1984 and 1991, the price of oral morphine sulfate has increased considerably in several countries. In some countries, such as Costa Rica in 1993, the importation of morphine was restricted to the government and then exclusively in ampules. In some cases, the unsanctioned administration of morphine to cancer patients is subject to the same fines and prison terms as the use of opioids by drug addicts (61). In Mexico in 1993, there was a severe limitation in obtaining morphine, resulting in a reliance on partial agonists and agonist/antagonists. This was so despite the evidence that opioids were used illicitly less than other drugs (62,63). In many countries, available formulations of morphine (e.g., 10-mg controlled-release formulations in the Philippines) predispose to underdosing (64). Opioid distribution and provision of hospice services in nations such as Uganda, where 94% of hospice referrals are for uncontrolled pain, were hampered by poorly developed infrastructures, damaged by prolonged civil strife (65).

In 1996, Joranson and Colleagues reported on the impact of a joint Chinese health ministry and WHO Collaborating Center plan to improve cancer pain management in China, a country with a high level of concern about the potential for opioid addiction (66). The 1993 per capita morphine consumption for China was 0.01 mg as compared with 66.53 mg for Denmark. The government has liberalized legislation limiting the availability of opioids, initiated joint ventures for the manufacture of opioids, and streamlined hospital policies allowing the availability of sufficient opioids. The Wisconsin Pain Research Group, in conjunction with the Chinese government, provided training seminars for health care professionals in five regional centers.

Data presented from the 1994 International Narcotics Control Board report demonstrated an increase in morphine consumption in countries that had initiated palliative care initiatives, including Argentina, Costa Rica, Mexico, and the Dominican Republic. Recommendations to increase opioid availability included the importation of morphine powder for the domestic manufacture of simple formulations of opioids. Governments were encouraged to reduce taxes and paper work restrictions on imported opioids. Members were encouraged to participate in training seminars of health care professionals, utilizing the International Association for the Study of Pain core curriculum as well as the involvement of pharmaceutical companies in these initiatives. Members were encouraged to lobby for a reduction in the information requested on special prescription forms, as well as restrictions on dosage, duration of therapy, concentration of opioids, and limitations on the storage of opioids by pharmacies.

Educational packages and rationalization of legislation are not sufficient to increase availability of essential drugs. Clearly, the huge disparities in per capita health expenditures suggest a role for reallocation of some of these resources. The allocation of development resources currently is often a function of strategic foreign policy rather than need. The disparities in governmental donations shown in Table 3.1 for development budgets suggest a role for mandatory contributions as a fixed percentage of gross domestic product as a precondition for membership in the United Nations.

Other barriers to effective cancer pain management

Clinician educational needs

Barriers to effective pain management are often conceptualized in terms of health care provider, patient, family, institutional, and societal. About 50% of physicians are reported as having erroneous assumptions about the use of opioids for cancer pain (67,68). These misconceptions include concerns about tolerance and addiction, the role of various routes of administration, and the prevalence

and management of side effects. As many as 20% thought of cancer pain as inevitable and something that could not be effectively managed (67,68). Other studies demonstrate clinician confusion about the difference between addiction and dependence and a belief that pain is an inevitable accompaniment of advanced cancer (29). Although nurses appear more aware of the prevalence and severity of patients' pain, there are similar knowledge gaps with regard to the efficacy of analgesia. More than one third of doctors and nurses in a U.S. survey of 971 nurses and physicians thought that opioid use should be restricted based on the stage of a patient's illness (68).

Knowledge deficits do not appear to correlate with the level of exposure to cancer patients and training in palliative care. A survey of 320 North American radiation oncologists suggested that up to 87% did not use standard assessment techniques (32). A survey of 897 oncologists suggested a tendency to ration the use of strong opioids based on clinician prediction of survival of a patient (16).

Studies conducted in a variety of countries are consistent in demonstrating a disparity between the perception of physicians of their knowledge of pain management

Table 3.1. *International per capita opioid consumption and health care resources*

Country	Per capita opioid consumption[a]	Per capita health care expenditure[b] ($1990)		Aid flow allocation to health care[c] ($1990)	Annualized government donor expenditure[d] ($1990)
Australia	41.16 (282)	1331	7.7% GDP		
Canada	36.46 (652)	1945	9.1% GDP		360 million (0.26%)
Denmark	80.19 (266)	1580	6.3% GDP		295 million (0.53%)
Iceland	26.56 (2)	N/A			N/A
Ireland	24.02 (74)	876	7.1% GDP		9 million (0.05%)
New Zealand	33.85 (71)	925	7.2% GDP		26.3 million (0.17%)
Sweden	50.12 (216)	2343	8.8% GDP		515 million (0.62%)
Norway	20.40 (77)	1835	7.4% GDP		220 million (0.39%)
United Kingdom	29.90 (1351)	1039	6.1% GDP		1.05 billion (0.24%)
United States	22.17 (3373)	2763	12.7% GDP		11.6 billion (0.84%)
Malaysia	0.574 (2)	67	3% GDP	100K/million	
Mexico	0.10 (1)	89	3.2% GDP	800K/million	
Cuba	0.9038 (1)	N/A		300K/million	
Bulgaria	0.9091 (3)	131	5.4% GDP	N/A	
India	0.10 (83)	21	6% GDP	300K/million	
Nicaragua	0.10 (0)	35	8.6% GDP	N/A	
Kenya	N/A (0)	16	4.3% GDP	3500K/million	
Albania	0.5928 (0)	26	4% GDP	N/A	
Zambia	N/A (0)	14	3.2% GDP	700K/million	
Bangladesh	N/A (0)	7	3.2% GDP	1200K/million	

Abbreviation: GDP, gross domestic product.

[a] Preliminary reports to the International Narcotics Control Board (INCB) on per capita milligram morphine consumption 1996. The figures in parentheses represent the total morphine consumption in 1991 reported to the INCB.

[b] Annual health care expenditures for 1991 at 1990 exchange rates.

[c] That portion of foreign development aid that is allocated to health care expenditure per million people.

[d] Annualized governmental development budgets based on allocations between 1970 and 1989. This is represented in parentheses as a percentage of total government expenditure reported in 1991.

and actual knowledge of WHO guidelines (60,69). There is also a mismatch between knowledge level and actual practice. A survey of 500 pharmacists in the United States indicated that although respondents recognized that physicians and nurses often undertreat cancer pain, fewer than 30% of respondents counseled patients on pain management (70). Knowledge deficits extend to the use of adjuvant analgesics for neuropathic pain (32,71). There also appear to be deficits based on specialty of physicians with general practitioners less knowledgeable than oncologists (26,72). Physicians display a reluctance to use validated assessment instruments, and this may be predictive of undertreatment of pain (32).

Patient and family barriers mirror these provider barriers. Many patients have unrealistic concerns about taking pain medications and inadequate knowledge about cancer pain management. When interviewed with self-report measures, 37%–85% of patients had concerns, including fear of addiction; 45% thought that they would not be a "good" patient if they talked about their pain with their doctor (73). Opioids are often regarded as a last resort medication (74). Patient barriers appear to correlate directly with patient age and inversely with income and education level (73). Family caregiver barriers to effective pain management are found to be inversely proportional to their knowledge of pain medications and their side effects (75,76). Frequent family concerns include fear of addiction and fear that the use of opioid medications represents disease progression (76).

Several studies enumerate attempts to educate physicians and nurses on an institutional and regional basis. They support the role of education in improving physician and nurse attitudes and knowledge toward pain management, as well as patient satisfaction with pain control (77,78). Tailored education programs of patients by nurses and the use of printed educational materials have been shown to improve patient adherence to pain medications (79).

Undertreatment and economic considerations

Obstacles to effective pain management include limited reimbursement for costs incurred by patients for analgesic medications. Internationally, palliative care services, including the provision of cancer pain management, are funded by a mixture of public funding, private funding, and charitable support (80).

The Medicare benefit in the United States exemplifies the impact of such cost shifting to patients. The Medicare system provides primary insurance to most elderly people and many people with chronic medical conditions. Medicare benefits do not cover most outpatient prescription medication (81).

In the United States, Medicaid programs cover prescription pain medications but with limitations on availability of drugs, restrictions on the number of refills on prescriptions, and number of medications covered in a month or quantity of medication. Soumerai et al. (82) reported on the impact of New Hampshire's Medicaid restriction to three prescriptions a month. This resulted in a severe reduction in the use of many medications, including anti-inflammatory drugs and opioids. The impact of this cap was felt most by a subgroup including women, the elderly, and the disabled. Replacement of this cap with a $1 co-payment resulted in a return to near previous levels of consumption. Soumerai et al. (82) also demonstrated that that Medicaid prescription caps resulted in an increased rate of admission to nursing homes for chronically ill outpatients.

Reimbursement for opioid medications in many other countries is similarly limited. In Latin American countries, such as Argentina, the cost per month for oral morphine can be very high; at a dose of 180 mg/day, the cost is $580 per month, in a country where the average industrial monthly wage is $400. Most health insurance policies do not reimburse for palliative care professional services, increasing the burden on voluntary support (83).

Internationally, the availability of palliative care beds and access to pain specialists is often limited. In Germany, where estimated need for palliative care beds in 1996 was about 4000 beds, only 230 beds were provided. Patients with cancer pain were reported to spend, on average, 2 years with pain, including 60 inpatient days, and to see five different physicians before having access to a pain clinic (84).

Although 80%–95% of patients with insurance by U.S. health maintenance organizations (HMOs) have comprehensive prescription coverage, HMOs may limit dispensing, substitute generic products, and apply rider policies denying coverage for certain medications. Ironically, Medicare and most insurers will cover for home infusions and patient-controlled analgesia pumps, but not for oral medications (85). Populations particularly vulnerable to the impact of this cost shifting to patients include the elderly, who may be forced to restrict their dose intake to keep down cost (86).

In the Netherlands, where the cost of home infusions and home care is covered by state insurance, it has been calculated that home infusions (intravenous and intraspinal) of analgesics costs $250 to $300 a day, in comparison with $750 per hospital day. Even at the latter cost, home infusion would be a projected saving of $14 million over inpatient management (87).

The unintended shifting to parenteral administration of opioids has had a variety of negative effects. It can place considerable strain on the budget of hospice units in most countries. Relatively high costs are seen even in the home setting, especially given the requirement for visits by a skilled nurse (88).

In the United States, the American Association of Retired Persons reports that only 40% of patients older than 75 have prescription coverage, in contrast to 75% of those in the 45- to 54-age brackets (89). Home parenteral infusions, which may be needed if the cost of oral drugs cannot be borne, add as much as $50,000 to the annual cost of a patient's care (90). Clinicians frequently are unaware of the cost when prescribing medication. In one study, 25% of physicians surveyed predicted accurately the cost of opioid medications (91).

Internationally, there is an impetus to transfer care of patients with cancer pain into the community. Little work has been performed on the impact of cost shifting to family caregivers. Studies in other health care delivery systems, such as the United Kingdom, suggest that families caring for patients with cancer pain sustain considerable out-of-pocket non-medical expenditures, which may account for significant portions of the weekly income. Research in Australia demonstrated that the availability of a local specialist palliative home care service did not result in a significant reduction in the use of hospital resources or costs to the local health authorities. The authors suggested that the removal of a local policy preventing access "after hours" to opioid analgesics could result in unnecessary hospital admissions, with the potential to allow cost containment (92). In other countries, lack of reimbursement for home nursing results in unnecessary hospital admissions for pain and symptom management (93,94).

Unscheduled admissions for uncontrolled pain accounted for 4% of admissions to the City of Hope National Medical Center (85). The average daily hospital cost was $1771 and the total annual cost was $5.1 million, suggesting a huge potential for cost saving by ensuring coverage for effective opioid delivery systems for outpatients. Some of these unscheduled admissions resulted in the parenteral delivery of opioids to justify hospital admissions. Alternatively, parenteral home delivery systems may be used by clinicians as a means of justifying home nursing care (85).

The U.S. Medicare Hospice is mandated by law to provide high quality pain and palliative care even if the cost of this care exceeds the per diem rate of reimbursement. The rising costs of opioids, and the expense associated with long-acting formulations, increases the cost of prescription medications for U.S. hospices. The per diem benefit is similarly threatened by the costs associated with intravenous and subcutaneous delivery systems. Waste of opioids may occur when a patient dies; opioids cannot be used lawfully for other patients or returned to the pharmacy stock and must be destroyed. Some of this cost could be avoided by pharmacies dispensing limited quantities of a prescription at intervals and by federal regulations permitting a pharmacist to partially dispense if a patient is resident in a long-term care facility or has a documented terminal illness. Patients receiving conventional care who are covered by Medicare are, in contrast, liable for the cost of this medication (95).

Conclusion

Cancer pain is highly prevalent and associated with significant morbidity. Greater efforts are needed to implement existing standards for pain management as well as improvements in education targeted to all phases of professional development for health care professionals. These programs should focus on deficits in professional knowledge and behaviors that have been found to create barriers to pain management in the existing body of research.

References

1. Stjernsward J. WHO cancer pain relief: an important global public health issue. In: Field HL, Dubner R, Cervero F, eds. Advances in pain research and therapy, Vol. 9. New York: Raven Press, 1985:555–8.
2. Chaplin JM, Morton RP. A prospective longitudinal study of pain in head and neck cancer patients. Head Neck 21(6):531–7, 1999.
3. Caraceni A. Clinicopathological correlates of common cancer pain syndromes. Hematol Oncol Clinic North Am 1:57–8, 1996.
4. Coyle N, Adelhardt J, Foley KM, Portenoy RK. Character of terminal illness in the advanced cancer patient: pain and other symptoms in the last 4 weeks of life. J Pain Symptom Manage 5:83–93, 1990.
5. Greenwald HP, Bonica JJ, Bergner M. The prevalence of pain in four cancers. Cancer 60:2563–9, 1987.
6. Daut RL, Cleeland CS. The prevalence and severity of pain in cancer. Cancer 50(19):13–8, 1982.
7. Kelsen DP, Portenoy RK, Thaler HT, et al. Pain and depression in patients with newly diagnosed pancreas cancer. J Clin Oncol 13:748–55, 1995.
8. Portenoy RK, Thaler HT, Kornblith AB, et al. The Memorial Symptom Assessment Scale: an instrument for the evaluation

of symptom prevalence, characteristics and distress. Eur J Cancer 30A(9):1326–36, 1994.

9. Twycross RG, Fairfield S. Pain in far advanced cancer. Pain 14:303–10, 1982.

10. Grond S, Zech D, Diefenbach C, et al. Assessment of cancer pain: a prospective evaluation in 2266 cancer patients referred to a pain service. Pain 64(1):107–14, 1996.

11. Caraceni A, Portenoy RK. An international survey of cancer pain characteristics and syndromes. IASP Task Force on Cancer Pain. Pain 82 (3):263–74, 1999.

12. Zeppetella G, O'Doherty CA, Collins S. Prevalence andcharacteristics of breakthrough pain in cancer patients admitted to a hospice. J Pain Symptom Manage 20(2):87–9, 2000.

13. Petzke F, Radbruch L, Zech D, et al. Temporal presentation of chronic cancer pain: transitory pains on admission to a multidisciplinary pain clinic. J Pain Symptom Manage 17(6):391–401, 1999.

14. Greer DS, Mor V. An overview of the National Hospice Study findings. J Chron Dis 39(1):5–7, 1986.

15. Ingham J, Portenoy RK. Symptom assessment. In: Cherny NI, Foley KM, eds. Hematol Oncol Clin North Am 21–39, 1996.

16. Von Roenn JH, Cleeland CS, Gonin R, et al. Pain and its treatment in outpatients with metastatic cancer. N Engl J Med 330:592–6, 1994.

17. Larue F, Colleau SM, Brasseur L, Cleeland CS. Multicentre study of cancer pain and its treatment in France. Br Med J 310:1034–7, 1995.

18. Saltzburg D, Breitbart W, Fishman B, et al. The relationship of pain and depression to suicidal ideation in cancer patients [abstract]. Proceedings ASCO 8:1215, 1989.

19. Spiegel D, Sands S, Koopman C. Pain and depression in patients with cancer. Cancer 74(9):2570–8, 1994.

20. Chochinov HM, Wilson KG, Enns M, et al. Desire for death in the terminally ill. Am J Psychiatry 152:1185–91, 1995.

21. Chochinov HM, Wilson KG, Enns M, Lander S. Depression, hopelessness, and suicidal ideation in the terminally ill. Psychosomatics 39(4):366–70, 1998.

22. Portenoy RK, Miransky J, Thaler HT, et al. Pain in ambulatory patients with lung or colon cancer. Prevalence, characteristics and effect. Cancer 70(6):1616–24, 1992.

23. Cherny N, Frager G, Ingham J, et al. Opioid pharmacotherapy in the management of cancer pain. Cancer 76(7):1283–93, 1995.

24. Solomon MZ, O'Donnell L, Jennings B. Decisions near the end of life: professionals views on life sustaining treatments. Am J Public Health 83(1):14–43, 1993.

25. Portenoy RK, Kanner RM. Patterns of analgesic prescription and consumption in an university-affiliated community hospital. Arch Intern Med 145:439–41, 1985.

26. Vainio A. Treatment of terminal cancer pain in France: a questionnaire study. Pain 62:155–62, 1995.

27. Zenz M, Zenz T, Tryba M, Strumpf M. Severe undertreatment of cancer pain: a 3 year survey of the German situation. J Pain Symptom Manage 10:187–90, 1995.

28. Vainio A. Treatment of terminal cancer pain in Finland: a second look. Acta Anaesthesiol Scand 36(1): 89–95, 1992.

29. Rawal J, Hylander J, Arner S. Management of terminal cancer in Sweden: a nationwide survey. Pain 54:169–79, 1993.

30. White ID, Hoskin PJ, Hanks GW, Bliss JM. Analgesics in cancer pain: current practice and beliefs. Br J Cancer 63:271–4, 1991.

31. Bernabei R, Gambassi I, Lapane KF. Pain management in elderly patients with cancer. JAMA 279(23):1877–82, 1998.

32. Cleeland CS, Janjan N, Scott CB, et al. Cancer pain management by radiotherapists: a survey of radiation oncology group physicians. Intl J Radiat Oncol Biol Phys 47(1):203–8, 2000.

33. Desbiens NA, Wu AW, Broste SK, et al. Pain and satisfaction with pain control in seriously hospitalized adults: findings from the SUPPORT research investigations. Crit Care Med 24(12):1953–61, 1996.

34. World Health Organization: Health of the elderly. Technical Report Series 779. Geneva: World Health Organization, 1989:7–30.

35. World Bank: World Development Report 1993. New York: Oxford University Press, 1993.

36. Hazzard WR, Bierman EL, Blass JP, eds. Pain the elderly. In: Principles of geriatric medicine and gerontology. New York: McGraw-Hill, 1994.

37. Kareholt I, Brattberg G. Pain and mortality risk among elderly persons in Sweden. Pain 77:271–8, 1998.

38. Brock DB, Holmes MB, Foley DJ, Holmes D. Methodological issues in a survey of the last days of life: the epidemiological study of the elderly. In: Wallace RB, Woolson RF, eds. New York: Oxford University Press, 1992:315–32.

39. Stein WJ. Cancer pain in the elderly hospice patient. J Pain Symptom Manage 8(7):474–88, 1993.

40. McGrath PA, de Veber LL, Hearn MT. Multidimensional pain assessment in children. In: Fields HL, Dubner R, Cervero F, eds. Advances in pain research and therapy, Vol. 9. New York: Raven Press, 1985:387–93.

41. Ljungman G, Kreuger A, Gordh T, et al. Treatment of pain in pediatric oncology: a Swedish nationwide survey. Pain 68(2–3):385–94, 1996.

42. Miser AW, McCalla J, Dothage JA, et al. Pain as a presenting symptom in children and young adults with newly diagnosed malignancy. Pain 29(1):85–90, 1987.

43. Miser AW, Dothage JA, Wesley RA, Miser JS. The prevalence of pain in a pediatric and young adult cancer population. Pain 29(1):73–83, 1987.

44. Elliott SC, Miser AW, Dose AM, et al. Epidemiological features of pain in pediatric cancer patients: a co-operative community-based study. North Central Cancer Treatment Group and Mayo Clinic. Clin J Pain 7(4):263–8, 1991.

45. Ljungman G, Gordh T, Sorensen S, Kreuger A. Pain variations during cancer treatment in children: a descriptive survey. Pediatr Hematol Oncol 3:211–21, 2000.

46. Cornalgia C, Massimo L, Haupt R, et al. Incidence of pain in children with neoplastic disease. Pain 2:S28, 1984.

47. Finley GA, McGrath PJ, Forward SP, et al. Parents' management of children's pain following "minor" surgery. Pain 64(1):83–7, 1996.

48. Romsing J, Hertel S, Harder A, Rasmussen M. Examination of acetaminophen for outpatient management of postoperative pain in children. Pediatr Anaesth. 8(3):235–9, 1998.

49. Borge A, Nordhagen R, Moe B, et al. Prevalence and persistence of stomachache and headache among children. Follow-up of a cohort of Norwegian children. Acta Pediatr 83:433–7, 1994.

50. Cleeland CS, Gonna R, Baez L, et al. Pain and treatment of pain in minority patients with cancer. Ann Intern Med 127:813–16, 1997.

51. Anderson KO, Mendoza TR, Valero V, et al. Minority cancer patients and their providers: pain management attitudes and practice. Cancer 88(8):1929–38, 2000.

52. McDonald DD. Gender and ethnic stereotyping and narcotic analgesic administration. Res Nurs Health 17:45–9, 1994.

53. Ramer L, Richardson JL, Cohen MZ, et al. Multimeasure pain assessment in an ethnically diverse group of patients with cancer. J Transcult Nurs 10(2):94–101, 1999.

54. Saxena A, Mendoza T, Cleeland CS. The assessment of cancer pain in North India: the validation of the Hindi Brief Pain Inventory–BPI-H. J Pain Symptom Manage 17(1):27–41, 1999.

55. United States Department of Health and Human Services. Agency for Health Care Policy and Research. Clinical Practice guideline for management of cancer pain. AHCPR Publication No 94-0592. Washington, D.C., US Government Printing Office, 1994.

56. Palos G. The influence and assessment of culture on cancer pain. Nursing Interventions in Oncology, 9:8–12. 1997.

57. Stjernsward J, Teoh N. Current status of the global cancer control program of the World Health Organization. J Pain Symptom Manage 8(6):340–7, 1993.

58. United Nations International Narcotics Control Board. Narcotic drugs: estimated world requirements for 1993, statistics for 1991. Vienna: United Nations, 1992.

59. International Narcotics Control Board. Report of the International Narcotics Control Board for 1995; availability of opiates for medical needs. New York: United Nations, 1996.

60. Bruera E. Palliative care in Latin America. J Pain Symptom Manage 8(6):365–8, 1993.

61. De Lima L, Bruera E, Joranson D. Opioid availability in Latin America: the Santa Domingo Report. Progress since the Declaration of Florinapolis. J Pain Symptom Manage 13(4):213–19, 1997.

62. Ortiz A, Romano M, Soriano A. Development of an information reporting system on illicit drug use in Mexico. Bull Narc 41(1–2):41–52, 1989.

63. Colleau S, Plancarte R, Bruera E. Mexico. Cancer Pain Release 6(2–3):7, 1993.

64. Laudico AV. The Phillipines: status of cancer pain and palliative care. J Pain Symptom Manage 12(2):133–5, 1996.

65. Merriman A. Uganda: status of cancer pain and palliative care. J Pain Symptom Manage 12(2):141–3, 1996.

66. Zhang H, Wei-ping G, Joranson DE, Cleeland CS. People's Republic of China: status of cancer pain and palliative care. J Pain Symptom Manage 12(2):124–6, 1996.

67. Fife BL, Irick N, Painter JD. A comparative study of the attitudes of physicians and nurses towards the management of cancer pain. J Pain Symptom Manage 8:132–9, 1993.

68. Elliott TE, Elliott BA. Physician attitudes and beliefs about use of morphine for cancer pain. J Pain Symptom Manage 7:141–8, 1992.

69. Sapir R, Catance R, Strauss-Liviatan N, Cherny NI. Cancer pain: knowledge and attitudes of physicians in Israel. J Pain Symptom Manage 17(4):266–76, 1999.

70. McCaffrey M, Ferrell B. Nurses knowledge about cancer pain: a survey of five countries. J Pain Symptom Manage 10(5):56–69, 1995.

71. Sjogren P, Banning N, Jensen M, et al. Management of cancer pain in Denmark: a nationwide questionnaire study. Pain 62:155–62, 1995.

72. O'Brien S, Dalton JA, Konsler G, Carlson J. The knowledge and attitudes of experienced oncology nurses regarding the management of cancer related pain. Oncol Nurs Forum 23(3):515–21, 1996.

73. Ward SE, Goldberg V, Miller-McCauley C, et al. Patient related barriers to management of cancer pain. Pain 52:319–24, 1993.

74. Wills BS, Wootton YS. Concerns and misconceptions about pain among Hong Kong Chinese patients with cancer. Cancer Nurs 22(6):408–13, 1999.

75. Elliott BA, Elliott TE, Murray DM, et al. Patients and family members: the role of knowledge and attitudes in cancer pain. J Pain Symptom Manage 12:209–20, 1996.

76. Berry PE, Ward SE. Barriers to pain management in hospice: a study of family caregivers. Hospice J 10:19–33, 1995.

77. Bookbinder M, Coyle N, Kiss M, et al. Implementing national standards for cancer pain management. J Pain Symptom Manage 12(6):334–47, 1996.

78. Janjan NA, Martin CG, Payne R, et al. Teaching cancer pain management: durability of educational effects of a role model program. Cancer 77:996–1001, 1996.

79. Rimer B, Levy MH, Keinitz MK, et al. Enhancing cancer pain control regimens through patient education. Patient Educ Couns 10:267–77, 1987.

80. Contracting with the National Health Service. Revised guidelines for voluntary hospices. National Council for Hospice and Specialist Palliative Care Services. Occasional Paper 6. 1994.

81. Gross DJ, Alecxib L, Gibson MJ, et al. Out-of-pocket health spending by poor and near-poor elderly Medicare beneficiaries. Health Serv Res 34(1):241–5, 1999.

82. Soumerai SB, Avorn J, Ross Degnan D, Gortmaker R. Payment restrictions for prescription medications under Medicaid. N Engl J Med 317:550–6, 1987.

83. Wenk R, Ochoa J. Argentina: status of cancer pain and palliative care. J Pain Symptom Manage 12(2):97–8, 1996.

84. Strumpf M, Zenz M, Donner B. Germany: status of cancer pain and palliative care. J Pain Symptom Manage 12(2):109–11, 1996.

85. Ferrell B. Cost issues surrounding the treatment of cancer-related pain. J Pharm Care Pain Symptom Control 1:9–23, 1993.

86. Special Committee on Aging, United States Senate. A status report on accessibility and affordability of prescription drugs for older Americans. Washington, D.C.: US Senate, 1992.

87. Witteveen PO, Van Groenestijn MAC, Blijham GH, Schrijvers AJP. Use of resources and costs of palliative care with parenteral fluids and analgesics in the home setting for patients with end-stage cancer. Ann Oncol 10:161–5, 1999.

88. McGettrick S, Rodgers J. Cost of administering controlled drugs in a hospice ward. Health Bull 54(6):441–2, 1996.

89. American Association for Retired People. Older people are pinched by drug costs. AARP Bull 33:3, 1996.

90. Joranson DE. Are health-care reimbursement policies a barrier to acute and cancer pain management? J Pain Symptom Manage 9(4):244–53, 1994.

91. Hoffman J, Barefield FA, Ramamurthy S. A survey of physician knowledge of drug costs. J Pain Symptom Manage 10(6):432–5, 1996.

92. Aristides M, Shiell A. The effects on hospital use and costs of a domiciliary palliative care nursing service. Aust Health Rev 16(4):405–13, 1993.

93. Bodkin CM, Pigott TJ, Mann JR. Financial burden of childhood cancer. Br Med J 284:1542–4, 1982.

94. Cherny N. Israel: status of cancer pain and palliative care. J Pain Symptom Manage 12(2):116–17, 1996.

95. Emanuel EJ. Cost savings at the end of life. What do the data show? JAMA 275(24):1907–14, 1996.

SECTION II ASSESSMENT AND SYNDROMES

4 The assessment of cancer pain

KAREN O. ANDERSON AND CHARLES S. CLEELAND
The University of Texas M. D. Anderson Cancer Center

Introduction

Regular pain assessment and pain management should have the highest priority in the routine care of the patient with cancer. Between 60% and 80% of patients with advanced cancer will need pain treatment. Pain is also a problem for many patients earlier and intermittently during the course of their disease. In addition, cancer survivors who are cured of their cancer may have persistent chronic pain as a result of the disease or its treatment.

When pain is present, the quality of life of patients and their family members is adversely affected. However, the majority of patients with cancer-related pain can obtain pain relief if the pain is adequately assessed and appropriate treatment is provided. Numerous guidelines for the management of cancer pain have been endorsed by governmental organizations, professional associations, and the World Health Organization (WHO). Research studies evaluating the WHO's guidelines for cancer pain relief (1,2) indicate that 70% to 90% of patients obtain good pain relief when this protocol for oral analgesic medications is followed (3–6). Other pain management therapies can provide pain control when oral analgesics are not effective.

In spite of the availability of effective pain treatments, multiple studies document undertreatment of pain (7–10). A study completed in the Eastern Cooperative Oncology Group (ECOG) surveyed more than 1300 outpatients with recurrent or metastatic cancer (7). A total of 67% of the patients had pain or were being treated for pain with daily analgesics. Among the patients with pain, 42% were prescribed analgesics that were less potent than those recommended by the WHO guidelines. One of the most important predictors of undertreatment of pain was the discrepancy between the patient and physician in their estimates of pain intensity.

Inadequate pain assessment is a major barrier to good pain control for the patient with cancer. Pain must be identified to be treated, and pain whose severity is underestimated will not be treated aggressively enough. More than 800 ECOG-affiliated physicians completed a survey designed to assess their knowledge and practice of cancer pain management (11). The physicians ranked a list of potential barriers to pain management to indicate barriers that hindered pain treatment in their practice settings. The most frequently identified barrier was inadequate pain assessment; 76% of the physicians rated poor assessment as one of the top four barriers to good pain management. Patient reluctance to report pain, closely related to inadequate assessment, was the next most frequently cited barrier. Similarly, recent surveys of physicians in the Radiation Therapy Oncology Group and health care providers treating minority cancer patients found that poor pain assessment and patient reluctance to report pain were identified as top barriers to optimal pain management (12,13).

Why is pain assessment so often inadequate in many cancer care settings? Most health care providers do not have the training and skills necessary to adequately assess pain and its impact. Accurate appraisal of pain may be even more difficult when the providers are not of the same gender or ethnic background as the patients (7,12,14). Moreover, pain assessment is not a standard part of patient appointments, and it is often up to patients to volunteer that they have pain, or that their current pain treatment is not working. Unfortunately, several studies have shown that patients are reluctant to be assertive in reporting their pain (15–17). When physicians and nurses do ask about pain, they often fail to document pain severity, characteristics, or etiology. Also, health care providers usually do not assess the impact of pain on the daily lives of the patient and the family.

In this chapter we will review the methodological and clinical issues involved in the assessment of cancer pain. Figure 4.1 provides an overview of the pain assessment process and indicates areas that need to be evaluated in a patient with cancer-related pain. The role of the medical evaluation and how pain assessment provides the information needed for pain treatment planning and evaluation are discussed, as well as the importance of determining pain severity and the relation of severity to treatment. Standardized pain scales and questionnaires that can facilitate the assessment process are described. Strategies for determining pain characteristics and the impact of pain on patients' lives are presented. The use of pain assessment procedures in special populations, quality assurance, and innovative technologies are also examined.

Medical and neurological evaluation

The assessment of cancer-related pain calls for a careful medical evaluation, including a thorough medical history, physical and neurological examination, and appropriate diagnostic procedures. A retrospective survey of cancer patients referred for pain assessment found that two-thirds of the patients had new and often treatable pathology diagnosed as a result of a neurological evaluation (18). Appropriate laboratory and imaging studies also may be necessary to evaluate the etiology of the patient's pain. Establishing the physical cause of the pain is an important goal of assessment and will influence the choice of treatment.

Pain in cancer patients can be due to the cancer itself or to cancer therapies, or related to non-cancer illnesses or conditions (19,20). A prospective study of more than 2000 patients referred to a pain service found that 70% of the patients had pain resulting from multiple sources (21). The most frequent sources of pain were soft tissue invasion, bone pain, nerve damage or infiltration, and visceral pain. Other studies found that bone pain and visceral pain were the most common etiologies of cancer pain (22–24). Cancer therapies such as surgery, chemotherapy, or radiation therapy also produce significant pain in many patients (21,23,25). Pain related to cancer therapy may have a short duration, or a chronic pain syndrome such as peripheral neuropathy may develop.

Assessment of pain severity

Pain severity is the dominant factor determining the effects of pain on the patient and the urgency of the treatment process. Many adults with mild cancer-related pain function quite effectively with pain that does not seriously impair their activities of daily living. As pain severity increases, however, it typically disrupts many areas of the patient's life (26). Guidelines for cancer pain treatment from the Agency for Health Care Policy and Research, the American Pain Society, the National Comprehensive Cancer Network, and the WHO all use a determination of pain severity as the primary item of information in specifying treatment (2,27–29). Thus, it is crucial to assess accurately the patient's pain severity.

Several reliable and valid methods for scaling the severity or intensity of pain have been developed. Verbal descriptor scales (VDS) have a long history in pain research (30). Patients are asked to pick a category, such as "none," "mild," "moderate," "severe," or "excruciating," that best describes their pain intensity. Pain relief can be rated in a similar way, using categories such as "none," "slight," "moderate," and "complete." Although VDS have proven useful in research and clinical settings, these scales assume that patients comprehend the meaning of the descriptors and define them in the same way. This assump-

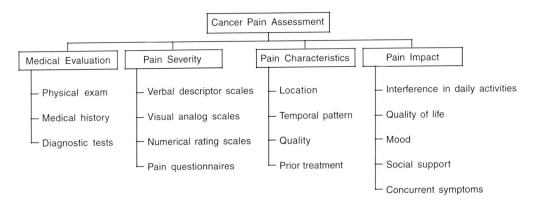

Fig. 4.1. Overview of cancer pain assessment.

tion is questionable when patients have diverse educational, cultural, or linguistic backgrounds (31).

Visual analog scales (VAS) are often used in clinical and research settings (32). The patient is asked to determine how much of the VAS, usually a straight line, is equivalent to or analogous with the severity of the pain. One end of the line represents "no pain," and the other end represents a concept such as "pain as bad as you can imagine." The VAS have proven useful in studies comparing the effectiveness of analgesic drugs and other pain treatments; however, the VAS concept may be difficult for some patients to comprehend (33).

Numerical rating scales (NRS) measure pain intensity by asking the patient to select a number to represent their pain severity. The most commonly used NRS uses an 11-point scale of 0 to 10. The numbers are typically arrayed along a horizontal line, with 0 on the left labeled as "no pain" and 10 on the right labeled with a phrase such as "pain as bad as you can imagine." As pain intensity resulting from cancer is often variable, patients can be asked to rate their pain at the time of responding to the scale, and also at its "worst," "least," and "average" over the last 24 hours. Numerical scales are often more easily understood by patients than VAS or VDS. The use of numbers may remove some sources of cultural and linguistic variation (34). In addition, the use of NRS is recommended in many pain treatment guidelines (27).

Ratings of pain intensity obtained using the NRS, VDS, and VAS are highly intercorrelated, with the NRS and VAS most highly correlated with one another (35–37). The NRS has been found to be more reliable than the VAS in clinical trials, especially with less-educated patients (33). Oral versions of the NRS are easily administered to very sick patients who are unable to write.

Pain questionnaires

Many standardized pain questionnaires assess pain severity and also other factors related to pain. Using pain assessment instruments minimizes many patient reporting biases and assists health care professionals in obtaining complete information. Using pain scales that assign a metric to pain intensity and interference makes pain an "objective" symptom, similar to other signs and symptoms such as blood pressure and heart rate. By making pain "objective," standard questions allow patients to feel free to report its presence and severity, and also to report treatment efficacy (38). Patients are often less concerned about acknowledging the failure of a treatment on a questionnaire than in response to questions put to them by their health care providers.

Three pain questionnaires are short enough to be considered for repeated clinical or research administration to cancer patients. The Memorial Pain Assessment Card (MPAC) includes visual analog scales that have been adapted for regular clinical use (39). The MPAC consists of one verbal descriptor scale and three VAS measuring pain intensity, pain relief, and mood. A short form of the McGill Pain Questionnaire (SF-MPQ) uses verbal descriptor scales to assess the sensory and affective components of pain (40). The SF-MPQ includes 15 descriptors that are rated on a 4-point severity scale. Three pain scores are derived from the sum of the intensity ratings of the sensory, affective, and total descriptors. The SF-MPQ also includes the Present Pain Intensity index of the standard MPQ and a VAS. The SF-MPQ and the MPAC provide valuable information, but the descriptor and VAS scales may be difficult for some patients to comprehend.

The Brief Pain Inventory (BPI) (34) was designed to assess pain in cancer patients. Using 0 to 10 NRS, the BPI asks patients to rate the severity of their pain at its "worst," "least," "average," and "now," the time the rating is made. Using 11-point NRS with anchors of "no interference" and "interferes completely," the BPI also assesses how much pain interferes with mood, walking, general activity, work, relations with others, sleep, and enjoyment of life. The BPI asks patients to mark the location of their pain on a pain drawing, and includes other questions about pain treatment and the extent of pain relief. The BPI also provides a list of descriptors to help the patient describe pain quality. A short form of the BPI is frequently used for regular pain assessment in clinical and research settings (Fig. 4.2).

Simple pain scales or questionnaires make it possible to assess pain on each outpatient contact with the patient and at least once every 24 hours for a patient in the hospital, or more frequently if pain is identified as a problem. Because pain in cancer is variable and often progressive, pain assessment must be repeated regularly to achieve and maintain optimal pain control.

Levels of pain intensity

Categorizing a pain severity rating as "mild," "moderate," or "severe" is a crucial step in the assessment process and determines the urgency of the treatment process. The guidelines for cancer pain treatment from the WHO, American Pain Society, Agency for Health Care Policy and Research, and National Comprehensive Cancer Network (NCCN) all recommend varying treatment approaches for these three categories of pain sever-

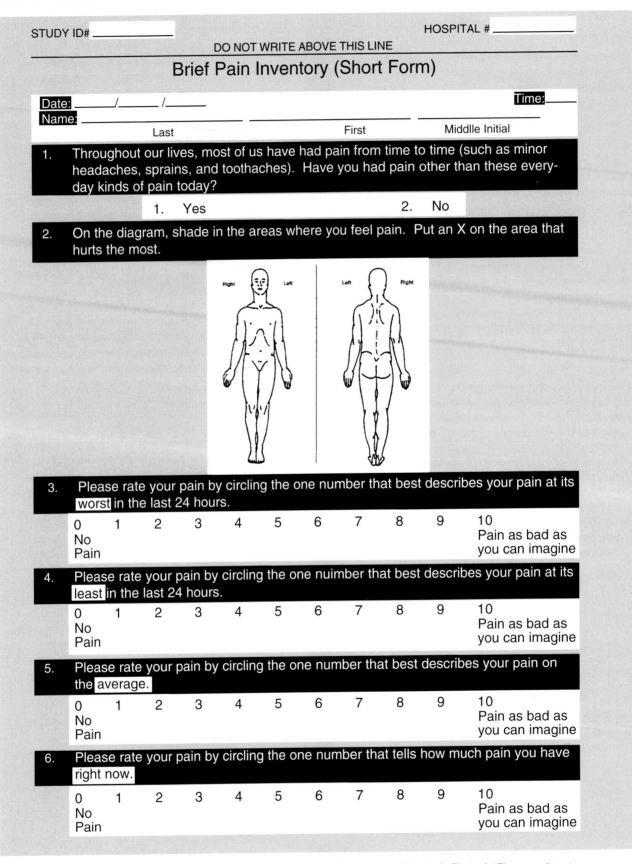

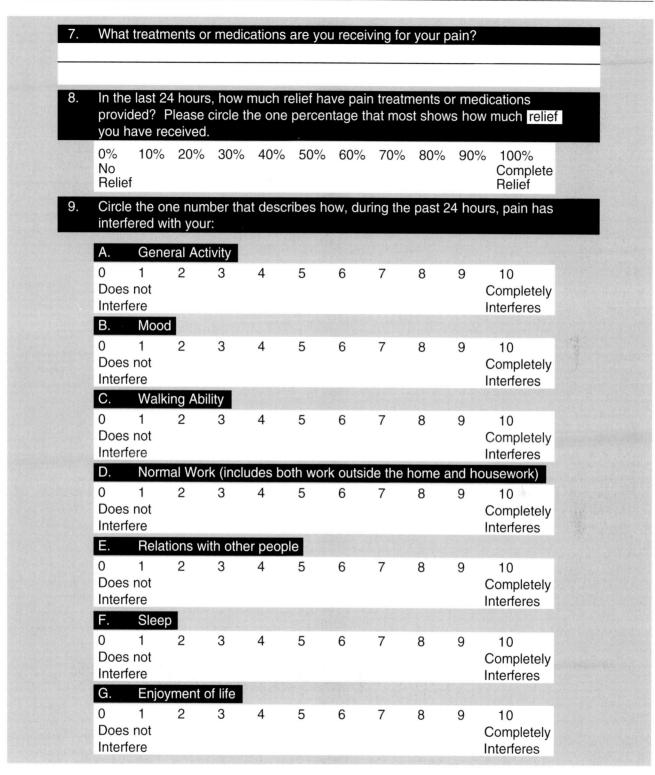

7. What treatments or medications are you receiving for your pain?

8. In the last 24 hours, how much relief have pain treatments or medications provided? Please circle the one percentage that most shows how much relief you have received.

0%	10%	20%	30%	40%	50%	60%	70%	80%	90%	100%
No Relief										Complete Relief

9. Circle the one number that describes how, during the past 24 hours, pain has interfered with your:

A. General Activity

0	1	2	3	4	5	6	7	8	9	10
Does not Interfere										Completely Interferes

B. Mood

0	1	2	3	4	5	6	7	8	9	10
Does not Interfere										Completely Interferes

C. Walking Ability

0	1	2	3	4	5	6	7	8	9	10
Does not Interfere										Completely Interferes

D. Normal Work (includes both work outside the home and housework)

0	1	2	3	4	5	6	7	8	9	10
Does not Interfere										Completely Interferes

E. Relations with other people

0	1	2	3	4	5	6	7	8	9	10
Does not Interfere										Completely Interferes

F. Sleep

0	1	2	3	4	5	6	7	8	9	10
Does not Interfere										Completely Interferes

G. Enjoyment of life

0	1	2	3	4	5	6	7	8	9	10
Does not Interfere										Completely Interferes

Fig. 4.2 *(Continued)*

ity. For example, the three-step analgesic ladder in the WHO guidelines recommends a family of analgesic drugs based on the three categories of pain intensity (1,2). The NCCN guidelines include a treatment algo-rithm that also is based on the categorization of pain as mild, moderate, or severe (27). For example, severe pain is considered a pain emergency that mandates rapid titra-tion of a short-acting opioid, as well as prevention of common side effects of opioids and psychosocial support. The recommended treatment of moderate pain includes an opioid medication, prevention of side effects, patient education, and psychosocial support (if indicated).

Thus, the implementation of cancer pain treatment guidelines necessitates the categorization of pain intensity. "Mild," "moderate," and "severe" pain can be defined as ranges of patient responses to a numerical rating of pain at its "worst" on an 11-point scale. The ranges for each category of pain severity are based on the degree of interference with function associated with each category (26).

Mild pain (1–4 "worst pain") will most often call for a "mild" analgesic (acetaminophen or a non-steroidal anti-inflammatory drug) or a "moderate" analgesic such as oxycodone or hydrocodone (28). Mild pain typically causes the least interference with function. However, patients with mild pain can benefit from education about the need to report pain when it occurs, when it gets worse, or if it is not relieved by current treatment.

Moderate pain (5–6 "worst pain") calls for a more aggressive analgesic program and thorough assessment of the impact of the pain on the patient's life. Because pain at this level is impairing multiple areas of a patient's function, a follow-up contact should be made within 24 to 72 hours to assess the efficacy of the pain treatment provided.

Severe pain (7–10 "worst pain") mandates very aggressive analgesic treatment with a "strong" opioid such as morphine. Follow-up contact for reassessment should occur within 24 hours after the initial assessment. A comprehensive assessment of the impact of the pain is necessary to determine if the patient needs psychosocial support or other behavioral treatments.

Assessing pain characteristics

In addition to measuring pain severity, the assessment of cancer pain should include the determination of other pain characteristics that will help to guide treatment choices. Much of this information can be obtained through the use of standardized questionnaires, which assess the patient's subjective reports of pain characteristics. A clinical interview can be used to collect additional information.

Pain location

Information on the location of the pain is helpful in determining the etiology of the pain. For example, patients may draw the pain in the distribution of a particular nerve, suggesting that the pain is neuropathic in origin. The location of the pain can be assessed by asking the patient to provide a graphic representation of the pain location. Some pain questionnaires, including the BPI, contain a human figure drawing for the patient to use. Pain location may also help to determine why pain is exacerbated by particular movements or positions.

Temporal pattern of the pain

Cancer pain does not always remain at the same intensity over a 24-hour period, and it is important to capture the temporal pattern of pain. Is it constant or episodically more severe? Are the episodes spontaneous or do they occur with specific movements or in response to other aggravating factors? The temporal pattern of pain is often clearly described by the patient in the initial interview. It may be necessary, however, to have patients rate their pain and analgesic use in a home diary to determine its pattern.

Assessment of the temporal pattern will help to determine if the patient experiences significant incident pain, exacerbation of pain with movement. Incident pain is common when the pathologic process responsible for the pain is influenced by movement or position. Some types of pain (e.g., neuropathic pain) may have periods when pain spontaneously becomes more severe. These periodic increases in pain are often referred to as "breakthrough pain," defined as a transitory increase in pain occurring in the context of stable baseline pain (41).

Cancer pain treatment guidelines recommend additional analgesics for the patient to take during breakthrough or incident episodes, or before episodes if it is possible to anticipate when they will occur. For some patients, however, the presence of breakthrough pain may indicate that the dose or potency of the routine analgesic prescribed for pain management is inadequate (42).

Pain quality

The etiology of the pain influences the patient's subjective report of the quality of the pain. For example, neuropathic pain is often described as "numb," "pins and needles," or "burning." Pain from tumor destruction of soft tissue or bone is often described as "aching." People may find it difficult to spontaneously describe their pain in a clinical interview. Word lists of potential descriptors help the patient to report pain quality. Some questionnaires, such as the BPI and the SF-MPQ, include lists of descriptors for the patient to select.

Evaluating the quality of the pain is an important part of pain assessment and will help to determine the etiology of the pain and the recommended treatments. For example, neuropathic pain often is less responsive to opioid analgesics than nociceptive pain and may be relieved by other types of medications such as antidepressants or anticonvulsants.

Response to prior treatment

The patient's history of pain therapies and their outcomes are additional variables that need to be assessed. When determining response to prior analgesics, patients' adherence to their prescribed medications must be determined. A recent study of outpatients with cancer-related pain found that patients adhered to their opioid therapy only 62% to 72% of the time (43). Non-adherence was a significant predictor of symptom distress and impaired quality of life. The most frequent reasons for non-adherence were side effects of the medications and concerns about addiction. In a study of minority cancer patients, the inability to understand instructions was associated with non-adherence to analgesic medications (44). Thus, it is important to assess adherence to analgesic regimens and the reasons for any non-adherence. Careful assessment can identify possible targets for patient education and/or the need to treat analgesic side effects or change medication regimens.

Results of recent studies indicate that a majority of cancer patients use some type of non-traditional or alternative approaches (e.g., spiritual practices, nutritional supplements) to treat their disease or its symptoms (45). Similarly, studies of cancer patients experiencing pain found that many patients use non-traditional treatment approaches (e.g., herbal teas, prayer) for their pain (17,44,46). Assessment of the patient's pain treatment history should include the evaluation of alternative treatment approaches and whether these approaches interfere with or supplement the prescribed analgesics. If possible and medically indicated, the patient's alternative approaches can be incorporated into the pain management program.

Assessment of barriers to pain control

Patients with cancer frequently underreport pain and pain severity. A number of patient-related barriers to the assessment of cancer pain have been identified (47–49). Patients with cancer often do not want to be labeled as complainers, do not want to distract their health care provider from treating the cancer, or are afraid that their pain means that their cancer is progressing (15,48). Some patients are fatalistic and believe that pain is an inevitable part of having cancer and must be accepted. Patients are often concerned about having to take potent

opioids because they fear that they will become addicts or will have unmanageable side effects (17). Not surprisingly, other frequently reported barriers include forgetting to take pain medications and the belief that one should be able to tolerate pain without medication (47). Some patients are also concerned that, if they take pain medication, they will become tolerant to the effects of analgesics when their disease progresses (16,48,50).

Barriers to pain control may be assessed in a clinical interview or by using a standardized measure such as the Barriers Questionnaire (49). After the barriers for a patient have been identified, then appropriate education can be initiated. Patients should be active partners in their pain assessment and treatment. They have to be reassured that, in most instances, pain relief can be obtained and that it is part of the health care professional's role to provide that relief. Educating patients about cancer pain can improve the outcome of pain treatment. Several randomized clinical trials with cancer patients experiencing pain found that education on pain management produced significant reductions in pain intensity ratings (51,52).

Assessing pain impact

Comprehensive assessment of cancer pain should include the measurement of pain interference with areas of the patient's life and functioning. Information on the impact of pain will contribute to specific treatment recommendations. An optimal treatment plan for pain control is based on evaluation of more than pain severity and pain etiology. The assessment of pain impact includes the measurement of quality of life, mood, and social support systems.

Quality of life

Health-related quality of life (QOL) is defined as the perceived value of life as modified by impairments, functional states, perceptions, and social opportunities influenced by disease, injury, treatment, or policy (53). Measures of QOL typically include evaluation of physical functioning, psychological status, social relationships, and symptoms (54–56). It is beyond the scope of this chapter to review the field of instruments available to measure QOL. Some of the QOL instruments that have been used successfully with cancer patients include the EORTC-Quality of Life Questionnaire (57); the Functional Living Index—Cancer (58); the Functional Assessment of Cancer Therapy (FACT) measurement system (59); and the Medical Outcomes Study (MOS) Short Form-36 (SF-36) and Short

Form-12 (SF-12) Health Surveys (60–62). All of these QOL questionnaires have demonstrated adequate reliability and validity in clinical research. One drawback to the repeated use of QOL measures is the time required for patients to complete the questionnaires and for clinicians to score and interpret the results.

The BPI provides a synopsis of areas of pain interference with functioning. For patients with cancer-related pain, this synopsis is a useful alternative to more lengthy QOL measures. A recent study of Chinese cancer patients found that pain interference ratings on the BPI were significantly correlated with ratings on a standardized QOL questionnaire (63). Moreover, pain intensity ratings were a significant predictor of QOL, even after controlling for disease severity. The BPI interference items provide valuable information related to QOL and may be adequate in many cases. However, the BPI does not indicate the extent to which functioning or QOL is impaired by non-pain factors. One of the preceding QOL measures can provide a good screening tool to determine the need for further assessment.

Mood

The majority of cancer patients adjust to the stress of the disease and its treatment without developing clinical depression, anxiety disorders, or any other psychiatric condition (64,65). However, patients with pain are more likely to report depression or anxiety than those without pain (66–68). Significant mood disorders among cancer patients are difficult to identify because of the similarity of some mood symptoms and common disease-related symptoms, such as fatigue, weight loss, sleep disturbance, and impaired concentration. The BPI or one of the QOL measures can be used to screen for a possible mood disorder. If a mood disorder is suggested, then additional assessment can be performed using a standardized mood questionnaire or a clinical interview.

The Profile of Mood States is one of the more commonly used measures of mood in cancer patients (69,70). The scale is relatively easy for patients to understand and complete. In addition, the scale is sensitive to change over a brief period of time, making it ideal for studying responsiveness to treatment. However, the 65-item standard version, and even the 30-item "short form," is lengthy for very ill patients to complete. Consequently, a shorter 11-item version has been developed for cancer patients (71).

The well-validated State-Trait Anxiety Inventory (STAI) has been used to measure anxiety in cancer patients (72). The STAI that assesses present levels of anxiety is usually most appropriate for patients with can-

cer (73). The Beck Depression Inventory (74,75) is a reliable, valid, and frequently used measure of clinical depression. The clinician or researcher needs to look closely at content of the items endorsed by the patient in addition to the overall score (76,77). Examination of responses to the somatic, cognitive, and affective items may help to differentiate symptoms that are related to cancer (e.g., weight loss) from symptoms related to depression (e.g., sadness).

Social support

Social support makes an important contribution to the functioning and well-being of cancer patients but is difficult to measure (78–80). For an abbreviated evaluation of social interactions, the BPI and the QOL measures include items on the impact of pain, illness, or general health on social relationships. If the BPI or a QOL measure suggests difficulty with social support, then further assessment is warranted. The Multidimensional Pain Inventory (MPI) includes subscales assessing social support and the perceived responses (negative, solicitous, distracting) to pain of the spouse or significant other (81). A recent study comparing the MPI responses of patients with and without cancer found that patients with cancer reported more support and solicitous behavior from spouses or significant others than patients without cancer (82).

The Family Relations Index, a brief form of the Family Environment Scale (83), provides a measure of family functioning style that may inform the clinician of the family's level of conflict, cohesiveness, and expressiveness as perceived by the patient. Scores on this scale have been shown to relate to physical and psychological outcomes in cancer patients (84,85).

Concurrent symptoms

Cancer patients with pain usually have symptoms other than pain that need to be assessed and treated. The disease itself often produces fatigue, weakness, cachexia, and cognitive deficits. Cancer treatments frequently cause nausea, vomiting, fatigue, and other physical, cognitive, or affective symptoms. The negative side effects of analgesic medications may include constipation, nausea, fatigue, and sedation. Common symptoms of cancer and cancer treatment significantly impair the daily function and quality of life of patients. Thus, it is important to assess symptoms routinely and develop appropriate treatment plans.

A checklist of potential concurrent symptoms such as the M. D. Anderson Symptom Inventory (MDASI) can be used to assess the presence and intensity of symptoms (86). The MDASI consists of a core list of symptoms that are common across all cancer diagnoses and treatments, plus modules of additional symptoms that can be included for patients who are at risk for symptoms not highly prevalent in oncology patients in general. The core MDASI consists of 13 symptoms: pain, fatigue, nausea, sleep disturbance, emotional distress, shortness of breath, lack of appetite, drowsiness, dry mouth, sadness, vomiting, difficulty remembering, and numbness or tingling (Fig. 4.3). Each symptom is rated on

Date: _____

Subject Initials: _____

Study Subject #: _____

Institution:_____

Hospital Chart #:_____

M. D. Anderson Symptom Inventory (MDASI) Core Items

Part I. How **severe** are your symptoms?

People with cancer frequently have symptoms that are caused by their disease or by their treatment. We ask you to rate how severe the following symptoms have been **in the last 24 hours.** Please fill in the circle below from 0 (symptom has not been present) to 10 (the symptom was as bad as you can imagine it could be) for each item.

	Not Present 0	1	2	3	4	5	6	7	8	9	As Bad As You Can Imagine 10
1. Your **pain** at its WORST?	○	○	○	○	○	○	○	○	○	○	○
2. Your **fatigue (tiredness)** at its WORST?	○	○	○	○	○	○	○	○	○	○	○
3. Your **nausea** at its WORST?	○	○	○	○	○	○	○	○	○	○	○
4. Your **disturbed sleep** at its WORST?	○	○	○	○	○	○	○	○	○	○	○
5. Your feelings of being **distressed (upset)** at its WORST?	○	○	○	○	○	○	○	○	○	○	○
6. Your **shortness of breath** at its WORST?	○	○	○	○	○	○	○	○	○	○	○
7. Your problem with **remembering things** at its WORST?	○	○	○	○	○	○	○	○	○	○	○
8. Your problem with **lack of appetite** at its WORST?	○	○	○	○	○	○	○	○	○	○	○
9. Your feeling **drowsy (sleepy)** at its WORST?	○	○	○	○	○	○	○	○	○	○	○
10.Your having a **dry mouth** at its WORST?	○	○	○	○	○	○	○	○	○	○	○

Fig. 4.3. The M. D. Anderson Symptom Inventory (MDASI). The core MDASI consists of 13 symptoms and 6 interference items. Courtesy of MD Anderson Cancer Center. *(Figure continues)*

Date: _____   Institution: _____

Subject Initials: _____   Hospital Chart #: _____

Study Subject #: _____

	Not Present										As Bad As You Can Imagine
	0	1	2	3	4	5	6	7	8	9	1 0
11. Your feeling **sad** at its WORST?	○	○	○	○	○	○	○	○	○	○	○
12. Your **vomiting** at its WORST?	○	○	○	○	○	○	○	○	○	○	○
13. Your **numbness or tingling** at its WORST?	○	○	○	○	○	○	○	○	○	○	○

Part II. How have your symptoms interfered with your life?

Symptoms frequently interfere with how we feel and function. How much have your symptoms interfered with the following items in the last 24 hours:

	Did Not Interfere										Interefered Completely
	0	1	2	3	4	5	6	7	8	9	1 0
14. General activity?	○	○	○	○	○	○	○	○	○	○	○
15. Mood?	○	○	○	○	○	○	○	○	○	○	○
16. Work (including work around the house)?	○	○	○	○	○	○	○	○	○	○	○
17. Relations with other people?	○	○	○	○	○	○	○	○	○	○	○
18. Walking?	○	○	○	○	○	○	○	○	○	○	○
19. Enjoyment of life?	○	○	○	○	○	○	○	○	○	○	○

Fig. 4.3 *(Continued)*

an 11-point scale, with 0 being "not present" and 10 being "as bad as you can imagine." The MDASI also contains six items that describe how much the symptoms have interfered with areas of the patient's life during the past 24 hours: general activity, mood, walking ability, normal work (including work outside the home and housework), relations with other people, and enjoyment of life.

The core symptom items on the MDASI can be used to monitor patients' symptoms in routine clinical care. Subsets of additional symptom items can be added to the basic MDASI for patients who are receiving aggressive treatments (e.g., bone marrow transplantation) or who have cancer diagnoses associated with specific symptoms (e.g, lung cancer and coughing). As with pain, it is important to evaluate these symptoms over time to monitor changes in severity and response to treatment.

Pain assessment in children with cancer

Historically, pain assessment in children with cancer has received less attention than pain in adults (87). However, adequate care of children with cancer must include a plan for the assessment and management of any cancer-related pain. The WHO has developed guidelines for the assessment and treatment of cancer-related pain in children (88). The guidelines recommend regular assessment and documentation of the child's pain level as an essential vital sign that guides treatment recommendations.

Developmentally appropriate pain intensity measures should be used with all children. Assessment of pain in infants often relies on physiological measures and observer reports of behaviors that indicate probable pain. A variety of pain intensity measures are available for toddlers and preschool children, including pain thermometers (89), color scales (90), and faces scales (91). Children over the age of 5 years usually are able to complete standard numeric and visual analog scales (92).

The child's self-report of pain should be considered the "gold standard" of pediatric pain assessment and used whenever possible. However, behavioral observations are necessary for pain assessment in very young children and in children who do not have the ability to report their pain because of disability or disease. A number of reliable, valid behavioral observation methods have been developed for the assessment of pediatric behaviors related to pain, such as crying, clinging, reduction in normal activity, and social withdrawal (93–96).

Two standardized interviews for school-aged children and adolescents can provide valuable information regarding the impact of cancer pain on the child's daily life: the Children's Comprehensive Pain Questionnaire (97) and the Varni-Thompson Pediatric Pain Questionnaire (98). In addition, a special panel of the American Academy of Pediatrics has suggested that a Pain Problem List be included in the medical record of every child with cancer (92). The goal of this list is to identify pain problems and appropriate pain management strategies.

Pain assessment in elderly patients with cancer

Sixty percent of all cancers occur in persons aged 65 years and older (99). Several recent studies found that elderly patients with cancer are at risk for undertreatment of cancer-related pain. In a survey of outpatients with metastatic cancer who were experiencing pain, Cleeland and colleagues (7) found that patients 70 years of age and older were more likely to receive inadequate analgesics than younger patients. Similarly, a survey of more than 13,000 nursing home residents with cancer found that 26% of the patients experiencing daily pain received no analgesics (100). Only about half of the patients in pain received opioids, and only 13% of patients more than 85 years old received strong analgesics.

Lack of pain assessment or inadequate assessment contributes to the undertreatment of cancer pain in the elderly. In the nursing home study by Bernabei and colleagues (100), regular pain assessments were not included in most patient charts. However, 86% of the patients, including cognitively impaired individuals, were able to verbally report pain to the research staff. Similarly, Ferrell and colleagues (101) found that 83% of elderly patients in a nursing home setting could complete at least one of the four pain intensity scales administered. Other studies have documented that elderly patients with mild to moderate cognitive impairment can complete simple pain rating scales (102,103). However, many elderly patients require careful instruction in the use of pain assessment instruments.

Before pain is assessed, all elderly patients should be screened to identify any sensory, motor, or cognitive deficits that affect their ability to report pain. Pain scales can be printed with large letters and scales for patients with limited visual abilities. The Faces Pain Scale for the elderly can be used for individuals who have difficulty understanding numerical or VAS formats (104). Pain assessment instruments also can be administered in an interview format for patients who have visual or motor impairments that prevent completion of paper and pencil measures. Clinicians and researchers should be aware of possible hearing impairments and assess whether elderly patients are able to comprehend oral instructions (105). When cognitive deficits are severe and prevent self-report of pain, observation of pain-related behaviors is an alternative strategy. An observation system to assess pain behaviors in elderly nursing home patients is a promising approach that needs further development (106).

Pain measurement for quality assurance

The development of specific practice guidelines for pain management has led to quality assurance standards for pain treatment (28,29). In addition, the Joint Committee on Accreditation of Healthcare Organizations has developed standards for the assessment and management of pain in health care organizations. Hospitals and other health care facilities will be expected to demonstrate compliance with these standards when they are reviewed for accreditation. The standards include regular assessment and recording of patients' pain levels. Pain assessment tools provide a method for routine monitoring and charting of pain in the hospital or clinic setting. Numerical scales seem best suited for easy tracking of pain for this purpose.

Innovative educational programs have been developed to improve pain assessment and treatment in health care institutions. A model pain management program to implement quality assurance guidelines for the treatment of cancer pain was evaluated recently at a tertiary care cancer center (107). The program included the formation of a quality improvement team, staff education on pain assessment and management, pain rounds, and focus groups to discuss issues related to cancer pain. After implementation of the model program, improvements were found in patients' satisfaction with pain treatment and nurses' knowledge of and attitudes toward pain management.

The Cancer Pain Role Model Program, developed by the Wisconsin Cancer Pain Initiative in 1990, has trained more than 1000 health care professionals in the United States (108–110). Health care professionals who participate in the program receive intensive education in cancer pain assessment and treatment. Then the professionals are asked to develop an action plan to facilitate improved pain assessment and treatment in their own institutions.

Innovative trends in pain assessment

Recent developments in computer and communications technology offer new opportunities for the assessment of patients' pain and other symptoms. Handheld computers and other electronic recording devices have been used for the assessment of pain in patients' home and work environments (111). Given that memory for pain and other symptoms is often poor, the "real time" assessment of symptoms can provide accurate data regarding symptom patterns and changes over time; however, not all patients are comfortable using handheld computers or other small automated devices. In addition, patients have to remember to use the devices every day and to transmit the symptom data to their health care providers.

The development of telephone interactive voice response (IVR) technology provides an exciting option for two-way communication with the provider that is acceptable to most patients. Telephone systems have been widely used in outpatient health care settings for communicating with patients. However, traditional telephone communica-

tion requires considerable staff time and is not feasible for assessing symptoms on a regular basis. Using IVR technology that combines touch-tone telephones with computers and the Internet may be an effective way to follow patients who have symptoms like pain that need to be monitored closely while away from the clinic or hospital (112). A patient can respond to spoken instructions by using the keypad of a touch-tone phone. For example, a patient might be asked to rate his/her pain at its worst in the last day from 0 (no pain) to 10 (pain as bad as you can imagine). Information obtained in this way can be used to update a patient file on an Internet or intranet site. The system also can be configured to alert physicians and other health care providers. In a pilot study at M.D. Anderson Cancer Center, the system paged a provider when patients reported that the severity of their worst pain in the last 24 hours was 7 or greater (113).

An IVR system should be especially helpful for assessing symptoms such as pain that patients may be reluctant to report to their busy treatment team. Accurate and regular symptom assessment, with data provided to the patients' physicians, should facilitate symptom management. The IVR system can also provide an innovative means of assessing patients' symptoms in their home and work environments.

Conclusions

Inadequate pain assessment is the most common reason for undertreatment of cancer-related pain. Oncology health care professionals often lack training in pain assessment and are focused on treating the cancer. Patients may hesitate to report their pain because of a variety of reasons, including concerns about the meaning of pain, their hesitancy to complain, a reluctance to distract their physician from treating the cancer, and concerns about pain medications. Accurate and regular assessment of patients' pain is essential for effective treatment planning and evaluation. Pain assessment measures designed for the patient with cancer can facilitate the assessment process. Pain severity and interference in daily activities caused by pain are important targets for pain assessment. Assessment based on questionnaires needs to be supplemented by patient interview and medical-neurological examination.

When deficits in quality of life, mood, or social support are indicated by patients' questionnaire or interview responses, additional evaluation is suggested. Pain is typically associated with other cancer-related symptoms that require regular assessment. Pain assessment should be repeated frequently to monitor treatment efficacy and to identify any changes in patients' pain related to treatments or disease progression. Pain assessment of pediatric and geriatric patients requires special considerations. Patients can benefit from education regarding cancer pain and effective pain management treatments. Quality assurance standards require the regular use of pain assessment measures in oncology treatment settings. Recent innovations in computer and communications technology provide new approaches to pain assessment in patients' daily environments.

Acknowledgments

Preparation for this chapter was supported by Public Health Service grants CA26582, CA64766, and CA85228 from the National Cancer Institute and SIG #21 from the American Cancer Society.

References

1. World Health Organization. Cancer pain relief. Geneva: Author, 1986.
2. World Health Organization. Cancer pain relief and palliative care. Geneva: Author, 1986.
3. Grond S, Radbruch L, Meuser T, et al. Assessment and treatment of neuropathic cancer pain following WHO guidelines. Pain 79:15–20, 1999.
4. Schug SA, Zech D, Dorr U. Cancer pain management according to WHO analgesic guidelines. J Pain Symptom Manage 5:27–32, 1990.
5. Ventafridda V, Tamburini M, Caraceni A, et al. A validation study of the WHO method for cancer pain relief. Cancer 59:850–6, 1987.
6. Zech DFJ, Grond S, Lynch J, et al. Validation of World Health Organization Guidelines for cancer pain relief: a 10-year prospective study. Pain 63:65–76, 1995.
7. Cleeland CS, Gonin R, Hatfield AK, et al. Pain and its treatment in outpatients with metastatic cancer. N Engl J Med 330:592–4, 1994.
8. Vainio A, Auvinen A. Prevalence of symptoms with advanced cancer: an international collaborative study. J Pain Symptom Manage 12:3–10, 1996.
9. Zenz M, Zenz T, Tryba M, Strumpf M. Severe undertreatment of cancer pain: a 3-year survey of the German situation. J Pain Symptom Manage 10:187–91, 1995.
10. Zhukovsky DS, Gorowski E, Hausdorff J, et al. Unmet analgesic needs in cancer patients. J Pain Symptom Manage 10:113–119, 1995.
11. von Roenn JH, Cleeland CS, Gonin R, et al. Physician attitudes and practice in cancer pain management. A survey from the Eastern Cooperative Oncology Group. Ann Intern Med 119:121–6, 1993.
12. Anderson KO, Mendoza TR, Valero V, et al. Minority cancer patients and their providers—pain management attitudes and practice. Cancer 88:1929–38, 2000.
13. Cleeland CS, Janjan NA, Scott CB, et al. Cancer pain management by radiotherapists: a survey of Radiation Therapy Oncology Group physicians. Int J Radiat Oncol Biol Phys 47:203–8, 2000.
14. Cleeland CS, Gonin R, Baez L, et al. Pain and treatment of pain in minority outpatients with cancer. The Eastern Cooperative Oncology Group minority outpatient pain study. Ann Intern Med 127:813–6, 1997.
15. Hodes RL. Cancer patients' needs and concerns when using narcotic analgesics. In: Hill CS, Fields WS, eds. Advances in pain research and therapy, Vol. 11. New York: Raven Press, 1989:91–9.
16. Dar R, Beach CM, Barden PL, Cleeland CS. Cancer pain in the marital system: a study of patients and their spouses. J Pain Symptom Manage 7:87–93, 1992.
17. Anderson KO, Richman SP, Hurley J, et al. Cancer pain management among underserved minority outpatients—perceived needs and barriers to optimal control. Cancer 94:2295–304, 2002.
18. Gonzales GR, Elliott KJ, Portenoy RK, Foley KM. The impact of a comprehensive evaluation in the management of cancer pain. Pain 47:141–4, 1991.
19. Payne R. Pathophysiology of cancer pain. In: Foley KM, Bonica JJ, Ventafridda V, Callaway MV, eds. Advances in pain research and therapy, Vol. 16. New York: Raven Press, 1990:13–26.
20. Portenoy RK, Lesage P. Management of cancer pain. Lancet 353(9165):1695–700, 1999.
21. Grond S, Zech D, Diefenbach C, et al. Assessment of cancer pain: a prospective evaluation in 2266 cancer patients referred to a pain service. Pain 64:107–14, 1996.
22. Banning A, Sjogren P, Henriksen H. Pain causes in 200 patients referred to a multidisciplinary cancer pain clinic. Pain 45:45–8, 1991.
23. Caraceni A, Portenoy RK, Working group of the IASP Task Force on Cancer Pain. An international survey of cancer pain characteristics and syndromes. Pain 82:263–74, 1999.
24. Foley KM. Pain syndromes in patients with cancer. In: Bonica JJ, Ventafridda V, eds. Advances in pain research and therapy, Vol. 2. New York: Raven Press, 1979:59–75.
25. Chapman CR, Kornell JA, Syrjala KL. Painful complications of cancer diagnosis and therapy. In: Yarbro CH, McGuire DB, eds. Cancer pain: nursing management. Orlando, FL: Grune & Stratton, 1987:47–67.
26. Serlin RC, Mendoza TR, Nakamura Y, et al. When is cancer pain mild, moderate or severe? Grading pain severity by its interference with function. Pain 61:277–84, 1995.
27. Grossman SA, Benedetti C, Payne R, Syrjala KL. NCCN Practice Guidelines for cancer pain. Oncology 13(11A): 33–44, 1999.
28. Jacox A, Carr DB, Payne R, et al. Management of cancer pain. Clinical practice guideline No. 9. AHCPR Publication no. 94-0592. Rockville MD: Agency for Health Care Policy

and Research, U.S. Department of Health and Human Services Public Health Service, 1994.

29. American Pain Society. Principles of analgesic use in the treatment of acute pain and cancer pain. Glenview IL: Author, 1999.

30. Lasagna L. Analgesic methodology: a brief history and commentary. J Clin Pharmacol 20:373–6, 1980.

31. Cleeland CS. Research in cancer pain: what we know and what we need to know. Cancer 67(Suppl 3):823–7, 1991.

32. Wallenstein S. Measurement of pain and analgesia in cancer patients. Cancer 53(Suppl 10):2260–4, 1984.

33. Ferraz MB, Quaresma MR, Aquino LR, et al. Reliability of pain scales in the assessment of literate and illiterate patients with rheumatoid arthritis. J Rheumatol 17:1022–4, 1990.

34. Cleeland CS. Measurement of pain by subjective report. In Chapman CR, Loeser JD, eds. Issues in pain measurement. New York: Raven Press, 1989.

35. De Conno F, Caraceni A, Gamba A, et al. Pain measurement in cancer patients: a comparison of six methods. Pain 57:161–6, 1994.

36. Jensen MP, Karoly P, Braver S. The measurement of clinical pain intensity: a comparison of six methods. Pain 27:117–26, 1986.

37. Syrjala KL. The measurement of pain: cancer pain management. Orlando, FL: Grune & Stratton, 1987.

38. Cleeland CS. Assessment of pain in cancer: Measurement issues. In: Foley KM, Bonica JJ, Ventafridda V, Callaway MV, eds. Advances in pain research and therapy, Vol. 16. New York: Raven Press, 1990:47–55.

39. Fishman B, Pasternak S, Wallenstein SL, et al. The Memorial Pain Assessment Card. A valid instrument for the evaluation of cancer pain. Cancer 60:1151–8, 1987.

40. Melzack R. The short-form McGill Pain Questionnaire. Pain, 30:191–7, 1987.

41. Portenoy RK, Hagen NA. Breakthrough pain: definition, prevalence and characteristics. Pain 41:273–81, 1990.

42. Petzke F, Radbruch L, Zech D, et al. Temporal presentation of chronic cancer pain: transitory pains on admission to a multidisciplinary pain clinic. J Pain Symptom Manage 17:391–401, 1990.

43. Du Pen SL, Du Pen AR, Polissar N, et al. Implementing guidelines for cancer pain management: results of a randomized controlled clinical trial. J Clin Oncol 17:361–70, 1999.

44. Juarez G, Ferrell B, Borneman T. Influence of culture on cancer pain management in Hispanic patients. Cancer Practice 6:262–9, 1998.

45. Richardson MA, Sanders T, Palmer JL, et al. Complementary/alternative medicine use in a comprehensive cancer center and the implications for oncology. J Clin Oncol 18:2505–14, 2000.

46. Wilkie DJ, Keefe FJ. Coping strategies of patients with lung cancer-related pain. Clin J Pain 7:292–9, 1991.

47. Thomason TE, McCune JS, Bernard SA, et al. Cancer pain survey: patient-centered issues in control. J Pain Symptom Manage 15:275–84, 1998.

48. Ward SE, Goldberg N, Miller-McCauley V, et al. Patient-related barriers to management of cancer pain. Pain 52:319–24, 1993.

49. Ward SE, Hernandez L. Patient-related barriers to management of cancer pain in Puerto Rico. Pain 58:233–8, 1994.

50. Cleeland CS. Pain control: public and physicians' attitudes. In: Hill Jr CS, Fields WS, eds. Advances in pain research and therapy, Vol. 11. New York: Raven Press, 1989:81–9.

51. De Wit R, van Dam F, Zandbelt L, et al. A pain education program for chronic cancer pain patients: follow-up results from a randomized controlled trial. Pain 73:55–69, 1997.

52. Syrjala KL, Abrams JR, Cowan J, et al. Is educating patients and families the route to relieving cancer pain? Presented at the International Association for the Study of Pain 8th World Congress on Pain, Vancouver, BC, Canada, 1996.

53. Patrick DL, Erickson P. Assessing health-related quality of life for clinical decision-making. In: Walker SR, Rosser RM, eds. Quality of life assessment: key issues for the 1990s. London: Kluwer Academic Press, 1993:11–64.

54. Cella DF. Quality of life: concepts and definitions. J Pain Symptom Manage 9:186–92, 1994.

55. Gill TM, Feinstein AR. A critical appraisal of the quality-of-life measurements. JAMA 272:619–26, 1994.

56. O'Boyle CA, Waldron D. Quality of life issues in palliative medicine. J Neurol 244 (Suppl 4):18–25, 1997.

57. Aaronson NK, Ahmedzai S, Bergman B, et al. The European Organization for Research and Treatment of Cancer QLQ-C30: a quality-of-life instrument for use in international clinical trials in oncology. J Nat Cancer Inst 85:365–76, 1993.

58. Schipper H, Clinch J, McMurray A, Levitt M. Measuring the quality of life of cancer patients: the Functional Living Index-Cancer: development and validation. J Clin Oncol 2:472–83, 1984.

59. Cella DF, Tulsky DS, Gray G, et al. The Functional Assessment of Cancer Therapy scale: development and validation of the general measure. J Clin Oncol 11:570–9, 1993.

60. Stewart AL, Hays RD, Ware JE. The MOS Short-form General Health Survey: reliability and validity in a patient population. Medical Care 26:724–35, 1988.

61. Ware JE, Sherbourne CS. The MOS 36-item Short-form Health Survey (SF-36). I. Conceptual framework and item selection. Medical Care 30:473–83, 1992.

62. Ware JE, Kosinski M, Keller SD. SF-12: how to score the SF-12 Physical and Mental Health Summary Scales. Boston, MA: The Health Institute, New England Medical Center, 1995.

63. Wang XS, Cleeland CS, Mendoza TR, et al. The effects of pain severity on health-related quality of life. Cancer 86:1848–55, 1999.

64. Derogatis LR, Morrow GR, Fetting J, et al. The prevalence of psychiatric disorders among cancer patients. JAMA 249:751–7, 1983.

65. Shacham S, Dar R, Cleeland CS. The relationship of mood state to the severity of clinical pain. Pain 18:187–97, 1984.

66. Ahles TA, Blanchard EB, Ruckdeschel JC. The multidimensional nature of cancer-related pain. Pain 17:277–88, 1983.

67. Glover J, Dibble SL, Dodd MS, Miaskowski C. Mood states of oncology outpatients: does pain make a difference? J Pain Symptom Manage 10:120–8, 1995.

68. Heim HM, Oei TPS. Comparison of prostate cancer patients with and without pain. Pain 53:159–62, 1993.

69. McNair DM, Lorr M, Droppleman LF. EdITS Manual for the Profile of Mood States. San Diego, CA: Educational and Industrial Testing Service, 1971.

70. McNair DM, Lorr M, Droppleman LF. EdITS Manual for the Profile of Mood States. San Diego, CA: Educational and Industrial Testing Service, 1992.

71. Cella DF, Jacobson PB, Orav EJ, et al. A brief POMS measure of distress for cancer patients. J Chronic Dis 40:939–42, 1987.

72. Spielberger CD. Manual for the State-Trait Anxiety Inventory. Palo Alto, CA: Consulting Psychologists Press, 1983.

73. Shumaker SA, Anderson RT, Czajkowski SM. Psychological tests and scales. In: Spilker B, ed. Quality of life assessments in clinical trials. New York: Raven Press, 1990:95–113.

74. Beck AT, Ward CH, Mendelson M, et al. An inventory for measuring depression. Arch General Psychiatry 4:561–71, 1961.

75. Beck AT, Steer RA. Beck Depression Inventory manual. San Antonio: Harcourt Brace Jovanovich, 1987.

76. Novy DM, Nelson DV, Berry LA, Averill PM. What does the Beck Depression Inventory measure in chronic pain? A reappraisal. Pain 61:261–70, 1995.

77. Williams AC, Richardson PH. What does the Beck Depression Inventory measure in chronic pain? Pain 55:259–66, 1993.

78. Dunkel-Schetter C. Social support and cancer: findings based on patient interviews and their implications. J Social Issues 40:77–98, 1984.

79. Moinpour CM, Feigl P, Metch B, et al. Quality of life end points in cancer clinical trials: review and recommendations. J Nat Cancer Inst 81:485–95, 1989.

80. Wortman CB. Social support and the cancer patient: conceptual and methodological issues. Cancer 53(Suppl 10):2339–60, 1984.

81. Kerns RD, Turk DC, Rudy TE. The West Haven-Yale Multidimensional Pain Inventory (WHYMPI). Pain 23:345–56, 1985.

82. Turk DC, Sist TC, Okifuji A, et al. Adaptation to metastatic cancer pain, regional/local cancer pain and non-cancer pain: role of psychological and behavioral factors. Pain 74:247–56, 1998.

83. Moos RH, Moos BS. Family Environment Scale—Manual, 2nd ed. Palo Alto, CA: Consulting Psychologists Press, 1986.

84. Bloom J, Spiegel D. The relationship of two dimensions of social support to the psychological well-being and social functioning of women with advanced breast cancer. Social Sci Med 19:831–7, 1984.

85. Syrjala KL, Chapko MK, Vitaliano PP, et al. Recovery after allogeneic marrow transplantation: prospective study of predictors of long-term physical and psychosocial functioning. Bone Marrow Transplant 11:319–27, 1988.

86. Cleeland CS, Mendoza TR, Wang XS, et al. Assessing symptom distress in cancer: the M. D. Anderson Symptom Inventory. Cancer 89:1634–46, 2000.

87. Ljungman G, Kreuger A, Gordh T, et al. Treatment of pain in pediatric oncology: a Swedish nationwide study. Pain 68:385–94, 1996.

88. World Health Organization. Cancer pain relief and palliative care in children. Geneva: Author, 1998.

89. Jay SM, Ozolins M, Elliott CH, Caldwell S. Assessment of children's distress during painful medical procedures. Health Psychol 2:133–47, 1983.

90. Eland JM. Minimizing pain associated with pre-kindergarten intramuscular injections. Issues in Comprehensive Pediatric Nursing 5:362–72, 1981.

91. McGrath PJ, Seifert CE, Speechley KN, et al. A new analogue scale for assessing children's pain: an initial validation study. Pain 64:435–43, 1996.

92. McGrath PJ, Beyer J, Cleeland CS, et al. American Academy of Pediatrics Report of the Subcommittee on Assessment and Methodologic Issues in the Management of Pain in Childhood Cancer. Pediatrics 86:814–7, 1990.

93. Gauvain-Piquard A, Rodary C, Francois P, et al. Validity assessment of DEGR^R scale for observational rating of 2-6-year-old child pain. J Pain Symptom Manage 6:171, 1991.

94. Krane EJ, Jacobson LE, Lynn AM, et al. Caudal morphine for postoperative analgesia in children: a comparison with caudal bupivacaine and intravenous morphine. Anesth Analg 66:647–53, 1987.

95. McGrath PJ, Johnson G, Goodman JT, et al. CHEOPS: a behavioral scale for rating postoperative pain in children. In: Fields HL, Dubner R, Cervero F, Jones LE, eds. Advances in pain research and therapy, Vol. 9. New York: Raven Press, 1985:395–402.

96. Tarbell SE, Cohen IT, Marsh JL. (1992). The Toddler-Preschooler Postoperative Pain Scale: an observational scale for measuring postoperative pain in children aged 1–5. Preliminary report. Pain 50:273–80, 1992.

97. McGrath PJ. Pain in children. New York: Guilford, 1990.

98. Varni JW, Thompson KL, Hanson V. The Varni/Thompson Pediatric Pain Questionnaire. I. Chronic musculoskeletal pain in juvenile rheumatoid arthritis. Pain 28:27–38, 1987.

99. Yancik R. Cancer burden in the aged. An epidemiologic and demographic overview. Cancer 80:1273–83, 1997.

100. Bernabei R, Gambassi G, Lapane K, et al. Management of pain in elderly patients with cancer. JAMA 279:1877–82, 1998.

101. Ferrell BA, Ferrell BR, Rivera L. Pain in cognitively impaired nursing home patients. J Pain Symptom Manage 10:591–8, 1995.

102. Parmalee PA. Pain in cognitively impaired older persons. Clin Geriatr Med 12:473–8, 1996.

103. Parmalee PA, Smith B, Katz IR. Pain complaints and cognitive status among elderly institution residents. J Am Geriatr Soc 31:517–22, 1993.

104. Herr KA, Mobily PR, Kohout FJ, Wagenaar D. Evaluation of the Faces Pain Scale for use with the elderly. Clin J Pain 14:29–38, 1998.

105. Herr KA, Mobily PR. Pain assessment in the elderly: clinical considerations. J Gerontol Nurs 17:12–19, 1991.

106. Weiner D, Peterson B, Keefe F. Chronic pain associated behaviors in the nursing home: resident versus caregiver perceptions. Pain 80:577–88, 1999.

107. Bookbinder M, Coyle N, Kiss M, et al. Implementing national standards for cancer pain management: program model and evaluation. J Pain Symptom Manage 12:334–47, 1996.

108. Janjan NA, Martin CG, Payne R, et al. Teaching cancer pain management: durability of educational effects of a role model program. Cancer 77:996–1001, 1996.

109. Weissman DE, Dahl JL. Update on the cancer pain role model education program. J Pain Symptom Manage 10:292–7, 1995.

110. Weissman DE, Griffie J, Gordon DB, Dahl JL. A role model program to promote institutional changes for management of acute and cancer pain. J Pain Symptom Manage 14:274–9, 1997.

111. Lewis B, Lewis D, Cumming G. Frequent measurement of chronic pain: an electronic diary and empirical findings. Pain 60:341–7, 1995.

112. Cleeland CS. Cancer-related symptoms. Semin Radiat Oncol 10:175–90, 2000.

113. Chandler SW, Payne R. Computerized tools to assess and manage cancer pain. Highlights in Oncology Practice 14(4):114–7, 1997.

5 Multidimensional assessment: pain and palliative care

PETER G. LAWLOR
University of Alberta

Introduction

Pain occurs in the majority of patients with advanced cancer (1,2) and is associated with multiple other symptoms (3,4), which in combination are manifested with increasing frequency toward the last days of life (5). Although the pursuit of World Health Organization (WHO) guidelines can achieve adequate pain relief for 80%–90% of patients with cancer (6,7), there is evidence to suggest that this is not achieved in clinical practice (6,8,9). Although there are many potential explanations, the failure to conduct a multidimensional assessment is likely to play a significant role in this undertreatment (8,10,11). A multidimensional approach incorporates the assessment of pain in the context of other variables, including other symptoms, therapeutic interventions, and the domains of physical, psychosocial, and spiritual functioning (12,13). This contrasts with the unidimensional approach, which attributes all aspects of the pain experience (including use of analgesics and psychological distress) to the patient's reported pain intensity.

More than 30 years ago, Melzack and Casey conceptualized pain as being composed of three major dimensions: *sensory-discriminative, motivational-affective,* and *cognitive-evaluative* (14). However, there is relatively limited literature reference to the multidimensional nature of cancer pain before the publication of a study by Ahles et al in 1983 (15). This study demonstrated that pain occurring in association with cancer consisted of the following general components: *sensory* (including characteristics such as site, radiation, intensity, and quality), *affective* (including mood disturbance and anxiety), *cognitive* (including the influence of pain on thought processes, and the meaning of pain), and *behavioral* (including use of analgesic medication, and relationship of pain to activities of daily living). The International Association for the Study of Pain has defined pain as "an unpleasant sensory and emotional

experience associated with actual or potential tissue damage, or described in terms of such damage" (16). There is evidence therefore to support the concept, and a high level of consensus regarding the multidimensional nature of pain. The educational efforts of WHO have in the last decade sought to promote multidimensional assessment by broadening its original cancer pain program into cancer care and palliative care (1).

Major steps in the pain experience

The basic components of the pain construct are represented in Fig. 5.1, using nociceptive pain as an example. First, the productive or nociceptive input stage involves activation of peripheral nociceptors and the arrival of impulses in the dorsal horn of the spinal cord. Neuropathic pain is associated with nerve injury or damage and can occur without peripheral nociceptor activation. Second, the actual perception of pain occurs at brain level. The extent to which the message is relayed from the spinal cord to higher brain centers comes under the influence of descending modulatory circuits, in addition to the action of endogenous and exogenous opioids in the dorsal horn. Third, the stage of expression is the measurable component of the pain experience. This expression is derived from multiple inputs. Pain is ultimately not only a sensory phenomenon; it also is an emotional experience, owing to input from various cognitive and affective factors (15,17) grouped under the headings of psychosocial milieu and emotional distress in the model described in Fig. 5.1.

Pain and quality of life: an overview

The interaction of pain and other domains contributing to the global quality of life construct is represented in the matrix in Fig. 5.2. In most of these interactions, there is

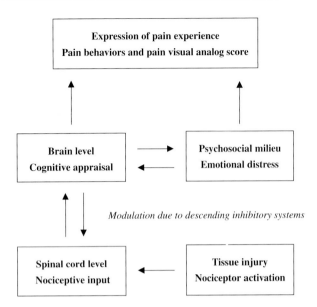

Fig. 5.1. Production, perception, and expression components of the pain construct.

potential for bidirectional influence. The degree of concomitant disturbance in the physical, psychological, and social functioning domains; the impact of pain and other symptoms; the role of spiritual and existential distress; the subtle contribution of cultural influences; and the relative interplay of all these factors is complex and relatively unique for each individual. For cancer patients without effective disease-modifying treatments, the illness trajectory usually entails an inexorable disease progression. The interrelationships and the relative roles of pain, other symptoms, and the various other domains in Fig. 5.2 are therefore subject to potential change over time. This temporal dynamic can be associated with varying levels of suffering, coping, and adjustment, which in turn influence the overall quality of life. At this stage, the palliative focus of care assumes primary importance.

In the case of patients with cancer pain that is difficult to control using conventional strategies such as that pro-

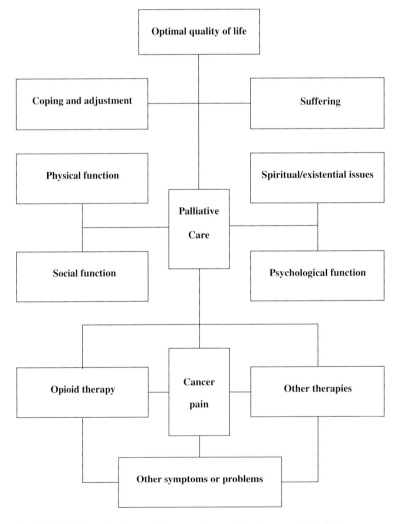

Fig. 5.2. Multidimensional matrix incorporating pain in the context of palliative care.

posed by the WHO (1), or other agencies (18), the need for a multidimensional assessment assumes even greater importance. These patients and others with varying care needs are often referred to pain specialists and practitioners in palliative care. Palliative care is concerned with the provision of care to patients with progressive incurable illness, and their families. The goal of palliative care is to achieve optimal quality of life with the emphasis on provision of comfort toward the end of life, as opposed to pursuit of primarily curative strategies. The provision of comfort entails pain relief in addition to alleviation of distress in relation to various social, psychological, existential, and spiritual issues, as well as the many other symptoms that emerge with advanced disease. The recognition and relief of distress in the many domains contributing to the multidimensional quality of life construct serve to enhance adjustment and adaptive coping, and reduce the global distress and potential suffering associated with terminal illness. Not surprisingly, therefore, the palliative care model in its usual capacity incorporates a multidisciplinary team approach.

Pivotal role of cognitive status

The presence of cognitive impairment, whether as a result of delirium or dementia, presents a major impediment in the assessment of pain and other symptoms in patients with advanced cancer (19). The chapter on cancer pain in the elderly (Chapter 20) addresses the challenges of pain assessment in patients with dementia. Although dementia occurs predominantly in the elderly, delirium occurs in all age groups with cancer (20). The frequency of delirium in advanced cancer patients varies from 28%–40% on admission (20,21), and the vast majority have delirium in the hours to days before death (20,22). The diagnosis of delirium is made on the basis of cognitive impairment, particularly disordered attention, along with other features such as altered awareness, perceptual disturbance, acute onset, and fluctuation in course (23). The Minimental State Examination (MMSE) (24) is widely used to screen for cognitive impairment, as a component of delirium. Normal population-based scores have been established for this instrument in relation to age and educational level (25). The diagnosis of delirium is frequently missed, particularly if no objective cognitive testing such as the MMSE is carried out (26–28). Regular screening with an instrument such as the MMSE therefore aids the detection of delirium and, in turn, provides useful information regarding the reliability of patient-rated pain assessment scores (29).

Based on the level of psychomotor activity, hyperactive and hypoactive subtypes of delirium have been proposed (30,31). A recent study suggests that a mixed subtype is the most common in patients with advanced cancer (32). The emotional lability, disinhibition, and psychomotor agitation components of the delirium syndrome are frequently interpreted as worsening pain by relatives, and sometimes by medical and nursing staff (33), especially in the absence of any objective cognitive testing. Family members with the best of intentions advocate for more analgesia for their relative, whom they see as being in excruciating pain. Fainsinger and colleagues (34) refer to the "destructive triangle" created as a result of the family's misinterpretation of the patient's delirium as pain, and their consequent advocacy for nursing and, in turn, physician efforts to "do something." In an effort to relieve the patient's distress, the physician often increases the opioid dose without taking the time to conduct a disciplined multidimensional assessment. The increase in opioid in turn tends to further aggravate the agitation, particularly when the opioid is already implicated as a precipitant (34,35). A multidimensional assessment in this setting would have embodied cognitive testing and the recognition of delirium. This assessment may suggest more appropriate interventions, such as an opioid switch or dose reduction, in addition to prescribing a neuroleptic for the symptomatic treatment of delirium.

A recent study suggests that the circadian distribution of opioid analgesic breakthrough use in advanced cancer patients with delirium differs from that of cancer patients without delirium (36). Patients in delirium used more breakthrough doses in the evening and night, compared to non-delirious patients, who used more breakthrough doses during the day. One potential explanation offered by the authors is that delirium-associated psychomotor agitation occurring in the "sundown" period could be misinterpreted by family and staff as worsening of pain, hence resulting in administration of a greater number of breakthrough doses.

Assessing other symptoms: relevance to the pain presentation

A study of 90 cancer patients in their last month of life reported a range of one to nine symptoms; 71% of patients described three or more symptoms (37). The symptom priority level ascribed by the patient in terms of distress can vary over time, and pain is not always associated with the highest level of distress. The presence of multiple other symptoms and problems besides pain therefore warrants serial assessment and monitoring of these symptoms or problems as part of the multidimensional assessment of both pain and other symptoms.

Clinical example

The interrelationships of pain, constipation, and its associated symptoms and problems represent a typical example from clinical practice, which highlights the need for evaluation of the patient's whole symptom profile (Fig. 5.3). Although there are usually multiple factors associated with constipation, asthenia with reduced physical activity, opioids, and hypercalcemia are among the most common causes. Constipation can produce nausea, which in turn can lead to decreased fluid intake, and consequently dehydration can occur. Dehydration can then contribute to or aggravate problems such as asthenia, opioid toxicity, and hypercalcemia. Similarly, constipation can produce abdominal pain or aggravate incident pain, in turn leading to a possible increase in opioid consumption, which perpetuates this cycle.

Constipation is a frequent, distressing, underestimated, yet highly treatable and preventable complication in advanced cancer patients (38). A plain abdominal radiograph, which allows for the assessment of stool in the colonic quadrants and the generation of a constipation score, has been suggested as a useful and reliable method for assessing this problem (39).

Optimal use of symptom assessment tools

The Memorial Symptom Assessment Scale (MSAS), the Symptom Distress Scale (SDS), and the Edmonton Symptom Assessment System (ESAS) are examples of instruments that have been developed to monitor multiple symptoms in the setting of advanced cancer. The MSAS is a validated, patient-rated instrument that assesses the frequency, intensity, and distress level associated with 32 physical and psychological symptoms. It contains specific subscales that capture physical, psychological, and global symptom distress (40). The SDS is a patient-rated instrument that assesses fre-

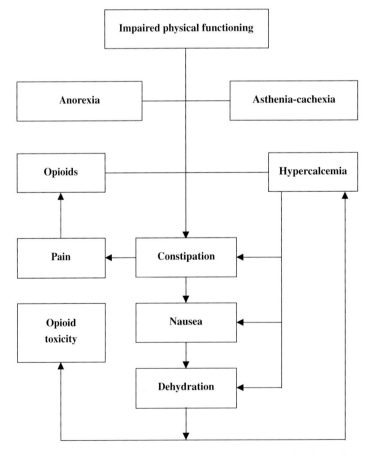

Fig. 5.3. Interrelationships of pain, constipation, and other symptoms in advanced cancer.

quency, intensity, and distress level of nine physical and two psychological symptoms (41).

The ESAS consists of a series of nine visual analog scales that evaluate a mix of psychological and physical symptoms, in addition to a global sense of well-being (Fig. 5.4A) (42,43). The visual analog scales are rated by patients who are cognitively intact, and the resulting scores are then transferred to a graphical representation in the patient's chart (Fig. 5.4B). In the case of patients with mild cognitive impairment, the ratings are conducted in association with family or staff. For patients with moderate or severe cognitive impairment, especially toward the last days of life (43,44), the family or staff provides the ratings. The graphical representations of the patient's ESAS symptom profile can visually portray dif-

ferent score patterns depending on the varying predominance of physical or psychosocial symptom complexes. Discordance can occur between pain intensity levels recorded on the ESAS and the patient's verbal pain descriptions, the patient's use of opioid, or other pain behaviors manifested by the patient. This discordance, which can be associated with apparent underreporting or overreporting of pain can be explored with the patient and family and thereby facilitate the identification of other dimensions associated with the pain experience, such as opioid phobia or somatization of psychological distress.

Although clear differences are likely to exist between patient and proxy raters of the ESAS (45), a recent study assessing the reliability of patient, nurse, and family

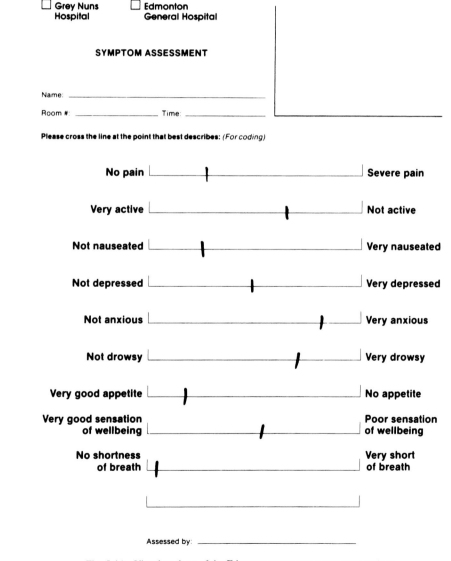

Fig. 5.4A. Visual analogs of the Edmonton symptom assessment system.

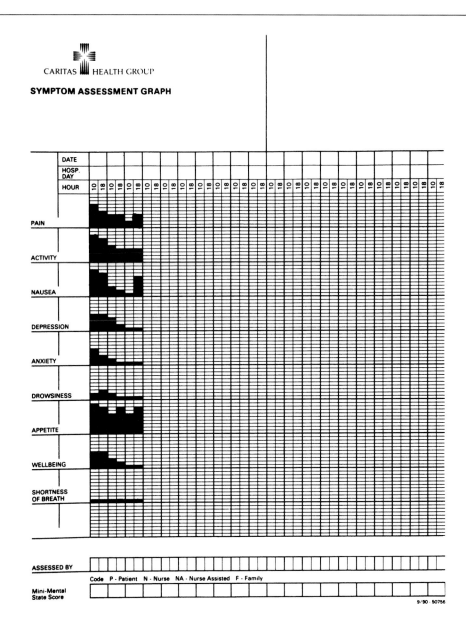

Fig. 5.4B. Graphical representation of the Edmonton Symptom Assessment System.

caregiver ESAS ratings suggested that an integrated approach incorporating proxy and patient ratings led to increased reliability (46). Although the patient's self-report has traditionally been regarded as the "gold standard," discordance arising between the patient and proxy ratings could potentially serve as a useful marker for further exploration of the meaning, for example, of unexpectedly high or low patient-reported pain scores.

A study examining the clinical utility of the ESAS showed that although 84% of patients were able to rate the ESAS items on admission to a palliative care unit, 83% of the assessments before death were rated by either a nurse or relative (42). In addition to having high levels of interrater reliability, the ESAS items (excluding activity level) show a high level of correlation with the Support Team Assessment Schedule, a validated, multidimensional clinician-assessment instrument (47). A recent validation study suggests that the ESAS has a satisfactory level of internal consistency, criterion validity, and concurrent validity (48). The ESAS has been widely used in palliative care research (49,50).

In a prospective study of delirium in patients with advanced cancer, patients who were able to rate their own ESAS scores had both higher pain scores and total ESAS scores during delirium than when delirium was absent (50). Here, the ESAS scoring appeared to capture the "crescendo pain" previously reported in association with the presence of delirium (33).

Prognostic factors for poor relief of cancer pain

Even when WHO guidelines are followed (1), 10%–20% of patients do not achieve satisfactory pain relief (6,7). Some authors have proposed descriptors in these instances such as "opioid-poorly-responsive pain" or "opioid-irrelevant pain" (51). Therefore, there is a need, both in clinical practice and in the standardized comparison of research findings, for a systematic approach to identifying and categorizing those factors associated with a poor prognosis.

Staging cancer pain: speaking a common language

The development of staging systems for the extent of cancer disease has helped to provide a basis for differential prognoses (52,53). It has also allowed a systematic and standardized approach in the comparison of research findings and, in turn, facilitated the development of evidence-based clinical management protocols. Using a somewhat analogous rationale, the Edmonton Staging System (ESS) for cancer pain has established different prognoses associated with the presence or absence of specific prognostic factors (54,55). In the most recent version, the new ESS, factors from various pain or patient attributes are associated with either a good (Stage 1) or poor (Stage 2) prognosis for achieving pain relief (Table 5.1) (55). The ESS acknowledges the multidimensional nature of pain in advanced cancer, and represents an attempt to establish a common language among researchers, both for study design and, in turn, for interpretation of research findings. As further developments emerge in our knowledge of these and possibly other prognostic variables, this system

Table 5.1. *Prognostic factors for analgesia as identified in the Edmonton Staging System*[55]

	Analgesic prognosis for specific factors	
Prognostic factor grouping	Good (Stage 1)	Poor (Stage 2)[a]
Pain mechanism	Visceral Bone or soft tissue	Neuropathic Mixed Unknown
Specific pain characteristics	Non-incidental	Incidental
Pharmacological tolerance	No evidence of tolerance	Evidence of tolerance
Psychological distress	Somatization absent	Somatization present
Chemical coping history (Drug or alcohol abuse)	Negative history	Positive history

[a] Presence of any one of these factors suggests a poorer prognosis for pain relief.

will need further modification and validation. These prognostic factors, along with other influences, are discussed in the following sections.

Pain mechanisms and specific characteristics

Various pain mechanisms and characteristics have been studied in relation to their associated prognosis for achievement of pain relief (Table 5.1) (54,55).

Neuropathic pain

Neuropathic pain is associated with neural dysfunction or pathological change in the peripheral or central nervous system. It is characterized by dysesthetic or lancinating components, and sometimes with the presence of hyperalgesia or allodynia. Studies have suggested that neuropathic pain is either not responsive to opioids (56), or more likely, less responsive to opioids (57–59). A recent survey in 593 cancer patients, however, could not demonstrate that the categorization of pain as neuropathic ($n = 32$), mixed ($n = 181$), or nociceptive ($n = 380$) predicted the outcome of pain treatment (60). In the ESS, the mixed pain mechanism category has been included as a poor prognostic indicator (Stage 2) for achieving analgesia. When the pain mechanism is still unknown after assessment with clinical history, physical examination, and imaging techniques, the unknown category applies, and this too results in a Stage 2 classification.

Incident pain

Incident pain results in a Stage 2 classification in the ESS. Incident pains are characterized by paroxysmal and transient pain exacerbations, typically but not exclusively related to movement (61). Other precipitants of incident pain include coughing, swallowing, urination, or defecation. Attempts to increase opioid doses to treat these incidental pain episodes can result in toxicity, such as undue sedation between episodes, when the pain is not present. Also, clinical experience suggests that some of these incident pains often subside themselves, either through cessation of movement or a decrease in other precipitating stimuli. This often occurs before an effective dose of opioid could be administered orally and absorbed, with the exception perhaps of oral transmucosal fentanyl (62).

Breakthrough pain

Incident pain is considered as one type of "breakthrough" pain, where a transitory flare of pain occurs against a tolerable background of pain (63). A recent survey of breakthrough pain characteristics suggested that breakthrough pain occurs in approximately 50% of cancer patients (the majority had metastatic disease), and although 61% of these patients could identify a precipitant, almost 50% reported that they were never able to predict its occurrence (64). The presence of breakthrough pain was associated with a higher intensity and greater frequency of background pain. The impact of breakthrough pain was reflected in a greater degree of pain-related functional impairment, worse mood, and greater anxiety levels in patients with breakthrough pain. Furthermore, multivariate analysis suggested that breakthrough pain was independently associated with impaired physical functioning and psychological distress. A recent international survey also identified breakthrough pain as an independent predictor of intense pain (9). However, this latter study also highlighted the large differences in the diagnosis of breakthrough pain across the world, perhaps indicating some ambiguity regarding definition.

Issues in the use of opioid and adjuvant analgesics

The salient pharmacotherapeutic issues that warrant consideration in multidimensional assessment are summarized in Table 5.2.

Myths and misconceptions

Misconceptions regarding opioid side effects, addiction, and other problems are held by some physicians and can be reflected both in failure to prescribe and inadequate dosing (65,66). Similar fears are held by some patients, who may underreport their pain because of fear of the associated implication of disease progression, or because of the desire to be a "good" patient and not complain (67,68). Clinical experience suggests that these factors can result in poor compliance with the opioid administra-

Table 5.2. *Pharmacotherapeutic issues requiring assessment in cancer pain*

Appropriate opioid dosing
Compliance
Choice of administrative route and opioid absorption
Opioid toxicity and metabolite accumulation
Opioid tolerance
Responsiveness to individual opioids
Opioid cross-tolerance
Dose calculation for opioid switches
Appropriate use of adjuvants

tion schedule, or the failure to use breakthrough doses of opioid. Ultimately, these patient and physician factors in combination can contribute to poor pain control (67).

Absorption and change of route

A change in the route of opioid administration is necessary in approximately 80% of patients before death (69). As the oral route is generally preferred, a change in route is usually made in response to concerns regarding absorption, as in the case of nausea, or because of dysphagia, delirium, or dyspnea. Miscalculation of opioid doses in the process of changing route of administration occasionally occurs, giving rise to incorrect dosing and consequently resulting in either inadequate pain control or opioid toxicity.

Opioid toxicity and metabolite accumulation

In the last decade, there has been increasing concern regarding the neurotoxic side effects of opioids (70–72). These side effects include delirium, myoclonus, hyperalgesia, allodynia, and seizures. Many of the reports concerning opioid neurotoxicity relate to patients on high-dose opioids (35,73,74). Often opioid neurotoxicity occurs in the presence of impaired renal function, in association with either high opioid doses (73,75) or standard opioid doses (76). Elevation of the morphine metabolites, morphine-3-glucuronide (M-3-G) and morphine-6-glucuronide (M-6-G) has been noted in association with renal impairment (76,77) and advancing age (78). M-6-G binds to opioid receptors and is recognized as a potent analgesic (79), whereas M-3-G has poor affinity for opioid receptors and is devoid of analgesic activity (80). Animal studies have demonstrated neuroexcitation and functional antagonism of morphine analgesia in association with M-3-G (81), and a neuroexcitatory state in association with hydromorphone-3-glucuronide (82) and normorphine (83), another morphine metabolite.

Agitation often occurs in association with opioid neurotoxicity (35,73,84). Recognition of this syndrome is essential to avoid further inappropriate escalation of opioid doses, with the consequent potential to aggravate the presentation. Dehydration often accompanies opioid toxicity, and accumulation of opioid metabolites in association with dehydration-induced hypovolemia has been postulated as the basis of some of this toxicity (20). Although the precise role of opioid metabolites in the generation of opioid toxicity remains to be established, assessment of symptoms and signs of both opioid toxicity and dehydration, often in addition to laboratory investigation of renal biochemistry, is an integral part of the multidimensional assessment of cancer pain.

Opioid tolerance and responsiveness to individual opioids

Opioid tolerance is one of the prognostic factors included in Stage 2 of the ESS (Table 5.1). Tolerance is defined as the decrease in a drug affect, such as analgesia or an adverse effect, as a result of exposure to the drug. Although tolerance could account for increasing opioid dose requirements (85), the occurrence of tolerance in humans is controversial (86) because disease progression could give rise to similar findings (87). In addition, potentially complex interplay can exist between various pharmacokinetic and pharmacodynamic factors (85).

Recent advances in molecular biology and receptor pharmacology have helped to elucidate some of the underlying mechanisms of opioid tolerance in animal or laboratory models. A shared mechanism for both the generation of opioid tolerance and hyperalgesia has been proposed, based on the central role of the N-methyl-D-aspartate (NMDA) receptor (88).

Targeting the NMDA receptor with NMDA antagonists raises the possibility of improving pain control. Methadone is a competitive antagonist of the NMDA receptor (89). This property has been postulated to explain its greater-than-expected potency in relation to morphine, when morphine has been used on a chronic basis before switching to methadone (90). Furthermore, some authors use it as a potential explanation for their clinical experience of obtaining superior results when methadone was used to treat neuropathic pain (91). Although there are no randomized trials demonstrating the special role of methadone in the case of tolerance or neuropathic pain, many case reports and retrospective surveys suggest such a role (92–101). A multidimensional assessment that identifies opioid tolerance and the nature of the pain syndrome, therefore, can assist in the process of opioid selection and help determine the appropriateness of a switch to methadone in these specific situations.

In estimating the level of tolerance, the ESS guidelines suggest calculating the percentage daily increase of oral equivalent morphine dose over a given time period (7 days was used in the study) (55). This is calculated as initial dose/(difference between final and initial daily dose) × 100/number of days of treatment. An increase of 5% or greater of the initial dose/day is considered to represent evidence of tolerance. Again, however, progressive dis-

ease or other factors, rather than tolerance, may drive dose escalation in the setting of cancer pain.

Switching opioids: dose calculation

The phenomenon of incomplete cross-tolerance is often apparent when switching or rotating opioids (85). Opioid rotation is used in the event of opioid toxicity, especially when accompanied by inadequate pain control. The rationale for opioid rotation is that the balance between analgesia and toxicity undergoes a favorable shift on the newly substituted opioid (102,103). This often occurs at a dose that is considerably less than that equianalgesic dose predicted by the standard reference tables, which were largely derived from single-dose studies (85). As part of a comprehensive assessment, the physician needs to assess the appropriateness of dose calculations used in any recent or proposed opioid switches. To account for incomplete cross-tolerance, clinical experience suggests that a dose reduction of 25%–50% be made in the equianalgesic dose derived from current tables (104,105). In the case of methadone, the ratio has been shown to vary in relation to the dose of the previous opioid (90,92,98,99), and the use of different dose ratios for different dose ranges of the previous opioid would appear to offer the safest approach.

Prior use and potential role of adjuvant analgesics

The use of adjuvant analgesics is of particular importance in neuropathic pain, where the response to opioid alone is likely to be less favorable than in the case of other pain syndromes. There is good evidence to support the efficacy of some adjuvants in the treatment of neuropathic pain, including antidepressants (106), anticonvulsants (107), and corticosteroids (108). Some of this evidence is derived from studies of chronic non-malignant pain. Similarly, pain resulting from metastatic bone disease can be effectively treated with bisphosphonates (109,110); in the case of clodronate, the subcutaneous route can be used for administration (111). A careful assessment should establish the levels of success, dosing, and side effects associated with previously tried adjuvants.

Assessing the prior use, role, and impact of other therapies

Although pain in patients with advanced cancer is most commonly due to the disease process, it must be remembered that pain has been attributed to antineoplastic treatment in 17%–35% of cases (9,112,113). This includes pain associated with chemotherapy, such as peripheral neuropathy (114,115), and postsurgical pains, such as postneck dissection or postmastectomy pain (116–118).

Palliative chemotherapy and radiation therapy

The potential therapeutic role of other therapies in palliation must always be borne in mind. Examples include palliative chemotherapy for small cell lung cancer (119,120) and other tumors, and palliative radiation therapy for most cancers, particularly painful bony metastases (121,122). There can be a time lag of many weeks for pain relief after completion of radiation treatment, but 50% of patients with bone metastases experience relief within 2 weeks (123). A radiation oncology referral should be considered to assess the feasibility of palliative radiation therapy. Within limits, retreatment of painful bony metastases can be undertaken if pain recurs after treatment (124). Assessments by other members of the multidisciplinary palliative care team, such as physiotherapy and occupational therapy, can also help to identify potential areas for their involvement in optimizing control of pain and other symptoms.

Complementary therapies

The increasing use of alternative or complementary medicine in palliative care warrants recognition. A recent systematic review of the use of complementary or alternative therapies in cancer patients yielded an average prevalence of 31.4% (125). Patients may not disclose this information to conventional practitioners in many cases, but express a lower level of satisfaction with conventional treatment (126). A recent study of alternative medicine use by women with early stage breast cancer, who had prior conventional treatment, suggested that use of alternative medicine could be a marker for greater psychosocial distress and worse quality of life (127). Communication regarding use of alternative or complementary therapies warrants inclusion in the patient's multidimensional assessment, not only from a drug safety perspective but also in relation to the patient's coping and quality of life.

Pain, physical function, and activity level

Physical activity is recognized as a common precipitant of pain in cancer patients (64,128). The presence of pain in turn tends to curtail physical activity. Studies examining the circadian use of breakthrough doses of opioid analgesics have found that in the absence of delirium, the highest numbers of breakthrough doses are used in the daytime, possibly associated with the time of highest physical activity (36,129).

The Brief Pain Inventory is an instrument designed to measure both the intensity of pain and the degree to which it interferes with patient functioning, including physical activity (130). Using this instrument, Serlin et al. (131) found a nonlinear correlation between pain severity and its interference with functioning, including physical activity. Although there was a difference between "mild" (0–4) and either "moderate" (5–6) or "severe" (7–10) pain, the nonlinear correlation was reflected by the lack of difference in the level of impairment in physical activity between moderate and severe pain levels. These findings were replicated in another study (132). The pain-related curtailment of physical activity may be further amplified by the fatigue and cachexia that accompany progression of the cancer. In combination, pain and other symptom severity, in addition to pre-existing impairment, contribute in varying degrees to the impairment in functional status in patients with progressive disease (133).

Assessment of physical function

In the assessment of physical function in cancer patients, the Karnofsky Performance Scale and the Eastern Cooperative Oncology Group scale have been used widely (134,135). In patients with advanced cancer in the palliative care setting, however, assessments with these instruments tend to generate clustering of scores at the extreme end of impairment. Consequently, newer instruments such as the Edmonton Functional Assessment Tool (EFAT) (136) and the Palliative Performance Scale (PPS) (137) have been developed. The EFAT includes domains such as pain, mental alertness, sensory function, communication, and respiratory function, in addition to domains that more directly reflect physical function, such as balance, mobility, wheelchair mobility, activity, activities of daily living, and dependence in performance status. An initial validation study demonstrated good reliability and validity for the EFAT (136). The PPS is essentially a modification of the Karnofsky Performance Scale and assesses ambulation, activity, self-care, intake, and conscious level (137). Although validation studies have not yet been published, the relative simplicity of administration of the PPS in the palliative care population is appealing.

An objective assessment of physical functioning constitutes an important part of the multidimensional assessment of pain in palliative care. Discrepancies between functional status performance and visual analog scores for pain warrant further exploration, as these might reflect somatization of distress in some patients. Impairment in physical functioning and distressing physical symptoms such as pain has the potential to adversely affect psychosocial function (15,64,138–140).

Pain and the multiple facets of psychosocial distress

Given the ever-increasing technological focus of the biomedical model of care, it is perhaps not surprising that medical staff often fail to recognize and address issues arising in the psychosocial and spiritual domains. Studies suggest that psychosocial (141) and spiritual distress (142) are underrecognized in oncology centers. In a multicenter study of advanced cancer patients, Kaasa et al. (143) found that 70% screened positive for psychological distress, which was associated with the presence of pain and impaired functional performance status. Portenoy et al. (140) found that 40%–80% of patients across a variety of cancers reported symptoms particularly suggestive of psychological distress, and greater symptom prevalence was associated with poorer Karnofsky Performance status. Cella et al. (144) examined associations between extent of disease, performance status, and psychological distress in patients with lung cancer. Both poorer performance status and more advanced disease were together associated with greater levels of psychological distress.

Other studies similarly have suggested a positive correlation between negative affect and various pain and general symptom factors including pain severity (145–147), pain duration (145), the presence of breakthrough pain (113), and overall symptom severity (148). A study of existential distress in cancer patients suggested an association between pain intensity and other factors including anxiety and fears concerning both the future in general and pain progression; fear of future pain was also associated with younger age and the duration of pain (149). Collectively, these data support the idea that in cancer patients, features such as the chronicity, severity, attributable psychosocial distress, impairment in physical function, and meaning of pain are particularly associated with impairment in quality of life (150).

Pain has been traditionally viewed from a dichotomous perspective as being either somatogenic or psychogenic. This view simply related pain intensity to the level of tissue damage, and in the absence of tissue damage, pain was deemed to be psychogenic in origin. However, incongruity between tissue damage and pain intensity level has been demonstrated in cancer patients, as in the case of asymptomatic bone metastases (151). Failure to explain the pain experience on the basis of tissue damage alone was first highlighted in the gate theory of pain (152), which advanced the idea that nociceptive input can be modulated. Brain areas involved in cognition or the regulation of mood can have an impact on this modulatory process (Fig. 5.1). Thus, the patient's subjective pain experience has multiple facets. The currently recommended assessment of a patient's report of pain therefore involves an integrated perspective that recognizes not only physical pathology and reported pain intensity but also the specific constitution of an individual patient's psychosocial and spiritual milieu (153,154).

In cancer patients, the interaction between physical symptom distress and distress in the psychosocial and spiritual domains is extremely complex, especially regarding the relative contributions of these two major sources of distress to each other and, in turn, to the negative impact on overall quality of life. Negative affect can occur as an enduring trait with or without clinical depression and as a transient or "state" form of mood disturbance. Negative affect is a frequent accompaniment of somatic distress such as pain (155,156). Various psychological models have been described to explain the relationship of negative affect and somatic symptoms (156). These include the psychosomatic model, which emphasizes the psychological origin of physical symptoms; a disability model proposing the reverse; and a symptom perception model, which emphasizes the importance of the cognitive appraisal of somatic symptoms in relation to level of negative affect. In the symptom perception model, features of negative affect, such as introspection and hypervigilance, are considered to contribute to an exaggerated cognitive appraisal of somatic sensations.

The level of reporting of somatic symptoms in cancer patients has been shown to have a highly positive association with negative affect and experienced social stigma (157), and a moderately negative association with social desirability (158). Fear of appearing weak might therefore contribute to the underreporting of pain in an attempt to maintain social desirability. Conversely, in some situations, displaying pain behavior can be used to engender a response from others or achieve gains in some other ways, a process referred to as secondary gain.

A constellation of concerns and emotions relating to issues in the existential, spiritual, and social domains has the potential to contribute to psychological distress (Table 5.3). These issues include the future, dying, finances, occupational matters, altered body image, the meaning of illness, illness as a punishment, retrospective life analysis, impaired physical function and associated loss of independence, provision of health care, guilt concerning the burden of care, anger concerning diagnosis, concern regarding the family, and family conflict (139,149,159–163). The relevance of distress arising in the psychosocial and spiritual domains to the pain presentation is discussed further, mainly in relation to the concepts of coping and suffering. Other maladaptive coping patterns and psychopathology are discussed separately.

The concepts of coping and suffering

The phenomenon of suffering, to a varying extent, can constitute part of both the "normal" burden and some of the psychopathological conditions arising toward the end of life, such as depression. Yet suffering differs from depression in that it represents a broader and more inclusive concept (164). Suffering is also distinct from pain (155,163), yet it is invariably closely related to it in the context of advanced disease. It has been described by Cassell as "an impending destruction of the person" or "a threat to personal integrity" (160,165), and by Chapman and Gavrin as "perceived damage to the integrity of the self" (164). Suffering has also been referred to as "total pain (166)" and "soul pain" (167). Despite these emotive terms and compelling definitions, suffering is often not recognized in advanced disease, "even when it stares physicians in the face" (165). Cassell proposed that, as physicians, our failure to recognize suffering relates to our preoccupation with objective findings and focusing our attention on the body without recognizing the personalized impact or meaning of pain and other symptoms for the person. Although cancer pain is a recognized source of suffering, it is rarely the sole cause. It is important to appreciate that suffering can arise in relation to any of the existential, spiritual, or social issues, as outlined in Table 5.3.

How does cancer pain result in suffering? An explanatory coping model, derived from a stress coping model (168,169) and adapted to the context of advanced cancer, is proposed in Fig. 5.5. This model outlines the processes of effective coping versus suffering in relation to pain, other symptoms, and the multiple other stressors captured under the heading of global distress. The model is based on the core features of primary appraisal, which results in perceived threat to self, and secondary appraisal, which refers to the perceived ability to cope with this threat in the light of available resources or strategies. Studies have suggested that the meaning of

Table 5.3. *Sources of distress in the patient's existential, spiritual, and social milieu*

Existential issues	Change in body image and function
	Dependency and loss of both autonomy and role
	Retrospective review of life losses
	Guilt: previous negligence, current care burden
	Fears: death and dying, future pain
	Anger: cancer diagnosis, treatment failures
	Concern for family or loved ones
Spiritual issues	Perception of illness as punishment
	Search for meaning
Social issues	Financial distress and insurance issues
	Occupational arrangements
	Conflict within the family
	Provision of care: fears, costs, conflict

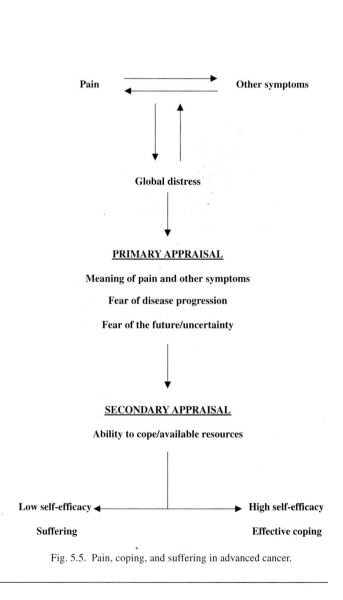

Fig. 5.5. Pain, coping, and suffering in advanced cancer.

cancer pain for the patient—for example, the threat of disease progression, the fear of disability, or the potential loss of social role—plays a major role in the genesis of psychological distress (139,170,171). Conversely, ascribing a transcendent or spiritual meaning to the threat associated with pain or any other source of distress, can facilitate coping and adaptation (160).

The concept of self-efficacy is also included in the model represented in Fig. 5.5. This concept is defined as the perceived sense of personal control or ability to enact coping strategies in the face of threat (172). The perception of low self-efficacy is associated with less effective coping (173), poorer pain control (174), and poorer quality of life (172,175). The patient with low self-efficacy, therefore, is more likely to become overwhelmed by a sense of vulnerability and suffering. Such patients are more likely to hold dysfunctional pain-related attitudes, such as catastrophizing, and also to underestimate the availability and value of their coping resources (163).

What impact does suffering have on the cancer pain presentation? A complex relationship can exist that involves existential concerns, the pain experience, and the pain expression. However, negative affect and anxiety often exist as common denominators in association with both pain and existential distress. Chapman and Gavrin (164) highlight the role of the stress response in the generation of suffering as a result of pain or any other stressors. They propose that neuroendocrine changes occurring in response to an acute stressor often confer adaptive advantage in the short term and help to maintain homeostasis; however, chronicity or persistence of the stressor can result in these neuroendocrine changes becoming maladaptive. An accompanying state of exhaustion, dysphoria, hypervigilance, and suffering can develop in the face of a chronic or persistent threat. Somatization, broadly defined as the somatic manifestation (such as pain) of psychological distress, could conceivably occur under these circumstances. This concept is discussed further in the section on other maladaptive coping patterns and psychopathology.

Assessment of psychosocial and spiritual distress

Recognition of suffering and other levels of psychosocial and spiritual distress in association with pain is essential to the conduct of good palliative care. This recognition helps to identify the need for cognitive behavioral and other psychotherapeutic interventions to address these components of the pain experience, which, in turn, complements the judicious use of opioids to alleviate the sen- sory or nociceptive component of pain. Hence, inadequate assessment and failure to recognize these psychosocial and spiritual dimensions can result in inappropriate opioid use and compound patient and family distress and staff frustration, especially when such a unidimensional management approach frequently results in opioid toxicity (35).

One of the difficulties in assessing the level of psychological distress in cancer patients is the degree of reluctance on the part of the patient to disclose information relating to distress in this domain (176). Failure to disclose this information can reflect failure on the part of the patient to appreciate the significance of such concerns, or it may reflect a repressive coping style (177). Alternatively, poor interviewing skills on the part of the health care professional can also inhibit disclosure of such information (178). Evidence suggests that interview skills that facilitate disclosure of information can be taught and learned (178,179).

The general interview approach involves an assessment of the patient's attitudes, beliefs, concerns, and behaviors. Given the intimacy of much of this information, an empathic approach is essential to establish a sense of rapport and trust (165). Patients and family are often interviewed together, but also separately to facilitate disclosure of their respective concerns. Visual analog scores on an instrument such as the ESAS—for example those for depression, anxiety, fatigue, and well-being— warrant clarification from the patient's perspective. Maguire et al. (178) demonstrated that patient disclosure of information pertaining to psychological distress was enhanced by the use of open directive questions that focused on psychological aspects, in addition to educated guesses and empathic statements, aiming to clarify and summarize the information from the patient's perspective. Meanwhile, the use of leading questions that focused on physical aspects and premature offering of advice and reassurance inhibited patient disclosure.

Various scales and questionnaires are available to screen for psychosocial and spiritual distress (180–182). Although these scales allow the researcher to systematically collect data, their actual role in the clinical practice of palliative care is less clear. One study found that a screening question "Are you depressed" had diagnostic potential similar to the use of a structured clinical interview for depression (183).

Time constraints, a lack of confidence in effectiveness, and some uncertainty regarding their role are major reasons given by physicians for their failure to more comprehensively address psychological and spiritual issues in cancer patients (142). The multidisciplinary team approach constitutes an important part of the management strategy in the palliative care model. In the assessment of psychosocial distress, utilization of skills and input from social workers, psychologists, pastoral care providers, physiotherapists, and occupational therapists is of vital importance and complements the contributions from the more traditional players such as nurses and physicians. Team conferencing allows the sharing of information across these disciplines and, in turn, facilitates a consistent team approach with the patient and family. Family conferences also allow further exploration of distressing psychosocial issues

Recognizing other maladaptive coping patterns and psychopathology

Psychiatric disorders occur in about 50% of cancer patients (21,184). In the Psychosocial Collaborative Oncology Group study, the 47% prevalence rate of psychiatric disorder included adjustment disorder in 68%, major affective disorder in 13%, organic mental disorder in 8%, personality disorder in 7%, and anxiety disorders in 4% (184). These percentages depend on the stage of disease; for example, delirium has a very high prevalence in the last days of life. The significance of these disorders relates to their associated distress, their impact on the pain presentation, and the potential to apply effective treatments in many cases. Maladaptive coping patterns, such as chemical coping and somatization of suffering, potentially increase the risk of opioid toxicity (35). The common psychiatric disorders, along with maladaptive coping patterns, are summarized in Table 5.4.

Somatization

It is important to distinguish between somatization in a general sense, as previously defined, and the definitive psychiatric condition, referred to as "somatization disorder" in the somatoform disorders section of DSM-IV

Table 5.4. *Psychopathological factors in advanced cancer*

Anxiety
Adjustment disorder
Somatization
Depression
Chemical-coping
Cognitive dysfunction and delirium
Personality disorder

(185). The somatoform disorders section also includes "pain disorder," which, like somatization disorder and the other somatoform disorders, has a restrictive set of criteria. Although the somatoform disorders, including pain disorder, occur in cancer patients, these rather specific disorders are likely to be far less common than somatization in the broader sense. In a large international primary care study, somatization disorder in the restrictive sense was generally an uncommon finding, whereas the less restrictively defined somatization process was more common (186). Somatization has been identified in the ESS as one of the poor prognostic indicators for achieving analgesia in the treatment of cancer pain (Table 5.1) (55).

The general process of somatization or the somatic manifestation of psychological distress occurs commonly across a variety of medical conditions (187) and cultures (188) and exhibits a wide spectrum of severity (189,190) ranging from a transient association with stressful life events to a severe persistent disorder. Despite the recognition of its generally high frequency (albeit at varying levels of severity) its protean manifestations (191), and its frequent association with depression (192,193), there is a dearth of data regarding the phenomenology of somatization, both in relation to pain and other somatic symptoms, in the advanced cancer population.

In cancer patients, studies suggest that somatization is associated with both depressive and anxiety disorder, in addition to a past history of atypical somatoform disorder (193,194). Given both the unique nature of the psychological distress and the concurrent presence of pain in the cancer population, caution must be exercised in attempting to extrapolate the findings of studies that examined characteristics of the somatization process in other populations to the cancer population.

Lipowski (190) suggested that there are three essential components to the somatization process. First, there is the experiential or perceptual component, which can refer to any distressing bodily sensation. Second, the cognitive component refers to the appraisal of the distressing perception and the attribution of meaning to it. Third, the behavioral manifestation includes communication of the patient's appraisal of the distressing perception in verbal and nonverbal modes, which, in the estimate of medical staff, is likely to be inconsistent with the degree of physical disease or dysfunction. When the somatization process involves pain, the patient might report a visual analog score of 9/10 for pain, yet the observed distress level or functional incapacity might appear to medical staff to be inconsistent with this. Hence the management approach in this situation would emphasize functional achievement, rather than the aggressive administration of opioids to treat pain that is largely opioid insensitive (35).

Ethnocultural influences on the pain experience are complex. Although studies have largely demonstrated consistency across cultures in the reporting of certain aspects of cancer pain (131,195), studies of somatization levels in different cultures suggest that differences exist (188,196,197). Cultural differences also exist regarding the degree of disclosure of the cancer diagnosis (198,199). A recent study from Taiwan suggested that nondisclosure of the cancer diagnosis was associated with higher levels of pain and pain interference and lower levels of satisfaction with the level of pain management provided by physicians (198). The authors suggested that lower levels of anxiety and distress in patients who are made aware of their diagnosis could account for the lower levels of pain and pain interference in this group.

In clinical practice of palliative care, patients with suspected somatization often present physicians with a dilemma. On one hand, the physician does not wish to precipitate opioid toxicity by inappropriately treating the somatization or opioid-insensitive pain component with opioids, but on the other hand, the physician does not wish to misdiagnose the nociceptive component of pain as somatization, inadvertently underprescribe opioids, and thereby expose the patient to unnecessary pain. Making an error in either direction can result in patient distress and have a negative effect on quality of life. To avoid making such errors in the resolution of this dilemma, a comprehensive and multidimensional assessment is essential. This assessment should place particular emphasis on the identification of psychosocial distress, particularly anxiety, suffering, depression, and also the recognition of a mismatch between reported pain intensity and impairment levels of physical and functional activity.

Chemical coping

A history of chemical coping, which refers to a history of drug or alcohol abuse, has been identified in the ESS as a prognostic indicator of poor pain control (Table 5.1) (55). The CAGE (cut down, annoy, guilt, eye-opener) (200) alcohol questionnaire is frequently used as a brief screening tool for the detection of alcohol abuse (Table 5.5). Bruera et al. (201) reported a positive CAGE score of 2/4 or more in 27 out of 100 (27%) cancer patients who were admitted to a palliative care unit. Patients with a positive CAGE Score had a higher mean morphine equivalent

Table 5.5. *Questions asked in the CAGE questionnaire*

- Have you ever felt you ought to *c*ut down on your drinking?
- Have people *a*nnoyed you by criticizing your drinking?
- Have you ever felt bad or *g*uilty about your drinking?
- Have you ever had a drink first thing in the morning to steady your nerves or get rid of a hangover (*e*ye-opener)?

daily dose of opioid, both on day 2 after admission and during their entire admission period. Physician's detection rate of alcohol abuse without conducting a screening test, such as the CAGE, varies from 25%–50%, depending on the physician's specialty. In a more recent retrospective study of 3380 cancer patients, we reported a positive CAGE score of 2 or more in 640 patients (18.9%) (202). Given the frequent occurrence of positive screening for alcohol abuse in the cancer population, and the associated difficulties in both achieving good pain control and dealing with the consequences of a maladaptive chemical coping style, the identification of patients with a history of alcohol abuse assumes great importance. Once identified, these patients can be monitored more carefully for their coping style and targeted for more intensive counseling. Furthermore, most psychiatric disorders are more common in patients with a history of alcohol abuse (203). The brevity and associated low burden of the CAGE make it a particularly useful instrument for use in the advanced cancer population.

Anxiety, adjustment disorder, and depression

In patients with advanced cancer, the distinction is often difficult to make between the "normal" psychological burden that exists in relation to physical and psychosocial distress and certain aspects of psychopathology such as anxiety, adjustment disorder, and depression. Hence varying degrees of anxiety, adjustment difficulty, and depressed mood can exist, which might not meet the psychiatric criteria for anxiety disorder, adjustment disorder, or major depression, respectively. Therefore, a wide spectrum of psychological distress can exist. Adjustment disorder is the most common psychiatric disorder occurring in cancer patients (184). Depressed mood or anxiety symptoms (not meeting the criteria for major depression or anxiety disorder) can occur in association with adjustment disorder (204).

The relationship of pain to major depression, anxiety, and adjustment disorder was largely addressed under the broad term psychological distress in this chapter's sections on suffering, coping, and somatization. Maladaptive coping is associated with later onset depression in cancer patients (171). The specific association of cancer pain with anxiety (149,205), depression (145,147), or a combination of both (206) is well recognized. There is some evidence to suggest that the presence of cancer pain is a risk factor for the development of depression (147). However, the temporal or causal relationship between pain and depression is complex, owing to the likelihood of a considerable degree of bi-directional impact. Given the potential for depression to respond to psychostimulants or other antidepressants, it is important that the physician search for and treat depression in the patient with cancer pain.

Personality disorder

Coping with the remarkable combination of physical and psychosocial stressors that accompany advanced cancer is invariably an enormous task for those who are psychologically well. Patients with a personality disorder are obviously less well equipped to address this task. Recognition or suspicion of personality disorder, especially the borderline type, is, therefore, important in the palliative management of these patients (207). The unique challenges in assessment and management often require specialist palliative and psychological or psychiatric consultation.

Personality disorders are broadly categorized into Clusters A, B, and C (208). Borderline personality disorder is included in Cluster B, and as its name suggests, is borderline between the psychotic-like group in Cluster A and the neurotic-like group in Cluster C. Borderline personality is characterized by a number of features: desperate efforts to avoid abandonment, manipulative and impulsive behavior, recurrent suicidal threats and behavior, a pattern of unstable interpersonal relationships, unstable self-image, intense mood swings, and difficulty controlling anger. A detailed account of its features is beyond the scope of this chapter. In the palliative care setting, when faced with terminal illness, borderline features may become more pronounced. From a pain assessment and management perspective, it is important to recognize the potential of these patients to split staff members, leading to disagreement over levels of pain control. There is a need for consistency in addressing this problem by possibly limiting the prescribing of analgesics to one physician (209).

Conclusion

The traditional unidimensional model of pain views the expression of pain, whether in the form of pain behaviors or patient ratings on a visual analog, as exclusively nociceptive or sensory in origin, and therefore responsive to opioid pharmacotherapy. This approach fails to appreciate the other dimensions of the pain experience: the impact of other symptoms, the positive and negative aspects of therapeutic interventions, and the input from the psychosocial milieu such as depression, somatization, and distress relating to financial, spiritual, and existential issues. This input is particularly important to recognize in the case of suffering or total pain, maladaptive coping, and other psychopathology. Hence, a multidimensional approach to pain assessment is essential to assess the interaction between pain and these factors.

Problems associated with a unidimensional approach include the potential for excessive reliance on pharmacological agents, especially opioids, and underutilization of non-pharmacological treatments. This in turn potentially increases the risk of opioid neurotoxicity and toxicities associated with other pharmacological agents. Recognition and relief of psychosocial and spiritual distress in the terminally ill patient are one of the fundamental tenets of the multidisciplinary palliative care model, whose ultimate objective is the relief of pain and global patient distress, thereby helping to provide an optimal quality of life. Future research studies should enable us to better characterize the phenomena of coping, suffering, somatization, and depression in the palliative care setting.

References

1. World Health Organization. Cancer pain relief and palliative care. Report of a WHO expert committee. World Health Organization Technical Report Series, 804. Geneva, World Health Organization, 1990:1–75.
2. Vainio A, Auvinen A. Prevalence of symptoms among patients with advanced cancer: an international collaborative study. Symptom Prevalence Group. J Pain Symptom Manage 12:3–10, 1996.
3. Grond S, Zech D, Diefenbach C, Bischoff A. Prevalence and pattern of symptoms in patients with cancer pain: a prospective evaluation of 1635 cancer patients referred to a pain clinic. J Pain Symptom Manage 9:372–82, 1994.
4. Donnelly S, Walsh D. The symptoms of advanced cancer. Semin Oncol 22:67–72, 1995.
5. Fainsinger R, Miller MJ, Bruera E, et al. Symptom control during the last week of life on a palliative care unit. J Palliat Care 7:5–11, 1991.
6. Zech DF, Grond S, Lynch J, et al. Validation of World Health Organization Guidelines for cancer pain relief: a 10-year prospective study. Pain 63:65–76, 1995.
7. Jadad AR, Browman GP. The WHO analgesic ladder for cancer pain management. Stepping up the quality of its evaluation. JAMA 274:1870–3, 1995.

8. Cleeland CS, Gonin R, Hatfield AK, et al. Pain and its treatment in outpatients with metastatic cancer. N Engl J Med 330:592–6, 1994.

9. Caraceni A, Portenoy RK. An international survey of cancer pain characteristics and syndromes. IASP Task Force on Cancer Pain. International Association for the Study of Pain. Pain 82:263–74, 1999.

10. Anderson KO, Mendoza TR, Valero V, et al. Minority cancer patients and their providers: pain management attitudes and practice. Cancer 88:1929–38, 2000.

11. Sloan PA, Donnelly MB, Schwartz RW, Sloan DA. Cancer pain assessment and management by housestaff. Pain 67:475–81, 1996.

12. Portenoy RK, Lesage P. Management of cancer pain. Lancet 353:1695–700, 1999.

13. Bruera E, Lawlor P. Cancer pain management. Acta Anaesthesiol Scand 41:146–53, 1997.

14. Melzack R, Casey KL. Sensory, motivational and central control determinants of pain: a new conceptual model. In: Kenshalo D, ed. The skin senses. Springfield, IL: Charles C Thomas, 1968:423–39.

15. Ahles TA, Blanchard EB, Ruckdeschel JC. The multidimensional nature of cancer-related pain. Pain 17:277–88, 1983.

16. Merskey H, Bogduk N. Classification of chronic pain. Seattle: IASP Press, 1994:210.

17. Price DD, Harkins SW, Baker C. Sensory-affective relationships among different types of clinical and experimental pain. Pain 28:297–307, 1987.

18. Jacox A, Carr DB, Payne R. Pharmacologic management. In: Clinical practice guidelines: management of cancer pain. Rockville, MD: U.S. Department of Health and Human Services, 1994:39–74.

19. Ingham J, Breitbart W. Epidemiology and clinical features of delirium. In: Portenoy RK, Bruera E, eds. Topics in palliative care, Vol 1. New York: Oxford University Press, 1997:7–19.

20. Lawlor PG, Gagnon B, Mancini IL, et al. Occurrence, causes, and outcome of delirium in advanced cancer patients: a prospective study. Arch Intern Med 160:786–94, 2000.

21. Minagawa H, Uchitomi Y, Yamawaki S, Ishitani K. Psychiatric morbidity in terminally ill cancer patients. A prospective study. Cancer 78:1131–7, 1996.

22. Massie MJ, Holland J, Glass E. Delirium in terminally ill cancer patients. Am J Psychiatry 140:1048–50, 1983.

23. American Psychiatric Association. Delirium, dementia and amnestic and other cognitive disorders. In: Diagnostic and Statistical Manual of Mental Disorders. Washington, DC: American Psychiatric Association, 1994:123–33.

24. Folstein MF, Folstein S, McHugh PR. "Mini-mental state:" a practical method for grading the cognitive state of patients for the clinician. J Psychiatr Res 12:189–98, 1975.

25. Crum R, Anthony JC, Bassett SS, Folstein MF. Population-based norms for the Mini-Mental State Examination by age and educational level. JAMA 269:2386–91, 1993.

26. Inouye SK. The dilemma of delirium: clinical and research controversies regarding diagnosis and evaluation of delirium in hospitalized elderly medical patients. Am J Med 97:278–88, 1994.

27. Armstrong SC, Cozza KL, Watanabe KS. The misdiagnosis of delirium. Psychosomatics 38:433–9, 1997.

28. Lipowski ZJ. Delirium in the elderly patient. N Engl J Med 320:578–82, 1989.

29. Pereira J, Hanson J, Bruera E. The frequency and clinical course of cognitive impairment in patients with terminal cancer. Cancer 79:835–42, 1997.

30. Lipowski ZJ. Transient cognitive disorders (delirium, acute confusional states) in the elderly. Am J Psychiatry 140:1426–36, 1983.

31. Ross CA, Peyser CE, Shapiro I, Folstein MF. Delirium: phenomenologic and etiologic subtypes. Int Psychogeriatr 3:135–47, 1991.

32. Lawlor P, Gagnon B, Mancini I, et al. Phenomenology of delirium and its subtypes in advanced cancer patients: a prospective study. Presented at the 12th International Congress on Care of The Terminally Ill. Montreal, September 13–17, 1998. J Palliat Care 14:106 (Abstract), 1998.

33. Coyle N, Breitbart W, Weaver S, Portenoy R. Delirium as a contributing factor to "crescendo" pain: three case reports. J Pain Symptom Manage 9:44–7, 1994.

34. Fainsinger RL, Tapper M, Bruera E. A perspective on the management of delirium in terminally ill patients on a palliative care unit. J Palliat Care 9:4–8, 1993.

35. Lawlor P, Walker P, Bruera E, Mitchell S. Severe opioid toxicity and somatization of psychosocial distress in a cancer patient with a background of chemical dependence. J Pain Symptom Manage 13:356–61, 1997.

36. Gagnon B, Lawlor PG, Mancini IL, et al. Delirium impacts on the circadian patterns of breakthrough analgesia in advanced cancer patients. Presented at the 35th Annual Meeting of the American Society of Clinical Oncology. Atlanta. May 12–14 1999. Abstract published in Proceedings of the 35th Annual Meeting of the American Society of Clinical Oncology, 1999.

37. Coyle N, Adelhardt J, Foley KM, Portenoy RK. Character of terminal illness in the advanced cancer patient: pain and other symptoms during the last four weeks of life. J Pain Symptom Manage 5:83–93, 1990.

38. Mancini I, Bruera E. Constipation in advanced cancer patients. Support Care Cancer 6:356–64, 1998.

39. Bruera E, Suarez-Almazor M, Velasco A, et al. The assessment of constipation in terminal cancer patients admitted to a palliative care unit: a retrospective review. J Pain Symptom Manage 9:515–19, 1994.

40. Portenoy RK, Thaler HT, Kornblith AB, et al. The Memorial Symptom Assessment Scale: an instrument for the evaluation of symptom prevalence, characteristics and distress. Eur J Cancer 30A:1326–36, 1994.

41. McCorkle R, Young K. Development of a symptom distress scale. Cancer Nurs 1:373–8, 1978.

42. Bruera E, Kuehn N, Miller MJ, et al. The Edmonton Symptom Assessment System (ESAS): a simple method for the assessment of palliative care patients. J Palliat Care 7:6–9, 1991.

43. Bruera E. Patient assessment in palliative cancer care. Cancer Treat Rev 22(Suppl A):3–12, 1996.

44. Rees E, Hardy J, Ling J, et al. The use of the Edmonton Symptom Assessment Scale (ESAS) within a palliative care unit in the UK. Palliat Med 12:75–82, 1998.

45. Nekolaichuk CL, Bruera E, Spachynski K, et al. A comparison of patient and proxy symptom assessments in advanced cancer patients. Palliat Med 13:311–23, 1999.

46. Nekolaichuk CL, Maguire TO, Suarez-Almazor M, et al. Assessing the reliability of patient, nurse, and family caregiver symptom ratings in hospitalized advanced cancer patients. J Clin Oncol 17:3621–30, 1999.

47. Bruera E, Macdonald S. Audit methods: The Edmonton Symptom Assessment System. In: Higginson I, ed. Clinical audit in palliative care. Oxford, Radcliffe Medical Press, 1993:61–77.

48. Chang VT, Hwang SS, Feuerman M. Validation of the Edmonton Symptom Assessment Scale. Cancer 88:2164–71, 2000.

49. Chochinov HM, Tataryn D, Clinch JJ, Dudgeon D. Will to live in the terminally ill. Lancet 354:816–19, 1999.

50. Gagnon B, Lawlor PG, Mancini I, et al. The impact of delirium on the expression of pain and other symptoms in advanced cancer patients. Presented at the 9th World Congress of the International Association for The Study of Pain. Vienna, August 22–27, 1999. Abstract published in Proceedings of the 9th World Congress of the International Association for The Study of Pain, 1999.

51. Hanks GW, Forbes K. Opioid responsiveness. Acta Anaesthesiol Scand 41:154–8, 1997.

52. American Joint Committee for Cancer Staging and End Result Reporting. Manual for staging of cancer. Chicago: American Joint Committee, 1977.

53. Paterson AHG. Clinical staging and its prognostic significance. In: Stall B, ed. Pointers to cancer prognosis. Dordecht: Martinus Nijhoff, 1988:37–48.

54. Bruera E, Macmillan K, Hanson J, MacDonald RN. The Edmonton staging system for cancer pain: preliminary report. Pain 37:203–9, 1989.

55. Bruera E, Schoeller T, Wenk R, et al. A prospective multi-center assessment of the Edmonton staging system for cancer pain. J Pain Symptom Manage 10:348–55, 1995.

56. Arner S, Meyerson BA. Lack of analgesic effect of opioids on neuropathic and idiopathic forms of pain. Pain 33:11–23, 1988.

57. Portenoy RK, Foley KM, Inturrisi CE. The nature of opioid responsiveness and its implications for neuropathic pain: new hypotheses derived from studies of opioid infusions. Pain 43:273–86, 1990.

58. Cherny NI, Thaler HT, Friedlander-Klar H, et al. Opioid responsiveness of cancer pain syndromes caused by neuropathic or nociceptive mechanisms: a combined analysis of controlled, single-dose studies. Neurology 44:857–61, 1994.

59. Jadad AR, Carroll D, Glynn CJ, et al. Morphine responsiveness of chronic pain: double-blind randomised crossover study with patient-controlled analgesia. Lancet 339:1367–71, 1992.

60. Grond S, Radbruch L, Meuser T, et al. Assessment and treatment of neuropathic cancer pain following WHO guidelines. Pain 79:15–20, 1999.

61. McQuay HJ, Jadad AR. Incident pain. Cancer Surveys 21:17–24, 1994.

62. Portenoy RK, Payne R, Coluzzi P, et al. Oral transmucosal fentanyl citrate (OTFC) for the treatment of breakthrough pain in cancer patients: a controlled dose titration study. Pain 79:303–12, 1999.

63. Portenoy RK, Hagen NA. Breakthrough pain: definition, prevalence and characteristics. Pain 41:273–81, 1990.

64. Portenoy RK, Payne D, Jacobsen P. Breakthrough pain: characteristics and impact in patients with cancer pain. Pain 81:129–34, 1999.

65. Larue F, Colleau SM, Fontaine A, Brasseur L. Oncologists and primary care physicians' attitudes toward pain control and morphine prescribing in France. Cancer 76:2375–82, 1995.

66. Warncke T, Breivik H, Vainio A. Treatment of cancer pain in Norway. A questionnaire study. Pain 57:109–16, 1994.

67. Grossman SA. Undertreatment of cancer pain: barriers and remedies. Support Care Cancer 1:74–8, 1993.

68. Ward SE, Goldberg N, Miller-McCauley V, et al. Patient-related barriers to management of cancer pain. Pain 52:319–24, 1993.

69. Cherny NJ, Chang V, Frager G, et al. Opioid pharmacotherapy in the management of cancer pain: a survey of strategies used by pain physicians for the selection of analgesic drugs and routes of administration. Cancer 76:1283–93, 1995.

70. Olsen AK, Sjogren P. Neurotoxic effects of opioids. Eur J Palliat Care 3(4):139–42, 1996.

71. Lawlor PG, Bruera E. Side-effects of opioids in chronic pain treatment. Curr Opin Anaesthesiol 11:539–45, 1998.

72. Daeninck PJ, Bruera E. Opioid use in cancer pain. Is a more liberal approach enhancing toxicity? Acta Anaesthesiol Scand 43:924–38, 1999.

73. Hagen N, Swanson R. Strychnine-like multifocal myoclonus and seizures in extremely high-dose opioid administration: treatment strategies. J Pain Symptom Manage 14:51–8, 1997.

74. Sjogren P, Jonsson T, Jensen NH, et al. Hyperalgesia and myoclonus in terminal cancer patients treated with continuous intravenous morphine. Pain 55:93–7, 1993.

75. Sjogren P, Dragsted L, Christensen CB. Myoclonic spasms during treatment with high doses of intravenous morphine in renal failure. Acta Anaesthesiol Scand 37:780–2, 1993.

76. Ashby M, Fleming B, Wood M, Somogyi A. Plasma morphine and glucuronide (M3G and M6G) concentrations in hospice inpatients. J Pain Symptom Manage 14:157–67, 1997.

77. Faura CC, Collins SL, Moore RA, McQuay HJ. Systematic review of factors affecting the ratios of morphine and its major metabolites. Pain 74:43–53, 1998.

78. McQuay HJ, Carroll D, Faura CC, et al. Oral morphine in cancer pain: influences on morphine and metabolite concentration. Clin Pharmacol Ther 48:236–44, 1990.

79. Osborne R, Thompson P, Joel S, et al. The analgesic activity of morphine-6-glucuronide. Br J Clin Pharmacol 34:130–8, 1992.

80. Gong QL, Hedner J, Bjorkman R, Hedner T. Morphine-3-glucuronide may functionally antagonize morphine-6-glucuronide induced antinociception and ventilatory depression in the rat. Pain 48:249–55, 1992.

81. Smith MT, Watt JA, Cramond T. Morphine-3-glucuronide—a potent antagonist of morphine analgesia. Life Sci 47:579–85, 1990.

82. Wright AW, Nocente ML, Smith MT. Hydromorphone-3-glucuronide: biochemical synthesis and preliminary pharmacological evaluation. Life Sci 63:401–11, 1998.

83. Smith GD, Smith MT. The excitatory behavioral and antianalgesic pharmacology of normorphine-3-glucuronide after intracerebroventricular administration to rats. J Pharmacol Exp Ther 285:1157–62, 1998.

84. MacDonald N, Der L, Allan S, Champion P. Opioid hyperexcitability: the application of alternate opioid therapy. Pain 53:353–5, 1993.

85. Lawlor P, Pereira J, Bruera E. Dose ratios among different opioids: update on the use of the equianalgesic table. In: Portenoy RK, Bruera E, eds. Topics in palliative care, Vol. 5. New York: Oxford University Press, 2001:247–76.

86. Colpaert FC. Drug discrimination: no evidence for tolerance to opiates. Pharmacol Rev 47:605–29, 1995.

87. Portenoy RK. Tolerance to opioid analgesics: clinical aspects. Cancer Surv 21:49–65, 1994.

88. Mao J, Price DD, Mayer DJ. Mechanisms of hyperalgesia and morphine tolerance: a current view of their possible interactions. Pain 62:259–74, 1995.

89. Ebert B, Andersen S, Krogsgaard-Larsen P, et al. Ketobemidone, methadone and pethidine are non-competitive N-methyl-D-aspartate (NMDA) antagonists in the rat cortex and spinal cord. Neurosci Lett 187:165–8, 1995.

90. Lawlor PG, Turner KS, Hanson J, Bruera ED. Dose ratio between morphine and methadone in patients with cancer pain: a retrospective study. Cancer 82:1167–73, 1998.

91. Makin MK, Ellershaw JE. Substitution of another opioid for morphine. Methadone can be used to manage neuropathic pain related to cancer. BMJ 317:81, 1998.

92. Bruera E, Pereira J, Watanabe S, et al. Opioid rotation in patients with cancer pain. A retrospective comparison of dose ratios between methadone, hydromorphone, and morphine. Cancer 78:852–7, 1996.

93. Crews JC, Sweeney NJ, Denson DD. Clinical efficacy of methadone in patients refractory to other mu-opioid receptor agonist analgesics for management of terminal cancer pain. Case presentations and discussion of incomplete cross-tolerance among opioid agonist analgesics. Cancer 72:2266–72, 1993.

94. Fainsinger RL, Louie K, Belzile M, et al. Decreased opioid doses used on a palliative care unit. J Palliat Care 12:6–9, 1996.

95. Lawlor P, Turner K, Hanson J, Bruera E. Dose ratio between morphine and hydromorphone in patients with cancer pain: a retrospective study. Pain 72:79–85, 1997.

96. Manfredi PL, Borsook D, Chandler SW, Payne R. Intravenous methadone for cancer pain unrelieved by morphine and hydromorphone: clinical observations. Pain 70:99–101, 1997.

97. Morley JS, Makin MK. The use of methadone in cancer pain poorly responsive to other opioids. Pain Rev 5:51–8, 1998.

98. Ripamonti C, De Conno F, Groff L, et al. Equianalgesic dose/ratio between methadone and other opioid agonists in cancer pain: comparison of two clinical experiences. Ann Oncol 9:79–83, 1998.

99. Ripamonti C, Groff L, Brunelli C, et al. Switching from morphine to oral methadone in treating cancer pain: what is the equianalgesic dose ratio? J Clin Oncol 16:3216–21, 1998.

100. Thomas Z, Bruera E. Use of methadone in a highly tolerant patient receiving parenteral hydromorphone. J Pain Symptom Manage 10:315–17, 1995.

101. Williams PI, Sarginson RE, Ratcliffe JM. Use of methadone in the morphine-tolerant burned paediatric patient. Br J Anaesth 80:92–5, 1998.

102. De Stoutz ND, Bruera E, Suarez-Almazor M. Opioid rotation for toxicity reduction in terminal cancer patients. J Pain Symptom Manage 10:378–84, 1995.

103. Mercadante S. Opioid rotation for cancer pain, rationale and clinical aspects. Cancer 86:1856–66, 1999.

104. Cherny NI, Foley KM. Nonopioid and opioid analgesic pharmacotherapy of cancer pain. Hematol Oncol Clin North Am 10:79–102, 1996.

105. Derby S, Chin J, Portenoy RK. Systemic opioid therapy for chronic cancer pain. Practical guidelines for converting drugs and routes of administration. CNS Drugs 9:99–109, 1998.

106. McQuay HJ, Tramer M, Nye BA, et al. A systematic review of antidepressants in neuropathic pain. Pain 68:217–27, 1996.

107. McQuay H, Carroll D, Jadad AR, et al. Anticonvulsant drugs for management of pain: a systematic review. BMJ 311:1047–52, 1995.

108. Kingery WS. A critical review of controlled clinical trials for peripheral neuropathic pain and complex regional pain syndromes. Pain 73:123–39, 1997.

109. Koeberle D, Bacchus L, Thuerlimann B, Senn HJ. Pamidronate treatment in patients with malignant osteolytic bone disease and pain: a prospective randomized double-blind trial. Support Care Cancer 7:21–7, 1999.

110. Ernst DS, MacDonald RN, Paterson AH, et al. A double-blind, crossover trial of intravenous clodronate in metastatic bone pain. J Pain Symptom Manage 7:4–11, 1992.

111. Walker P, Watanabe S, Lawlor P, Bruera E. Subcutaneous clodronate. Lancet 348:345–6, 1996.

112. Grond S, Zech D, Diefenbach C, et al. Assessment of cancer pain: a prospective evaluation in 2266 cancer patients referred to a pain service. Pain 64:107–14, 1996.

113. Portenoy RK, Payne D, Jacobsen P. Breakthrough pain: characteristics and impact in patients with cancer pain. Pain 81:129–34, 1999.

114. Amato AA, Collins MP. Neuropathies associated with malignancy. Semin Neurol 18:125–44, 1998.

115. Pace A, Bove L, Nistico C, et al. Vinorelbine neurotoxicity: clinical and neurophysiological findings in 23 patients. J Neurol Neurosurg Psychiatry 61:409–11, 1996.

116. Foley KM. Pain assessment and cancer pain syndromes. In: Doyle D, Hanks GWC, Macdonald N, eds. Oxford textbook of palliative medicine. Oxford: Oxford University Press, 1995:148–65.

117. Vecht CJ. Arm pain in the patient with breast cancer. J Pain Symptom Manage 5:109–17, 1990.

118. Vecht CJ, Hoff AM, Kansen PJ, et al. Types and causes of pain in cancer of the head and neck. Cancer 70:178–84, 1992.

119. Ihde DC. Chemotherapy of lung cancer. N Engl J Med 327:1434–41, 1992.

120. Carney DN, Grogan L, Smit EF, et al. Single-agent oral etoposide for elderly small cell lung cancer patients. Semin Oncol 17:49–53, 1990.

121. Arcangeli G, Giovinazzo G, Saracino B, et al. Radiation therapy in the management of symptomatic bone metastases: the effect of total dose and histology on pain relief and response duration. Int J Radiat Oncol Biol Phy 42:1119–26, 1998.

122. Hoskin PJ. Radiotherapy for bone pain. Pain 63:137–9, 1995.

123. Price P, Hoskin PJ, Easton D, et al. Prospective randomised trial of single and multifraction radiotherapy schedules in the treatment of painful bony metastases. Radiother Oncol 6:247–55, 1986.

124. Mithal NP, Needham PR, Hoskin PJ. Retreatment with radiotherapy for painful bone metastases. Int J Radiat Oncol Biol Phy 29:1011–14, 1994.

125. Ernst E, Cassileth BR. The prevalence of complementary/alternative medicine in cancer: a systematic review. Cancer 83:777–82, 1998.

126. Begbie SD, Kerestes ZL, Bell DR. Patterns of alternative medicine use by cancer patients. Med J Aust 165:545–8, 1996.

127. Burstein HJ, Gelber S, Guadagnoli E, Weeks JC. Use of alternative medicine by women with early-stage breast cancer. N Engl J Med 340:1733–9, 1999.

128. McQuay HJ, Jadad AR. Incident pain. Cancer Sur 21:17–24, 1994.

129. Bruera E, Macmillan K, Kuehn N, Miller MJ. Circadian distribution of extra doses of narcotic analgesics in patients with cancer pain: a preliminary report. Pain 49:311–314, 1992.

130. Cleeland CS. Measurement of pain by subjective report. In: Advances in pain research and therapy, Vol. 12, Issues in pain measurement. New York: Raven Press, 1989:391–403.

131. Serlin RC, Mendoza TR, Nakamura Y, et al. When is cancer pain mild, moderate or severe? Grading pain severity by its interference with function. Pain 61:277–84, 1995.

132. Wang XS, Cleeland CS, Mendoza TR, et al. The effects of pain severity on health-related quality of life: a study of Chinese cancer patients. Cancer 86:1848–55, 1999.

133. Kurtz ME, Kurtz JC, Stommel M, et al. Predictors of physical functioning among geriatric patients with small cell or non-small cell lung cancer 3 months after diagnosis. Support Care Cancer 7:328–31, 1999.

134. Yates JW, Chalmer B, McKegney FP. Evaluation of patients with advanced cancer using the Karnofsky Performance Status. Cancer 45:2220–4, 1980.

135. Osoba D, MacDonald N. Principles governing the use of cancer chemotherapy in palliative care. In: Doyle D, Hanks GWC, MacDonald N, eds. Oxford textbook of palliative medicine. Oxford: Oxford University Press, 1998:249–67.

136. Kaasa T, Loomis J, Gillis K, et al. The Edmonton Functional Assessment Tool: preliminary development and evaluation for use in palliative care. J Pain Symptom Manage 13:10–19, 1997.

137. Anderson F, Downing GM, Hill J, et al. Palliative performance scale (PPS): a new tool. J Palliat Care 12:5–11, 1996.

138. Ingham J, Portenoy RK. The measurement of pain and other symptoms. In: Doyle D, Hanks GWC, MacDonald N, eds. Oxford textbook of palliative medicine. Oxford: Oxford University Press, 1998:203–19.

139. Heaven CM, Maguire P. The relationship between patients' concerns and psychological distress in a hospice setting. Psychooncology 7:502–7, 1998.

140. Portenoy RK, Thaler HT, Kornblith AB, et al. Symptom prevalence, characteristics and distress in a cancer population. Qual Life Res 3:183–9, 1994.

141. Bredart A, Didier F, Robertson C, et al. Psychological distress in cancer patients attending the European Institute of Oncology in Milan. Oncology 57:297–302, 1999.

142. Kristeller JL, Zumbrun CS, Schilling RF. 'I would if I could': how oncologists and oncology nurses address spiritual distress in cancer patients. Psychooncology 8:451–8, 1999.

143. Kaasa S, Malt U, Hagen S, et al. Psychological distress in cancer patients with advanced disease. Radiother Oncol 27:193–7, 1993.

144. Cella DF, Orofiamma B, Holland JC, et al. The relationship of psychological distress, extent of disease, and performance status in patients with lung cancer. Cancer 60:1661–7, 1987.

145. Glover J, Dibble SL, Dodd MJ, Miaskowski C. Mood states of oncology outpatients: does pain make a difference? J Pain Symptom Manage 10:120–8, 1995.

146. Shacham S, Reinhardt LC, Raubertas RF, Cleeland CS. Emotional states and pain: intraindividual and interindividual measures of association. J Behav Med 6:405–19, 1983.

147. Spiegel D, Sands S, Koopman C. Pain and depression in patients with cancer. Cancer 74:2570–8, 1994.

148. Kurtz ME, Kurtz JC, Stommel M, et al. The influence of symptoms, age, comorbidity and cancer site on physical functioning and mental health of geriatric women patients. Women Health 29:1–12, 1999.

149. Strang P. Existential consequences of unrelieved cancer pain. Palliat Med 11:299–305, 1997.

150. Portenoy RK. Pain and quality of life: clinical issues and implications for research. Oncology 4:172–8, 1990.

151. Front D, Schneck SO, Frankel A, Robinson E. Bone metastases and bone pain in breast cancer. Are they closely associated? JAMA 242:1747–8, 1979.

152. Melzack R, Wall P. Pain mechanisms: a theory. Science 150:971–9, 1965.

153. Turk DC, Okifuji A. Assessment of patients' reporting of pain: an integrated perspective. Lancet 353:1784–8, 1999.

154. Tope DM, Ahles TA, Silberfarb PM. Psycho-oncology: psychological well-being as one component of quality of life. Psychother Psychosom 60:129–47, 1993.

155. Chapman CR, Gavrin J. Suffering and its relationship to pain. J Palliat Care 9:5–13, 1993.

156. Watson D, Pennebaker JW. Health complaints, stress, and distress: exploring the central role of negative affectivity. Psychol Rev 96:234–54, 1989.

157. Koller M, Kussman J, Lorenz W, et al. Symptom reporting in cancer patients: the role of negative affect and experienced social stigma. Cancer 77:983–95, 1996.

158. Koller M, Heitmann K, Kussmann J, Lorenz W. Symptom reporting in cancer patients II: relations to social desirability, negative affect, and self-reported health behaviors. Cancer 86:1609–20, 1999.

159. Chaturvedi SK. Exploration of concerns and role of psychosocial intervention in palliative care—a study from India. Ann Acad Med Singapore 23:256–60, 1994.

160. Cassell EJ. The nature of suffering and the goals of medicine. N Engl J Med 306:639–45, 1982.

161. Dalton JA, Feuerstein M. Biobehavioral factors in cancer pain. Pain 33:137–47, 1988.

162. Cherny NI, Coyle N, Foley KM. Suffering in the advanced cancer patient: a definition and taxonomy. J Palliat Care 10:57–70, 1994.

163. Fishman B. The treatment of suffering in patients with cancer pain. Cognitive-behavioral approaches. In: Foley KM, Bonica JJ, Ventafridda V, eds. Adv Pain Res Ther, vol. 16. New York: Raven Press, 1990:301–16.

164. Chapman CR, Gavrin J. Suffering: the contributions of persistent pain. Lancet 353:2233–7, 1999.

165. Cassell EJ. Diagnosing suffering: a perspective. Ann Intern Med 131:531–4, 1999.

166. Saunders C. The philosophy of terminal care. In: Saunders C, ed. The management of terminal malignant disease. Baltimore: Arnold, 1984:232–41.

167. Kearney M. Mortally wounded. Stories of soul pain, death, and healing. New York: Scribner, 1996.

168. Folkman S, Lazarus RS, Dunkel-Schetter C, et al. Dynamics of a stressful encounter: cognitive appraisal, coping, and encounter outcomes. J Pers Soc Psychol 50:992–1003, 1986.

169. Lazarus RS. Coping with the stress of illness. WHO Regional Publications European Series 44:11–31, 1992.

170. Barkwell DP. Ascribed meaning: a critical factor in coping and pain attenuation in patients with cancer-related pain. J Palliat Care 7:5–14, 1991.

171. Parle M, Jones B, Maguire P. Maladaptive coping and affective disorders among cancer patients. Psychol Med 26:735–44, 1996.

172. Bandura A: Self-efficacy: toward a unifying theory of behavioral change. Psychol Rev 84:191–215, 1977.

173. Lin CC. Comparison of the effects of perceived self-efficacy on coping with chronic cancer pain and coping with chronic low back pain. Clin J Pain 14:303–10, 1998.

174. Syrjala KL, Chapko ME. Evidence for a biopsychosocial model of cancer treatment-related pain. Pain 61:69–79, 1995.

175. Cunningham AJ, Lockwood GA, Cunningham JA. A relationship between perceived self-efficacy and quality of life in cancer patients. Patient Educ Counsel 17:71–8, 1991.

176. Maguire P. Barriers to psychological care of the dying. Br Med J Clin Res Educ 291:1711–13, 1985.

177. Myers LB. Repressors' responses to health-related questionnaires. Br J Health Psychol 2:245–57, 1900.

178. Maguire P, Faulkner A, Booth K, et al. Helping cancer patients disclose their concerns. Eur J Cancer 32A:78–81, 1996.

179. Platt FW, Keller VF. Empathic communication:a teachable and learnable skill. J Gen Intern Med 9:222–6, 1994.

180. Beck A, Ward C, Mendelson M, et al. An inventory for measuring depression. Arch Gen Psychiatry 4:561–71, 1961.

181. Holland JC, Kash KM, Passik S, et al. A brief spiritual beliefs inventory for use in quality of life research in life-threatening illness. Psychooncology 7:460–9, 1998.

182. Zigmond AS, Snaith PR. The hospital anxiety and depression scale. Acta Psychiatr Scand 67:360–70, 1983.

183. Chochinov HM, Wilson KG, Enns M, Lander S. "Are you depressed?" Screening for depression in the terminally ill. Am J Psychiatry 154:674–6, 1997.

184. Derogatis LR, Morrow GR, Fetting J, et al. The prevalence of psychiatric disorders among cancer patients. JAMA 249:751–7, 1983.

185. American Psychiatric Association. Somatoform disorder. In: Diagnostic and statistical manual of mental disorders. Washington, DC: American Psychiatric Association, 1994:445–65.

186. Gureje O, Simon GE, Ustun TB, Goldberg DP. Somatization in cross-cultural perspective: a World Health Organization study in primary care. Am J Psychiatry 154:989–95, 1997.

187. Guthrie E. Emotional disorder in chronic illness: psychotherapeutic interventions. Br J Psychiatry 168:265–73, 1996.

188. Kirmayer LJ, Young A. Culture and somatization: clinical, epidemiological, and ethnographic perspectives. Psychosom Med 60:420–30, 1998.

189. Katon W, Lin E, Von Korff M, et al. Somatization: a spectrum of severity. Am J Psychiatry 148:34–40, 1991.

190. Lipowski ZJ. Somatization: a borderland between medicine and psychiatry. Canadian Medical Association Journal 135:609–14, 1986.

191. Lipowski ZJ. Somatization: the concept and its clinical application. Am J Psychiatry 145:1358–68, 1988.

192. Simon GE, VonKorff M, Piccinelli M, et al. An international study of the relation between somatic symptoms and depression. N Engl J Med 341:1329–35, 1999.

193. Chaturvedi SK, Maguire GP. Persistent somatization in cancer:a controlled follow-up study. J Psychosom Res 45:249–56, 1998.

194. Chaturvedi SK, Hopwood P, Maguire P. Non-organic somatic symptoms in cancer. Eur J Cancer 29A:1006–8, 1993.

195. Cleeland CS, Nakamura Y, Mendoza TR, et al. Dimensions of the impact of cancer pain in a four country sample: new information from multidimensional scaling. Pain 67:267–73, 1996.

196. Erbil P, Razavi D, Farvacques C, et al. Cancer patients psychological adjustment and perception of illness: cultural differences between Belgium and Turkey. Support Care Cancer 4:455–61, 1996.

197. Farooq S, Gahir MS, Okyere E, et al. Somatization: a transcultural study. J Psychosom Res 39:883–8, 1995.

198. Lin CC. Disclosure of the cancer diagnosis as it relates to the quality of pain management among patients with cancer pain in Taiwan. J Pain Symptom Manage 18:331–7, 1999.

199. Hamadeh GN, Adib SM. Cancer truth disclosure by Lebanese doctors. Soc Sci Med 47:1289–94, 1998.

200. Ewing JA. Detecting alcoholism. The CAGE questionnaire. JAMA 252:1905–7, 1984.

201. Bruera E, Moyano J, Seifert L, et al. The frequency of alcoholism among patients with pain due to terminal cancer. J Pain Symptom Manage 10:599–603, 1995.

202. Lawlor PG, Quan H, Hanson J, Bruera E. Screening for alcohol abuse in an advanced cancer population. Presented at the 12th MASCC International Symposium. Washington DC. March 23–25, 2000 (abstract). Support Care Cancer 8:253, 2000.

203. Helzer JE, Pryzbeck TR. The co-occurrence of alcoholism with other psychiatric disorders in the general population and its impact on treatment. J Stud Alcohol 49:219–24, 1988.

204. American Psychiatric Association: Adjustment disorders. In: Diagnostic and statistical manual of mental disorders. Washington, DC: American Psychiatric Association, 1994:623–7.

205. Velikova G, Selby PJ, Snaith PR, Kirby PG. The relationship of cancer pain to anxiety. Psychother Psychosom 63:181–4, 1995.

206. Strang P. Emotional and social aspects of cancer pain. Acta Oncol 31:323–6, 1992.

207. Hay JL, Passik SD. The cancer patient with borderline personality disorder: suggestions for symptom-focussed management in the medical setting. Psychooncology 9:91–100, 2000.

208. American Psychiatric Association. Personality disorders. In: Diagnostic and statistical manual of mental disorders. Washington DC: American Psychiatric Association, 1994:629–73.

209. Passik SD, Hay JL. Symptom control in patients with severe character pathology. In: Portenoy RK, Bruera E, eds. Topics in palliative care, Vol. 3. New York: Oxford University Press, 1998:213–27.

6 Cancer pain syndromes

RUSSELL K. PORTENOY
Albert Einstein College of Medicine

MARIA CONN
Harlem Hospital Center

Introduction

Pain can undermine quality of life, leading to psychological distress and a decline in physical function and social interaction (1,2). Surveys have demonstrated that 30%–60% of cancer patients experience pain during active anticancer therapy and that this prevalence rises to more than two thirds among those with advanced disease (3). Uncontrollable pain is a major risk factor in cancer-related suicide (4–10).

Given the pervasiveness of acute and chronic pain in the cancer population and its propensity to cause psychological distress and decreased physical functioning, all treating health care professionals should become skilled in pain management (11–14). Unfortunately, cancer pain continues to be undertreated by clinicians (11,15). Among the reasons for this inadequate treatment is poor assessment (16,17). The problematic nature of poor assessment was highlighted in a study of the concordance of pain reports between patient and clinician; in 73% of cases, oncologists stated pain as less severe than did the patients themselves (16).

The first step in cancer pain assessment involves characterization of the pain complaint. This includes description of the pain syndrome and inferences about the pathophysiology of the pain. Second, it is imperative to properly evaluate the impact of pain on every aspect of the individual's functioning.

A description of pain intensity clarifies the urgency of relief and guides selection of medication, route of administration, and rate of dose titration (18). Assessment of pain intensity also may help elucidate the pain mechanism and underlying syndrome.

The quality of pain is used empirically to help infer pathophysiology. For instance, somatic nociceptive pain may be localized, sharp, aching, and/or throbbing with a pressure sensation. Conversely, visceral nociceptive pain is commonly diffuse and may be crampy or gnawing sec-

ondary to obstruction of a viscus or aching, sharp, or throbbing because of the involvement of organ capsules or mesentery (19,20). Neuropathic pains may be described as burning or shock-like.

Temporal descriptions of cancer pain are helpful diagnostically and are used to classify syndromes (see later). Cancer pain may be acute or chronic. The appearance of overt pain behaviors such as moaning, grimacing, anxiety, and signs of sympathetic hyperactivity is consistent with acute pain, but may or may not occur. Chronic pain persists beyond the healing of the inciting event or occurs in association with a nonhealing lesion. Chronic cancer pain may be associated with symptoms such as asthenia, anorexia, and sleep disturbance (21–24).

The association of particular pain characteristics and physical signs with specific consequences of the underlying disease or its treatment define the cancer pain syndromes. These syndromes have distinct etiologies and pathophysiologies, as well as important prognostic and therapeutic implications. Cancer pain syndromes can be either acute (Table 6.1) or chronic (Table 6.2) (25). Diagnostic and therapeutic interventions are primarily responsible for the acute pain syndromes. Chronic cancer pain usually results from direct tumor infiltration. Adverse effects of cancer therapy, including surgery, chemotherapy, and radiation therapy, also may be responsible for chronic cancer pain syndromes, and a small number of chronic pain syndromes are caused by factors unrelated to either cancer or the cancer therapy (26–31).

Acute pain syndromes

Acute pain associated with diagnostic interventions

Lumbar puncture headache
Lumbar puncture headache is characterized as a positional headache developing after a lumbar puncture. This

Table 6.1. *Acute cancer pain syndromes*

Acute Pain Associated with Diagnostic Interventions
Examples: Lumbar puncture headache
            Needle biopsy

Acute Pain Associated with Therapeutic Interventions
Examples: Postoperative pain
            Cryosurgery of the cervix
            Other interventions

Acute Pain Following Analgesic Interventions
Acute Pain Associated with Anticancer Therapies
Acute pain associated with chemotherapy infusion techniques
Examples: Intravenous infusion pain
            Hepatic artery infusion pain
            Intraperitoneal chemotherapy pain
            Intravesical chemotherapy or immunotherapy
Acute pain associated with chemotherapy toxicity
Examples: Mucositis
            Painful peripheral neuropathy
            Methotrexate- and L-asparaginase-induced
               headaches
            Headache and diffuse bone pain with trans-retinoic
               therapy
            Arthralgia and myalgia caused by paclitaxel
            5-Fluorouracil-induced angina
            Palmar-plantar erythrodysesthesia syndrome
            Postchemotherapy gynecomastia
            Postchemotherapy acute ischemia
Acute pain syndromes following hormonal therapy
Examples: Flare syndrome in prostate cancer
            Flare syndrome in breast cancer
Acute pain associated with immunotherapy
Acute pain associated with growth factors
Radiotherapy pain syndromes
Examples: Oropharyngeal mucositis
            Acute radiation enteritis
            Transient brachial plexopathy
            Acute and subacute radiation-induced myelitis
            Radiopharmaceutical pain flare

Acute Pain Associated with Infection
Example: Acute herpetic neuralgia

Acute Pain Associated with Vascular Events
Example: Acute thrombosis pain

Table 6.2. *Chronic cancer pain syndromes*

Tumor-Related Somatic Pain Syndromes
Examples: Bone pain
                  Multifocal bone pain
                  Vertebral syndromes
                     Atlantoaxial destruction and odontoid fracture
                     C7–T1 syndrome
                     T12–L1 syndrome
                     Sacral syndrome
                     Pain secondary to epidural compression
            Arthritides
                  Hypertrophic pulmonary osteoarthropathy
            Muscle and soft tissue pain
                  Primary and secondary tumors
                  Cramps
            Headache and facial pain
                  Intracerebral tumor
                  Leptomeningeal metastases
                  Base of skull metastases
                     Orbital syndrome
                     Parasellar syndrome
                     Middle cranial fossa syndrome
                     Jugular foramen syndrome
                     Occipital condyle syndrome
                     Clivus syndrome
                     Sphenoid sinus syndrome
                  Ear and eye pain syndromes
                     Otalgia
                     Eye pain

Tumor-Related Neuropathic Pain
Examples: Painful cranial neuralgias
                  Glossopharyngeal neuralgia
                  Trigeminal neuralgia
            Painful radiculopathy
            Cervical plexopathy
            Malignant brachial plexopathy
            Malignant lumbosacral plexopathy
            Painful peripheral mononeuropathies

**Pain Syndromes of the Viscera and Miscellaneous
   Tumor-Related Syndromes**
Examples: Hepatic distention syndrome
            Midline retroperitoneal syndrome
            Chronic intestinal obstruction
            Peritoneal carcinomatosis
            Malignant perineal pain
            Adrenal pain syndrome
            Ureteric obstruction

Chronic Pain Syndromes Associated with Cancer Therapy
Examples: Postchemotherapy pain syndromes
                  Painful peripheral neuropathy
                  Avascular (aseptic) necrosis of the femoral or
                     humeral head
                  Plexopathy
                  Raynaud's syndrome
            Chronic pain associated with hormonal therapy
            Chronic postsurgical pain syndromes
                  Breast surgery pain syndromes
                  Postradical neck dissection pain
                  Postthoracotomy pain
                  Postoperative frozen shoulder
                  Stump pain and phantom pain

(continues)

headache commences and worsens with upright posture. The syndrome results from ongoing leakage of cerebrospinal fluid through the defect in the dural sheath and dilation of intracerebral veins (32). There is a decrease in the incidence of lumbar puncture headache when a small-gauge needle is used with longitudinal insertion of the needle bevel (32–35). A lumbar puncture headache most commonly starts hours to several days after a lumbar puncture. Patients usually describe this headache as a dull occipital discomfort that radiates to the frontal region or to the shoulders (32,35–37). If pain escalates, it may be accompanied by diaphoresis and nausea (38). The duration

Table 6.2. *(continued)*

Chronic Pain Syndromes Associated with Cancer Therapy
(continued)
    Chronic postradiation pain syndromes
      Radiation-induced brachial plexopathy
      Radiation-induced lumbosacral plexopathy
      Chronic radiation myelopathy
      Chronic radiation enteritis and proctitis
      Lymphedema pain
      Burning perineum syndrome
      Osteoradionecrosis

of the headache is typically 1 to 7 days (38). Routine management includes bed rest, hydration, and analgesics. If the headache is not alleviated by these standard modes of treatment, an epidural blood patch may be used. Also, severe headaches have been known to respond to treatment with intravenous or oral caffeine (32).

Needle biopsy

Although a biopsy of an intrathoracic mass is a relatively small procedure, a severe transitory pain may result. This has been reported, for example, from biopsy of neurogenic tumor (39).

An important procedure in the diagnosis and management of prostate cancer is the transrectal, ultrasound-guided prostate biopsy. A prospective study showed that 16% of patients reported pain of moderate or greater severity during this procedure (40). Transrectal, ultrasound-guided prostatic neural blockade can decrease the pain associated with this procedure (41).

Acute pain associated with therapeutic interventions

Postoperative pain

Acute postoperative pain is universal and needs prompt and adequate treatment. Unfortunately, postoperative pain continues to be undertreated despite the availability of adequate medications and interventions (42,43). Persistent postoperative pain often indicates further evaluation for the possibilities of infection and other complications.

Cryosurgery of the cervix

Cryosurgery is used in the management of intraepithelial neoplasm of the cervix. This procedure can produce an acute cramping pain syndrome. The duration of the freeze period is directly proportional to the severity of pain. It has been noted that a prophylactic nonsteroidal anti-inflammatory drug is not helpful (44).

Other interventions

Tumor embolization techniques (45,46) and chemical pleurodesis (47,48) are routine invasive procedures in cancer therapy. Both can cause acute severe pain that is typically transitory and can be effectively managed if anticipated.

Acute pain after analgesic interventions

Occasionally, opioid administration may cause a generalized headache, often with vascular features. This may be due to opioid-induced histamine release.

Intradermal, subcutaneous, and intramuscular injections may be painful. For example, intradermal and subcutaneous injection of lidocaine causes a transient burning pain before the lidocaine can take effect (49). Intramuscular opioid administration in cancer patients is not recommended if a repetitive dosing schedule is needed (42,50). The pain associated with subcutaneous injection is influenced by both volume and the drug. After subcutaneous opioid injection, a painful subdermal reaction may develop. This reaction occurs more frequently with methadone (51). The addition of a small amount of a steroid to the opioid may lessen the reaction (52).

High neuraxial opioid doses can cause pain and hyperalgesia; this syndrome may be associated with myoclonus, piloerection, and priapism (53–55). Occasionally, epidural drug delivery can cause compression or irritation of nerve roots, with back, pelvic, or leg pain (56).

Acute pain associated with anticancer therapies

Acute pain associated with chemotherapy infusion techniques

Intravenous Infusion Pain Venous spasm, chemical phlebitis, vesicant extravasation, and anthracycline-associated flare may cause pain at the site of chemotherapy infusion. Venous spasm may be lessened by the application of a warm compress or by decreased infusion rate. It is not accompanied by inflammation. Phlebitis may be caused by many drugs (57–59), by potassium chloride infusion, and by hyperosmolar solutions (60). Vesicant extravasation produces extreme pain along with linear erythema, desquamation, and ulceration (61,62). A venous flare reaction manifests with local urticaria and pain and may appear after the administration of an anthracycline or doxorubicin (63,64).

Hepatic artery infusion pain For patients with hepatic metastases, a hepatic artery cytotoxic infusions may be part of standard therapy. Side effects include diffuse abdominal pain, gastric ulcerations, or cholangitis (65). If the infusion is stopped, the pain typically disappears, and some patients tolerate reinfusion at a lower rate (66).

Intraperitoneal chemotherapy pain Intraperitoneal chemotherapy can cause abdominal pain (67). If severe, it is usually secondary to the presence of chemical serositis or infection (68). Serositis may follow treatment with mitoxantrone (69), doxorubicin (70), or paclitaxel (71). The presence of fever or leukocytosis in blood and peritoneal fluid suggests infectious peritonitis (72).

Intravesical chemotherapy or immunotherapy Bladder irritability characterized by frequency and/or painful micturition can be caused by the administration of intravesical bacillus Calmette-Guérin therapy for transitional cell carcinoma (73,74). Intravesical doxorubicin often causes a painful cystitis (75).

Acute pain associated with chemotherapy toxicity

Mucositis Mucositis typically follows dose intense chemotherapy, particularly the myeloablative chemotherapy before bone marrow transplantation (76–78). The mucosal membranes of the oral cavity, pharynx, esophagus, and stomach or intestine may be involved. Symptoms include pain, odynophagia, dyspepsia, or diarrhea. Mucosal surfaces can become superinfected with candida, herpes simplex, or other organisms. Numerous therapies have been attempted to reduce the incidence of mucositis, including cryotherapy (79,80), surface coating agents (81), antiviral agents (82,83), and disinfectant mouthwashes (84). None are yet established. Once mucositis reaches a severe stage, treatment usually combines these local measures and opioid analgesics (85–87).

Painful peripheral neuropathy Cis-platinum, paclitaxel, and vinca alkaloids can produce a dose-related peripheral neuropathy. Vincristine can cause a typical painful polyneuropathy or more focal pains in the jaw and face, legs, arms, or abdomen. The orofacial pain is self-limiting and starts 2 to 3 days after treatment starts (88).

Methotrexate- and L-asparaginase-induced headaches Headache is common after treatment with intrathecal methotrexate for leukemia or leptomeningeal disease. Pain may be associated with vomiting, nuchal rigidity, fever, irritability, and lethargy. There may be an associated cerebrospinal fluid pleocytosis. Patients may experience these symptoms hours after administration of methotrexate, and the syndrome may last for several days. It may occur once and not recur with repeated administration (89,90).

L-asparaginase, which is used in the treatment of acute lymphoblastic leukemia, may produce thrombosis of cerebral veins or dural sinuses in 1%–2% of patients (91). The thrombosis of cerebral veins or dural sinuses may be confirmed by angiography or gradient echo sequences on MRI scan (92). The syndrome is associated with severe headache and, at times, focal neurological deficits.

Headache and diffuse bone pain with trans-retinoic Therapy Trans-retinoic acid is used to treat acute promyelocytic leukemia and may cause pseudotumor cerebri (93) or transitory diffuse bone pain (94,95). There also may be a transient neutrophilia, most likely secondary to bone marrow expansion (96).

Arthralgia and myalgia caused by paclitaxel A total of 10%–20% of patients treated with paclitaxel experience diffuse joint and muscle pain (97,98). These unexplained arthralgias and myalgias appear 1 to 4 days after paclitaxel infusion and may last up to a week, and sometimes longer.

5-Fluorouracil-Induced angina Continuous 5-fluorouracil (5-FU) infusion causes a threefold increase in cardiac ischemic episodes, which presumably result from vasospasm. These episodes are more common among patients with known coronary artery disease (99–101).

Palmar-plantar erythrodysesthesia syndrome Palmar-plantar erythrodysesthesia syndrome is a painful rash on palms and soles that may follow chemotherapy infusion. The rash may progress to bulla formation and desquamation. It is self-limited and may be attenuated by co-administration of pyridoxine. The syndrome has been associated with continuous low-dose infusions of 5-FU (102,103), liposomal doxorubicin (104,105), and other drugs.

Postchemotherapy gynecomastia Chemotherapy for testicular cancer and sometimes other neoplasms may be associated with a painful, usually transitory, gynecomastia (106,107). If a patient with a history of testicular cancer has painful gynecomastia, tumor-related gynecomastia must be excluded (108,109).

Postchemotherapy acute ischemia Bleomycin, vinblastine, and *cis*-platinum are known to cause Raynaud's phenomenon or transient ischemia of the toes (110). Bleomycin also has been reported to cause a rare irreversible digital ischemia progressing to gangrene (111).

Acute pain syndromes after hormonal therapy

Flare syndrome in prostate cancer A total of 5%–25% of prostate cancer patients who receive leutenizing hormone-releasing factor (LHRF) experience an exacerbation of bone pain or urinary retention (112,113). Rarely, spinal cord compression and sudden death complicate this therapy (114). This syndrome occurs with initial dose of LHRF and is thought to be caused by the stimulation of leutenizing hormone before it is suppressed. Androgen antagonist therapy during the initiation of LHRF administration may prevent these phenomena.

Flare syndrome in breast cancer Hormonal therapy for metastatic breast cancer can produce diffuse musculoskeletal pain, skin erythema, change in liver function studies, and hypercalcemia. (115,116). The mechanism of this syndrome is not understood.

Acute pain associated with immunotherapy

Patients who receive interferon may experience myalgias, arthralgias, and headache. These symptoms may be accompanied by fever and severe fatigue and appear shortly after initial dosing. They decrease in severity after repeated dosing. Acetaminophen given before treatment may be useful in lowering the intensity (117).

Acute pain associated with growth factors

Colony-stimulating factors (CSFs) stimulate the production, maturation, and function of blood elements. Bone pain, fever, headache, and myalgias may follow treatment with granulocyte-macrophage CSF, granulocyte CSF, and interleukin-3 (118,119). Erythropoietin injection may cause pain at the subcutaneous injection site (120–122).

Radiotherapy pain syndromes

Oropharyngeal mucositis Radiation oropharyngeal mucositis occurs with doses above 1000 cGy to the head and neck. Ulceration is common at doses above 4000 cGy. Pain may escalate to a point that patients are unable to eat. The pain from the mucositis can linger several weeks after completion of the radiotherapy (77,123).

Acute radiation enteritis Fifty percent of patients undergoing pelvic and/or abdominal radiation experience abdominal cramping, nausea, and vomiting (124). After pelvic radiotherapy, a patient may experience tenesmoid pain with diarrhea, mucus discharge, and bleeding (125).

Transient brachial plexopathy Retrospective studies have shown that approximately 1.4%–20% of breast cancer patients receiving radiation develop a transient brachial plexopathy (126,127). Most patients experience symptoms during radiotherapy or immediately after completion. Patients usually present with paresthesias, pain,

and weakness in the shoulder, arm, and hand. The syndrome is self-limited. A subacute syndrome also occurs.

Acute and subacute radiation-induced myelitis Radiation that includes spinal cord can result in acute or subacute syndromes. The acute syndrome usually involves worsening at sites of existing spinal cord injury. The subacute type takes the form of a Lhermitte's sign, shock-like pains in the neck and back that are precipitated by neck flexion. The pain begins weeks to months after treatment and is usually gone in 3 to 6 months (128,129).

Radiopharmaceutical pain flare Strontium-89, rhenium-186, and samarium-153 are systemically administered beta-emitting radiopharmaceuticals that are taken up by bone in areas of osteoblastic activity. These drugs decrease bony pain secondary to blastic bone metastases (130). A flare response, characterized by worsening of pain 1 to 2 days after administration of radiopharmaceutical agents, occurs in as many as 20% of patients (131). The pain flare is transitory but can be intense.

Acute pain associated with infection

Acute herpetic neuralgia

Herpes zoster infections occur at an increased rate among cancer patients, particularly those with hematological or lymphoproliferative malignancies (132,133). Pain or an itch usually precedes the rash by several days, and the dermatomal location of the infection is often associated with the site of malignancy (133). For instance, patients with breast or lung carcinomas tend to present with thoracic lesions. Because of the risk of viral dissemination, patients with an acute zoster should be treated with adequate doses of an antiviral drug.

Acute pain associated with vascular events

Acute thrombosis pain

Thrombosis is extremely common among cancer patients. It can be the presenting sign of malignancy (134) and is the second leading cause of death in those with metastatic disease (135). Patients with advanced pelvic tumors (136), pancreatic cancer (137), gastric cancer, advanced breast cancer (138), and brain tumors (139) are at the greatest risk for thrombosis. Chemotherapy and hormonal therapy increase the risk further.

Lower extremity deep vein thrombosis presents with pain and swelling of the lower extremity. Pain may vary and is characterized as a dull cramp or diffuse heaviness.

The most common site of pain is the calf. Physical examination reveals swelling, warmth, dilation of superficial veins, and with pain induced by stretching (140,141). The diagnosis may be confirmed by ultrasound, impedance plethysmography, and venography. If there is a variance between the results of the noninvasive test and clinical suspicion, however, a venography should be used to confirm the diagnosis (141). Rarely, deep venous thrombosis may progress to a phlegmasia cerulea dolens (142), a syndrome characterized by severe pain, extensive edema, and cyanosis of the legs. Gangrene can occur unless the obstruction is relieved (143).

Deep venous thrombosis in the upper extremity is uncommon (144). The diagnosis is suggested by edema, dilated collateral circulation, and pain (145). Extrinsic compression of venous outflow by tumor is a common cause for an upper extremity thrombosis. Anticoagulation controls intrinsic damage to vessels; however, pain and swelling may persist secondary to the extrinsic compression (146).

Superior vena cava syndrome obstruction is most commonly caused by extrinsic compression from enlarged mediastinal lymph nodes (147). This syndrome is most common in lung cancer and lymphomas. Intravascular devices also can cause the syndrome (147). Patients present with facial swelling, dilated neck and chest wall veins.

Chronic pain syndromes

Approximately three fourths of chronic cancer pain syndromes result from the direct invasion of pain-sensitive structures by the neoplasm. Others result from the therapies administered to treat the disease or from disorders unrelated to the disease or its treatment.

Tumor-related somatic pain syndromes

Tumor spread to bone, joint, muscle, or connective tissue can cause persistent somatic pain (25). Bone metastases are the most common cause of chronic pain in cancer patients (26,27,31,148,149).

Bone pain
More than 25% of patients with bony metastases do not feel pain, and patients with multiple bony lesions typically report pain in only a few sites. Endosteal or periosteal nociceptor activation, mechanical distortion or release of chemical mediators, or tumor growth may be involved in the conversion of a painless bone metastasis into one associated with pain (150).

Multifocal bone pain Multifocal bone pain is caused by widespread bone metastases. Hematogenous malignancies rarely produce a similar syndrome secondary to bone marrow expansion. In contrast to bone metastases, there are no radiological abnormalities when pain is caused by bone marrow expansion.

Vertebral syndromes More than two thirds of vertebral metastases are located in the thoracic spine; lumbosacral and cervical metastases account for approximately 10%–20%, respectively. Early recognition of tumor invasion into vertebral bodies is important to prevent compression of adjacent neural structures and hence neurological deficits.

Atlantoaxial destruction and odontoid fracture. Nuchal or occipital pain that often radiates over the posterior aspect of the skull is a typical presentation of destruction of the atlas or fracture of the odontoid process. This type of pain is exacerbated by neck flexion (151). The syndrome can evolve into compression of the spinal cord with subluxation at the cervicomedullary junction. Patients usually present with insidious neurological deficits in one or more extremities. Upper extremity involvement is more prominent at early stages. MRI is probably the best method for imaging this region of the spine.

C7-T1 syndrome. A patient with tumor invasion of a C7 or T1 vertebra can experience pain in the interscapular region. This phenomenon implies that patients with pain at this site should have extensive radiograph evaluation of both the cervical and thoracic spine.

T12-L1 syndrome. A T12 or L1 vertebral metastatic lesion may refer pain to the ipsilateral iliac crest or sacroiliac joint. Imaging procedures directed at pelvic bone may miss the metastatic lesion.

Sacral syndrome. Pain radiating to buttocks, perineum, or posterior thighs may indicate destruction of sacrum (152–154). Sitting exacerbates the pain. The neoplasm may spread laterally into the pyriformis and cause incident pain with hip motion. Pyriformis syndrome is characterized by buttock or posterior leg pain that is exacerbated by internal rotation of the hip.

Pain secondary to epidural compression. Epidural compression (EC) of the spinal cord or cauda equina is the second most common neurological complication of cancer (155). EC usually is caused by posterior extension of a vertebral body metastasis into the epidural space. On occasion, tumor extends from the posterior arch of the vertebra or grows through the intervertebral foramen from a paraspinal location. The presenting sign of EC usually is back pain. Pain may precede neurological impairment by weeks or months. Accurate diagnosis at this stage is crucial so that effective treatment may begin. Treatment may prevent or retard the progression of neurological impairment. In all 75% of patients who begin treatment while they are ambulating will not develop further neurological impairment (156–163).

Imaging of the epidural space is needed to promptly diagnose epidural compression. The choices for imaging include MRI, myelography, and computed tomography (CT)-myelography. MRI is preferred because it is noninvasive and offers soft tissue imaging and multiplanar views. However, CT-myelography and MRI have the same specificity and sensitivity for the detection of epidural lesions.

Treatment for EC includes corticosteroids and radiotherapy. Surgical decompression may be appropriate for patients with radioresistant tumors, those who have received maximal radiation therapy, and those with spinal instability or posterior displacement of bony fragments (155,164,165).

Management algorithms have been developed in an effort to ensure that appropriate treatment is given sufficiently early to optimize the likelihood of good outcomes for patients with EC. The most useful algorithms outline the urgency and course of evaluation for cancer patients with back pain. In one approach (166), patients with emerging symptoms and signs indicative of spinal cord or cauda equina dysfunction are treated with a high dose of intravenous steroids, such as an initial bolus of dexamethasone 100 mg followed by 96 mg/day in divided doses. These patients are imaged and then treated urgently. Patients with signs of radiculopathy or stable or mild signs of spinal cord or cauda equina syndrome are usually treated with a lower dose of corticosteroid and scheduled for definitive imaging of the epidural space as soon as possible. Patients with back pain and no signs or symptoms suggesting EC should undergo MRI if pain is rapidly progressive or worsens with recumbency or Valsalva maneuver. In the absence of these ominous characteristics, plain spine radiographs may be helpful to define the risk of EC. If greater than 50% vertebral collapse is present, an imaging study to evaluate the epidural space is needed. It should be recognized, however, that the absence of vertebral collapse does not exclude EC. In fact, 60% of patients with EC caused by lymphoma had normal radiographs in one study (167,168).

Arthritides

Hypertrophic pulmonary osteoarthropathy Hypertrophic pulmonary osteoarthropathy is a paraneoplastic syndrome that includes clubbing of fingers, periostitis of long bones, and occasionally a rheumatoid-like polyarthritis (169). The syndrome has been associated with lung cancer, breast cancer, mesothelioma, and other neoplasms (170,171). The diagnosis is supported by pain, tenderness, and swelling in the knees, wrists, and ankles; and confirmation is provided by physical findings, radiological appearance, and radionuclide scan (169,172,173). The syndrome can precede diagnosis of the underlying malignancy by months.

Muscle and soft tissue pain

Primary and secondary tumors Soft tissue, sarcomas can arise from fat, fibrous tissue, or skeletal muscle. Pain is common in these lesions. Metastatic lesions are rarely found in skeletal muscles, but when present can cause a dull aching muscle pain (174,175).

Cramps Muscular cramps in cancer patients are usually caused by a neural, muscular, or biochemical abnormality (176). In a study of 50 cancer patients, 22 had a peripheral neuropathy, 17 had root or plexus pathology, 2 had polymyositis, and 1 had low serum magnesium levels.

Headache and facial pain

Among cancer patients, headache may arise from traction, inflammation, or infiltration of pain-sensitive structures in the head and/or neck region (174,175). Headache may also be due to increased intracranial pressure or vascular lesions (see previously).

Intracerebral tumor The prevalence of headache in patients with brain primary tumors or metastases is approximately 60%–90% (177,178). Traction on pain-sensitive vascular and dural structures is responsible for these headaches. Multifocal metastases and posterior fossa metastases produce both focal and generalized headaches (177). Patients with supratentorial lesions often have unilateral headaches (178). Headache may occur without other symptoms or signs (179).

Headaches associated with intracranial space-occupying lesions usually are most severe in the morning. Headaches often fluctuate during the day and, when intracranial hypertension is severe, some of the fluctuation may be related to so-called "plateau waves." These waves of massively increased pressure can occur spontaneously or be induced by movement or by Valsalva maneuver. They may be associated with nausea, vomiting, photophobia, lethargy, and transient neurological deficits. They may produce brainstem herniation when severe (180,181).

Leptomeningeal metastases Leptomeningeal metastases are diffuse or multifocal involvement of the subarachnoid space by metastatic tumor (182). This complication can occur with any neoplasm and is most common in non-Hodgkin's lymphoma, acute lymphocytic leukemia, and cancers of the breast and lung (183).

Leptomeningeal metastases may present with headache, or neck or back pain, and with focal or multifocal neurological symptoms and/or signs at any level of the neuraxis (182,184). Significant pain occurs in fewer than one fourth of patients. Seizures, radicular pain, mental status changes, nausea, vomiting, and memory loss also can occur (184–186).

Leptomeningeal metastases can be confirmed via analysis of the cerebrospinal fluid. The cerebrospinal fluid may reveal elevated pressure, elevated protein, depressed glucose, and/or lymphocytic pleocytosis. False-negative rate after a single lumbar puncture may be as high as 55% and decreases significantly after the third lumbar puncture (184,185,187). Tumor markers, such as lactic dehydrogenase isoenzymes (184), carcinoembryonic carcinoma, beta-2-microglobulin (188), tissue polypeptide antigen (189), and others may help establish the diagnosis or monitor for recurrence. Imaging studies also may aid in confirming the diagnosis. MRI of the cranium and spinal cord with gadolinium enhancement is most sensitive (190).

Treatment of leptomeningeal metastases may ameliorate symptoms and prolong life. Treatment options include radiation therapy, corticosteroids, intraventricular or intrathecal chemotherapy, and systemic chemotherapy (191).

Base of skull metastases Cancers of the breast, lung, and prostate are most commonly associated with base of skull metastases (192). Base of skull metastases cause headache associated with well-described clinical features. Varied syndromes are named according to the site of metastatic involvement. When metastases are suspected, the diagnosis may be confirmed using axial CT imaging with bone windows or MRI. MRI is more sensitive for assessing soft tissue extension.

Orbital syndrome. Cancer patients with orbital metastases present with increasing pain in the retroorbital and supraorbital region of the affected eye. Associated problems include blurred vision, diplopia, proptosis, chemosis of the involved eye, external ophthalmoparesis, ipsilateral papilledema, and decreased sensation in the ophthalmic division of the trigeminal nerve.

Parasellar syndrome. Patients with neoplastic invasion in the parasellar region can develop unilateral supra-

orbital and frontal headache, as well as diplopia (193). Ophthalmoparesis or papilledema and/or a visual field cut may be present.

Middle cranial fossa syndrome. Facial numbness, paresthesias, or pain with a referral pattern to the cheek or jaw are the presenting signs of middle cranial fossa syndrome (194). The pain is typically described as dull continual ache. Physical examination may reveal hypesthesia in the trigeminal nerve distribution, signs of weakness in the ipsilateral muscles of mastication, and abducens palsy (192,195).

Jugular foramen syndrome. Patients with a jugular foramen syndrome can develop hoarseness, dysphagia, deep aching in the ipsilateral mastoid region, and glossopharyngeal neuralgia with or without syncope (192). Additionally, there also may be referred neck and shoulder pain. Neurological signs on examination may include ipsilateral Horner's syndrome; weakness of the palate, sternocleidomastoid or trapezius; and ipsilateral paresis of the tongue.

Occipital condyle syndrome. The occipital condyle syndrome presents with unilateral occipital pain that is worsened with neck flexion (196,197). Physical examination may reveal a head tilt, limited movement of the neck, and tenderness to palpation over the occipitonuchal junction. Neurological signs include ipsilateral hypoglossal nerve paralysis and sternocleidomastoid weakness.

Clivus syndrome. The clivus syndrome is characterized by vertex headache, which is exacerbated by neck flexion. Lower cranial nerve (VI–XII) dysfunction usually occurs later.

Sphenoid sinus syndrome. A sphenoid sinus metastasis often presents with bifrontal and retrorbital pain. This pain may radiate to the temporal regions (198). Patients may have associated nasal congestion and diplopia caused by unilateral or bilateral sixth nerve paresis.

Ear and eye pain syndromes
Otalgia. Otalgia, ear pain, may originate in an area far removed from the ear. The ear has a sensory innervation from four different cranial nerves and two cervical nerves that supply other areas in the head, neck, thorax, and abdomen. Ear pain may be caused by cancer of the oropharynx or hypopharynx (199,200), acoustic neuroma (201), and metastases to the temporal bone or infratemporal fossa (202,203)

Eye pain. Eye pain and blurry vision are the two most common symptoms of choridal metastases (204–206). Chronic eye pain can occur from metastases to the bony orbit or intraorbital structures such as the rectus muscle (207,208) or optic nerve (209).

Tumor-related neuropathic pains

Neuropathic pain syndromes caused by neoplastic invasion of peripheral nerve include cranial neuralgias, radiculopathy, plexopathy, mononeuropathy, or peripheral neuropathy.

Painful cranial neuralgias

Cranial neuralgias can occur from metastases in the base of the skull or leptomeninges (210). Other lesions result from cancer in the soft tissue of the head or neck, or sinuses.

Glossopharyngeal neuralgia Neuralgia of the ninth cranial nerve has been seen in patients with leptomeningeal metastases, jugular foramen, or head or neck malignancies (192,211–214). Patients have severe pain in the throat or neck, which may radiate to the ear and mastoid region. Pain may be initiated by swallowing and may be associated with sudden orthostasis and syncope.

Trigeminal Neuralgia Trigeminal neuralgia may produce pain that is paroxysmal or constant. Tumors of the middle or posterior fossa may mimic classic trigeminal neuralgia (195,215–217). Pain on a continuous basis may be an early sign of acoustic neuroma (218).

Painful radiculopathy

Any process that compresses, distorts, or inflames nerve roots may cause radiculopathy or a polyradiculopathy. If a patient presents with painful radiculopathy, an epidural tumor or leptomeningeal disease must be suspected.

Cervical plexopathy

Ventral rami of the upper four cervical spinal nerves join to form the cervical plexus between the deep anterior and lateral muscles of the neck. The cutaneous branches emerge from the posterior border of the sternocleidomastoid. Tumor invasion or compression of the cervical plexus may be due to direct extension of a primary head and neck malignancy or neoplastic involvement of the cervical lymph nodes (219). Pain may be experienced in the periauricular, postauricular, or anterior neck. Additionally, pain may be referred to the lateral aspect of the face or head or shoulder. Pain may be aching and burning and may worsen by neck movement or swallowing. Patients with this syndrome may also present with Horner's or hemidiaphragmatic paralysis.

Malignant brachial plexopathy

Malignant brachial plexopathy is most common in patients with lymphoma, lung cancer, or breast cancer. Tumor may invade from nodes in the axillary, cervical, or supraclavicular chains or from the superior sulcus of the lung (Pancoast lesion) (220). Pain is the presenting sign of malignant brachial plexopathy in 85% of patients. Neurological signs follow. Lower plexus involvement (C7, C8, and TI) presents with pain in the elbow, medial forearm, or fourth and fifth fingers. Some patients may experience lancinating dysesthesias along the ulnar aspect of the forearm. Upper plexus involvement is characterized by pain in the shoulder girdle lateral arm and hand.

Cross-sectional imaging is essential with symptoms or signs compatible with a plexopathy. CT scanning has 80%–90% sensitivity in detecting tumor infiltration (221). MRI allows multiplanar views.

Malignant lumbosacral plexopathy

The lumbar plexus is formed by the ventral rami L1–4. The sacral plexus forms in the sacroiliac notch from the ventral rami of S1–3 and the lumbosacral trunk (L4–5) which courses caudally over the sacral ala to join the plexus (222). Colorectal, cervical, breast, sarcoma, and lymphoma are the primary tumors associated with lumbosacral plexopathy. One fourth of the cases are attributed to direct extension from the intrapelvic neoplasm. In one study, two thirds of the patients developed plexopathy within 3 years of their primary diagnosis and one third had symptoms within 1 year (223).

Similar to brachial plexopathy, the initial symptom of lumbosacral plexopathy is pain. Pain may be followed by numbness, paresthesias, or weakness weeks to months later. Sensory loss in a dermatomal fashion, reflex asymmetry, focal tenderness, leg edema, and positive direct or reverse straight leg raising signs also may occur.

Lower lumbosacral plexopathy usually occurs from direct extension of rectal cancer, gynecological tumors, or a pelvic sarcoma. Pain may be focal in buttocks and perineum. It may also be referred to the posterolateral thigh and leg. Associated symptoms and signs conform to an L4–S1 distribution. Physical examination may reveal weakness or sensory changes in the L5 and S1 dermatomes. There may also be some leg edema and bladder and bowel dysfunction.

An upper lumbosacral plexopathy may occur from neoplastic extension to the pelvic sidewall or lumbar paraspinal region. Pain is experienced in the anterolateral thigh, knee, and proximal leg. Physical examination can demonstrate neurological deficits from L4 to S2.

Sacral plexopathy may be secondary to midline tumors, usually arising from the rectum or prostate. Patients may experience dysesthesias in the buttocks, perineum, or posterior legs. Pain is often severe while sitting, less severe while standing, and least severe while standing or walking.

Panplexopathy involvement in L1–S3 distribution occurs in almost one fifth of patients with a lumbosacral plexopathy. Pain may be anywhere from the lower abdomen, back, buttocks, or perineum. Referred pain can be experienced anywhere in the distribution of the plexus. Leg edema is a common finding. Neurological findings can occur anywhere along the L1–S3 distribution.

Autonomic dysfunction such as anhydrosis and vasodilation has been associated with plexus and peripheral nerve injuries (224). Focal autonomic neuropathy can suggest an anatomic site (225).

Cross-sectional MRI or CT is the usual diagnostic procedure to evaluate lumbosacral plexopathy. Limited data suggest that MRI may be more sensitive than CT (226).

Painful peripheral mononeuropathies

Tumor-related mononeuropathy usually results from compression or infiltration of a nerve from tumor arising in an adjacent bony structure. Patients experience dysesthesias in the area of sensory loss. Examples include intercostal nerve injury from rib metastases, sciatica associated with tumor invasion of the sciatic notch, and peroneal palsy associated with primary bone tumors of the proximal fibula. Patients rarely develop common types of nerve entrapment, such as carpal tunnel syndrome, secondary to compression by tumor (227).

Paraneoplastic painful peripheral neuropathy can be related to injury to the dorsal root ganglion or to the peripheral nerves. These painful neuropathies can be the initial manifestation of an underlying malignancy. Subacute sensory neuropathy caused by injury to the dorsal root ganglion is characterized by pain, paresthesias, sensory loss in the extremities, and severe sensory ataxia (228). This neuropathy is most commonly associated with small-cell carcinoma of the lung. Other tumor types associated with this neuropathy are breast cancer and Hodgkin's lymphoma (229,230).

A painful sensorimotor peripheral neuropathy has been associated with many tumor types. The peripheral neuropathies associated with multiple myeloma, Waldenstrom's macroglobulinemia, and small fiber amyloid neuropathy are thought to be due to antibodies that cross-react with constituents of peripheral nerves (228,231,232).

Pain syndromes of the viscera and miscellaneous tumor-related syndromes

Pain may be caused by the pathology involving the hollow organs of gastrointestinal or genitourinary tracts, the parenchymal organs, the peritoneum, or other retroperitoneal soft tissues.

Hepatic distention syndrome

Pain-sensitive structures in the region of the liver include the liver capsule, vessels, and biliary tract (233). Nociceptive afferents that innervate these structures travel via the celiac plexus, phrenic nerve, and lower right intercostal nerves. Extensive intrahepatic metastases, or gross hepatomegaly associated with cholestasis, may produce discomfort in the right subcostal region, and less commonly in the right scapular region (232,234,235). Patients usually experience dull aching pain. CT imaging will help identify the presence of space-occupying lesions.

Midline retroperitoneal syndrome

Retroperitoneal pathology may produce pain by injury to deep somatic structure of the posterior abdominal wall, connective tissue distortion, local inflammation, and direct infiltration of the celiac plexus. The most common causes are pancreatic cancer (236–238) and retroperitoneal lymphadenopathy (239). Pain is experienced in the epigastrium, low thoracic region of the back, or in both locations. It is diffuse in nature and character.

Chronic intestinal obstruction

Abdominal pain may be a sign of chronic intestinal obstruction associated with abdominal or pelvic cancers (240,241). The mechanisms responsible for this pain include smooth muscle contractions, mesenteric tension, and mural ischemia. Obstructive symptoms may be due primarily to the tumor or a combination of mechanical obstruction and other processes. Pain may be both continuous and colicky and may be referred to the dermatomes represented by the spinal segments supplying the affected viscera. Vomiting, anorexia, and constipation are important associated symptoms. Abdominal radiographs taken both in the supine and erect positions may demonstrate the presence of air-fluid levels and intestinal distention. CT or MRI scanning of the abdomen may be able to reveal the extent and intra-abdominal neoplasm.

Peritoneal carcinomatosis

Peritoneal carcinomatosis cause peritoneal inflammation, mesenteric tethering, malignant adhesions, and ascites, all of which can cause pain. Pain and abdominal distention are the most common presenting symptoms. CT scanning may demonstrate evidence of ascites, omental infiltration, and peritoneal nodules (242).

Malignant perineal pain

Tumors of the colon or rectum, female reproductive tract, and distal genitourinary system are most commonly responsible for perineal pain (243,244). Pain may be aggravated by sitting or standing and may be associated with tenesmus or bladder spasms (245).

Adrenal pain syndrome

Large adrenal metastases can produce unilateral flank and abdominal pain (246). The pain can radiate into the ipsilateral upper and lower quadrants of the abdomen.

Ureteric obstruction

Ureteric obstruction usually is caused by tumor compression or infiltration within the true pelvis (247,248). This type of obstruction is associated with cancers of the cervix, ovary, prostate, and rectum. If pain occurs, it is usually in the flank region and may radiate into the inguinal region or genitalia. Diagnosis can usually be confirmed by demonstration of hydronephrosis on renal sonography, and pyleography can identify the level of obstruction. CT scanning techniques will usually demonstrate the etiology of the obstruction (249).

Chronic pain syndromes associated with cancer therapy

Most treatment-related pains are caused by tissue-damaging procedures. These pains are acute and self-limited. Chronic treatment-related pain syndromes are associated with either persistent tissue injury or neuropathic mechanisms.

Postchemotherapy pain syndromes

Painful peripheral neuropathy Although painful peripheral neuropathy resulting from cytotoxic therapy usually subsides over time, some patients develop persistent pain. The neuropathy associated with cis-platinum may progress for a prolonged period after therapy has concluded (250,251).

Avascular (aseptic) necrosis of femoral or humeral head Avascular necrosis of the femoral or humeral head may occur as a complication of corticosteroid therapy (252,253). Osteonecrosis may be unilateral or bilateral. Involvement of the femoral head is most common and causes pain in the hip, thigh, or knee. Pain is exacerbated by movement and relieved by rest. Radiological changes on MRI or CT may not appear for a few months after the initiation of pain.

Plexopathy Lumbosacral or brachial plexopathy may follow chemotherapy infusion into the iliac artery (254) or axillary artery (255), respectively. Patients develop pain, weakness, and paresthesias within 48 hours after infusion. The mechanism of action is thought to be secondary to small vessel damage and infarction of the plexus.

Raynaud's syndrome Raynaud's phenomenon is observed in approximately 20%–30% of patients with germ cell tumors treated with cis-platinum, vincristine, and bleomycin (256). It has been speculated that this reaction is related to a deranged sympathetic nervous system (257).

Chronic pain associated with hormonal therapy

Chronic gynecomastia and breast tenderness are complications of antiandrogen therapies for prostate cancer. This syndrome is associated with diethyl stilbesterol (258) and bicalutamide (259); it is less common with flutamide (260) and cyproterone (261), and is uncommon among patients receiving LHRF agonist therapy (112,113).

Chronic postsurgical pain syndromes

Breast surgery pain syndromes Chronic neuropathic pain after surgery for breast cancer is common. Pain may follow breast-conserving treatments, mastectomy (262), or axillary dissection (263–266). It may occur immediately after the surgery, but more often begins after a delay of weeks to months. Onset later than 18 months after surgery is very uncommon. The pain is characterized as a constricting and burning discomfort that is localized to the medial arm, axilla, and anterior chest wall (266–270). On examination, there is often an area sensory loss within the region of pain (269). The etiology of this syndrome is believed to be related to surgical injury to the intercostobrachial nerve (266,269).

Postradical neck dissection pain A persistent neuropathic pain can develop weeks to months after surgical injury to the neck. Patients may experience burning or lancinating dysesthesias in the area of sensory loss. Another syndrome can result from musculoskeletal imbalance in the shoulder girdle after surgical removal of neck muscles. There may also be thoracic outlet syndrome or suprascapular nerve entrapment. The suprascapular nerve entrapment is associated with selective weakness and wasting of supraspinatus and infraspinatus muscles (271). Escalating pain may signify recurrent tumor or soft tissue infection.

Postthoracotomy pain Postthoracotomy pain refers to pain in the chest wall after surgery. Recurrent neoplasm is the major concern in the differential diagnosis and must be excluded.

Postthoracotomy frozen shoulder Postthoracotomy or postmastectomy patients are at risk for the development of a frozen shoulder (264). This lesion may become an independent focus of pain, particularly if complicated by complex regional pain syndrome. It is imperative to have adequate postoperative analgesia and active range of motion of the shoulder joint.

Stump pain and phantom pain Stump pain can follow the amputation of any body part. This pain is secondary to a neuroma formation in the region of the amputation. Although the pain can be continuous, there may also be periods of exacerbations. The location of the pain in the stump distinguishes it from phantom pain, which is experienced in the area of the missing body part.

Chronic postradiation pain syndromes

Chronic pain complicating radiation therapy tends to occur late in the course of a patient's illness. These syndromes must be distinguished from recurrent tumor.

Radiation-induced brachial plexopathy Early onset transient plexopathy can occur anywhere from a few weeks to 6 months after radiation. Delayed-onset progressive plexopathy can occur 6 months to 20 years after a course of radiotherapy that included the plexus in the radiation portal. The presenting signs are weakness and sensory changes that predominate in C5–C6 distribution (265,272,273). Radiation changes in the skin and lymphedema are commonly associated. CT scan reveals diffuse infiltration and cannot be distinguished from tumor infiltration. MRI shows increased T2 signal in or near the brachial plexus and is also seen in malignant plexopathy (274). Electromyography may demonstrate myokymia (272,275,276).

Radiation-induced lumbosacral plexopathy Radiation fibrosis of the lumbosacral plexus may occur from 1 to 30 years after radiation treatment. Its presenting symptom is progressive weakness and leg swelling (277,278). CT scan may show a nonspecific diffuse infiltration of the tissues. Electromyography may show myokimic discharges (278).

Chronic radiation myelopathy Chronic radiation myelopathy is a late complication of spinal cord irradiation. It may develop 1 to many years after radiation. It most often presents as a transverse myelopathy at the cervicothoracic level, sometimes in a Brown-Séquard pattern (279). Sensory symptoms, including pain, typically precede the development of progressive motor and autonomic dysfunction. The pain is usually characterized as a burning dysesthesia and is localized to the area of spinal cord damage or below. MRI allows the clinician to exclude an epidural lesion and demonstrates the nature and extent of intrinsic cord pathology. The course of chronic radiation myelopathy is described by steady progression over months followed by a subsequent phase of slow progression or stabilization.

Chronic radiation enteritis and proctitis Chronic enteritis and proctitis occur as a late complication in 2%–10% of patients who undergo abdominal or pelvic radiation therapy (280,281). The rectum and rectosigmoid are more commonly involved than the small bowel. It typically causes colicky abdominal pain, which can be associated with chronic nausea or malabsorption. Barium studies may reveal tubular bowel segment resembling Crohn's disease or ischemic colitis.

Lymphedema pain One third of patients with lymphedema of the arm experience pain and tightness (282). Some patients develop entrapment syndromes involving the median nerve in the carpal tunnel or the brachial plexus (265,283). Severe or progressive pain in the lymphedematous arm is strongly suggestive of tumor recurrence or progression of disease.

Burning perineum syndrome Perineal discomfort is a rare delayed complication of pelvic radiotherapy. It can develop approximately 6 to 18 months after radiation therapy. The pain is burning in nature and localized to perianal region. The pain may extend anteriorly to involve the vagina or scrotum (284).

Osteoradionecrosis Osteoradionecrosis can complicate radiotherapy to bone. Bone necrosis occurs as a result of endarteritis obliterans. Overlying tissue breakdown can occur without cause or because of trauma such as dental extraction.

Conclusion

Recognition and proper assessment of pain continue to challenge health care providers. Although strides have been made to accept pain as the fifth vital sign, it is still ignored or undertreated by many clinicians. Cancer patients develop complex pain syndromes. Proper recognition and assessment can guide therapy. Optimal pain treatment is an essential component of cancer care.

References

1. Cleeland CS, Nakamura Y, Mendoza TR, et al. Dimensions of the impact of cancer pain in a four country sample: new information from multidimensional scaling. Pain 67:267–73, 1996.
2. Tanaka K, Akechi T, Okuyama T, et al. Impact of dyspnea, pain and fatigue on daily life activities in ambulatory patients with advanced lung cancer. J Pain Symptom Manage 23:417–423, 2002.
3. Bonica JJ, Ventafridda V, Twycross RG. Cancer pain. In: Bonica JJ, ed. The management of pain, 2nd ed., vol. 1. Philadelphia: Lea & Febiger, 1990:400–60.
4. Allebeck P, Bolund C. Suicides and suicide attempts in cancer patients. Psychol Med 21(4):979–84, 1991.
5. Baile WF, DiMaggio JR, Schapira DV, Janofsky JS. The request for assistance in dying. The need for psychiatric consultation. Cancer 72(9):2786–91, 1993.
6. Breitbart W. Cancer pain and suicide. In: Foley KM, Bonica JJ, Ventafridda V, eds. Second International Congress on Cancer Pain. Advances in pain research and therapy, vol. 16. New York: Raven Press, 1990:399–412.
7. Cleeland CS. The impact of pain on the patient with cancer. Cancer 54(11 Suppl):2635–41, 1984.
8. Goldstein FJ. Inadequate pain management: a suicidogen (Dr. Jack Kevorkian: friend or foe?). J Clin Pharmacol 37(1):1–3, 1997.
9. Henderson JM, Ord RA. Suicide in head and neck cancer patients. J Oral Maxillofac Surg 55(11):1217–22, 1997.
10. Van Duynhoven V. Patients need compassionate pain control. An alternative to physician-assisted suicide. Oregon Nurse 59(3):11, 1994.
11. Cherny NI, Catane R. Professional negligence in the management of cancer pain. A case for urgent reforms [editorial; comment]. Cancer 76(11):2181–5, 1995.
12. Edwards RB. Pain management and the values of health care providers. In: Hill CS, Fields WS, eds. Drug treatment of cancer pain in a drug oriented society. Advances in pain research and therapy, vol. 11. New York: Raven Press, 1989:101–12.
13. Emanuel EJ. Pain and symptom control. Patient rights and physician responsibilities. Hematol Oncol Clin North Am 10(1):41–56, 1996.
14. Haugen PS. Pain relief. Legal aspects of pain relief for the dying. Minn Med 80(11):15–8, 1997.
15. Stjernsward J, Colleau SM, Ventafridda V. The World Health Organization Cancer Pain and Palliative Care Program. Past, present, and future. J Pain Symptom Manage 12(2):65–72, 1996.
16. Grossman SA, Sheidler VR, Swedeen K, et al. Correlation of patient and caregiver ratings of cancer pain. J Pain Symptom Manage 6(2):53–7, 1991.
17. Von Roenn JH, Cleeland CS, Gonin R, et al. Physician attitudes and practice in cancer pain management. A survey from the Eastern Cooperative Oncology Group. Ann Intern Med 119(2):121–6, 1993.
18. Cherny NJ, Chang V, Frager G, et al. Opioid pharmacotherapy in the management of cancer pain: a survey of strategies used by pain physicians for the selection of analgesic drugs and routes of administration. Cancer 76(7):1283–93, 1995.
19. Cervero F. Visceral nociception: peripheral and central aspects of visceral nociceptive systems. Philos Trans R Soc Lond B Biol Sci 308(1136):325–37, 1985.
20. Giamberardino MA, Vecchiet L. Visceral pain, referred hyperalgesia and outcome: new concepts. Eur J Anaesthesiol Suppl 10:61–6, 1995.
21. Coyle N, Adelhardt J, Foley KM, Portenoy RK. Character of terminal illness in the advanced cancer patient: pain and other symptoms during the last four weeks of life. J Pain Symptom Manage 5(2):83–93, 1990.
22. Reuben DB, Mor V, Hiris J. Clinical symptoms and length of survival in patients with terminal cancer. Arch Intern Med 148(7):1586–91, 1988.
23. Ventafridda V, Ripamonti C, De Conno F, et al. Symptom prevalence and control during cancer patients' last days of life. J Palliat 6(3):7–11, 1990.
24. Caraceni A, Portenoy RK. An international survey of cancer pain characteristics and syndromes. IASP Task Force on Cancer Pain. Pain 82:263–74, 1999.
25. Portenoy RK. Pain syndromes in patients with cancer and HIV/AIDS. In: Portenoy RK, ed. Contemporary diagnosis and management of pain in oncologic and AIDS patients, 3rd ed. Newtown, PA: Handbooks in Healthcare Co., 2000:49–78.
26. Banning A, Sjogren P, Henriksen H. Pain causes in 200 patients referred to a multidisciplinary cancer pain clinic. Pain 45(1):45–8, 1991.
27. Grond S, Zech D, Diefenbach C, et al. Assessment of cancer pain: a prospective evaluation in 2266 cancer patients referred to a pain service. Pain 64(1):107–14, 1996.
28. Miaskowski C, Dibble SL. The problem of pain in outpatients with breast cancer. Oncol Nurs Forum 22(5):791–7, 1995.
29. Portenoy RK, Miransky J, Thaler HT, et al. Pain in ambulatory patients with lung or colon cancer. Prevalence, characteristics, and effect. Cancer 70(6):1616–24, 1992.
30. Twycross R. Cancer pain classification. Acta Anaesthesiol Scand 41(1 Pt 2):141–5, 1997.
31. Twycross R, Harcourt J, Bergl S. A survey of pain in patients with advanced cancer. J Pain Symptom Manage 12(5):273–82, 1996.
32. Morewood GH. A rational approach to the cause, prevention and treatment of postdural puncture headache [see comments]. CMAJ 149(8):1087–93, 1993.
33. Fink BR. Postspinal headache [letter]. Anesth Analg 71(2):208–9, 1990.

34. Kempen PM, Mocek CK. Bevel direction, dura geometry, and hole size in membrane puncture: laboratory report. Reg Anesth 22(3):267–72, 1997.

35. Leibold RA, Yealy DM, Coppola M, Cantees KK. Post-dural-puncture headache: characteristics, management, and prevention. Ann Emerg Med 22(12):1863–70, 1993.

36. Bonica JJ. Headache and other visceral disorders of the head and neck. In: Bonica JJ, ed. The management of pain, 1st ed. Philadelphia: Lea & Febiger, 1983: 1263–309.

37. Evans RW. Complications of lumbar puncture. Neurol Clin 16(1):83–105, 1998.

38. Lybecker H, Djernes M, Schmidt JF. Postdural puncture headache (PDPH): onset, duration, severity, and associated symptoms. An analysis of 75 consecutive patients with PDPH. Acta Anaesthesiol Scand 39(5):605–12, 1995.

39. Jones HM, Conces DJ Jr, Tarver RD. Painful transthoracic needle biopsy: a sign of neurogenic tumor. J Thorac Imag 8(3):230–2, 1993.

40. Irani J, Fournier F, Bon D, et al. Patient tolerance of transrectal ultrasound-guided biopsy of the prostate. Br J Urol 79(4):608–10, 1997.

41. Nash PA, Bruce JE, Indudhara R, Shinohara K. Transrectal ultrasound guided prostatic nerve blockade eases systematic needle biopsy of the prostate. J Urol 155(2):607–9, 1996.

42. Agency for Health Care Policy and Research. Acute Pain Management Panel. Acute pain management: operative or medical procedures and trauma. Clinical practice guidelines. Washington, DC: U.S. Dept. of Health and Human Services, 1992.

43. Ready LB. The treatment of post-operative pain. In: Bond MR, Charlton JE, Woolf CJ, eds. Proceedings of the VIth World Congress on Pain. Pain Research and Clinical Management, vol. 4. Amsterdam: Elsevier, 1991:51–8.

44. Harper DM. Pain and cramping associated with cryosurgery. J Fam Pract 39(6):551–7, 1994.

45. Chen C, Chen PJ, Yang PM, et al. Clinical and microbiological features of liver abscess after transarterial embolization for hepatocellular carcinoma. Am J Gastroenterol 92(12):2257–9, 1997.

46. Sanz-Altamira PM, Spence LD, Huberman MS, et al. Selective chemoembolization in the management of hepatic metastases in refractory colorectal carcinoma: a phase II trial. Dis Colon Rectum 40(7):770–5, 1997.

47. Prevost A, Nazeyrollas P, Milosevic D, Fernandez-Valoni A. Malignant pleural effusions treated with high dose intrapleural doxycycline: clinical efficacy and tolerance. Oncol Rep 5(2):363–6, 1998.

48. Walker-Renard PB, Vaughan LM, Sahn SA. Chemical pleurodesis for malignant pleural effusions [see comments]. Ann Intern Med 120(1):56–64, 1994.

49. Palmon SC, Lloyd AT, Kirsch JR. The effect of needle gauge and lidocaine pH on pain during intradermal injection. Anesth Analg 86(2):379–81, 1998.

50. Agency for Health Care Policy and Research: Management of cancer pain: adults. Cancer Pain Guideline Panel. Agency for Health Care Policy and Research. Am Fam Physician 49(8):1853–68, 1994.

51. Bruera E, Fainsinger R, Moore M, et al. Local toxicity with subcutaneous methadone. Experience of two centers. Pain 45(2):141–3, 1991.

52. Shvartzman P, Bonneh D. Local skin irritation in the course of subcutaneous morphine infusion: a challenge. J Palliat Care 10(1):44–5, 1994.

53. Cartwright PD, Hesse C, Jackson AO. Myoclonic spasms following intrathecal diamorphine. J Pain Symptom Manage 8(7):492–5, 1993.

54. De Conno F, Caraceni A, Martini C, et al. Hyperalgesia and myoclonus with intrathecal infusion of high-dose morphine. Pain 47(3):337–9, 1991.

55. Glavina MJ, Robertshaw R. Myoclonic spasms following intrathecal morphine. Anaesthesia 43(5):389–90, 1988.

56. De Castro MD, Meynadier MD, Zenz MD. Regional opioid analgesia. Developments in critical care medicine and anesthesiology, vol. 20. Dordrecht: Kluwer Academic Publishers, 1991.

57. Hundrieser J. A non-invasive approach to minimizing vessel pain with DTIC or BCNU. Oncol Nurs Forum 15(2):199, 1988.

58. Mrozek-Orlowski M, Christie J, Flamme C, Novak J. Pain associated with peripheral infusion of carmustine. Oncol Nurs Forum 18(5):942, 1991.

59. Rittenberg CN, Gralla RJ, Rehmeyer TA. Assessing and managing venous irritation associated with vinorelbine tartrate (Navelbine). Oncol Nurs Forum 22(4):707–10, 1995.

60. Pucino F, Danielson BD, Carlson JD, et al. Patient tolerance to intravenous potassium chloride with and without lidocaine. Drug Intell Clin Pharm 22(9):676–9, 1988.

61. Bertelli G. Prevention and management of extravasation of cytotoxic drugs. Drug Saf 12(4):245–55, 1995.

62. Boyle DM, Engelking C. Vesicant extravasation: myths and realities. Oncol Nurs Forum 22(1):57–67, 1995.

63. Curran CF, Luce JK, Page JA. Doxorubicin-associated flare reactions. Oncol Nurs Forum 17(3):387–9, 1990.

64. Vogelzang NJ. "Adriamycin flare:" a skin reaction resembling extravasation. Cancer Treat Rep 63(11–12):2067–9, 1979.

65. Batts KP. Ischemic cholangitis. Mayo Clin Proc 73(4):380–5, 1998.

66. Kemeny N. Review of regional therapy of liver metastases in colorectal cancer. Semin Oncol 19(2 Suppl 3):155–62, 1992.

67. Almadrones L, Yerys C. Problems associated with the administration of intraperitoneal therapy using the Port-A-Cath system. Oncol Nurs Forum 17(1):75–80, 1990.

68. Markman M. Cytotoxic intracavitary chemotherapy. Am J Med Sci 291(3):175–9, 1986.

69. Topuz E, Aydiner A, Saip P, et al. Intraperitoneal cisplatin—mitoxantrone in ovarian cancer patients with minimal residual disease. Eur J Gynaecol Oncol 18(1):71–5, 1997.

70. Deppe G, Malviya VK, Boike G, Young J. Intraperitoneal doxorubicin in combination with systemic cisplatinum and

cyclophosphamide in the treatment of stage III ovarian cancer. Eur J Gynaecol Oncol 12(2):93–7, 1991.

71. Francis P, Rowinsky E, Schneider J, et al. Phase I feasibility and pharmacologic study of weekly intraperitoneal paclitaxel: a Gynecologic Oncology Group pilot Study. J Clin Oncol 13(12):2961–7, 1995.

72. Kaplan RA, Markman M, Lucas WE, et al. Infectious peritonitis in patients receiving intraperitoneal chemotherapy. Am J Med 78(1):49–53, 1985.

73. Kudo S, Tsushima N, Sawada Y, et al. [Serious complications of intravesical bacillus Calmette-Guerin therapy in patients with bladder cancer]. Nippon Hinyokika Gakkai Zasshi 82(10):1594–1602, 1991.

74. Uekado Y, Hirano A, Shinka T, Ohkawa T. The effects of intravesical chemo-immunotherapy with epirubicin and bacillus Calmette-Guerin for prophylaxis of recurrence of superficial bladder cancer: a preliminary report. Cancer Chemother Pharmacol 35(Suppl):S65–68, 1994.

75. Matsumura Y, Akaza H, Isaka S, et al. The 4th study of prophylactic intravesical chemotherapy with adriamycin in the treatment of superficial bladder cancer: the experience of the Japanese Urological Cancer Research Group for Adriamycin. Cancer Chemother Pharmacol 30(Suppl):S10–14, 1992.

76. Dose AM. The symptom experience of mucositis, stomatitis, and xerostomia. Semin Oncol Nurs 11(4):248–55, 1995.

77. Rider CA. Oral mucositis. A complication of radiotherapy. NY State Dental J 56(9):37–9, 1990.

78. Verdi CJ. Cancer therapy and oral mucositis. An appraisal of drug prophylaxis. Drug Saf 9(3):185–95, 1993.

79. Cascinu S, Fedeli A, Fedeli SL, Catalano G. Oral cooling (cryotherapy), an effective treatment for the prevention of 5-fluorouracil-induced stomatitis. Eur J Cancer B Oral Oncol 30B(4):234–36, 1994.

80. Rocke LK, Loprinzi CL, Lee JK, et al. A randomized clinical trial of two different durations of oral cryotherapy for prevention of 5-fluorouracil-related stomatitis. Cancer 72(7):2234–8, 1993.

81. Loprinzi CL, Ghosh C, Camoriano J, et al. Phase III controlled evaluation of sucralfate to alleviate stomatitis in patients receiving fluorouracil-based chemotherapy. J Clin Oncol 15(3):1235–8, 1997.

82. Feld R. The role of surveillance cultures in patients likely to develop chemotherapy-induced mucositis. Support Care Cancer 5(5):371–5, 1997.

83. Redding SW, Montgomery MT. Acyclovir prophylaxis for oral herpes simplex virus infection in patients with bone marrow transplants. Oral Surg Oral Med Oral Pathol 67(6):680–3, 1989.

84. Spijkervet FK, van Saene HK, van Saene JJ, et al. Mucositis prevention by selective elimination of oral flora in irradiated head and neck cancer patients. J Oral Pathol Med 19(10):486–9, 1990.

85. Chapman CR, Donaldson GW, Jacobson RC, Hautman B. Differences among patients in opioid self-administration during bone marrow transplantation. Pain 71(3):213–23, 1997.

86. Chapman CR, Hill HF. Prolonged morphine self-administration and addiction liability. Evaluation of two theories in a bone marrow transplant unit. Cancer 63(8):1636–44, 1989.

87. Coda BA, O'Sullivan B, Donaldson G, et al. Comparative efficacy of patient-controlled administration of morphine, hydromorphone, or sufentanil for the treatment of oral mucositis pain following bone marrow transplantation. Pain 72(3):333–46, 1997.

88. McCarthy GM, Skillings JR. Jaw and other orofacial pain in patients receiving vincristine for the treatment of cancer. Oral Surg Oral Med Oral Pathol 74(3):299–304, 1992.

89. Weiss HD, Walker MD, Wiernik PH. Neurotoxicity of commonly used antineoplastic agents (first of two parts). N Engl J Med 291(2):75–81, 1974.

90. Weiss HD, Walker MD, Wiernik PH. Neurotoxicity of commonly used antineoplastic agents (second of two parts). N Engl J Med 291(3):127–33, 1974.

91. Priest JR, Ramsay NK, Steinherz PG, et al. A syndrome of thrombosis and hemorrhage complicating L-asparaginase therapy for childhood acute lymphoblastic leukemia. J Pediatr 100(6):984–9, 1982.

92. Schick RM, Jolesz F, Barnes PD, Macklis JD. MR diagnosis of dural venous sinus thrombosis complicating L-asparaginase therapy. Comput Med Imag Graph 13(4):319–27, 1989.

93. Visani G, Bontempo G, Manfroi S, et al. All-trans-retinoic acid and pseudotumor cerebri in a young adult with acute promyelocytic leukemia: a possible disease association [see comments]. Haematologica 81(2):152–4, 1996.

94. Castaigne S, Chomienne C, Daniel MT, et al. All-trans retinoic acid as a differentiation therapy for acute promyelocytic leukemia. I. Clinical results [see comments]. Blood 76(9):1704–9, 1990.

95. Ohno R, Yoshida H, Fukutani H, et al. Multi-institutional study of all-trans-retinoic acid as a differentiation therapy of refractory acute promyelocytic leukemia. Leukaemia Study Group of the Ministry of Health and Welfare. Leukemia 7(11):1722–7, 1993.

96. Hollingshead LM, Goa KL. Recombinant granulocyte colony-stimulating factor (rG-CSF). A review of its pharmacological properties and prospective role in neutropenic conditions. Drugs 42:300–30, 1991.

97. Muggia FM, Vafai D, Natale R, et al. Paclitaxel 3-hour infusion given alone and combined with carboplatin: preliminary results of dose-escalation trials. Semin Oncol 22(4 Suppl 9):63–6, 1995.

98. Rowinsky EK, Chaudhry V, Cornblath DR, Donehower RC. Neurotoxicity of taxol. J Natl Cancer Inst Monogr (15):107–15, 1993.

99. Eskilsson J, Albertsson M. Failure of preventing 5-fluorouracil cardiotoxicity by prophylactic treatment with verapamil. Acta Oncol 29(8):1001–3, 1990.

100. Freeman NJ, Costanza ME. 5-Fluorouracil-associated cardiotoxicity. Cancer 61(1):36–45, 1988.

101. Rezkalla S, Kloner RA, Ensley J, et al. Continuous ambulatory ECG monitoring during fluorouracil therapy: a prospective study. J Clin Oncol 7(4):509–14, 1989.

102. Leo S, Tatulli C, Taveri R, et al. Dermatological toxicity from chemotherapy containing 5-fluorouracil. J Chemother 6(6):423–6, 1994.

103. Lokich JJ, Moore C. Chemotherapy-associated palmar-plantar erythrodysesthesia syndrome. Ann Intern Med 101(6):798–99, 1984.

104. Alberts DS, Garcia DJ. Safety aspects of pegylated liposomal doxorubicin in patients with cancer. Drugs 54(Suppl 4):30–5, 1997.

105. Uziely B, Jeffers S, Isacson R, et al. Liposomal doxorubicin: antitumor activity and unique toxicities during two complementary phase I studies. J Clin Oncol 13(7):1777–85, 1995.

106. Aki FT, Tekin MI, Ozen H. Gynecomastia as a complication of chemotherapy for testicular germ cell tumors. Urology 48(6):944–6, 1996.

107. Trump DL, Pavy MD, Staal S. Gynecomastia in men following antineoplastic therapy. Arch Intern Med 142(3):511–3, 1982.

108. Saeter G, Fossa SD, Norman N. Gynaecomastia following cytotoxic therapy for testicular cancer. Br J Urol 59(4):348–52, 1987.

109. Trump DL, Anderson SA. Painful gynecomastia following cytotoxic therapy for testis cancer: a potentially favorable prognostic sign? J Clin Oncol 1(7):416–20, 1983.

110. Aass N, Kaasa S, Lund E, et al. Long-term somatic side-effects and morbidity in testicular cancer patients. Br J Cancer 61(1):151–5, 1990.

111. Elomaa I, Pajunen M, Virkkunen P. Raynaud's phenomenon progressing to gangrene after vincristine and bleomycin therapy. Acta Med Scand 216(3):323–6, 1984.

112. Chrisp P, Goa KL. Goserelin. A review of its pharmacodynamic and pharmacokinetic properties, and clinical use in sex hormone-related conditions. Drugs 41(2):254–88, 1991.

113. Chrisp P, Sorkin EM. Leuprorelin. A review of its pharmacology and therapeutic use in prostatic disorders. Drugs Aging 1(6):487–509, 1991.

114. Thompson IM, Zeidman EJ, Rodriguez FR. Sudden death due to disease flare with luteinizing hormone-releasing hormone agonist therapy for carcinoma of the prostate [see comments]. J Urol 144(6):1479–80, 1990.

115. Plotkin D, Lechner JJ, Jung WE, Rosen PJ. Tamoxifen flare in advanced breast cancer. JAMA 240(24):2644–6, 1978.

116. Reddel RR, Sutherland RL. Tamoxifen stimulation of human breast cancer cell proliferation in vitro: a possible model for tamoxifen tumour flare. Eur J Cancer Clin Oncol 20(11):1419–24, 1984.

117. Quesada JR, Talpaz M, Rios A, et al. Clinical toxicity of interferons in cancer patients: a review. J Clin Oncol 4(2):234–43, 1986.

118. Veldhuis GJ, Willemse PH, van Gameren MM, et al. Recombinant human interleukin-3 to dose-intensify carboplatin and cyclophosphamide chemotherapy in epithelial ovarian cancer: a phase I trial. J Clin Oncol 13(3):733–40, 1995.

119. Vial T, Descotes J. Clinical toxicity of cytokines used as haemopoietic growth factors. Drug Saf 13(6):371–406, 1995.

120. Frenken LA, van Lier HJ, Gerlag PG, et al. Assessment of pain after subcutaneous injection of erythropoietin in patients receiving haemodialysis. BMJ 303(6797):288, 1991.

121. Morris KP, Hughes C, Hardy SP, et al. Pain after subcutaneous injection of recombinant human erythropoietin: does Emla cream help? Nephrol Dial Transplant 9(9):1299–1301, 1994.

122. Alon US, Allen S, Rameriz Z, et al. Lidocaine for the alleviation of pain associated with subcutaneous erythropoietin injection. J Am Soc Nephrol 5(4):1161–2, 1994.

123. Epstein JB, Stewart KH. Radiation therapy and pain in patients with head and neck cancer. Eur J Cancer B Oral Oncol 29B(3):191–9, 1993.

124. Yeoh E, Horowitz M. Radiation enteritis. Br J Hosp Med 39(6):498–504, 1988.

125. Babb RR. Radiation proctitis: a review. Am J Gastroenterol 91(7):1309–11, 1996.

126. Pierce SM, Recht A, Lingos TI, et al. Long-term radiation complications following conservative surgery (CS) and radiation therapy (RT) in patients with early stage breast cancer [see comments]. Int J Radiat Oncol Biol Phys 23(5):915–23, 1992.

127. Salner AL, Botnick LE, Herzog AG, et al. Reversible brachial plexopathy following primary radiation therapy for breast cancer. Cancer Treat Rep 65(9–10):797–802, 1981.

128. Ang KK, Stephens LC. Prevention and management of radiation myelopathy. Oncology 8(11):71–82, 1994.

129. Schultheiss TE. Spinal cord radiation tolerance [editorial]. Int J Radiat Oncol Biol Phys 30(3):735–6, 1994.

130. McEwan AJ. Unsealed source therapy of painful bone metastases: an update. Semin Nucl Med 27(2):165–82, 1997.

131. Robinson RG, Preston DF, Schiefelbein M, Baxter KG. Strontium 89 therapy for the palliation of pain due to osseous metastases. JAMA 274(5):420–4, 1995.

132. Portenoy RK, Duma C, Foley KM. Acute herpetic and postherpetic neuralgia: clinical review and current management. Ann Neurol 20(6):651–64, 1986.

133. Rusthoven JJ, Ahlgren P, Elhakim T, et al. Varicella-zoster infection in adult cancer patients. A population study. Arch Intern Med 148(7):1561–6, 1988.

134. Agnelli G. Venous thromboembolism and cancer: a two-way clinical association. Thromb Haemost 78(1):117–20, 1997.

135. Donati MB. Cancer and thrombosis. Haemostasis 24(2):128–31, 1994.

136. Clarke-Pearson DL, Olt G. Thromboembolism in patients with Gyn tumors: risk factors, natural history, and prophylaxis. Oncology 3(1):39–48, 1989.

137. Heinmoller E, Schropp T, Kisker O, et al. Tumor cell-induced platelet aggregation in vitro by human pancreatic cancer cell lines. Scand J Gastroenterol 30(10):1008–16, 1995.

138. Levine M, Hirsh J, Gent M, et al. Double-blind randomised trial of a very-low-dose warfarin for prevention of thromboembolism in stage IV breast cancer [see comments]. Lancet 343(8902):886–9, 1994.

139. Sawaya RE, Ligon BL. Thromboembolic complications associated with brain tumors. J Neurooncol 22(2):173–81, 1994.

140. Criado E, Burnham CB. Predictive value of clinical criteria for the diagnosis of deep vein thrombosis. Surgery 122(3):578–83, 1997.

141. Wells PS, Hirsh J, Anderson DR, et al. Comparison of the accuracy of impedance plethysmography and compression ultrasonography in outpatients with clinically suspected deep vein thrombosis. A two centre paired-design prospective trial. Thromb Haemost 74(6):1423–7, 1995.

142. Hirschmann JV. Ischemic forms of acute venous thrombosis. Arch Dermatol 123(7):933–66, 1987.

143. Perkins JM, Magee TR, Galland RB. Phlegmasia caerulea dolens and venous gangrene [see comments]. Br J Surg 83(1):19–23, 1996.

144. Nemmers DW, Thorpe PE, Knibbe MA, Beard DW. Upper extremity venous thrombosis. Case report and literature review. Orthop Rev 19(2):164–72, 1990.

145. Burihan E, de Figueiredo LF, Francisco J Jr, Miranda F Jr. Upper-extremity deep venous thrombosis: analysis of 52 cases. Cardiovasc Surg 1(1):19–22, 1993.

146. Donayre CE, White GH, Mehringer SM, Wilson SE. Pathogenesis determines late morbidity of axillosubclavian vein thrombosis. Am J Surg 152(2):179–84, 1986.

147. Escalante CP. Causes and management of superior vena cava syndrome. Oncology 7(6):61–77, 1993.

148. Daut RL, Cleeland CS. The prevalence and severity of pain in cancer. Cancer 50(9):1913–8, 1982.

149. Foley KM. Pain syndromes in patients with cancer. Med Clin North Am 71(2):169–84, 1987.

150. Mercadante S. Malignant bone pain: pathophysiology and treatment. Pain 69(1–2):1–18, 1997.

151. Phillips E, Levine AM. Metastatic lesions of the upper cervical spine. Spine 14(10):1071–7, 1989.

152. Feldenzer JA, McGauley JL, McGillicuddy JE. Sacral and presacral tumors: problems in diagnosis and management. Neurosurgery 25(6):884–91, 1989.

153. Hall JH, Fleming JF. The "lumbar disc syndrome" produced by sacral metastases. Can J Surg 13(2):149–56, 1970.

154. Porter AD, Simpson AH, Davis AM, et al. Diagnosis and management of sacral bone tumours [see comments]. Can J Surg 37(6):473–8, 1994.

155. Posner JB. Back pain and epidural spinal cord compression. Med Clin North Am 71(2):185–205, 1987.

156. Barcena A, Lobato RD, Rivas JJ, et al. Spinal metastatic disease: analysis of factors determining functional prognosis and the choice of treatment. Neurosurgery 15(6):820–7, 1984.

157. Gilbert RW, Kim JH, Posner JB. Epidural spinal cord compression from metastatic tumor: diagnosis and treatment. Ann Neurol 3(1):40–51, 1978.

158. Huddart RA, Rajan B, Law M, et al. Spinal cord compression in prostate cancer: treatment outcome and prognostic factors. Radiother Oncol 44(3):229–36, 1997.

159. Maranzano E, Latini P. Effectiveness of radiation therapy without surgery in metastatic spinal cord compression: final results from a prospective trial [see comments]. Int J Radiat Oncol Biol Phys 32(4):959–67, 1995.

160. Milross CG, Davies MA, Fisher R, et al. The efficacy of treatment for malignant epidural spinal cord compression. Australas Radiol 41(2):137–42, 1997.

161. Portenoy RK, Galer BS, Salamon O, et al. Identification of epidural neoplasm. Radiography and bone scintigraphy in the symptomatic and asymptomatic spine. Cancer 64(11):2207–13, 1989.

162. Rosenthal MA, Rosen D, Raghavan D, et al. Spinal cord compression in prostate cancer. A 10-year experience. Br J Urol 69(5):530–3, 1992.

163. Ruff RL, Lanska DJ. Epidural metastases in prospectively evaluated veterans with cancer and back pain. Cancer 63(11):2234–41, 1989.

164. Grant R, Papadopoulos SM, Sandler HM, Greenberg HS. Metastatic epidural spinal cord compression: current concepts and treatment. J Neurooncol 19(1):79–92, 1994.

165. Harris JK, Sutcliffe JC, Robinson NE. The role of emergency surgery in malignant spinal extradural compression: assessment of functional outcome. Br J Neurosurg 10(1):27–33, 1996.

166. Weinstein SM, Portenoy RK. Back pain in the cancer patient. In: Vecht CJ, ed. Handbook of clinical neurology, vol. 25(69): Neuro-Oncology, Part III. Amsterdam: Elsevier Science, 1997:57–70.

167. Haddad P, Thaell JF, Kiely JM, et al. Lymphoma of the spinal extradural space. Cancer 38(4):1862–6, 1976.

168. Perry JR, Deodhare SS, Bilbao JM, et al. The significance of spinal cord compression as the initial manifestation of lymphoma. Neurosurgery 32(2):157–62, 1993.

169. Martinez-Lavin M. Hypertrophic osteoarthropathy. Curr Opin Rheumatol 9(1):83–6, 1997.

170. Briselli M, Mark EJ, Dickersin GR. Solitary fibrous tumors of the pleura: eight new cases and review of 360 cases in the literature. Cancer 47(11):2678–89, 1981.

171. Shapiro JS. Breast cancer presenting as periostitis. Postgrad Med 82(4):139–40, 1987.

172. Greenfield GB, Schorsch HA, Shkolnik A. The various roentgen appearances of pulmonary hypertrophic osteoarthropathy. Am J Roentgenol Radium Ther Nucl Med 101(4):927–31, 1967.

173. Sharma OP. Symptoms and signs in pulmonary medicine: old observations and new interpretations. Dis Mon 41(9):577–638, 1995.

174. Araki K, Kobayashi M, Ogata T, Takuma K. Colorectal carcinoma metastatic to skeletal muscle. Hepatogastroenterology 41(5):405–8, 1994.

175. Sridhar KS, Rao RK, Kunhardt B. Skeletal muscle metastases from lung cancer. Cancer 59(8):1530–4, 1987.

176. Siegal T. Muscle cramps in the cancer patient: causes and treatment. J Pain Symptom Manage 6(2):84–91, 1991.

177. Forsyth PA, Posner JB. Headaches in patients with brain tumors: a study of 111 patients. Neurology 43(9):1678–83, 1993.

178. Suwanwela N, Phanthumchinda K, Kaoropthum S. Headache in brain tumor: a cross-sectional study. Headache 34(7):435–8, 1994.

179. Medina LS, Pinter JD, Zurakowski D, et al. Children with headache: clinical predictors of surgical space-occupying lesions and the role of neuroimaging. Radiology 202(3):819–24, 1997.

180. Hayashi M, Handa Y, Kobayashi H, et al. Plateau-wave phenomenon (I). Correlation between the appearance of plateau waves and CSF circulation in patients with intracranial hypertension. Brain 114(Pt 6):2681–91, 1991.

181. Matsuda M, Yoneda S, Handa H, Gotoh H. Cerebral hemodynamic changes during plateau waves in brain-tumor patients. J Neurosurg 50(4):483–8, 1979.

182. Grossman SA, Moynihan TJ. Neoplastic meningitis. Neurol Clin 9(4):843–56, 1991.

183. Jayson GC, Howell A. Carcinomatous meningitis in solid tumours. Ann Oncol 7(8):773–86, 1996.

184. Wasserstrom WR, Glass JP, Posner JB. Diagnosis and treatment of leptomeningeal metastases from solid tumors: experience with 90 patients. Cancer 49(4):759–72, 1982.

185. Kaplan JG, DeSouza TG, Farkash A, et al. Leptomeningeal metastases: comparison of clinical features and laboratory data of solid tumors, lymphomas and leukemias. J Neurooncol 9(3):225–9, 1990.

186. DeAngelis LM, Payne R. Lymphomatous meningitis presenting as atypical cluster headache. Pain 30(2):211–6, 1987.

187. Olson ME, Chernik NL, Posner JB. Infiltration of the leptomeninges by systemic cancer. A clinical and pathologic study. Arch Neurol 30(2):122–37, 1974.

188. Twijnstra A, Ongerboer de Visser BW, van Zanten AP. Diagnosis of leptomeningeal metastasis. Clin Neurol Neurosurg 89(2):79–85, 1987.

189. Bach F, Soletormos G, Dombernowsky P. Tissue polypeptide antigen activity in cerebrospinal fluid: a marker of central nervous system metastases of breast cancer. J Natl Cancer Inst 83(11):779–84, 1991.

190. Freilich RJ, Krol G, DeAngelis LM. Neuroimaging and cerebrospinal fluid cytology in the diagnosis of leptomeningeal metastasis. Ann Neurol 38(1):51–7, 1995.

191. Balm M, Hammack J. Leptomeningeal carcinomatosis. Presenting features and prognostic factors [see comments]. Arch Neurol 53(7):626–32, 1996.

192. Greenberg HS, Deck MD, Vikram B, et al. Metastasis to the base of the skull: clinical findings in 43 patients. Neurology 31(5):530–7, 1981.

193. Bitoh S, Hasegawa H, Ohtsuki H, et al. Parasellar metastases: four autopsied cases. Surg Neurol 23(1):41–8, 1985.

194. Lossos A, Siegal T. Numb chin syndrome in cancer patients: etiology, response to treatment, and prognostic significance [see comments]. Neurology 42(6):1181–84, 1992.

195. Bullitt E, Tew JM, Boyd J. Intracranial tumors in patients with facial pain. J Neurosurg 64(6):865–71, 1986.

196. Loevner LA, Yousem DM. Overlooked metastatic lesions of the occipital condyle: a missed case treasure trove. Radiographics 17(5):1111–21, 1997.

197. Moris G, Roig C, Misiego M, et al. The distinctive headache of the occipital condyle syndrome: a report of four cases. Headache 38(4):308–11, 1998.

198. Lawson W, Reino AJ. Isolated sphenoid sinus disease: an analysis of 132 cases. Laryngoscope 107(12 Pt 1):1590–5, 1997.

199. Aird DW, Bihari J, Smith C. Clinical problems in the continuing care of head and neck cancer patients. Ear Nose Throat J 62(5):230–43, 1983.

200. Talmi YP, Waller A, Bercovici M, et al. Pain experienced by patients with terminal head and neck carcinoma. Cancer 80(6):1117–23, 1997.

201. Morrison GA, Sterkers JM. Unusual presentations of acoustic tumours. Clin Otolaryngol 21(1):80–3, 1996.

202. Hill BA, Kohut RI. Metastatic adenocarcinoma of the temporal bone. Arch Otolaryngol 102(9):568–71, 1976.

203. Shapshay SM, Elber E, Strong MS. Occult tumors of the infratemporal fossa: report of seven cases appearing as preauricular facial pain. Arch Otolaryngol 102(9):535–8, 1976.

204. Hayreh SS, Blodi FC, Silbermann NN, et al. Unilateral optic nerve head and choroidal metastases from a bronchial carcinoma. Ophthalmologica 185(4):232–41, 1982.

205. Servodidio CA, Abramson DH. Presenting signs and symptoms of choroidal melanoma: what do they mean? Ann Ophthalmol 24(5):190–4, 1992.

206. Swanson MW. Ocular metastatic disease. Optom Clin 3(3):79–99, 1993.

207. Friedman J, Karesh J, Rodrigues M, Sun CC. Thyroid carcinoma metastatic to the medial rectus muscle. Ophthalmol Plast Reconstr Surg 6(2):122–5, 1990.

208. Weiss R, Grisold W, Jellinger K, et al. Metastasis of solid tumors in extraocular muscles. Acta Neuropathol (Berl) 65(2):168–71, 1984.

209. Laitt RD, Kumar B, Leatherbarrow B, et al. Cystic optic nerve meningioma presenting with acute proptosis. Eye 10(Pt 6):744–6, 1996.

210. Gupta SR, Zdonczyk DE, Rubino FA. Cranial neuropathy in systemic malignancy in a VA population [see comments]. Neurology 40(6):997–9, 1990.

211. Sozzi G, Marotta P, Piatti L. Vagoglossopharyngeal neuralgia with syncope in the course of carcinomatous meningitis. Ital J Neurol Sci 8(3):271–5, 1987.

212. Dykman TR, Montgomery EB Jr, Gerstenberger PD, et al. Glossopharyngeal neuralgia with syncope secondary to tumor. Treatment and pathophysiology. Am J Med 71(1):165–70, 1981.

213. Giorgi C, Broggi G. Surgical treatment of glossopharyngeal neuralgia and pain from cancer of the nasopharynx. A 20-year experience. J Neurosurg 61(5):952–5, 1984.

214. Metheetrairut C, Brown DH. Glossopharyngeal neuralgia and syncope secondary to neck malignancy. J Otolaryngol 22(1):18–20, 1993.

215. Barker FG II, Jannetta PJ, Babu RP, et al. Long-term outcome after operation for trigeminal neuralgia in patients with posterior fossa tumors. J Neurosurg 84(5):818–25, 1996.

216. Cheng TM, Cascino TL, Onofrio BM. Comprehensive study of diagnosis and treatment of trigeminal neuralgia secondary to tumors. Neurology 43(11):2298–302, 1993.

217. Hirota N, Fujimoto T, Takahashi M, Fukushima Y. Isolated trigeminal nerve metastases from breast cancer: an unusual cause of trigeminal mononeuropathy [In Process Citation]. Surg Neurol 49(5):558–61, 1998.

218. Payten RJ. Facial pain as the first symptom in acoustic neuroma. J Laryngol Otol 86(5):523–34, 1972.

219. Jaeckle KA. Nerve plexus metastases. Neurol Clin 9(4):857–66, 1991.

220. Kori SH. Diagnosis and management of brachial plexus lesions in cancer patients. Oncology 9(8):756–65, 1995.

221. Cascino TL, Kori S, Krol G, Foley KM. CT of the brachial plexus in patients with cancer. Neurology 33(12):1553–57, 1983.

222. Chad DA, Bradley WG. Lumbosacral plexopathy. Semin Neurol 7(1):97–107, 1987.

223. Jaeckle KA, Young DF, Foley KM. The natural history of lumbosacral plexopathy in cancer. Neurology 35(1):8–15, 1985.

224. Dalmau J, Graus F, Marco M. 'Hot and dry foot' as initial manifestation of neoplastic lumbosacral plexopathy. Neurology 39(6):871–2, 1989.

225. Evans RJ, Watson CPN. Lumbosacral plexopathy in cancer patients. Neurology 35:1392–3, 1985.

226. Taylor BV, Kimmel DW, Krecke KN, Cascino TL. Magnetic resonance imaging in cancer-related lumbosacral plexopathy. Mayo Clin Proc 72(9):823–9, 1997.

227. Desta K, O'Shaughnessy M, Milling MA. Non-Hodgkin's lymphoma presenting as median nerve compression in the arm. J Hand Surg [Br] 19(3):289–91, 1994.

228. Brady AM. Management of painful paraneoplastic syndromes. Hematol Oncol Clin North Am 10(4):801–9, 1996.

229. Peterson K, Forsyth PA, Posner JB. Paraneoplastic sensorimotor neuropathy associated with breast cancer. J Neurooncol 21(2):159–70, 1994.

230. Plante-Bordeneuve V, Baudrimont M, Gorin NC, Gherardi RK. Subacute sensory neuropathy associated with Hodgkin's disease. J Neurol Sci 121(2):155–8, 1994.

231. Kissel JT, Mendell JR. Neuropathies associated with monoclonal gammopathies. Neuromuscul Disord 6(1):3–18, 1996.

232. Dalmau JO, Posner JB. Paraneoplastic syndromes affecting the nervous system. Semin Oncol 24(3):318–28, 1997.

233. Coombs DW. Pain due to liver capsular distention. In: Ferrer-Brechner T, ed. Common problems in pain management. Common problems in anesthesia. Chicago: Year Book Medical Publishers, 1990:247–53.

234. De Conno F, Polastri D. [Clinical features and symptomatic treatment of liver metastasis in the terminally ill patient]. Ann Ital Chir 67(6):819–26, 1996.

235. Mulholland MW, Debas H, Bonica JJ. Diseases of the liver, biliary system and pancreas. In: Bonica JJ, ed. The management of pain, vol. 2. Philadelphia: Lea & Febiger, 1990:1214–31.

236. Grahm AL, Andren-Sandberg A. Prospective evaluation of pain in exocrine pancreatic cancer. Digestion 58(6):542–9, 1997.

237. Kelsen DP, Portenoy R, Thaler H, et al. Pain as a predictor of outcome in patients with operable pancreatic carcinoma. Surgery 122(1):53–9, 1997.

238. Kelsen DP, Portenoy RK, Thaler HT, et al. Pain and depression in patients with newly diagnosed pancreas cancer. J Clin Oncol 13(3):748–55, 1995.

239. Schonenberg P, Bastid C, Guedes J, Sahel J. [Percutaneous echography-guided alcohol block of the celiac plexus as treatment of painful syndromes of the upper abdomen: study of 21 cases]. Schweiz Med Wochenschr 121(15):528–31, 1991.

240. Baines MJ. Intestinal obstruction. Cancer Surv 21:147–56, 1994.

241. Ripamonti C. Management of bowel obstruction in advanced cancer. Curr Opin Oncol 6(4):351–7, 1994.

242. Archer AG, Sugarbaker PH, Jelinek JS. Radiology of peritoneal carcinomatosis. Cancer Treat Res 82:263–88, 1996.

243. Boas RA, Schug SA, Acland RH. Perineal pain after rectal amputation: a 5-year follow-up. Pain 52(1):67–70, 1993.

244. Hagen NA. Sharp, shooting neuropathic pain in the rectum or genitals: pudendal neuralgia. J Pain Symptom Manage 8(7):496–501, 1993.

245. Stillman M. Perineal pain: diagnosis and management, with particular attention to perineal pain of cancer. In: Foley KM, Bonica JJ, Ventafrida V, eds. Second International Congress on Cancer Pain. Advances in pain research and therapy, vol. 16. New York: Raven Press, 1990: 359–77.

246. Berger MS, Cooley ME, Abrahm JL. A pain syndrome associated with large adrenal metastases in patients with lung cancer. J Pain Symptom Manage 10(2):161–6, 1995.

247. Harrington KJ, Pandha HS, Kelly SA, et al. Palliation of obstructive nephropathy due to malignancy. Br J Urol 76(1):101–7, 1995.

248. Kontturi M, Kauppila A. Ureteric complications following treatment of gynaecological cancer. Ann Chir Gynaecol 71(4):232–8, 1982.

249. Greenfield A, Resnick MI. Genitourinary emergencies. Semin Oncol 16:516–20, 1989.

250. LoMonaco M, Milone M, Batocchi AP, et al. Cisplatin neuropathy: clinical course and neurophysiological findings. J Neurol 239(4):199–204, 1992.

251. Rosenfeld CS, Broder LE. Cisplatin-induced autonomic neuropathy. Cancer Treat Rep 68(4):659–60, 1984.

252. Ratcliffe MA, Gilbert FJ, Dawson AA, Bennett B. Diagnosis of avascular necrosis of the femoral head in patients treated for lymphoma. Hematol Oncol 13(3):131–7, 1995.

253. Thornton MJ, O'Sullivan G, Williams MP, Hughes PM. Avascular necrosis of bone following an intensified chemotherapy regimen including high dose steroids. Clin Radiol 52(8):607–12, 1997.

254. Castellanos AM, Glass JP, Yung WK. Regional nerve injury after intra-arterial chemotherapy. Neurology 37(5):834–7, 1987.

255. Kahn CE Jr, Messersmith RN, Samuels BL. Brachial plexopathy as a complication of intraarterial cisplatin chemotherapy. Cardiovasc Intervent Radiol 12(1):47–9, 1989.

256. Kukla LJ, McGuire WP, Lad T, Saltiel M. Acute vascular episodes associated with therapy for carcinomas of the upper aerodigestive tract with bleomycin, vincristine, and cisplatin. Cancer Treat Rep 66(2):369–70, 1982.

257. Hansen SW, Olsen N, Rossing N, Rorth M. Vascular toxicity and the mechanism underlying Raynaud's phenomenon in patients treated with cisplatin, vinblastine and bleomycin [see comments]. Ann Oncol 1(4):289–92, 1990.

258. Srinivasan V, Miree J Jr, Lloyd FA. Bilateral mastectomy and irradiation in the prevention of estrogen induced gynecomastia. J Urol 107(4):624–5, 1972.

259. Soloway MS, Schellhammer PF, Smith JA, et al. Bicalutamide in the treatment of advanced prostatic carcinoma: a phase II multicenter trial. Urology 47(1A Suppl):33–53, 1996.

260. Brogden RN, Chrisp P. Flutamide. A review of its pharmacodynamic and pharmacokinetic properties, and therapeutic use in advanced prostatic cancer. Drugs Aging 1(2):104–15, 1991.

261. Goldenberg SL, Bruchovsky N. Use of cyproterone acetate in prostate cancer. Urol Clin North Am 18(1):111–22, 1991.

262. Tasmuth T, von Smitten K, Hietanen P, et al. Pain and other symptoms after different treatment modalities of breast cancer. Ann Oncol 6(5):453–9, 1995.

263. Hladiuk M, Huchcroft S, Temple W, Schnurr BE. Arm function after axillary dissection for breast cancer: a pilot study to provide parameter estimates. J Surg Oncol 50(1):47–52, 1992.

264. Maunsell E, Brisson J, Deschenes L. Arm problems and psychological distress after surgery for breast cancer. Can J Surg 36(4):315–20, 1993.

265. Vecht CJ. Arm pain in the patient with breast cancer. J Pain Symptom Manage 5(2):109–17, 1990.

266. Vecht CJ, Van de Brand HJ, Wajer OJ. Post-axillary dissection pain in breast cancer due to a lesion of the intercostobrachial nerve. Pain 38(2):171–6, 1989.

267. Granek I, Ashikari R, Foley KM. Postmastectomy pain syndrome: clinical and anatomic correlates. Proceedings American Society of Clinical Oncology 3:Abstract 122, 1983.

268. Paredes JP, Puente JL, Potel J. Variations in sensitivity after sectioning the intercostobrachial nerve. Am J Surg 160(5):525–8, 1990.

269. van Dam MS, Hennipman A, de Kruif JT, et al. [Complications following axillary dissection for breast carcinoma (see comments)]. Ned Tijdschr Geneeskd 137(46):2395–8, 1993.

270. Wood KM. Intercostobrachial nerve entrapment syndrome. South Med J 71(6):662–3, 1978.

271. Brown H, Burns S, Kaiser CW. The spinal accessory nerve plexus, the trapezius muscle, and shoulder stabilization after radical neck cancer surgery. Ann Surg 208(5):654–61, 1988.

272. Mondrup K, Olsen NK, Pfeiffer P, Rose C. Clinical and electrodiagnostic findings in breast cancer patients with radiation-induced brachial plexus neuropathy. Acta Neurol Scand 81(2):153–8, 1990.

273. Olsen NK, Pfeiffer P, Mondrup K, Rose C. Radiation-induced brachial plexus neuropathy in breast cancer patients. Acta Oncol 29(7):885–90, 1990.

274. Thyagarajan D, Cascino T, Harms G. Magnetic resonance imaging in brachial plexopathy of cancer. Neurology 45(3 Pt 1):421–7, 1995.

275. Esteban A, Traba A. Fasciculation-myokymic activity and prolonged nerve conduction block. A physiopathological relationship in radiation-induced brachial plexopathy. Electroencephalogr Clin Neurophysiol 89(6):382–91, 1993.

276. Lederman RJ, Wilbourn AJ. Brachial plexopathy: recurrent cancer or radiation? Neurology 34(10):1331–5, 1984.

277. Stryker JA, Sommerville K, Perez R, Velkley DE. Sacral plexus injury after radiotherapy for carcinoma of cervix. Cancer 66(7):1488–92, 1990.

278. Thomas JE, Cascino TL, Earle JD. Differential diagnosis between radiation and tumor plexopathy of the pelvis. Neurology 35(1):1–7, 1985.

279. Schultheiss TE, Stephens LC. Invited review: permanent radiation myelopathy. Br J Radiol 65(777):737–53, 1992.

280. Nussbaum ML, Campana TJ, Weese JL. Radiation-induced intestinal injury. Clin Plast Surg 20(3):573–80, 1993.

281. Yeoh EK, Horowitz M. Radiation enteritis. Surg Gynecol Obstet 165(4):373–9, 1987.

282. Newman ML, Brennan M, Passik S. Lymphedema complicated by pain and psychological distress: a case with complex treatment needs. J Pain Symptom Manage 12(6):376–9, 1996.

283. Ganel A, Engel J, Sela M, Brooks M. Nerve entrapments associated with postmastectomy lymphedema. Cancer 44(6):2254–9, 1979.

284. Minsky BD, Cohen AM. Minimizing the toxicity of pelvic radiation therapy in rectal cancer. Oncology 2(8):21–9, 1988.

SECTION III PHARMACOLOGICAL TREATMENT

7 Pharmacology of analgesia: basic principles

CHARLES E. INTURRISI
Weill Medical College of Cornell University

Introduction

Opioid analgesic drugs are commonly prescribed for the management of pain resulting from cancer. During the last 20 years there has been a dramatic increase in our knowledge of the sites and mechanisms of action of opioids (1). The development of analytical methods has also been of great importance by facilitating pharmacokinetic studies of the disposition and fate of opioids in patients. These studies have begun to offer us a better understanding of some of the sources of interindividual variation in the response to opioids and to suggest ways to minimize some of their adverse effects (2,3). Although there are gaps in our knowledge of opioid pharmacology, the rational and appropriate use of these drugs is based on the knowledge of their pharmacological properties derived from well-controlled clinical trials (4).

Individualized dosage

The fundamental concept that underlies the appropriate and successful management of cancer pain by the use of opioid and non-opioid analgesics is individualization of analgesic therapy (4,5). This concept entails selection of the right analgesic, administered in the right dose and on the right schedule so as to maximize pain relief and minimize adverse effects (4–6). This comprehensive approach begins with the non-opioids or mild analgesics for mild pain (see Chapter 10). In patients with moderate pain that is not controlled by non-opioids alone, the so-called weak opioids alone or in combination should be prescribed. In patients with severe pain, a strong opioid is the drug of choice given alone or in combination (see Chapter 8). At all levels certain adjuvant drugs are used for specific indications (5–7) (see Chapter 11).

Opioid analgesics

The selection of an opioid analgesic is based on the need to treat moderate to severe pain. These drugs have been characterized by their important pharmacological differences that are derived from their complex interactions with three opioid receptor types (mu, delta, and kappa) (1). Recently, molecular genetic approaches have used gene targeting (knockout) technology to disrupt the genes that code for these three opioid receptors Mice that lack the mu receptor (MOR-deficient mice) do not respond to morphine with analgesia, respiratory depression, constipation, physical dependence, reward behaviors, or immunosuppression (8). These results confirm and extend previous pharmacological and receptor binding studies and demonstrate that the mu receptor mediates the analgesic and adverse effects of morphine. The morphine-like agonist drugs represent one end of the spectrum. They bind predominately to the mu opioid receptor and produce analgesia. The opioid antagonists represent the other end of the spectrum. These drugs bind to each of the three opioid receptor types with different affinities and therefore can block the effects of morphine-like agonists that do not have analgesic properties of their own. Between these two groups are the mixed agonist-antagonist drugs, which, depending on the patient circumstances (see below), can demonstrate agonist (at the kappa receptor) and antagonist (at the mu receptor) properties.

Morphine-like agonists

Morphine is the prototype and standard of comparison for opioid analgesics. The morphine-like agonists (Table 7.1) share with morphine a similar profile of pharmacodynamic effects both desirable and undesirable. However, they differ in factors critical in dosage selection (i.e., relative anal-

Table 7.1. *Opioid analgesics commonly used for severe pain*

Name	Equianalgesic i.m. dose[a]	i.m./p.o. potency	Starting oral dose range (mg)	Comments	Precautions
Morphine-like agonists					
Morphine	10	6	30–60[b]	Standard of comparison for opioid analgesics. Sustained-release preparations (MS Contin, OramorphSR, and Kadian)	Lower doses for aged patients; impaired ventilation; bronchial asthma; increased intracranial pressure; liver failure
Hydromorphone (Dilaudid)	1.5	5	4–8	Slightly shorter acting. HP refers to 10 mg/ml dosage form for tolerant patients	Like morphine
Methadone (Dolophine)	10	2	10–20	Good oral potency; long plasma half-life	Like morphine; may accumulate with repetitive dosing causing excessive sedation
Levorphanol (Levo-Dromoran)	2	2	2–4	Like methadone	Like methadone
Oxymorphone (Numorphan)	1	See comments	See comments	Not available orally Available as a rectal suppository	Like im morphine
Oxycodone	20	—	15–30	Immediate-release (Roxicodone and OxyIR) and sustained-release (OxyContin) forms. Also lower doses in combination with non-opioids for less severe pain	Like morphine
Meperidine (Demerol)	75	4	Not recommended	Slightly shorter acting Used orally for less severe pain	Normeperidine (toxic metabolite) accumulates with repetitive dosing causing CNS excitation; not for patients with impaired renal function or receiving monoamine oxidase inhibitors[c]
Codeine	130	1.5	See comments	Used orally for less severe pain	Like morphine
Fentanyl	0.1	—	—	Transdermal fentanyl (Duragesic). Also oral transmucosal fentanyl citrate for breakthrough pain	Transdermal creates skin reservoir of drug-12-hour delay in onset and offset. Fever increases absorption
Mixed agonist-antagonists					
Pentazocine (Talwin)	60	3	See comments	Used orally for less severe pain; mixed agonist-antagonist	May cause psychotomimetic effects; may precipitate withdrawal in opioid dependent patients; not for myocardial infarction
Nalbuphine (Nubain)	10	See comments	See comments	Not available orally; like im pentazocine but not scheduled	Incidence of psychotomimetic effects lower than with pentazocine
Butorphanol (Stadol)	2	See comments	See comments	Not available orally like im nalbuphine	Like nalbuphine
Partial agonists					
Buprenorphine (Buprenex)	0.4	See comments	See comments	Not available orally; sublingual preparation not yet in United States; does not produce psychotomimetic effects	May precipitate withdrawal in opioid-dependent patients; not readily reversed by naloxone; avoid in labor

Abbreviations: i.m., intramuscular; p.o., oral.
For these equianalgesic im doses (also see comments) the time of peak analgesia in nontolerant patients ranges from $1/2$ to 1 hour and the duration from 4 to 6 hours. The peak analgesic effect is delayed and the duration prolonged after oral administration.
[a] Recommended starting im doses from which the optimal dose for each patient is determined by titration and the maximal dose limited by adverse effects. For single iv bolus doses use half the im dose.
[b] A value of 3 is used when calculating an oral dosage regimen of q4h around-the-clock.
[c] Irritating to tissues on repeated administration.

gesic potency and oral to parenteral [im/po] analgesic potency). They also differ in pharmacokinetics (e.g., elimination half-life) and biotransformation to pharmacologically active metabolites (2,3). These latter characteristics are of particular importance when opioid administration is continued beyond 1 or 2 days. Much of this information is summarized in Table 7.1. This dosage information is, for the most part, derived from controlled clinical trials comparing single doses of opioids and morphine (2,3).

Morphine

The World Health Organization has requested that oral morphine be part of the essential drug list and made available throughout the world for cancer pain (6). Although its oral bioavailability varies from 35%–75%, its plasma half-life (2 to 3.5 hours) is somewhat shorter than its duration of analgesia (4–6 hours), which limits accumulation. Furthermore, with repetitive administration, its pharmacokinetics remain linear and there does not appear to be autoinduction of biotransformation even after large chronic doses (2). These pharmacokinetic properties contribute to the safe use of morphine. Morphine-6-glucuronide (M-6-G) is an active metabolite of morphine that appears to contribute to the analgesic activity of morphine (9). In addition, animal studies indicate that M-6-G produces pharmacological actions at what appear to be opioid receptors derived from splice variants of the cloned mu receptor where morphine is inactive (10). M-6-G is eliminated by the kidney and will accumulate relative to morphine in patients with renal insufficiency (11–13). The degree to which this accumulation of M-6-G contributes to the incidence and severity of adverse effects experienced by these patients has not been conclusively demonstrated (12,13). In a survey that measured steady-state morphine and M-6-G levels and adverse effects in 109 cancer patients, the presence of myoclonus or cognitive impairment was not associated with M-6-G accumulation (12). For a subset of the 20 patients with the highest M-6-G levels (>2000 μg/ml), the M-6-G level and concurrent organ failure were associated with the most severe toxicity (respiratory depression and/or obtundation) (12). It is appropriate to consider an alternative opioid for a patient receiving morphine who experiences a decrease in renal function and a concomitant increase in undesirable effects. M-3-G, the predominate metabolite of morphine in humans, is devoid of opioid activity but has excitatory effects in animals after direct injection into the central nervous system (CNS). This has led to the suggestion that M-3-G may be responsible for the neuroexcitatory effects sometimes seen with large chronic morphine dosing (14). This speculation awaits definitive studies in patients receiving morphine.

Based on single-dose studies in patients with either acute or chronic pain, the relative potency of intramuscular to oral morphine is 1:6. However, with repeated administration, when patients are dosed on a regular schedule (around the clock), the im/po ratio is reduced to 1:2 or 1:3 . Thus, for patients with acute pain who are being titrated using an as-needed schedule, the 1:6 ratio should be used initially with a lower ratio expected, if dosing continues and a steady-state develops.

The delayed-release morphine preparations provide analgesia with a duration of 8 to 12 hours (MSContin, Roxanol-SR) or 24 hours (Kadian) and allow the cancer patient a greater freedom from repetitive dosing, especially during the night. These preparations appear to be safe and efficacious. Patients should be initially titrated on immediate-release morphine and, once stabilized, converted to the delayed-release preparation according to either an 8- or 12-hour dosing schedule. To manage acute "breakthrough" pain, "rescue" medication (immediate-release morphine) should be made available to the patient receiving delayed-release preparations.

Table 7.1 lists other morphine-like agonists that may be substituted for morphine. An alternative opioid to morphine may be selected based on the need with a particular patient to overcome an adverse effect of morphine (e.g., vomiting or sedation). Other reasons include the patient's favorable prior experience with another opioid or even local availability of other morphine-like opioids. It must be emphasized that there is no evidence to suggest that any opioid has greater analgesic efficacy than morphine.

Hydromorphone

Hydromorphone is a short half-life opioid used as an alternative to morphine by the oral and parenteral routes. It is more soluble than morphine and available in a concentrated dosage form at 10 mg/ml. This preparation is intended for parenteral administration to the opioid-tolerant, cachectic patient where the volume of the opioid solution to be injected must be limited. In this regard hydromorphone serves the same role in cancer pain management in the United States as does heroin in those countries where it is available.

Levorphanol

Levorphanol, which is a long half-life opioid (Table 7.2), is also a useful alternative to morphine, but it must be

Table 7.2. *Plasma half-life values for opioids and their active metabolites*

	Plasma half-life (hours)
Short half-life opioids	
Morphine	2–3.5
Morphine-6-glucuronide	2
Hydromorphone	2–3
Oxycodone	2–3
Fentanyl	3.7
Codeine	3
Meperidine	3–4
Pentazocine	2–3
Nalbuphine	5
Butorphanol	2.5–3.5
Buprenorphine	3–5
Long half-life opioids	
Methadone	24
Levorphanol	12–16
Propoxyphene	12
Norpropoxyphene	30–40
Normeperidine	14–21

used cautiously to prevent accumulation. For patients who are unable to tolerate morphine and methadone, levorphanol represents a useful medication with a good oral/parenteral potency ratio of 1:2.

Oxymorphone

Oxymorphone, a congener of morphine, has had a limited but important role in the management of pain in cancer patients. It is currently most widely used in suppository form, infrequently used parenterally on a chronic basis, and is not available orally.

Methadone

Methadone's bioavailability is 85% and from single-dose studies its oral/parenteral potency ratio is 1:2. Its plasma half-life averages 24 hours (Table 7.2) but may range from 13 to 50 hours, whereas the duration of analgesia is often only 4 to 8 hours (2,3). Repetitive analgesic doses of methadone lead to drug accumulation because of the discrepancy between its plasma half-life and the duration of analgesia. Sedation, confusion, and even death can occur when patients are not carefully monitored (2,3) and dosage adjusted during the accumulation period that can last from 5 to 10 days (2). It is a useful alternative to morphine but requires greater sophistication in its clinical use as compared with morphine. Initial doses should be titrated carefully and as-needed dosing used during

the titration period. Ripamonti et al. (15) reported a prospective study of 38 consecutive cancer patients who were switched from morphine to oral methadone and titrated to effect so that the equianalgesic dose ratio (morphine/methadone) could be estimated. The dose ratio increased as a function of the prior morphine dose so that no single dose ratio was appropriate for naive patients or patients who were receiving various doses of morphine at the time they were switched to methadone. Data indicate that those patients who were receiving the highest doses of morphine were relatively more sensitive to the analgesic effects of methadone (i.e., they had the highest dose ratio). This unidirectional variability in the dose ratio may reflect incomplete cross-tolerance between morphine and methadone and further emphasizes the need for individualization of dose and careful titration to effect when switching to methadone (16).

The dosage form of methadone that is used clinically in most countries, including the United States, is a racemic mixture of equal amounts of the l-isomer, an opioid and the d-isomer, which lacks opioid activity (17–19). However, both the l- and d-isomers of methadone bind to the *N*-methyl-D-aspartate (NMDA) receptor and the d-isomer has functional NMDA receptor antagonist activity in animals, including antihyperalgesic activity and the ability to prevent the development of morphine tolerance (17,18,20). Some of the implications of these properties are discussed next.

NMDA receptor antagonists and pain management

A variety of compounds have been found to possess NMDA receptor antagonist activity in binding studies and/or in animal models. These include some opioids (methadone, meperidine, ketobemidone, and dextropropxyphene) and a diverse group of other compounds (e.g., racemic ketamine and its isomers, dextromethorphan and memantine) (17,18,20,21). These compounds have antihyperalgesic and antiallodynic activity in animal models of painful peripheral neuropathy (21) and in other models that also involve central sensitization (19). The clinical usefulness of some of these compounds (e.g., ketamine) as single-entity analgesics in neuropathic pain has been limited by adverse effects in most patients (22). Dextromethorphan is effective in painful diabetic neuropathy in patients who can tolerate high doses (22). Preclinical studies have also revealed that these same NMDA receptor antagonists can prevent or reverse the development of morphine tolerance (20). Taken together, these observations suggest that the combination of an opioid plus an NMDA receptor antagonist should be of particular value in pain states where the potency of the opioid has been reduced as a result of hyperalgesia and/or morphine tolerance (16,18). This new therapeutic strategy has led to the development of a morphine-dextromethorphan combination (Morphi-Dex), which is currently undergoing clinical trials (23–25), and it may be expected that other combinations will be evaluated. In this context, racemic methadone represents a naturally occurring combination of an opioid and isomers with NMDA receptor antagonist activity. Although subject to much speculation, the relative contributions of its opioid and NMDA receptor antagonist components have not been evaluated in patients with pain. A number of favorable therapeutic consequences could result from this type of combination and the initial clinical studies of Morphi-Dex have provided some insights. In single-dose studies, additive or synergistic analgesic effects are seen, so that a lower dose of morphine can be used with the combination (23). The combination does not result in an increase in respiratory depression or abuse liability (24). It remains to be determined whether the combination also results in a reduction in adverse effects or the prevention or reversal of morphine tolerance (25). We also need to learn whether the combination provides an increase in maximal efficacy that extends to conditions that are less responsive to opioids, such as neuropathic pain.

Meperidine

Studies of meperidine in cancer patients have demonstrated that repetitive dosing can lead to accumulation of its toxic metabolite, normeperidine, resulting in CNS hyperexcitability (2). This is characterized initially by subtle mood effects, followed by tremors, multifocal myoclonus, and occasionally seizures. This CNS hyperexcitability occurs commonly in patients with renal disease, but it can occur after repeated administration in patients with normal renal function (2).

Oxycodone

Oxycodone is available both as immediate-release and a continuous-release (8–12 hour duration) preparation (OxyContin), and these dosage forms can be used for moderate to severe pain. However, lower doses (e.g., 5 mg) in combination with nonopioids (aspirin, acetaminophen) are frequently used for mild to moderate pain. The fixed-dose oxycodone combinations should not be used chronically in large doses for more severe pain

because of the risk of dose-related toxicity from the nonopioid ingredients.

Fentanyl

Fentanyl is estimated to be approximately 80 to 100 times as potent as morphine (1,4). It is a highly lipophilic drug with shorter duration of action than parenteral morphine. Fentanyl is used for the management of postoperative pain by the intravenous and epidural routes of administration, and a transdermal patch device is used for chronic pain requiring opioid analgesia and a transmucosal dosage form is used for breakthrough cancer pain (see later).

Agonist-antagonist analgesics

The mixed agonist-antagonist analgesics (Table 7.1) include pentazocine, butorphanol, and nalbuphine. They produce analgesia in the non-tolerant patient but may precipitate withdrawal in patients tolerant-dependent to morphine-like drugs. Therefore, when used for chronic pain, they should be tried before repeated administration of a morphine-like agonist drug. There is a ceiling effect on the ability of the mixed agonist-antagonists to produce respiratory depression, and they have a significantly lower abuse liability than the morphine-like drugs. In therapeutic doses, they may produce certain self-limiting psychotomimetic effects in some patients, with pentazocine the most common drug associated with these effects (2,3). These drugs play a limited role in the management of chronic pain because the incidence and severity of the psychotomimetic effects increase with dose escalation (2,3) and because they are not available in convenient oral dosage forms. Thus, nalbuphine is available only for parenteral use, and the oral preparation of pentazocine is marketed in combination with naloxone. Butorphanol is available for both parenteral and intranasal use. However, recent single-dose studies indicate that women may derive more pain relief than men from kappa opioid analgesics (26,27), and this may stimulate the development of kappa opioids that can be administered by routes (oral, transdermal) appropriate for the management of persistent pain.

Partial agonist analgesics

The partial agonist buprenorphine (Table 7.1) has less abuse liability than the morphine-like drugs, but like the mixed agonist-antagonists, it may also precipitate withdrawal in patients who have received repeated doses of a morphine-like agonist and developed physical dependence. It does not produce the psychotomimetic effects seen with the mixed agonist-antagonists, however, and is available in both a sublingual and parenteral form. Only the latter dosage form is currently available in the United States. Buprenorphine's respiratory depressant effects are reversed only by relatively large doses of naloxone (28). It has been studied in cancer patients with pain and is useful for moderate to severe pain requiring an opioid analgesic; however, it should be used before the morphine-like agonists are introduced (2).

Opioid pharmacokinetics

As noted previously, the opioids differ significantly in one measure of drug elimination, the plasma half-life value (Table 7.2). Thus, although morphine and hydromorphone are short half-life opioids that on repeated dosing reach steady-state in 10 to 12 hours, levorphanol and methadone are long half-life opioids that on average may require 70 to 120 hours, respectively, to achieve steady-state. During dose titration the maximal (peak) effects produced by a change dose of a short half-life opioid will appear relatively quickly, whereas the peak effects resulting from a change in the dose of a long half-life opioid will be achieved after a longer accumulation period. For example, a patient who reports adequate pain relief after the initial doses of methadone may experience excessive sedation if this dosage is fixed and not modified as required during the accumulation period of 5 to 10 days.

Also, note that the active (toxic) metabolites, normeperidine and norpropoxyphene, have much longer plasma half-life values than their corresponding parents (meperidine and propoxyphene) so that administration of the parent on a schedule designed to produce continued pain relief results in accumulation of the metabolite (2,3).

Opioid pharmacokinetics are altered by certain drug and/or disease interactions (see reference 2).

Route of administration

Oral route

When given orally, the opioids differ substantially with respect to their presystemic elimination (i.e., the degree to which they are inactivated as they are absorbed from the gastrointestinal tract and pass through the liver into the systemic circulation). As indicated in Table 7.1, morphine, hydromorphone, and oxymorphone have ratios of oral to intramuscular potency of 1:5 to 1:12. Methadone, levorphanol, and oxycodone are subject to less presystemic elimination, resulting in an oral/intramuscular potency ratio of at least 1:2. Meperidine and pentazocine have intermediate ratios. The failure to recognize these differences often results in a substantial reduction in analgesia when the change from the parenteral to oral administration is attempted without upward titration of the dose. In general, orally administered drugs have a slower onset of action, delayed peak time, and a longer duration of effect, whereas drugs administered parenterally have a rapid onset of action but a shorter duration of effect.

Transdermal

The development of a transdermal system for the delivery of fentanyl through the skin (TTS-Fentanyl) provides a convenient mode of opioid administration that avoids frequent parenteral or oral dosing for patients with relatively constant cancer pain. This system is currently available in four dosage strengths that vary in drug delivery rate from 25 to 100 µg/hr and is to be applied at 72-hour intervals. The package insert provides estimates of the equivalence of morphine to TTS-Fentanyl. Donner et al. (29) found that cancer patients who were switched from oral morphine to transdermal fentanyl required approximately 25 µg/hr of fentanyl to replace 45 mg/day of oral morphine. The system creates a drug reservoir probably in the striatum corneum at the site of application of the system, so there is a lag in the systemic absorption of the fentanyl (30). A total of 12 to 16 hours are required to achieve a therapeutic effect and 48 hours to reach approximately steady-state blood levels (30). Therefore, patients should be titrated to adequate pain relief with short-acting opioids and then switched to transdermal fentanyl. In addition, supplemental short-acting opioids should be available for breakthrough pain. The tissue reservoir limits fluctuations in drug concentrations in blood over the dosing interval. However, after removal of the system, drug concentrations in blood decline relatively slowly so that pharmacodynamic effects may not diminish for many hours, and adverse effects must be monitored for an appropriate duration.

Intramuscular

This route provides a longer onset (30–60 minutes) compared to intravenous and a shorter duration than after the oral route. Intramuscular injections are often painful and, therefore, this route is not usually appropriate for the management of persistent pain.

Intravenous—bolus, continuous infusion, and patient-controlled analgesia

An intravenous bolus provides the most rapid onset and shortest duration of action. Time to peak effect correlates with the lipid solubility of the opioid, ranging from 2 to 5 minutes for methadone to 10 to 15 minutes for morphine. Opioids given by intravenous bolus can be used to titrate analgesia in patients with acute or escalating severe pain (31).

A continuous intravenous infusion is useful for some patients who cannot be maintained on oral opioids. This mode of administration allows for complete systemic absorption and can be supplemented with bolus injections to conveniently titrate opioid dosage in patients with rapidly escalating pain. Loading and maintenance doses can be estimated as described by Edwards and Breed (31).

Patient-controlled analgesia (PCA) is a mode of opioid administration that involves the concept of individualization of analgesic dosage wherein the patients, within limits, can titrate their analgesia requirements. PCA has been widely used for postoperative pain (32). Compared to as-needed intramuscular injections, PCA provides an improvement in analgesia without any increase in sedation (33). PCA has been effectively used for the short- and long-term management of cancer pain in adults (34), and those adolescents and children who are able to use the device correctly (35). Dosing guidelines for opioids administered by PCA are given in guidelines from the American Pain Society (4).

Continuous subcutaneous infusion

For patients who cannot absorb adequate amounts of orally administered opioids because of nausea and vomiting, gastrointestinal intolerance, or obstruction, the parenteral routes described previously can be used. In addition to circumventing oral absorption, however, the continuous subcutaneous infusion mode of opioid delivery avoids the problems associated with intramuscular/subcutaneous injection and the need for an intravenous access, and can be used by ambulatory patients. Most opioids available for parenteral use can be administered by continuous subcutaneous infusion (36).

Rectal

The rectal route is an alternative to the parenteral route for patients unable to take opioids orally. Rectal suppositories containing hydromorphone, oxymorphone, and morphine are available.

Epidural and intrathecal (intraspinal)

Opioid receptors are expressed on primary afferents, and spinal cord dorsal horn neurons are the target of intraspinal opioids. This relatively localized administration usually requires lower doses than systemic routes and can produce a segmental analgesia (37). These techniques are used to provide intraoperative and postoperative as well as obstetric pain relief. The two most commonly used opioids are morphine and fentanyl. Morphine is a hydrophilic compound that slowly distributes into tissues and therefore a substantial fraction remains in the CSF. This reservoir of drug results in a long duration of analgesia, but also allows for the rostral spread to supraspinal sites where sedation and, rarely, respiratory depression can occur. The much more lipid soluble fentanyl is rapidly taken up into tissues and cleared into the systemic circulation reducing the duration of action and the risk of supraspinally mediated adverse effects (37). Intraspinal opioids can be administered in single dose or by continuous infusion (38). Other issues and considerations include the contribution of an added local anesthetic to the degree of analgesia (39) and whether intraspinal opioids have an advantage over a well-managed systemic dosing regimen (40). Dosing guidelines for intraspinal opioids are given in guidelines from the American Pain Society (4).

Other routes and modes of administration—intranasal and transmucosal

Butorphanol is available for intranasal administration (41). Oral transmucosal fentanyl citrate (OTFC) is a solid dosage form of fentanyl that consists of fentanyl incorporated into a sweetened lozenge on a handle. With this dosage form, a portion of the fentanyl is rapidly absorbed through the oral mucosa, avoiding liver first pass biotransformation, and the rest is swallowed and absorbed through the gastrointestinal tract and exposed to the liver. Plasma concentrations peak approximately 5 to 10 minutes after consumption of OTFC that usually requires 15 minutes (4). OTFC is approved for the treatment of cancer-related breakthrough pain in patients receiving strong opioids (42).

Changing the route of administration

The slower onset of analgesia after oral administration often requires some adaptation on the part of a patient who is accustomed to the more rapid onset seen after a parenteral opioid. Problems associated with switching from the parenteral to the oral route of opioid administration can be minimized by slowly reducing the parenteral dose and increasing the oral dose over a 2- to 3-day period. When patients are switched from the intramuscular to intravenous or intravenous to intramuscular route, we have made the assumption that the equianalgesic doses by these two routes are the same. However, there are no studies of the relative potency of drugs comparing these routes.

When patients are switched from one opioid analgesic to another or from one route of administration to another, it is the lack of attention to the route-dependent differences in opioid dose that accounts for the common reports of undermedication of patients. In patients who have been receiving one opioid repeatedly to the point where some degree of tolerance has developed and are then switched to another opioid, half of the analgesic drug dose of the new drug should be given as the initial starting dose. This information has been gained empirically but is based on the concept that cross-tolerance is not complete among opioids and conforms to our recognition that the relative potency of some of the opioid analgesics may change with repetitive dosing, particularly those opioids with a long plasma half-life. In using Table 7.1, it becomes important to recognize that the equianalgesic dose estimates are based on the single-dose studies and they represent a useful reference point for the initiation of dose titration. They are not meant to be used as the standard dose for every patient.

Scheduled opioid administration

The schedule of opioid administration should be individualized for each patient. In general, patients with persistent pain should receive opioids on a regular schedule once the patient's dosage has been established by titration using an as-needed schedule. This approach is especially important when the dose titration involves a long half-life opioid such as methadone or levorphanol as discussed previously. A regular around-the-clock schedule of opioid administration can prevent severe pain from recurring and may allow for a reduction in the total opioid required per day. For some patients an as-needed order for a supplemental opioid dose (rescue) between the regularly scheduled doses may be required to provide adequate pain relief.

Drug combinations that enhance analgesia

Drug combinations can provide additive analgesia, may reduce adverse effects, and can reduce the rate of escalation of the opioid portion of the combination (2–5). Several combinations produce additive analgesic effects.

These include an opioid plus one of the following: a non-opioid analgesic (acetaminophen, a salicylate or a non-steroidal anti-inflammatory drug of either the mixed cyclo-oxygenase [COX] COX-1 and COX-2 or COX-2 inhibitor type), caffeine, hydroxyzine (an antihistamine), methotrimeprizine (a phenothiazine), or dextroamphetamine (a stimulant). Other adjuvant analgesics that are commonly used with opioids are the tricyclic antidepressants (amitriptyline, imipramine, nortriptyline and desipramine) and the anticonvulsants (gabapentin, phenytoin, carbamazepine, sodium valproate, and clonazepam) (see references 2–5 and Chapters 8,10, and 11).

Adverse effects of opioids

A number of side effects associated with the use of opioid analgesics can, depending on the circumstances, be categorized as desirable or undesirable (2–5, and see Chapter 9). It is the development of adverse effects that markedly limits the use of analgesics in cancer pain, and these limitations have been a major impetus in the development of novel routes of opioid administration such as epidural, intrathecal, or continuous subcutaneous infusion. The mechanisms that underlie these various adverse effects are only partly understood and, as discussed previously, appear to depend on a number of factors including the age, extent of disease and organ dysfunction, concurrent administration of certain drugs, prior opioid exposure, and the route of drug administration (2–5). Studies comparing the adverse effects of one opioid analgesic to another in this population are often lacking. Similarly, controlled studies comparing the adverse effects produced by the same opioid given by various routes of administration are also lacking. The most common adverse effects are sedation, nausea and vomiting, constipation, and respiratory depression. Other adverse effects include confusion, hallucinations, nightmares, urinary retention, multifocal myoclonus, dizziness, and dysphoria that have been reported by patients receiving these drugs (43).

Respiratory depression

Respiratory depression is potentially the most serious adverse effect. The morphine-like agonists act on brainstem respiratory centers to produce, as a function of dose, increasing respiratory depression to the point of apnea. In humans, death from overdose of a morphine-like agonist is nearly always due to respiratory arrest. Therapeutic doses of morphine may depress all phases of respiratory activity (rate, minute volume, and tidal exchange). However, as CO_2 accumulates, it stimulates central chemoreceptors, resulting in a compensatory increase in respiratory rate that masks the degree of respiratory depression. At equianalgesic doses, the morphine-like agonists produce an equivalent degree of respiratory depression. For these reasons individuals with impaired respiratory function or bronchial asthma are at greater risk of experiencing clinically significant respiratory depression in response to usual doses of these drugs. Respiratory depression and CO_2 retention result in cerebral vasodilation and an increase in cerebrospinal fluid pressure unless P_{CO_2} is maintained at normal levels by artificial ventilation. When respiratory depression occurs, it is usually in opioid-naive patients after acute administration of an opioid and is associated with other signs of CNS depression including sedation and mental clouding. Tolerance develops rapidly to this effect with repeated drug administration, allowing the opioid analgesics to be used in the management of chronic cancer pain without significant risk of respiratory depression. If respiratory depression occurs, it can be reversed by the administration of the specific opioid antagonist, naloxone. In patients chronically receiving opioids who develop respiratory depression, naloxone diluted 1:10 should be titrated carefully to prevent the precipitation of severe withdrawal symptoms while reversing the respiratory depression. An endotracheal tube should be placed in the comatose patient before administering naloxone to prevent aspiration-associated respiratory compromise with excessive salivation and bronchial spasm. In patients receiving meperidine chronically, naloxone may precipitate seizures by blocking the depressant action of meperidine and allowing the convulsant activity of the active metabolite, normeperidine, to be manifest (2). If naloxone is to be used in this situation, diluted doses slowly titrated with appropriate seizure precautions are advised.

The mixed agonist-antagonists and the partial agonist (buprenorphine) appear to differ in the dose-response characteristics of their respiratory depression curves from that of the morphine-like drugs, so that, although therapeutic doses of pentazocine produce respiratory depression equivalent to that of morphine, increasing the dose does not ordinarily produce a proportional increase in respiratory depression. Whether this apparent ceiling to respiratory depression offers any clinical advantage remains to be determined. Also the clinical symptoms of a large overdose of these drugs with particular respect to respiratory depression has not been well defined (28).

Nausea and vomiting

The opioid analgesics produce nausea and vomiting by an action on the medullary chemoreceptor trigger zone. The incidence of nausea and vomiting is markedly increased in ambulatory patients, suggesting that these drugs also alter vestibular sensitivity. The ability of opioid analgesics to produce nausea and vomiting appears to vary with drug and patient so that some advantage may result from switching to an equianalgesic dose of another opioid. Alternatively, an antiemetic may be used in combination with the opioid. For some patients initiating treatment by the parenteral route and then switching to the oral route may reduce the emetic symptoms (3).

Sedation

The opioid analgesics produce sedation and drowsiness. Although these effects may be useful in certain clinical situations (e.g., preanesthesia), they are not usually desirable concomitants of analgesia, particularly in ambulatory patients. The CNS-depressant actions of these drugs can be expected to be at least additive with the sedative and respiratory depressant effects of sedative-hypnotics such as alcohol, the barbiturates, and the benzodiazepines.

Although it has been suggested that methadone produces more sedation than morphine, this has not been supported by single-dose controlled trials or surveys in hospitalized patients (3). However, the half-life of methadone is substantially longer than morphine and can result in cumulative CNS depression after repeated doses. A reduction in dose and interval, so that a lower dose is given more frequently, may counteract excessive sedation. In addition, other CNS depressants including sedative-hypnotics and antianxiety agents that potentiate the sedative effects of opioids should be discontinued. Concurrent administration of dextroamphetamine in 2.5 to 5.0 mg oral doses twice daily has been reported to reduce the sedative effects of opioids. Tolerance usually develops to the sedative effects of opioid analgesics within the first several days of chronic administration.

Constipation

The most common adverse effect of the opioid analgesics is constipation. These drugs act at multiple sites in the gastrointestinal tract and spinal cord to produce a decrease in intestinal secretions and peristalsis, resulting in a dry stool and constipation. Tolerance develops slowly to the smooth muscle effects of opioids, so that constipation will persist when these drugs are used for chronic pain. At the same time that the use of opioid analgesics is initiated, provision for a regular bowel regimen, including cathartics and stool softeners, should be instituted to diminish this adverse effect.

Urinary retention

Because the opioid analgesics increase smooth muscle tone, they can cause bladder spasm and an increase in sphincter tone leading to urinary retention. This is most common in the elderly patient. Attention should be directed at this potential side effect, and catheterization may be necessary to manage this transient side effect.

Multifocal myoclonus

At high doses, all of the opioid analgesics can produce multifocal myoclonus (2,3,43). This complication is most prominent with the use of repeated administration of large parenteral doses of meperidine (e.g., 250 mg or more per day). As previously discussed, accumulation of normeperidine is responsible for this toxicity.

Immune function

In vitro assays and animal studies indicate that opioids such as morphine can suppress a number of immunological variables (see reference 44 for additional references). However, little information is available on the immunological effects of continuous opioid treatment in patients with persistent pain. Palm et al. (44) evaluated cellular and humoral immune variables in 10 pain patients (7 chronic non-cancer and 3 cancer-related) together with 8 normal, aged matched (untreated) control patients. Patients were studied before and at 1, 4, and 12 weeks during which they received oral sustained-release morphine for pain. Morphine treatment did not affect cellular immune function. Interestingly, these chronic pain patients produced smaller amounts of immunoglobulin (Ig) than controls, and Ig production was reduced further by morphine. Additional studies of the immunological effects of opioids in acute and chronic pain patients are required to determine the clinical significance of the effects observed on humoral immune function by pain itself and the use of opioids to relieve pain.

Interactions between immune-cell derived opioid peptides and opioid receptors located in the peripheral inflamed tissues can result in analgesia. Opioid receptors are present on peripheral sensory nerves and are upregulated during the development of inflammation. Opioid peptides are synthesized in circulating immune cells that migrate to sites of injury. Under stressful stimuli or in response to releasing agents (corticotropin-releasing factor or cytokines), these immunocytes can secrete endogenous opioids that activate peripheral opioid receptors by inhibiting either the excitability of sensory nerves or the release of pro-inflammatory neuropeptides (45). This information provides the basis for the development of opioids whose actions are confined to the periphery.

The opioid-tolerant patient

Tolerance develops when a given dose of an opioid produces a decreasing effect, or when a larger dose is required to maintain the original effect. Some degree of tolerance to analgesia appears to develop in most patients receiving opioid analgesics chronically (46). The hallmark sign of the development of tolerance is the patient's complaint of a decrease in the duration of effective analgesia. For reasons not yet understood, the rate of development of tolerance varies greatly among cancer patients so that some will demonstrate tolerance within days of initiating opioid therapy, whereas others will remain well controlled for many months on the same dose (47). A sudden dramatic increase in opioid requirements may represent a progression of the cancer rather than the development of tolerance per se. In these patients, objective evidence of progression of disease is sought and pain management techniques reevaluated accordingly (47).

With the development of tolerance, increasing the frequency and/or increasing the dose of the opioid is required to provide continued pain relief. Because the analgesic effect is a logarithmic function of the dose of opioid, a doubling of the dose may be required to restore full analgesia. There appears to be no limit to the development of tolerance and with appropriate adjustment of dose patients can continue to obtain pain relief.

In cancer patients with severe pain, opioid analgesics should not be used sparingly or "save to the last" out of the fear that an increasing opioid requirement represents a "loss of control." A number of strategies can be used to forestall the development of tolerance in patients with chronic cancer pain. Because tolerance development is a function of the dose and frequency of administration, it is not surprising that continuous intravenous administration of opioids often results in the rapid development of tolerance. For this and other reasons cited previously, the oral route of administration is preferred.

When the oral route cannot be used, the alternative is parenteral administration. In the tolerant patient, hydromorphone-HP can provide the flexibility required for dose titration. Combinations of opioids with non-opioids that enhance analgesia not only provide additive analgesia, but as tolerance does not develop to the non-opioid component of the mixture, the overall result is slower rate development of tolerance. From the start, a non-opioid (e.g., acetaminophen) should be used with the opioid. In the tolerant patient, methotrimeprazine, a non-opioid analgesic, can be substituted for part of the opioid analgesic requirement. Cross-tolerance among the opioid analgesics appears not to be complete and, therefore, advantage is gained by switching to an alternative opioid and selecting half the predicted equianalgesic dose from Table 7.1 as the starting dose. The use of bolus or continuous epidural local anesthetics in patients with localized pain, for example, perineal pain, can dramatically reduce the need for systemic opioids and thus reverse opioid tolerance.

The opioid dependent patient: definitions and misconceptions

Psychological and physical dependence

The properties of the opioid analgesics that are most likely to lead to their being misused or the patient mistreated are effects mediated in the CNS and seen after chronic administration, including psychological and physical dependence. It must be emphasized that although development of physical dependence and tolerance are predictable pharmacologic effects seen in humans and laboratory animals in response to repeated administration of an opioid, these effects are distinct from the behavioral pattern seen in some individuals and described by the terms *psychological dependence* or *addiction* (48). Psychological dependence is used to describe a pattern of drug use characterized by a continued craving for an opioid that is manifest as compulsive drug-seeking behavior leading to an overwhelming involvement with the use and procurement of the drug. Within these definitions, anyone who is addicted to opioids is likely to be physically dependent. However, the term *addiction* cannot be used interchangeably with physical dependence; that is, it is possible to be physically dependent on an opioid analgesic without being addicted. Fear of addiction is a major consideration limiting the use of appropriate doses of opioids in hospitalized patients in pain. Some patients are reluctant to take even small doses of opioids for fear of becoming addicted. Surveys in hospitalized medical patients (49)

and in burn patients (50) and an analysis of the recent medical use and abuse of opioid analgesics (51) suggested that medical use of opioids rarely, if ever, leads to drug abuse or iatrogenic opioid addiction. The most recent survey found that from 1990 to 1996, there were significant increases in the medical use of morphine (59%), fentanyl (1168%), oxycodone (23%), and hydromorphone (19%) without a significant increase in reports of drug abuse (mentions of drug abuse) as compiled by the Drug Abuse Warning Network (51).

Physical dependence is the term used to describe the phenomenon of withdrawal when an opioid is abruptly discontinued or if an opioid antagonist is administered. The severity of withdrawal is a function of the dose and duration of administration of the opioid just discontinued (i.e., the patient's prior opioid exposure). Administration of an opioid antagonist to a physically dependent individual produces an immediate precipitation of the withdrawal syndrome. Patients who have received repeated doses of a morphine-like agonist to the point where they are physically dependent may experience an opioid withdrawal reaction when given a mixed agonist-antagonist. Prior exposure to a morphine-like drug can be shown to greatly increase a patient's sensitivity to the antagonist component of a mixed agonist-antagonist. Therefore, when used for chronic pain, they should be tried before initiating prolonged administration of a morphine-like agonist.

The abrupt discontinuation of an opioid analgesic in a patient with significant prior opioid experience will result in signs and symptoms characteristic of the opioid withdrawal or abstinence syndrome. The onset of withdrawal is characterized by the patient's report of feelings of anxiety, nervousness and irritability, and alternating chills and hot flushes. A prominent withdrawal sign is "wetness" including salivation, lacrimation, rhinorrhea, and diaphoresis, as well as gooseflesh (48). At the peak intensity of withdrawal, patients may experience nausea, vomiting, abdominal cramps, insomnia, and, rarely, multifocal myoclonus. The time-course of the withdrawal syndrome is a function of the elimination half-life of the opioid to which the patient has become dependent. Abstinence symptoms will appear within 6 to 12 hours and reach a peak at 24 to 72 hours, after cessation of a short half-life drug such as morphine, whereas onset may be delayed for 36 to 48 hours with methadone, a long half-life drug. It is important, therefore, to emphasize that even in a patient in whom pain has been completely relieved by a procedure (e.g., a cordotomy), it is necessary to slowly decrease the opioid dose to prevent withdrawal (2,3).

Experience indicates that the usual daily dose required to prevent withdrawal is equal to one fourth of the previous daily dose. This dose, called for want of a better term, *the detoxification dose,* is given in four divided doses. The initial detoxification dose is given for 2 days and then decremented by half (administered in four divided doses) for 2 days until a total daily dose of 10 to 15 mg/day (in morphine equivalents) is reached, and after 2 days on this dose the opioid can be discontinued. Thus, a patient who had been receiving 240 mg/day of morphine for pain would require an initial detoxification dose of 60 mg given as 15 mg every 6 hours. Alternately, the patient may be switched to the equieffective oral analgesic dose of methadone, using one fourth of this dose as the initial detoxification dose and proceeding as described previously (2–4).

References

1. Reisine T, Pasternak GW. Opioid analgesics and antagonists. In: Goodman LS, Limbird LE, Milinoff, PB, eds. Goodman & Gilman's the pharmacological basis of therapeutics, 9th ed. New York: McGraw-Hill, 1996:521–55.
2. Inturrisi CE, Hanks GWC. Opioid analgesic therapy. In: Doyle D, Hanks GWC, MacDonald N, eds. Oxford textbook of palliative medicine. Oxford: Oxford University Press, 1993:166–82.
3. Foley KM. Problems of overarching importance, which transcend organ systems. In: Bennett JC, Plum F, eds. Cecil textbook of medicine. Philadelphia: WB Saunders, 1996:100–7.
4. American Pain Society. Principles of analgesic use in the treatment of acute pain and cancer pain, 4th ed. Glenview, IL: American Pain Society, 1999.
5. Jacox A, Carr DB, Payne R, et al. Management of cancer pain. Clinical Practice Guideline No. 9. AHCPR Publication No. 94-0592. U.S. Department of Health and Human Services, Public Health Service. Rockville, MD: Agency for Health Care Policy and Research, 1994.
6. World Health Organization. Cancer pain relief. Geneva: World Health Organization, 1986.
7. Portenoy RK. Adjuvant analgesic agents. Hematol Oncol Clin North Am 10:103–19, 1996.
8. Kieffer BL. Opioids: first lessons from knockout mice. Trends Pharmacol Sci 20:19–26, 1999.
9. Portenoy RK, Thaler HT, Inturrisi CE, et al. The metabolite morphine-6-glucuronide contributes to the analgesia produced by morphine infusion in patients with pain and normal renal function. Clin Pharmacol Ther 51:422–31, 1992.
10. Rossi GC, Brown GP, Leventhal L, et al. Novel receptor mechanisms for heroin and morphine-6-glucuronide analgesia. Neurosci Lett 216:1–4, 1996.
11. Portenoy RK, Foley KM, Stulman J, et al. Plasma morphine and morphine-6-glucuronide during chronic morphine therapy for cancer pain: plasma profiles, steady-state concentra-

tions and the consequences of renal failure. Pain 47:13–9, 1991.
12. Tiseo PJ, Thaler HT, Lapin J, et al. Morphine-6-glucuronide concentrations and opioid-related side effects: a survey in cancer patients. Pain 61:47–54, 1995.
13. Mercadante S. The role of morphine glucuronides in cancer pain. Palliat Med 13:95–104, 1999.
14. Smith MT. Neuroexcitatory effects of morphine and hydromorphone: evidence implicating the 3-glucuronide metabolites. Clin Exp Pharmacol Physiol 27:524–8, 2000.
15. Ripamonti C, Groff L, Brunelli C, et al. Switching from morphine to oral methadone in treating cancer pain: what is the equianalgesic dose ratio? J Clin Oncol 16:3216–21, 1998.
16. Foley KM, Houde RW. Methadone in cancer pain management: Individualize dose and titrate to effect. J Clin Oncol 16:3213–15, 1998.
17. Morley JS. New perspectives in our use of opioids. Pain Forum 8:200–5, 1999.
18. Inturrisi CE. Old dogs, new tricks. Pain Forum 8:210–12, 1999.
19. Davis AM, Inturrisi CE. d-Methadone blocks morphine tolerance and N-methyl-D-aspartate (NMDA)-induced hyperalgesia. J Pharmacol Exp Ther 289:1048–53, 1999.
20. Inturrisi CE. Preclinical evidence for a role of glutamatergic systems in opioid tolerance and dependence. Semin Neurosci 9:110–19, 1997.
21. Bennett GJ. Update on the neurophysiology of pain transmission and modulation: focus on the NMDA-receptor. J Pain Symptom Manage 19:S2–S6, 2000.
22. Sang CN. NMDA-receptor antagonists in neuropathic pain: experimental methods to clinical trials. J Pain Symptom Manage 9:S21–S25, 2000.
23. Caruso FS. MorphiDex pharmacokinetic studies and single-dose analgesic efficacy studies in patients with postoperative pain. J Pain Symptom Manage 19:S31–S36, 2000.
24. Jasinski DR. Abuse potential of morphine/dextromethorphan combinations. J Pain Symptom Manage 19:S26–S30, 2000.
25. Katz NP. MorphiDex (MS:DM) double-blind, multiple-dose studies in chronic pain patients. J Pain Symptom Manage 19:S37–S41, 2000.
26. Gear RW, Miaskowski C, Gordon NC, et al. Kappa-opioids produce significantly greater analgesia in women than in men. Natl Med 11:1248–50, 1996.
27. Gear RW, Gordon NC, Heller PS, et al. Gender difference in analgesic response to the kappa-opioid pentazocine. Neurosci Lett 205:207–9, 1996.
28. Gal TJ. Naloxone reversal of buprenorphine-induced respiratory depression. Clin Pharmacol Ther 45:66–71, 1989.
29. Donner B, Zenz M, Tryba M, Strumpf M. Direct conversion from oral morphine to transdermal fentanyl: a multicenter study in patients with cancer pain. Pain 64:527–34, 1996.
30. Portenoy RK, Southam MA, Gupta SK, et al. Transdermal fentanyl for cancer pain. Repeated dose pharmacokinetics. Anesthesiology 78:36–43, 1993.
31. Edwards WT, Breed RJ. Treatment of postoperative pain in the post anesthesia care unit. Anesthesiol Clin North Am 8:235–65, 1990.

32. White PF. Patient-controlled analgesia: an update on its use in the treatment of postoperative pain. Anesthesiol Clin North Am 7:63–78, 1989.

33. Citron ML, Johnston-Early A, Boyer M, et al. Patient-controlled analgesia for severe cancer pain. Arch Intern Med 146:734–6, 1986.

34. Kerr IG, Sone M, De Angelis C, et al. Continuous narcotic infusion with patient-controlled analgesia for chronic cancer pain in outpatients. Ann Intern Med 108:554–7, 1988.

35. Ferrante FM, Orav EJ, Rocco A, Gallo J. A statistical model for pain in patient-controlled analgesia and conventional intramuscular opioid regimens. Anesth Analg 67:457–61, 1988.

36. Coyle N, Mauskop A, Maggard J, Foley KM. Continuous subcutaneous infusions of opiates in cancer patients with pain. Oncol Nurs Forum 13:53–7, 1986.

37. Sabbe M, Yaksh T. Pharmacology of spinal opioid. J Pain Symptom Manage 5:191–203, 1990.

38. DeLeon-Casasola OA, Lema M. Postoperative epidural opioid analgesia: What are the choices? Anesth Analg 83:867–75, 1996.

39. Carr DB, Cousins MJ. Spinal route of analgesia: opioids and future options. In: Cousins MJ, Bridenbaugh PO, eds. Neural blockade in clinical anesthesia and the management of pain, 3rd ed. Philadelphia: Lippincott-Raven Publishers, Philadelphia, 1998:915–83.

40. Cousins MJ, Plummer JL. Design of studies of spinal opioids in acute and chronic pain. In: Max MB, Portenoy RK, Laska EM, eds. The design of analgesic clinical trials. Advances in pain research and therapy, vol. 18. New York: Raven Press, 1991:457–80.

41. Gillis JC, Benfield P, Goa KL. Transnasal butorphanol. A review of its pharmacodynamic and pharmacokinetic proper-ties, and therapeutic potential in acute pain management. Drugs 50:57–175, 1995.

42. Christie JM, Simmonds M, Patt R, et al. Dose titration: a multicenter study of oral transmucosal fentanyl citrate for the treatment of breakthrough pain in cancer patients using transdermal fentanyl for persistent pain. J Clin Oncol 16:3238–45, 1998.

43. Bruera E, Pereira J. Neuropsychiatric toxicity of opioids. In: Jensen TS, Turner JA, Wiesenfeld-Hallin Z, eds. Proceedings of the 8th World Congress on Pain, vol. 8. Seattle: IASP Press, 1997:717–38.

44. Palm S, Lehzen S, Mignat C, et al. Does prolonged oral treatment with sustained-release morphine tablets influence immune function? Anesth Anal 86:166–72, 1998.

45. Machelska H, Stein C. Pain control by immune-derived opioids. Clin Exp Pharmacol Physiol 27:533–6, 2000.

46. McQuay H. Opioids and pain management. Lancet 353:2229–32, 1999.

47. Kanner RM, Foley KM. Patterns of narcotic drug use in a cancer pain clinic. Ann NY Acad Sci 362:161–72, 1981.

48. O'Brien C. Drug addiction and drug abuse. In: Goodman LS, Limbird LE, Milinoff, PB, eds. Goodman & Gilman's the pharmacological basis of therapeutics, 9th ed. New York: McGraw-Hill, 1996:557–77.

49. Porter J, Jick H. Addiction rare in patients treated with narcotics. N Engl J Med 302:123, 1980.

50. Perry S, Heidrich G. Management of pain during debridement: a survey of U.S. burn units. Pain 13:267–80, 1982.

51. Joranson DE, Ryan KM, Gilson AM, Dahl JL. Trends in medical use and abuse of opioid analgesics. JAMA 283:1710–14, 2000.

8 Pharmacology of opioid analgesia: clinical principles

CARLA RIPAMONTI
National Cancer Institute of Milan

Introduction

According to the World Health Organization (WHO) guidelines, opioid analgesics are the mainstay of analgesic therapy and are classified according to their ability to control mild to moderate pain (codeine, tramadol, dextropropoxyphene) (second step of the WHO analgesic ladder) and to control moderate to severe pain (morphine, methadone, oxycodone, buprenorphine, hydromorphone, fentanyl, heroin) (third step of the WHO analgesic ladder) (1,2). Opioid analgesics can be associated with non-opioid drugs such as paracetamol or with nonsteroidal anti-inflammatory drugs (NSAIDs) and to adjuvant drugs (3).

The current recommended management of cancer pain consists of the regular administration of opioids and intermittent rescue doses of opioids or NSAIDs for excess pain. Individualized pain management should take into account the intensity of pain and its nature, concurrent medical conditions, and above all the subjective perception of the intensity of pain that is not proportional to the type or to the extension of the tissue damage but depends on the interaction of physical, cultural, and emotional factors.

Oral route of opioid administration remains the preferred one. However, in some clinical situations such as vomiting, dysphagia, confusion, and where rapid dose escalation is necessary, oral administration may be impossible, and alternative routes must be implemented (4,5). Table 8.1 shows the potential application of the different routes of opioid administration (6).

Intraindividual variability in response to different opioids is a common clinical phenomenon. Different explanations have been proposed such as the genetic makeup, tolerance to different opioid effects, the incomplete cross-tolerance among opioids selective for the same receptor subtype due to differential affinity for receptor

subtypes, the differences in profile of active metabolites between various opioids (7–12), and the pain mechanism (13). Neuropathic pain has been associated with a less favorable response to opioid analgesics in respect to other types of pain (14,15). However, opioids may also be effective in neuropathic pain even if high doses are often required (16–18).

Patients have an unpredictable predilection to develop adverse effects with opioids. Some patients may be able to tolerate very large doses of opioids without developing the common adverse effects such as sedation or nausea and vomiting, whereas others may do so at very small doses.

A regular and continuous assessment about the possible causes, frequency, intensity, and type of adverse effects is mandatory to obtain adequate symptomatic treatment. It is not always possible to distinguish if the symptom(s) referred by the patient is a consequence of opioid administration and/or if it is due to the presence or progression of the cancer or concomitant diseases. Thus it is important to evaluate if the administration of the opioid worsens the symptoms already present or if it provokes new symptoms. Before thinking that the opioid administration is the only and/or main cause of the symptom (s) in particular cognitive failure, a series of other factors must be ruled out (Table 8.2).

Over the last few years, data shows that in patients with cancer-related pain, the type of opioid analgesic and/or the route of administration must be changed once or more often (15,19,20) so that the therapy is tailor-made to face specific clinical circumstances, improve pain control (21–23), and/or reduce opioid toxicity (24).

This chapter considers the most used opioid analgesics in clinical practice, their administration routes, the co-administration of different opioids, the potential role of

Table 8.1. *Potential applications of the different routes of opioid administration*

Symptoms	Oral	Sublingual	Rectal	CSI	Intravenous	Transdermal[a]	Spinal
Vomiting	–	++	++	++	++	++	++
Bowel obstruction	–	++	++	++	++	++	++
Dysphagia	–	++	++	++	++	++	++
Cognitive failure	–	–	–	++	++	++	–
Diarrhea	–	++	–	++	++	++	++
Hemorrhoids Anal fissures	++	++	–	++	++	++	++
Coagulation disorders	++	++	++	–	++	++	–
Severe immunosuppression	++	++	++	–	++	++	–
Generalized edema	++	++	++	–	++	–	++
Frequent dose changes	++	++	–	++[b]	++[b]	–	+
Titration	++	++	+	++[b]	++[b]	–	–
Breakthrough pain	++[c]	++	++	++[b]	++[b]	–	–

Abbreviation: CSI, continuous subcutaneous infusion.
+ = may be indicated; ++ = is indicated; – = is contraindicated.
[a] Fentanyl.
[b] Patient controlled analgesia (PCA).
[c] Only immediate release formulations.
(Modified from Bruera[6]).

Table 8.2. *Main causes of cognitive impairment in cancer patients*

Metabolic/ Endocrine	Hypercalcemia, hyper/hypoglycemia, hypoxia, hyponatremia, hypomagnesemia, liver failure, renal failure, adrenal insufficiency, hyperthyroid/hypothyroid
Sepsis	Pneumonia, urinary tract infection, other
Brain involvement	Metastasis, edema, leptomeningeal involvement, encephalitis (bacterial, viral, fungal), cerebellar degeneration, limbic encephalitis, progressive multi-focal leucoencephalopathy, vascular disorders
Drugs Drugs/Interactions	Opioids, antidepressants, benzodiazepines, other psychoactive drugs, NSAIDs, ranitidine, ciprofloxacin, steroids, anticholinergics, IL-2
Withdrawals	Alcohol, opioids, benzodiazepines, barbiturates
Dehydration	Emesis, anorexia, bowel obstruction, decreased fluid intake
Psychological distress	Fear, anxiety, sleep deprivation, isolation, feeling of dependence, hopelessness, loss of dignity
Others	Severe constipation, fecal impaction, bladder distension

Abbreviations: NSAID, nonsteroidal anti-inflammatory drug; IL, interleukin.

opioid, as well as route switching in the management of opioid-related adverse effects.

Opioids for mild to moderate pain

Although the role of "strong" opioids is universally recognized in the treatment of moderate to severe pain, there is no common agreement regarding the role of "weak" opioids for mild to moderate pain. No significant differences in pain relief between non-opioids alone and non-opioids plus weak opioids have been reported in a meta-analysis of data from published randomized controlled trials (25). Different results were obtained by Moore et al. (26) in a systematic review of randomized controlled trials on analgesia obtained from single oral doses of paracetamol alone and in combination with codeine in postoperative pain. They found that 60 mg codeine added to paracetamol produced worthwhile additional pain relief even in single oral doses.

Uncontrolled studies show that the efficacy of the second step of the WHO ladder is limited in time to 30 to 40 days in the majority of the patients and that switching to strong opioids is mainly due to poor analgesia rather than to adverse effects (27–29). In a study of 944 patients treated with drugs of the second step, 24% of the patients still benefited after 1 month of treatment, and the percentage decreased to 4% after 90 days (28). This study evaluated several drugs, including oxycodone at low doses and buprenorphine, which are now considered drugs for moderate to severe pain (2). In a study of 745 home care cancer patients, more than 60% of those with pain were administered "weak" opioids until death with adequate pain relief and no need to switch to strong opioids (30).

Several authors have suggested abolishing the second step and initiating earlier low-dose morphine therapy (25,31,32). Controversial points regarding the use of second step are that 1) there are insufficient data regarding the effectiveness of the so-called "weak" opioids; 2) there are few studies showing a real advantage in their use compared with strong opioids; 3) the second-step drugs are often marketed in combination with a non-opioid such as paracetamol, aspirin, or NSAID and it is the latter component that limits the dose; and 4) these drugs are often expensive in respect to their potential benefits (cost-benefit ratio).

Codeine

Codeine is an opium alkaloid with a potency of about 1/10 in respect to morphine. The efficacy of codeine (200–400 mg/day) in moderate cancer-related pain has been confirmed in a controlled trial (33). Codeine is almost always commercially available in association with paracetamol. Codeine is a pro-drug of morphine with a biotransformation of about 10%. The pharmacodynamic effects of codeine are largely due to the production of its active metabolite morphine (34).

Codeine is metabolized to active drugs within the body by CYP2D6, an enzyme of the hepatic P450 microsomal enzyme system (34,35). Poor metabolizers produce no CYP2D6 or undetectable levels of it, thus preventing them from metabolizing drugs that are substrates of this enzyme. Without CYP2D6, codeine provides little or no analgesia (36,37). Data from an animal study shows that when the o-demethylation of codeine to morphine is blocked, codeine lacks significant analgesic activity (38). Moreover, a patient who takes codeine or its derivatives in combination with a high-affinity substrate or potent inhibitor of CYP2D6 (such as quinidine, paroxetine, fluoxetine) will experience attenuated analgesia, whether this person is a poor or an extensive metabolizer (39,40).

Dihydrocodeine

Dihydrocodeine is a semisynthetic analog of codeine with an oral bioavailability of about 20% (41) and the same equianalgesic when administered orally but a narrower therapeutic range. Palmer et al. (42) showed that 60 mg of dihydrocodeine produced greater analgesia than 30 mg,

but there was little difference in analgesia between doses of 60 and 90 mg; moreover, the adverse effects were dose related. When administered subcutaneously, 30 to 70 mg of dihydrocodeine are equivalent to 10 mg of morphine (42). Dihydrocodeine can produce severe toxicity when administered in patients with renal impairment (43).

Tramadol

Tramadol is a synthetic drug with opioid and non-opioid properties (44,45), the latter being correlated to inhibition of serotonin and noradrenalin reuptake. After repeated oral administration the bioavailability is about 90%–100%, the excretion is mostly via kidneys (90%). O-demethyl-tramadol is the active metabolite and is two to four times more potent than parent compound. The elimination time of this metabolite is double in patients with hepatic or renal impairment (45).

Oral tramadol (200–400 mg/day) is considered effective and safe in the treatment of cancer pain (46–48). Although tramadol is considered to be a drug at low risk of causing respiratory depression, two cases of severe respiratory depression after tramadol use have been described in children (45) and in one adult with cancer pain and renal insufficiency (49).

With respect to morphine, the potency is considered to be about 1/10 when administrated via parenteral route and 1/5 when administered orally (50). Other authors found morphine tramadol ratios ranging from 1:3.8 to 1:5.3 (46–48). In a retrospective study of a large number of patients, Grond et al. (51) found that a dose of tramadol up to 600 mg/day was effective and safe and was similar to 60 mg/day of oral morphine. Furthermore, patients on morphine received corticosteroids, laxatives, and antiemetics more often and experienced constipation, neuropsychological symptoms, and pruritus more frequently than patients treated with tramadol.

Osipova et al. (46) compared cancer patients treated with oral tramadol and morphine. Tramadol was effective and safe for 1 to 3 months in the majority of patients, at mean dose of about 370 mg/day. In comparison to tramadol, morphine produced better analgesia but was associated with more frequent and intense adverse effects such as nausea and constipation. Similar results have been reported by other authors (47,48).

Sindrup et al. (52) carried out a randomized, double-blind, placebo-controlled, crossover trial to evaluate the analgesic efficacy of tramadol in 34 patients with chronic painful polyneuropathy. Tramadol dose was increased to maximum 200 mg twice daily; however, 11 patients needed doses between 200 and 300 mg/day. Pain scores, paresthesia, and allodynia were significantly lower in the tramadol group than in the group receiving placebo. The authors suggest that the analgesic effect of tramadol is due to a reduction of central hyperexcitability. Similar positive results were obtained in a multicenter trial of tramadol in patients with diabetic neuropathy (53). Tramadol can be administered orally, rectally, intravenously, subcutaneously, or intramuscularly.

Dextropropoxyphene (DPP)

Propoxyphene is a synthetic derivative of methadone, and its analgesic properties are due to dextrogyral isomer called dextropropoxyphene. It is mu agonist and a weak *N*-methyl-D-aspartate (NMDA) antagonist receptor (54). DPP has a mean beta half-life of about 15 hours. When it is administered regularly, plasmatic concentration gradually increased with a plateau after 2 to 3 days. It is metabolized in the liver to nor-propoxyphene, which can accumulate in the body because of its long half-life (about 23 hours) and may produce central nervous system (CNS) toxicity. The analgesic effect of DPP hydrochloride in doses of 65 mg or more has been established in controlled studies (55).

In a prospective, randomized study comparing oral morphine and DPP, titrated doses of DPP were associated with a more favorable adverse effects-analgesia balance in opioid-naive patients, but this study did not exclude a similar result with lower doses of oral morphine (56) (Table 8.3).

Table 8.3. *Comparative studies between morphine and other opioids*

Author (Ref)	Study design	No. of patients	Opioid	Opioid	Results
Ventafridda et al. (82)	Prospective randomized	54	27 patients oral morphine	27 patients oral methadone for 2 weeks	Comparable analgesia Patients on methadone had significantly more headache Patients on morphine had significantly more dry mouth Dose escalation significantly lower with methadone
Mercadante et al. (83)	Prospective randomized	40	20 patients CR oral morphine	20 patients oral methadone	Comparable analgesia and adverse effects Dose escalation significantly lower with methadone
Mercadante et al. (56)	Prospective randomized	32 opioid naives	16 patients CR morphine 20 mg/day	16 patients DPP 20–240 mg/day	Patients on morphine had significantly more frequency and severity of drowsiness, vomiting, dry mouth 11 patients on DPP switched to CR morphine to increase analgesia 3 patients on morphine switched to DPP due to intolerable vomiting and drowsiness and had pain relief until death
Coda et al. (85)	Randomized double blind parallel-group	100 bone marrow transplant patients	PCA with IV morphine or hydromorphone	Sufentanil	Comparable analgesia Sedation, sleep, and mood disturbances were significantly lower in the morphine group than hydromorphone or sufentanil group Sufentanil dose requirement increased by 10-fold compared to morphine and hydromorphone (only 5-fold)
Miller et al. (84)	Randomized double blind	74	Morphine CSI Conversion rate: 5:1[a]	hydromorphone CSI	Comparable analgesia and adverse effects

Abbreviations: CR, controlled release; DPP, dextropropoxyphene; PCA, patient-controlled analgesia; IV, intravenous; CSI, continuous subcutaneous infusion.
[a] 5 mg morphine = 1 mg hydromorphone.

Opioids for moderate to severe pain

Oral morphine

Since 1977, oral morphine has been used by hospices and palliative care units as the drug of choice for the management of chronic cancer pain of a moderate to severe intensity (57,58) because it provides effective pain relief, is widely tolerated, is simple to administer, and is comparatively inexpensive. However, there are no studies showing the superiority of morphine to other strong opioids as far as analgesia and tolerability are concerned.

Important studies investigated the clinical pharmacology and pharmacokinetics of oral morphine (59–64). Morphine by mouth is not an especially effective pain-relieving drug when it is administered in a single dose, owing to its limited bioavailability (65). Conversely, the effectiveness of repeated doses seems to result from the presence of the enterohepatic circulation, which allows a recirculation of morphine and its metabolites (66).

The effective analgesic dose varies considerably among patients (64). This variability is due not only to a difference in pain severity and perception by the patient but also to other factors previously described. For this reason, it is necessary to administer it in an individualized dose and thoroughly monitor its analgesic effect, especially during the phase of titration. Morphine clearance decreases in patients over 50 years old, which helps to explain elderly patients' higher sensitivity to the drug (67). This clinical observation implies that younger patients may need larger doses of morphine to achieve the same analgesic effect (68). Experimental studies carried out on animals show that morphine is glucuronized in the liver and the intestinal mucosa (69). Morphine has three different metabolites: morphine 3-glucuronide (M-3-G), morphine-6-glucoronide (M-6-G), and normorphine (10,70–74). Morphine administered via oral, buccal, and sublingual routes resulted in higher metabolite production than routes of administration that avoid first-pass metabolism (75). M-6-G is an opioid-binding metabolite with analgesic properties (70). M-3-G is a non-opioid binding agent that has the ability to cause generalized hyperexcitability, myoclonus, and grand mal seizures in animals (10,72). Normorphine may also cause central hyperexcitability (73). M-6-G is known to accumulate during renal failure (70,74,76,77) and cause late opioid toxicity. Wolff et al. (78) found an accumulation of both morphine glucuronides in patients with elevated serum creatinine.

Oral morphine adverse effects are common to all opioids and may occur during both titration and the therapy maintenance phase (Table 8.4). Individual titration of dosages and

Table 8.4. *Side effects during morphine therapy*

Titration	Continuing
Nausea	Constipation
Vomiting	Sedation
Constipation	Xerostomia
Sedation	Hallucinations
Xerostomia	Hyperalgesia, allodynia
Pruritus	Myoclonus
Respiratory depression	Cognitive failure
	Respiratory depression

the prevention of some adverse effects (e.g., nausea, vomiting, constipation) are strongly recommended.

Ideally, two types of oral morphine formulation are required: immediate release (IR) and controlled release (CR) (5). An IR formulation is indicated for dose titration (every 4 hours) and for breakthrough pain (as required). The regular dose must be adjusted according to how many rescue doses have been administered. Most patients control their own pain by taking doses ranging from 5 to 30 mg every 4 hours. Some patients may need larger doses. Larger doses are acceptable, as morphine does not have a ceiling effect.

Once the optimal dose requirements for at least a 24-hour period have been established by titration, a CR formulation may be indicated for maintenance treatment to be administered every 12 hours or every 8 hours in association to immediate release morphine as rescue dose. In a double-blind, placebo-controlled, crossover study carried out on a group of 34 patients, Finn et al. (79) compared immediate release morphine formulation administered every 4 hours with a sustained release morphine formulation administered every 12 hours. No difference with respect to pain, adverse effects, or incidence of breakthrough pain was found.

Another controlled release formulation can provide up to 24 hours of pain relief with a single daily dose. In a controlled clinical study, Gourlay et al. (80) studied the pharmacokinetics and the pharmacodynamics of two controlled-release oral morphine formulations to be administered every 24 hours and 12 hours, respectively. No significant differences were found between the two formulations as regards analgesic effectiveness, adverse effects, the need of rescue doses, and the preference of treatment at the end of the study. Similar results were obtained by Smith et al. (81).

Table 8.3 shows the prospective, randomized, comparative studies between morphine and other opioids. Overlapping analgesia and adverse effect profile (nausea, vomiting, sedation) were found between morphine and methadone orally administered (82,83). However, the dose escalation in patients treated with methadone was significantly lower.

Morphine and hydromorphone administered via continuous subcutaneous infusion (CSI) showed comparable analgesia and tolerability (84). Patients treated with intravenous (IV) morphine achieved comparable analgesia but had significantly lower adverse effects compared with patients treated with IV hydromorphone and sufentanil (85).

A series of controlled studies compared the CR or IR morphine to analog formulations of oxycodone (86–89) (Table 8.5). Between the two drugs, the analgesia was similar in all the studies. Whereas some authors reported lower adverse effects during oxycodone treatment (86,88,89), Bruera et al. (87) found that the tolerability was comparable between CR morphine and CR oxycodone. Further studies are necessary to compare the adverse effect profile between these drugs as well as the dose ratio.

Other routes of morphine administration

Subcutaneous (SC), rectal, IV, and spinal (epidural and intrathecal) (4,5,90) are the most frequent alternative routes of morphine administration. Intermittent or frequent SC administration is associated with a "bolus effect" phenomenon characterized by acute toxicity and a brief analgesic efficacy caused by a transient high plasma drug concentration. To avoid a bolus effect as well as painful repeated injections, the CSI is recommended. A continuous infusion plus an intermittent bolus dose allows a patient to maintain a baseline level of opioid administration plus additional doses for breakthrough pain (patient-controlled analgesia [PCA]) (91). The blood levels of morphine during CSI is not subject to sudden changes (92) and are similar to continuous intravenous infusion (CII) (93). In a study by Coyle et al. (94), 13 of 15 patients undergoing CSI reported adequate pain control and were maintained on this route for 3 to 76 days. Ventafridda et al. (95) showed that the CSI of morphine can be used when nausea and vomiting make oral administration impossible, as well as when analgesia is difficult to obtain with oral morphine or by parenteral injection. In this study only 16% of the patients preferred CSI compared with 94% of patients studied by Bruera et al. (96). When switching from oral morphine to SC morphine, a conversion factor of 2:1 or 3:1 should be used (97–99) according to the pain relief reported before switching. An initial bolus dose equivalent to 2 hours of infusion is a way to reduce the time necessary to achieve plasmatic steady-state. Many different devices are avail-

Table 8.5. *Comparative studies between oral morphine and oxycodone*

Authors (Ref)	Study design	No. patients	Route	Route	Results
Lo Russo et al. (86)	Parallel-group study	101	CR morphine	CR oxycodone	Comparable efficacy and tolerability Two patients on CR morphine reported hallucinations and no patients on CR oxycodone
Bruera et al. (87)	Prospective double blind crossover	32 23 completed the study	CR morphine for 7 days	CR oxycodone	Comparable efficacy and tolerability Conversion rate from 1.5 to 2.3 Oxycodone > potent than morphine
Kalso et al. (88)	Double blind crossover	20	Oral morphine every 4 hr; 4.0 mg/ml after IV PCA for titration	Oral oxycodone every 4 hr 2.7 mg/ml after IV PCA for titration	Comparable pain relief Morphine caused more nausea Hallucinations occurred only during morphine treatment Both drugs produced sedation
Heiskanen et al. (89)	Double blind randomized crossover	27	CR morphine[a]	CR oxycodone	Comparable analgesia Significantly more vomiting with morphine Constipation more common with oxycodone Nightmares only with morphine (n.s.)

Abbreviations: CR, controlled release; IV, intravenous; PCA, patient-controlled analgesia.
[a] Opioid consumption ratio of oxy/morph was 2:3 when oxy was administered first and 3:4 when oxy was administered after morphine.

able for CSI. It is important to consider which of the different portable pumps is most suitable for a given patient. PCA devices permit the patient to choose an intermittent (demand) bolus, continuous infusion, or intermittent and continuous modes of administration.

Tables 8.6 and 8.7 show comparative studies of different routes of morphine administration. In the study of Drexel et al. (98), CSI of morphine produced significantly lower adverse effects compared to oral or SC morphine administered intermittently. In 164 patients who were switched from oral to SC morphine, significant improvements in pain relief, nausea, and vomiting were obtained (99) (Table 8.6). The rectal route of administration gives a better bioavailability of those opioids subject to first-pass liver metabolism (100,101). Rectal drug vehicles may be liquid or solid. In some countries, preparations of opioids in the form of suppositories are not commercially available. To overcome this situation, microenemas made up of parenteral formulation of morphine or other opioids may be prepared and then administered rectally as a bolus using a needless insulin-type syringe. The advantage of this approach is that absorption of aqueous and alcoholic solutions occurs rapidly (101). The colostomy administration route of opioids is not recommended (102).

The rectal route of drug administration may present some disadvantages when used chronically and when feces or diarrhea is present. This alternative route can be administered successfully in patients with breakthrough pain (defined as transient flares of severe or excruciating pain in patients already managed with analgesics) and in some clinical situations (Table 8.1). Studies comparing

Table 8.6. *Comparative studies on different routes of morphine administration*

Authors (Ref)	Study design	No. of patients	Route	Route	Results
Drexel et al. (98)	Prospective	36	Morphine 10–90 mg/day intermittent oral or SC	Morphine 5–48 mg/day CSI conversion rate 2:1	Significantly lower incidence of constipation, nausea, and drowsiness with CSI
MacDonald et al. (99)	Prospective	164 switched due to drowsiness, nausea, vomiting, not controlled pain, difficulty in swallowing	Oral morphine	Bolus SC morphine every 4 hr Conversion rate 2:1	Significant improvement in pain relief and significantly less nausea and vomiting but not drowsiness with SC
Bruera et al. (103)	Double-blind cross over	23	CR morphine sulfate suppository every 12 hr	SC morphine rect/parent ratio 2.5:1	Comparable analgesia and side effects
Babul et al. (104)	Double-blind crossover	27	CR morphine suppository every 12 hr	CR morphine tablets every 12 hr Conversion rate 1:1	No difference in pain and sedation Small but significant difference in nausea in favor of rectal administration
De Conno et al. (105)	Double-blind, double-dummy crossover single-dose study	34 opioid naives	Rectal morphine conversion rate 1:1	Oral morphine	Rectal morphine had a faster onset of action and longer duration of analgesia than an acute dose of oral morphine No significant difference in intensity of sedation, nausea, or number of vomiting episodes between the two routes
Bruera et al (106)	Randomized, double-blind crossover	12 6 evaluable	CR morphine sulfate suppository every 12 hr	CR morphine sulfate suppository every 24 hr	No significant difference between the q12 h and q24h treatment groups in symptom (pain, nausea, sedation), intensity, adverse effects, patient choice

Abbreviations: SC, subcutaneous; CSI, continuous subcutaneous infusion; CR, controlled release.

Table 8.7. *Studies on different routes of morphine administration*

Authors (Ref)	Study design	No. of patients	Route	Route	Results
Vainio and Tigerstedt (111)	Prospective randomized	30	Oral morphine 151 (24–480) mg/day	Epidural morphine 45 (2–800) mg/day	CNS side effects were less frequent and the KPS slightly superior in the epidural groups (n.s) Pain relief was similar and adequate in both groups For patients with neuropathic pain, double doses of oral morphine were needed for similar pain relief
Kalso et al. (21)	Randomized double blind cross over	10 switched due to adverse effects or not controlled pain	Oral morphine every 4 h median dose 225 mg switch to	CSI morphine median dose 327 mg CEI morphine median dose 106 mg	Pain at rest significantly less during CSI compared with oral morphine Pain when moving significantly less during both CSI and CEI compared with oral morphine No significant difference in pain relief between CSI and CEI Total amount of adverse effects (sum of VAS values) significantly higher during oral compared to CSI Median of the sum of adverse effects during CEI did not differ significantly from oral or CSI

Abbreviations: CNS, central nervous system; CSI, continuous subcutaneous infusion; CEI, continuous epidural infusion.

oral or SC morphine and morphine administered rectally (Table 8.6) showed comparable analgesia and adverse effects (103,104). In a single-doses study, De Conno et al. (105) found that IR rectal morphine had a faster onset and longer duration of analgesia than oral morphine. Patients who achieve stable pain control with suppositories every 12 hours could undergo a trial of a single daily dose (106).

For some time, many reports have described the successful spinal administration of morphine and other opioids to treat cancer pain, especially refractory pain (90, 107–109). The number of cancer patients with cancer pain requiring spinal analgesia has not been clearly defined. According to Zech et al. (110) only 1%–2% of patients need this treatment. There are no comparative trials between oral and intrathecal morphine, but two prospective trials have compared the analgesia and tolerability of morphine administered orally or by epidural (21,111) (Table 8.7). An improvement in pain control as well as in adverse effects was shown by switching from oral to epidural or continuous subcutaneous infusion of morphine (21). Of interest, Kalso showed no significant benefits, either in efficacy or in adverse effects, by administering morphine epidural compared with the SC route. The authors concluded that the co-administration of local anesthetic agents, alpha-2-adrenergic agonists or

NMDA antagonists may significantly improve the quality of epidural analgesia as compared with the SC route (21). Further studies are necessary to validate this hypothesis.

Oral methadone

Methadone is a synthetic opioid agonist developed more than 50 years ago. Although it has been used mostly for the maintenance drug for opioid addicts, methadone has also proved to be a powerful analgesic and a suitable drug in treating cancer pain (82,83,112–118).

Methadone is a mu and delta opioid receptor agonist with NMDA receptor antagonist affinity (119,120). Thus methadone may play a positive role with patients experiencing neuropathic pain; Data are still controversial (121,122).

After 50 years, because of its resurgence in the analgesic arena, methadone may still be considered one of the new analgesics based on impressive study results and clinical successes. Methadone has a number of unique characteristics including excellent oral and rectal absorption, no known active metabolites, high potency, and longer administration intervals, as well as an incomplete cross-tolerance with respect to other mu-opioid receptor agonist drugs (113,118). Methadone showed to control pain no longer responsive to morphine, hydromorphone, and fentanyl (123–127). Some data suggest that methadone may be less constipating than other opioids (128–130) but controlled studies have not been done to confirm this hypothesis. For different reasons, methadone has the potential of playing a major role in the treatment of cancer pain, as well as chronic non-malignant pain (131). However, its use is limited by the remarkably long and unpredictable half-life, large interindividual variations in pharmacokinetics, the potential for delayed toxicity, and above all by the limited knowledge of the correct administration intervals and the equianalgesic ratio with other opioids when administered chronically. The analgesic role of methadone in treating cancer-related pain remains relatively unknown to physicians, nurses, and administrators involved in hospice and palliative care primarily because of its low cost and consequent non-promotion by the pharmaceutical industry.

Different authors have suggested 8-, 12-, or 24-hour dosing intervals for methadone administration to avoid accumulation risk because of its long terminal half-life. Others have suggested titrating the analgesic therapy with an initial loading dose of methadone followed by progressive dose reduction during the first week of treatment.

In two randomized prospective studies on cancer patients (82,83) (Table 8.3), morphine and methadone, orally administered every 8 hours, showed comparable analgesia and side effect profile.

De Conno et al. (132) treated 196 advanced cancer patients with methadone in solution form administered every 8 hours. They analyzed the assessments carried out at T0 and then T7, 15, 30, 45, 60, and 90 days. After 3 months, 43 patients were on methadone again. In respect to T0 a significant reduction in pain score occurred at each time point. The mean dose of oral methadone ranged from 14 mg at T7 to 23.65 mg at T90. Only 11.2% of patients dropped out because of analgesic inefficacy and 6.6% because of methadone-related side effects.

Mercadante et al. (133) carried out a study of PCA with oral methadone in 24 patients with advanced cancer-related pain. A regimen of self-administered methadone with a fixed dose and flexible patient-controlled dosage intervals to achieve appropriate analgesia and to avoid the risk of toxicity from accumulation of methadone was prescribed. Opioid-naive patients took a fixed dose of 5 mg of methadone t.i.d. for 3 days, whereas patients switching from morphine received 50% of morphine equivalent of methadone for 3 days. From the fourth day, both groups received the fixed night dosage of oral methadone and another dose when the pain reappeared. When more than four administrations of methadone a day were used, an increase in dosage was prescribed. The methadone escalation index was about 2% a day, with a mean dosage increase of 0.3 mg/day for a mean of 60 days of treatment, with daily dosages ranging from 9 to 80 mg. A mean of 2.4 doses a day was reported (including the fixed night dose). The intensity of side effects was considered acceptable.

In a prospective, open trial of PCA with oral methadone, Sawe et al. (134) found that the 14 patients initially took from 30 to 80 mg over 24 hours at 3- to 7-hour intervals. After 1 week, these patients prolonged their dosing intervals to a mean of 10 hours with total oral doses of 10 to 40 mg/day.

Unlike morphine, which is glucuronidated, methadone is metabolized by the cytochrome P450 group of enzymes and does not produce active metabolites. The main enzyme mediating N-demethylation of methadone in the liver is CYP3A4, with lesser involvement of CYP1A2 and CYP2D6. Therefore, the most important interactions between methadone and other drugs are related to drugs that are able to induce or inhibit CYP3A4. In these circumstances, the methadone plasma concentrations will be reduced or increased, respectively. Moreover, it must be remembered that methadone strongly inhibits CYP2D6; as a result, it can reduce the hepatic biotransformation of drugs metabolized by this enzyme, such as the neuroleptics haloperidol, domperidone, and resperidone or the tricyclic antidepressants (118,135,136).

Other routes of methadone administration

Few data are available on the analgesia and tolerability of rectally administered methadone. A study evaluated the analgesic efficacy, tolerability, and absorption profile of 10 mg of methadone hydrochloride administered rectally (in the form of microenema) in six opioid-naive cancer patients with pain (137). The pharmacokinetics of rectal methadone showed rapid and extensive distribution phases followed by a slow elimination phase. The plasmatic concentrations presented a great intraindividual variability. Pain relief was statistically significant after 30 minutes and continued more than 8 hours after administration. Five patients required an analgesic only after 24 hours from the first administration of rectal methadone. In a prospective, randomized study, Bruera et al. (138) demonstrated that custom-made capsules and suppositories of methadone were safe, effective, and low cost in 37 advanced cancer patients with poor pain control receiving high doses of SC hydromorphone (mean daily dose 276 ± 163 mg). These patients had significant improvement in pain control with minimal toxicity, using doses of oral or rectal methadone higher than those reported in the literature. This study also demonstrated a large interindividual variation between methadone dosage and plasma level. Rectal methadone can be considered an effective, safe, and low-cost therapy for patients with cancer pain where oral and/or parenteral opioids are not indicated or available.

In most patients, continuous SC infusion of different doses of methadone produced inflammatory skin reactions at the injection site occurring within 24 to 72 hours (139,140). Mathew and Storey (140) confirmed the high incidence of local toxicity connected to the CSI of methadone in six patients. However, they were able to continue the parenteral methadone at a variable dose of 75 to 280 mg/24 hours, frequently changing the position of the needle. Adding dexamethasone in the same syringe driver allowed the extension of the number of days, averaging 4.9 in dexamethasone group and 2.6 in those receiving methadone alone.

The pharmacokinetics of IV methadone showed rapid and extensive distribution phases followed by a slow elimination phase (141). Manfredi et al. (124) described the dramatical beneficial effects of IV methadone in four patients in whom IV morphine and hydromorphone failed to produce adequate pain relief despite titration to dose-limiting side effects. All the patients had long-lasting pain relief without significant side effects at a methadone dose equal to 20% of the hydromorphone dose. Fitzgibbon and Ready (123) described the successful use of large doses of IV methadone administered by PCA and continuous infusion for pain refractory to large doses of IV morphine. Morphine was stopped, and treatment with methadone via PCA was initiated (incremental dose 10 mg every 6 minutes) with a continuous infusion of methadone at a rate of 40 mg/hr. On day 3, methadone was decreased to 200 mg, with good pain management and no adverse effects. The patient was discharged after 5 days with a dose of 220 mg/day (average daily methadone was approximately one-tenth that of morphine). After 6 weeks the dose was increased up to 400 mg/day with good pain control and no adverse effects.

Intravenous methadone administered by PCA was safe and effective in controlling cancer pain, sedation, and confusion in 18 patients previously treated with IV fentanyl. A conversion ratio of 25 µg/hr of fentanyl to 0.1 mg/hr of methadone was used to estimate the initial dose of methadone in all patients (0.25 ratio between fentanyl and methadone) (127). Self-administered bolus doses of IV methadone equal to 50%–100% of the hourly infusion rate were allowed every 20 minutes and additional boluses of 100%–200% of the hourly infusion rate every 60 minutes. To control pain, there was a 10% increase in the median hourly infusion dose of methadone from day 1 (64.45 mg) to day 2; after day 2 the median hourly infusion dose of methadone was the same and decreased to 54 mg on day 4.

The use of epidural methadone in the treatment of cancer pain is reported to be effective, devoid of adverse effects, and to have a lesser tendency to be associated with tolerance (142). In another study, methadone doses of 5, 10, and 20 mg administered by the intrathecal route were compared with 0.5 mg of intrathecal morphine after orthopedic surgery in 38 patients. Whereas the intrathecal morphine produced effective and prolonged analgesia, intrathecal methadone at all three doses produced effective analgesia for only 4 hours. Generalized pruritus, nausea, vomiting, and urinary retention were common, both among patients treated with morphine and in those treated with methadone. Respiratory depression occurred in three of eight patients treated with 20 mg methadone (143).

Equianalgesic potency between methadone and other opioids

Although morphine and methadone demonstrated approximately the same analgesic potency after single-dose administration (144), these results are not necessarily applicable to the management of patients with multiple repeated doses. A number of authors have reported major differences in the dose of methadone required to control pain in cancer patients as compared to other opioid agonists such as morphine and hydromorphone.

In all the reports, the dose of methadone required for maintaining an analgesic effect was lower (from 2.5 to 14 times) than the dose of the previous opioid agonist (82,115,117,138,145,146). In a prospective study of 38 patients with a good pain control, the median oral equivalent daily dose of morphine was 145 mg/day; after the switch to methadone the median equianalgesic oral methadone dose was 21 mg/day. A median time of 3 days (range 1 to 7 days) was necessary to achieve the equianalgesia with oral methadone (117). Results of retrospective and prospective studies show that methadone is a potent opioid, more potent than that suggested by single-dose studies. Also, the dose ratio between methadone and morphine and between methadone and hydromorphone is not a fixed number as proposed in the published equianalgesic tables but rather changes as a function of the previous dose exposure. This suggests the presence of partial development of tolerance between methadone and other opioid agonists (116,117,145,146). The results of a cross-sectional prospective study (117) carried out in patients who switched from morphine to oral methadone showed that dose ratios ranged from 2.5:1 to 14.3:1 (median 7.75:1). In respect to the equianalgesic tables, no patient presented a dose ratio of 1:1, whereas the dose ratios of 3:1 and 4:1 approached those obtained only in patients previously treated with low daily doses of morphine (30 to 90 mg). The dose ratio increased with the increase of the previous morphine dose with a much higher increase at low morphine doses. These results agree with those of Lawlor et al. (145) who retrospectively evaluated 14 patients with advanced cancer who switched from morphine to oral methadone and were treated with a median morphine daily dose eight times greater than that used in our study (117). The authors reported that the median dose ratio obtained was 11.36, which shows that methadone is much more potent than expected and the dose ratio correlates with the previous administered morphine dose.

With respect to the equianalgesic tables mentioned previously (117), Mercadante et al. (147) found that when patients with poor pain control and/or adverse effects from treatment with oral morphine were switched to methadone, it is necessary to increase the methadone dose by 20%–30%. On the basis of a preliminary study, Santiago-Palma et al. (127) suggested that when switching patients from IV fentanyl to methadone, a conversion ratio of 25 µg/hr of fentanyl to 0.1 mg/hr of methadone may be safe and effective. If the final mean hourly infusion dose of methadone were used to calculate the initial hourly infusion rate, a conversion of 25 µg/hr of IV fentanyl for 0.125 mg/hr of IV methadone would result. No significant correlation was found between the total dose of fentanyl before the switch and the ratio between the total daily dose of fentanyl before the switch and the total daily dose of methadone on day 4.

How to switch to methadone

Switching from an opioid agonist to methadone is not always easy and should be carried out by doctors experienced in treating cancer pain. Contrary to expectations, toxicity is more frequent in patients who were previously exposed to high doses of opioids with respect to those who received low doses; therefore more caution is necessary when patients are switched to methadone from higher doses of parenteral opioids. Although some authors have been able to change patients from low opioid doses to methadone in 1 day as outpatients (82,132,146, 148), reports on patients on high-dose opioids suggest that the change to methadone should occur in an inpatient setting over 3 to 6 days. Only Hagen and Wasylenko (149) found that cancer patients with advanced disease and severe pain can be safely and effectively switched to methadone in the outpatient setting; however, on average, it took 32 days to successfully switch to methadone in the outpatient setting. Different switching modalities have been reported.

Slow switching   At the Palliative Care Unit in Edmonton, Canada, and at the Symptom Control Division at the M.D. Anderson, Houston, Texas, the switching is performed over 3 days (116,145). The common practice consists in decreasing one third of the previous opioid dose over the first 24 hours and replacing it with methadone using an initial equianalgesic dose ratio estimating of 10:1 (i.e., a patient receiving 1000 mg/day of oral morphine will switch to 660 mg of oral morphine plus 33 mg oral methadone during the first day). Methadone will be administered orally every 8 hours. During the second day, if pain control is good, the patient will undergo a further 30% decrease in the dose of the previous opioid, but the dose of methadone will be increased only if the patient experiences moderate to severe pain. Transient episodes of pain will be managed with intermittent rescue doses of short-acting opioids. Finally, during day 3 the final one third of the previous opioid will be discontinued, and the patient will be maintained on regular methadone every 8 hours, plus approximately 10% of the daily methadone dose as an extra dose orally or rectally for breakthrough pain. Daily assessment of pain and methadone dose titration is necessary to obtain adequate pain relief.

Rapid switching   Mercadante et al. (146) prospectively studied 24 cancer patients treated with oral morphine switched to oral methadone at 20% (dose ratio between morphine and methadone 1:5) of the previous opioid dose while morphine was completely discontinued. The methadone daily dose was divided into three daily doses and a further dose as needed. Half the patients obtained good pain relief in the first 24 hours and the others within 3 days after switching. During the 3 days of the study, methadone dose was reduced in 6 patients who received higher presetting morphine doses (range 120–400 mg), increased in 11 patients who had received lower preswitching doses of morphine (range 30–90 mg), and remained stable in 7 who had received a mean preswitching morphine dose of 107 mg (range 30–180 mg). No serious complications were found among patients in this study. According to the authors, rapid switching between morphine and methadone can also be used for patients cared for at home if continuous monitoring is performed by an experienced team.

It is also our practice to stop morphine and immediately begin treatment with oral methadone every 8 hours using as guidelines the median dose ratio which we found in our previous study (117) of 4:1 (previously morphine dose of 30–90 mg/day), 8:1 (previously morphine dose of > 90 to 300 mg/day), and 12:1 (previously morphine dose < 300 mg/day), titrating the dose daily according to pain intensity (117).

According to Morley and Makin (125), the previous opiate should be stopped and replaced by a fixed dose of methadone that is one tenth of the actual or calculated equivalent oral morphine dose when the 24-hour dose is less than 300 mg, or a fixed dose of 30 mg of methadone when the 24-hour dose is greater than 300 mg. This fixed dose should then be administered orally as required, but not more frequently than every 3 hours for 6 days. On day 6, the amount of methadone administered over the previous 2 days is noted and converted into a regular 12-hour regimen. In this case, there is a wide range of doses, up to 300 mg of equivalent oral morphine dose, in which the equianalgesic dose between morphine and methadone is always 10:1. As can be seen in switching to methadone, there is no set standard modality.

Oral hydromorphone

Hydromorphone is an analog of morphine with similar pharmacokinetic and pharmacodynamic properties. It produces some metabolites, the principle one being hydromorphone-3-glucuronide, and like M-3-G, it is likely to be responsible for the neuroexcitatory adverse effects (150).

Immediate release formulation provides useful analgesia for about 4 hours, whereas sustained-release tablets may be administered twice a day or three times a day. In a double-blind, crossover, randomized study comparable analgesia and tolerability were found between CR hydromorphone and CR oxycodone (151) (Table 8.8).

Table 8.8. *Comparative studies on oxycodone administration*

Authors (Ref)	Study design	No. of patients	Route	Route	Results
Kaplan et al. (172)	Randomized, double blind	164	81 patients CR oxycodone	83 patients IR oxycodone	No difference in pain intensity Overall significantly fewer adverse events for CR Compared with IR oxycodone for digestive system
Leow et al. (162)	Open, crossover, single dose	12	Oral oxycodone 9.1 mg	IV oxycodone 4.6–9.1 mg	IV oxycodone had a faster onset of pain relief than oxycodone tablets but the duration of analgesia was the same (4 hours) IV oxycodone had a significantly higher incidence and severity of nausea, drowsiness, light-headedness than oral oxycodone
Leow et al. (163)	Open, crossover, single dose	12 11 opioid naives	Rectal oxycodone 30 mg	IV oxycodone 7.9 +/– 1.5 mg (mean)	IV oxycodone had faster onset of analgesia (5–8 min) with respect to the rectal route (0.5–1 hr) but had a shorter analgesic effect (4h IV vs. 8–12 hr rectal) No difference in incidence and severity of adverse effects
Hagen and Babul (151)	Double-blind, crossover, randomized	44 31 completed the study	CR oxycodone every 12 hr final dose 124 +/– 22 mg/day	CR hydromorphone every 12 hr 30 +/– 6 mg/day for 7 days	Comparable analgesic efficacy and tolerability Two patients had hallucinations on hydromorphone and no patients on oxycodone
Parris et al. (173)	Randomized, double-blind, parallel-group	111 66 completed the study	CR oxycodone every 12 hr	IR oxycodone every 6 hr	No differences in pain scores and tolerability

Abbreviations: CR, controlled release; IR, immediate release; IV, intravenous.

Wide variations in the equianalgesic dose ratio have been reported between morphine and hydromorphone (116,152,153). No correlation between the previous opioid dose has been found. The ratio may differ depending on whether the switch is from morphine to hydromorphone or from hydromorphone to morphine. A unified ratio of 4.2:1 (4.2 mg of morphine = 1 mg hydromorphone) has been suggested (152). The hydromorphone/methadone ratio is 5 to 10 times greater than previously reported (154) and varies significantly according to the previously administered dose of hydromorphone (138,152,155).

Other routes of hydromorphone administration

In some countries hydromorphone is available in rectal as well as injectable formulations for IV, SC, epidural, and intrathecal administration. Hydromorphone administered SC has some advantages compared to morphine because of its high solubility, the availability of a high-concentration preparation (10 mg/ml), and a bioavailability of about 78% (156).

In a double-blind, crossover study, CII and CSI of hydromorphone for chronic cancer pain were compared. No differences were reported in terms of side effects or analgesia. Plasma concentrations were also comparable, and after 24 and 48 hours, the two infusion methods showed a stable steady-state (156). In a prospective randomized trial (Table 8.3) hydromorphone administered via CSI showed comparable analgesia and adverse effects as compared to morphine (84). By the spinal route in opioid-naive patients, hydromorphone caused about 33% less pruritus than did morphine (157). In a case report (158) hydromorphone administered via continuous IV infusion and then orally was able to abolish itching present during oral and IV morphine administration (Table 8.9).

Oral oxycodone

Oxycodone (dihydrohydroxycodeine) hydrochloride is a semisynthetic opioid that is a derivative of tebaine, with an agonist action at mu and Kappa receptors. In in vitro binding studies, oxycodone showed a lower affinity for the mu opioid

Table 8.9. *Opioid switching for the treatment of adverse effects due to morphine administration*

Author (Ref)	Study design	No. patients	Opioid dose/route	Symptoms	Switching	Results
Katcher and Walsh (158)	Case report	1	CR oral morphine 15 mg t.i.d + 5 mg every 4hr then CII	Itching with both routes nonresponsive to drugs	Hydromorphone by CII then oral	Itching stopped within 24 hr of starting hydromorphone
Paix et al. (232)	Retrospective	4	Morphine 5–120 mg/day oral and CSI	Delirium, hallucinations	Fentanyl	Clinical improvement
de Stoutz et al. (233)	Retrospective	80	Multiple opioids: morphine, hydro-morphone, metha-done, diamorphine, fentanyl	Cognitive failure, hallucinations myoclonus	Multiple opioids	Clinical improvement in 73% of patients and also in pain control
Sjogren et al. (234)	Retrospective	4	Morphine 20 mg/day IV 60–300 mg/day CR morphine 150–960 mg/day IM	Hyperalgesia, allodynia, myoclonus	Methadone sufentanil ketobemidone + benzodiazepines or amitriptyline	Clinical improvement
Maddocks et al. (178)	Prospective	19	Oral or SC morphine	Acute delirium	Oxycodone CSI conversion 0.7:1	Attenuation of delirium significant improve-ment in nausea and vomiting
Lawlor et al. (235)	Case report	1	Morphine 14.400 mg/day IV lorazepam 8 mg/day	Myoclonus, delirium, hyperalgesia	Methadone	Clinical improvement
Mercadante et al. (147)	Prospective	50	Oral morphine from 90 to 300 mg/day	Uncontrolled pain and/or adverse effects	Oral methadone	Clinical improvement in 80% of the patients

Abbreviations: CR, controlled release; CII, continuous intravenous infusion; CSI, continuous subcutaneous infusion; IV, intravenous; IM, intramuscular; SC, subcutaneous.

Table 8.10. *Opioid switching for the treatment of adverse effects due to opioid administration*

Author (Ref)	Study design	No. patients	Opioid dose/route	Symptoms	Switching	Results
Eisendrath et al. (236)	Retrospective	6	Meperidine 300–1050 mg/day IM	Delirium seizure (2 patients)	Morphine	Clinical improvement
Steinberg et al. (237)	Case report	1 renal failure	Transdermal fentanyl 125 µg/hr	Delirium nonresponsive to haloperidol and lorazepam	Morphine	Clinical improvement
Szeto et al. (238)	Prospective	14	Meperidine 75–150 mg every 2–3 hr IM	Seizures, myoclonus	Morphine, levorphanol, and phenytoin	Clinical improvement
Kaiko et al. (239)	Prospective survey	67	Meperidine 240–540 mg/day	48/67 had symptoms of CNS excitation, 8 myoclonus, 2 seizures	Morphine, diazepam, or anticonvulsant for seizure	Clinical improvement
Parkinson et al. (240)	Case report	1	Hydromorphone/ morphine intrathecal/ epidural	Rhythmic jerking of the legs, spastic contractions of stomach and legs	IV morphine, IV sufentanil	Clinical improvement
MacDonald et al. (241)	Case reports	3	Hydromorphone 65–200 µg/hr	Myoclonus, delirium	Morphine, methadone	Clinical improvement
Santiago-Palma et al. (127)	Prospective	18	Fentanyl IV PCA	Pain, sedation, confusion	Methadone IV PCA	Clinical improvement

Abbreviations: IM, intramuscular; CNS, central nervous system; IV, intravenous; PCA, patient-controlled anesthesia.

receptor (88,159). Oxycodone has the same structural relationship to codeine but is nearly 10 times more potent (160). It is metabolized like codeine, that is, demethylated and conjugated in the liver to form oxymorphone in a reaction catalyzed by the enzyme cytochrome P450 2D6 (CYP2D6), and excreted in the urine (161). The bioavailability of oral oxycodone is higher than that of oral morphine (about 87% vs. 37%) (162). Different studies show marked interindividual variations in the pharmacokinetics and pharmacodynamic of oxycodone that support the need for individualized dosing regimens (162–166). The role of oxycodone metabolites such as noroxycodone and oxymorphone (165, 167–170) is not clear. According to Kaiko et al. (168) oxycodone, but not oxymorphone, is primarily responsible for pharmacodynamic and analgesic effects.

The half-life of oxycodone does not seem to be modified in patients with renal and hepatic impairment, which is why these patients may benefit from switching to oxycodone if toxicity is present (168).

Until 1995, the only commercial formulations available were made up of 5 mg of oxycodone hydrochloride in combination with a non-opioid drug. For this reason oxycodone has always been considered a weak opioid and classified in the second step of the WHO ladder. At present commercial preparations of oxycodone at different doses are also available as a single preparation.

In a controlled study of patients with postherpetic neuralgia (171), CR oxycodone was an effective analgesic for the management of steady pain, paroxysmal spontaneous pain, and allodynia when compared with a placebo. Comparative controlled trials between CR and IR oxycodone (172,173) showed no difference in pain scores. Parris (173) reported that tolerability between the two formulations was the same, but Kaplan et al. (172) found overall significantly fewer adverse effects for CR compared with IR oxycodone (Table 8.8).

Comparative studies between orally administered oxycodone and morphine are described in Table 8.5. The most interesting result is the absence of hallucinations during oxycodone administration compared with morphine. In one study (89) oxycodone produced constipation more frequently than morphine. The manufacturer and others recommend a conversion ratio of 2:1 from oral morphine to oral oxycodone (2 mg morphine = 1 mg oxycodone) (174). However, clinical experience supports the use of a 1:1 mg conversion ratio (88,175,176)

Different routes of oxycodone administration

Commercially prepared parenteral oxycodone is available in only a few countries. Gagnon et al. (176) treated 63 advanced cancer patients with intermitted SC injection of oxycodone. Local tolerance and systemic toxicity were evaluated prospectively. Intolerance at the injection site appeared in two patients who received a concentration of 50 and 60 mg/ml. Most patients were switched to oxycodone because of opioid toxicity and in 34% of them delirium was reversed. The conversion ratio used from oral to SC oxycodone was 2:1. Dose ratio between IM oxycodone and IM morphine is 3:2 (167,177). Maddocks et al. (178) showed that in patients with morphine-induced delirium, switching to oxycodone produced significant improvement in mental status, nausea, and vomiting. (Table 8.9).

Oxycodone pectinate suppositories are available in countries such as the United Kingdom and need to be given every 8 hours. The single-dose pharmacokinetics and pharmacodynamics of oxycodone administered by IV and rectal routes were determined in 12 cancer patients (163). Intravenous oxycodone was associated with a rapid onset of analgesia (5–8 minutes) compared with the rectal route (0.5–1 hour) but with a shorter analgesic effect (4 hours via IV route compared to 8–12 hours via rectal route) (Table 8.8). Oral and IV oxycodone were compared in a single-dose study (162). Although IV oxycodone produced a faster onset of pain relief, the duration of analgesia was about 4 hours with both routes of oxycodone administration; IV oxycodone produced significantly more adverse effects (Table 8.8).

Fentanyl

Fentanyl is a semisynthetic opioid and an established IV anesthetic and analgesic drug. It is not used orally because it rapidly undergoes extensive first-pass metabolism. Among analgesic opioid drugs, fentanyl citrate has a very high potency (about 75 times more than morphine) and is skin compatible, having a low molecular weight with good solubility and thus suitable for transdermal administration.

Other routes of fentanyl administration

Different studies show that the transdermal fentanyl patch is as effective as oral opioids in relieving cancer-related pain, with a safety and side effect profile equal to or better than that of oral opioids (179–188). In a randomized, open, two-period, crossover study comparing transdermal fentanyl with sustained-release oral morphine, transdermal therapeutic system (TTS) fentanyl was associated with significantly less constipation and less daytime drowsiness but greater sleep disturbance and shorter sleep duration than morphine (179). Donner et al. (180) evaluated the long-term therapy of 51 patients using transdermal fentanyl. Constipation and the need for laxatives were significantly reduced using TTS

compared with sustained release morphine in the prestudy phase (181). Korte and Morant (182) evaluated 20 patients on fentanyl TTS. Constipation was not a major problem; overall, laxatives were needed only during one third of all treatment days. In another study of 38 patients, Korte et al. (183) found that fentanyl TTS induced less constipation than might be expected. Laxatives were administered continuously in 8% of the patients and intermittently in 79% of them. Five (13%) patients did not need any laxative at all. Nine patients on CR release morphine and one patient on hydromorphone switched to fentanyl TTS. Constipation, appetite, drowsiness, and concentration were not statistically different between the two treatments (184). Zech et al. (185) carried out a pilot study to evaluate the efficacy and side effects of a combination of initial PCA for dose-finding with transdermal fentanyl administration in 20 cancer patients. In comparison with the prestudy situation (step 2 and 3 of the WHO), there was a slight decrease in the visual analog scale (VAS) scores for constipation, nausea, vomiting, anorexia, and fatigue, whereas other symptoms remained unchanged.

In an open prospective study Grond et al. (186) evaluated the combination of initial dose titration with PCA and long-term treatment with fentanyl TTS in 50 cancer patients requiring opioids for severe pain. The frequency of moderate or severe constipation was found in 40% of patients before the study, in 18% of patients during titration period (285 days), and in 10% of patients during long-term treatment (2979 days). The efficacy and tolerability of a combination of initial PCA for dose finding with fentanyl TTS were evaluated in 70 patients requiring strong opioids for severe cancer pain (187). A respiratory rate below 8 per minute during sleep was noted in three patients during the titration period. Comparing the incidence of major symptoms such as constipation, nausea, and vomiting on days 0 and 3, a marked reduction was present during fentanyl treatment, whereas other symptoms such as sweating, fatigue, dizziness, and pruritus were unchanged. In a large cross-sectional study Payne et al. (188) compared pain-related treatment satisfaction, side effects, functioning, and well-being in 504 patients with advanced cancer who were receiving either fentanyl TTS or sustained-release oral morphine. The fentanyl patients had lower functioning (they were significantly older) scores than did the oral morphine patients; however, despite this lower functioning, they reported many fewer side effects than patients treated with oral morphine. The level of analgesia was similar in the two groups.

Preclinical evidence support the relatively low incidence of intestinal side effects observed clinically with the use of fentanyl in comparison with morphine both after SC and oral administration (189). Some patients switching from oral or SC morphine to transdermal fentanyl may experience acute symptoms of morphine withdrawal, in spite of adequate pain control. It is not understood if this is the cause of reduced constipation when switching to TTS-fentanyl. Patients experienced severe abdominal symptoms with diarrhea, abdominal cramps, nausea, sweating, anxiety, and restlessness within 24 to 48 hours of switching from oral or parenteral morphine to TTS-fentanyl. Some patients were converted back to their usual dose of sustained-release morphine or the administration of 10 mg of morphine SC successfully, reporting that they fell back to their usual state after 48 hours (179,190–193). It is not known what induces the withdrawal syndrome. It may be due to different receptors, different receptor subtypes, different secondary messenger systems, different affinities, or different potencies of the two drugs at different receptors. It may be necessary to gradually reduce the dose of morphine to avoid withdrawal symptoms while switching from oral or SC (subacute) morphine to fentanyl.

For patients refractory to laxatives and general measures, a trial should be considered with a fentanyl patch or with continuous SC infusion of morphine. However, TTS-fentanyl should be used only in a stable situation where the patient has been titrated to good pain control using an IR opioid formulation. Further studies should be carried out to evaluate the degree of constipation of one opioid versus another when administered at equianalgesic doses.

Oral transmucosal fentanyl citrate is a synthetic opioid agonist manufactured in a matrix of sucrose and liquid glucose base and fitted onto a radiopaque plastic handle. Doses are available in six different strengths (200 μg, 400 μg, 600 μg, 800 μg, 1200 μg and 1600 μg). Absorption is via the oral mucosa. Administration of a drug through this route avoids the first-pass effect and allows easy and rapid dose titration. From the pharmacokinetic point of view, oral transmucosal fetanyl citrate (OTFC) is similar to IM and IV fentanyl, whereas the plasmatic concentrations are double those of oral fentanyl and are reached 86 minutes earlier oral fetanyl (194,195). Peak effect occurs in about 20 minutes. Approximately 25% of the dose of fentanyl goes directly into the bloodstream through mucosal absorption and accounts for 50% of the dose that reaches the plasma. Total bioavailability is approximately 50%, as duration of action ranges from 2.5 to 5 hours. The onset of analgesic effect is obtained within 5 to 15 minutes (196) compared to 30 to 60 minutes with normal-release oral opioids. A total of 76% of

patients with incident and breakthrough pain have experienced favorable results (197).

In a multicenter, randomized, double-blind, placebo-controlled trial of OTFC for cancer-related breakthrough pain carried out by Farrar et al. (198), OTFC produced significantly larger changes in pain intensity and better pain relief than placebo. In another controlled dose titration study (199) in cancer patients treated with OTFC, 74% were successfully titrated. Moreover, OTFC provided significantly greater analgesic effect at 15, 30, and 60 minutes, and a more rapid onset of effect than the usual rescue drug. There was no relationship between the total daily dose of the fixed schedule opioid regimen and the dose of OTFC required to manage breakthrough pain. As the optimal dose cannot be predicted, treatment should begin with a dose of 200 μg and increased at 15 minute intervals. It emerged from controlled and uncontrolled studies that the adverse effects of the OTFC were similar to other opioids and very few adverse events were severe or serious.

OTFC is approved by Food and Drug Administration solely for the management of breakthrough pain in opioid-tolerant cancer patients (200). It is not recommended for treating acute and/or postoperative pain. Future studies are required to establish the OTFC dose to be used as rescue dose in patients with breakthrough pain compared to type and dose of opioid taken by the patient.

Diamorphine

Diamorphine (diacetylmorphine) is an semisynthetic analog of morphine and a pro-drug that must be biotransformed to 6-acetylmorphine and morphine to produce the analgesic effect (201). It is available for clinical purposes only in Canada and the United Kingdom. Although there does not appear to be any difference between diamorphine and morphine when administered orally, diamorphine is about twice as potent as morphine when administered SC or IM (202). Moreover, diamorphine is more soluble than morphine when administered parenterally and shows a more rapid onset of analgesia and less vomiting but more sedation when administered IV (203). Diamorphine can also be administered through the spinal route (204–206).

Buprenorphine

Buprenorphine is a semisynthetic tebaine derivative. It is a potent partial agonist at the mu receptor. As a mu partial agonist, there is a ceiling to the morphine-like effects of the drug (207). Sublingual administration allows a direct drug absorption into the systemic circulation, thus avoiding the hepatic first-pass metabolism. The peak of morphine-like subjective effects occurs at a dose of approximately 1 mg SC buprenorphine, corresponding to 20 to 30 mg morphine (208). Patients previously treated with buprenorphine required a dose of morphine significantly higher than those treated with other opioids (codeine, oxycodone, dextropropoxyphene, pentazocine) to obtain the same pain relief (209). Like the mixed agonist-antagonists, buprenorphine may precipitate withdrawal in patients who have received repeated doses of a morphine-like agonist and developed physical dependence. Naloxone is relatively ineffective in reversing serious respiratory depression caused by buprenorphine (210).

Levorphanol

Levorphanol is a synthetic potent mu-opioid agonist and also binds delta and kappa receptors (211). It is readily absorbed from the gastrointestinal tract and has a favorable oral-to-parenteral ratio of approximately 1:1 (212). When administered parenterally, 2 mg of levorphanol is equianalgesic to 10 mg of morphine (211). It has a half-life of 12 to 30 hours and a duration of analgesia of 4 to 6 hours. Levorphanol is considered a useful alternative to morphine, hydromorphone, or fentanyl; however, it must be used cautiously to prevent accumulation (213). The kappa receptor binding may explain its high prevalence of psychotomimetic effects (delirium, hallucinations) compared with other opioids (211).

Co-administration of different opioids

It is well known that the association of opioid and non-opioid drugs, acting on different receptors, increase the analgesic efficacy through an additive effect (26,214). What is now emerging is that the co-administration of morphine and other opioids, which act on different receptors, not only produce an increase in the analgesic effect of morphine but also reduce CNS adverse effects and opioid tolerance, while offering a more balanced analgesia.

A review study (215) reported the results of in vivo and in vitro studies of co-treatment of morphine plus selective antagonists of a subset of opioid receptors that are coupled to an excitatory second-messenger system. Co-administration of morphine plus very low doses of opioid antagonists such as naloxone and naltrexone markedly enhances the intensity and duration of morphine-induced analgesia. At the same time, chronic co-treatment reduces opioid tolerance and dependence

through a direct competitive antagonism of Gs-coupled excitatory opioid receptor functions. In clinical studies, low-dose naloxone enhanced pentazocine analgesia (216) and morphine analgesia (217), whereas codeine analgesia is increased by low-dose naltrexone (218,219). Low-dose nalmefene, a potent opioid antagonist with a long duration of action, was able to enhance morphine analgesia in both animals and humans (215,220). In preclinical studies the marked increase in the analgesic effect of morphine through the co-administration of naltrexone did not produce an increase in morphine's depressant effects on respiratory system (219).

According to the studies of Ross and Smith (221), oxycodone is not a mu-opioid agonist, rather a kappa-opioid agonist. Ross et al. (222) conducted a study to evaluate whether the co-administration of sub-antinociceptive doses of morphine and oxycodone via intracerebroventricular and/or subacute or intraperitoneal produced synergistic pain relief in animals. When the drugs were administered separately there was no significant difference regarding pain in respect to basal time or placebo group of rats of both groups. However, a marked analgesic synergy, rapid onset of action (10 minutes), and duration of action lasting approximately 3 hours were observed when the drugs were administered concomitantly. Furthermore, the animals did not present the classic opioid-related CNS adverse effects that appeared when the opioids were administered separately.

Dextromethorphan (DM) is a low affinity NMDA receptor antagonist. When administered alone in low doses (90 mg/day or less), it was not able to relieve neuropathic pain (223,224); when administered at higher doses (400 mg/day or more) it was superior to placebo in patients with diabetic neuropathy, but not in those with postherpetic neuralgia (225).

Preclinical and clinical studies have been carried out to evaluate the role of DM on the enhancement of analgesia and on the prevention of tolerance development when administered in association with morphine. In rats treated with this oral combination of DM and morphine, there was prevention of opiate tolerance and dependence, and enhancement of the peak analgesic potency and duration of morphine-related analgesia without increasing side effects (226,227). In two double-blind, multidose clinical studies (228) carried out in patients with chronic pain, the co-administration of commercial preparations of morphine sulfate (MS) and DM (ratio 1:1) provided significantly greater analgesia than an equal dose of immediate release MS, with a faster onset and longer duration. To maintain satisfactory pain control over 4 weeks, patients in the MS group increased their daily dose but patients in the MS:DM group did not increase their dose, suggesting a reduced tolerance development for MS alone. Similar results have been obtained in single-dose studies in patients with postoperative pain using 60 mg of MS and 60 mg of DM (229).

The tolerability of MS:DM association appears to be good even after chronic treatment. The most common adverse effects reported in the multiple dose-controlled studies were nausea, dizziness, vomiting, somnolence, constipation, confusion, pruritus, and headache (230).

Future studies are needed to clarify the clinical implications of the co-administration of different opioid analgesics. In particular we need to know the effects of these preparations in the long term, what doses are required for treating breakthrough pain, the cost of these drugs, and their impact on the patient's quality of life.

Role of switching the opioid and/or the route of administration

In clinical practice, we can observe patients treated with oral morphine or another opioid who present with an imbalance between analgesia and unwanted effects. In particular, some clinical situations may be present: 1. Pain is controlled but there are some intolerable adverse effects for the patient; 2. Pain is not adequately controlled and it is impossible to increase the opioid dose because of adverse effects; or 3. Pain is not adequately controlled notwithstanding the continuous increase of the opioid dose which does not produce adverse effects.

Different therapeutic strategies may prevent or treat adverse effects: 1. General measures (reduce the opioid dose, hydrate the patient, correct abnormal biochemistry if present, reduce the number of pharmacological associations); 2. Administration of symptomatic drugs (adjuvant drugs); 3. Administration by an alternative route; 4. Administration of an alternative opioid; or 5. Switching to both an alternative opioid and route (231). Symptomatic drugs used to prevent or control opioid adverse effects are usually used in clinical practice. Nevertheless, there have been no studies to evaluate their possible toxicity when they are administered in association with opioids (for instance the increase of sedation when they act on the CNS like some antiemetics), their efficacy on a large sample of patients (above all for control of symptoms such as itching, myoclonus, hallucinations, delirium), and/or the patient's compliance when more drugs are prescribed. Data are not available to allow to us to compare the advantages and disadvantages of the different thera-

peutic strategies such as the use of drugs for symptom control (adjuvant drugs), the switching of opioid, and/or route of administration.

Patients who have poor analgesic efficacy or tolerability with one opioid will frequently tolerate another opioid well, although the mechanisms that underlie this variability in the response to different opioids are not known (13,15,23). According to Bruera et al. (87) the benefits of opioid switching are more likely to be related to subtle differences in pharmacology that emerge when a new opioid is substituted in a patient who has developed toxicity to another opioid than to overt differences in pharmacologic profile in patients in stable pain control. However, much more needs to be understood to answer these questions.

Tables 8.9 and 8.10 list a series of positive results from case reports, retrospective studies, and prospective uncontrolled studies on the role of opioid switching for the management of adverse effects resulting from morphine or other opioid administration (127,147,158,178, 232–241). Most authors switched the opioid in the presence of adverse CNS effects such as delirium, hallucinations, cognitive failure, myoclonus, seizure, hyperalgesia, and allodynia. Opioid switching was often effective where the use of symptomatic drugs for symptom control was not effective.

The selection of an alternative opioid is largely empirical. A pure opioid agonist such as oxycodone, methadone, hydromorphone, and fentanyl is recommended when morphine fails. Positive results in symptom control and pain relief were also obtained by switching the route of opioid administration. In the prospective study carried out by Mac Donald et al. (99) (Table 8.6), switching from oral to SC morphine produced significant improvement in pain relief and nausea and vomiting. Kalso et al. (21) (Table 8.7) carried out the only randomized double-blind crossover trial to evaluate the efficacy and tolerability of morphine in patients who switched from oral to epidural or SC administration. The positive results obtained indicate that this practice should be implemented in clinical practice.

There is no sound evidence from well-designed clinical trials of the superiority of one opioid over another regarding the side effect profile and/or analgesic profile. However, although conclusions drawn from observational studies and clinical trials must be interpreted with caution, they give some useful information.

Theoretically, there may be some benefit in opioid switching in any situation of unacceptable side effects with initial opioid (147,231,242,243). However, it is not possible to foresee such side effects in any individual. The goal is to personalize the therapy and reassess the patient continuously.

In the future, it will be necessary to evaluate the relative roles of adjuvant (symptomatic) drugs to treat the adverse effects compared to opioid and/or route switching, when patients suffer persistent adverse effect from an opioid. For each symptom we must consider the available therapeutic strategies in terms of symptomatic drugs, their efficacy and tolerability, or switching routes and/or opioid. The choice of one strategy over another should take into account the advantages, disadvantages, evidence, comparison of alternatives, and costs in different care settings.

Conclusion

Notwithstanding the number and types of opioid analgesic drugs available today, and the relatively simple and effective guidelines to treat cancer pain, too many people with cancer pain continue to suffer needlessly. The effective drugs available are probably not always used or are not used in the suitable way.

The horizon may hold promising new additions to the field of pain therapy. Possibilities include the isolation and development of analgesics or combinations that may minimize to an even greater extent the adverse effects that are often associated with the current therapeutic class of opioid analgesics. In addition, new strategies such as opioid and/or route switching for the management of adverse effects and the improvement of the analgesic benefits may offer therapeutic alternatives for the clinical community.

With clinical effort today focusing on assessment, evaluation, education, and application of the tools and therapies we currently have, we need to use the opioids available as well as look for new compounds that might offer greater safety and efficacy for the patient. In the new millennium, studies should be designed with solid research methodology and structured so that the analgesic benefit of a drug is paralleled by issues of tolerability, cost, and the impact on the cancer patient's quality of life.

References

1. World Health Organization. Cancer pain relief. Geneva: World Health Organization, 1986.
2. World Health Organization. Cancer pain relief, 2nd ed. Geneva: World Health Organization, 1996.
3. Portenoy RK. Adjuvant analgesics in pain management. In: Doyle D, Hanks GWC, MacDonald N, eds. Oxford text-

book of palliative medicine, 2nd ed. Oxford: Oxford University Press, 1998:361–90.
4. Ripamonti C, Zecca E, De Conno F. Pharmacological treatment of cancer pain: alternative routes of opioid administration. Tumori 84:289–300, 1998.
5. Hanks GW, De Conno F, Ripamonti C, et al. Morphine in cancer pain: modes of administration. Expert Working Group of the European Association for Palliative Care. BMJ 312:823–826, 1996.
6. Bruera E, Ripamonti C. Alternate routes of administration of opioids for the management of cancer pain. In: Patt R, ed. Cancer pain. Philadelphia: J.B. Lippincott, 11:161–84, 1993.
7. Gong Q-L, Hedner J, Bjorkman R, et al. Morphine-3-glucuronide may functionally antagonize morphine-6-glucuronide induced antinociception and ventilatory depression in the rat. Pain 48:249–55, 1992.
8. Ekblom M, Gardmark M, Hannarlund-Udenaes M. Pharmacokinetics and pharmacodynamics of morphine-3-glucuronide in rats and its influence on the antinociceptive effect of morphine. Biopharm Drug Dispos 14:1–11, 1993.
9. Pasternak GW, Bodnar RJ, Clark JA, et al. Morphine-6-glucuronide, a potent mu agonist. Life Sci 41:2845–9, 1987.
10. Smith MT, Watt JA, Cramond T. Morphine-3-glucuronide: a potent antagonist of morphine analgesia. Life Sci 47:579–85, 1990.
11. Yaksh TL, Harty LG, Onofrio BM. High doses of spinal morphine produced a nonopiate receptor-mediated hyperesthesia: clinical and theoretic implications. Anesthesiology 71:936–40, 1989.
12. Dale AP, Riegler FX, Albrecht RF. Ventilatory effects of fourth cerebroventricular infusions of morphine-6- or morphine-3-glucuronide in the awake dog. Anesthesiology 71:936–40, 1989.
13. Watanabe S. Intraindividual variability in opioid response: a role for sequential opioid trials in patient care. In: Portenoy RK, Bruera E, eds. Topics in palliative care, vol 1. New York: Oxford University Press, 10:195–203, 1997.
14. Hanks GW, Forbes K. Opioid responsiveness. Acta Anaesthesiol Scand 41:154–8, 1997.
15. Cherny NJ, Chang V, Frager G, et al. Opioid pharmacotherapy in the management of cancer pain: a survey of strategies used by pain physicians for the selection of analgesic drugs and routes of administration. Cancer 76:1283–93, 1995.
16. Sindrup SH, Jensen TS. Efficacy of pharmacological treatments of neuropathic pain: an update and effect related to mechanism of drug action. Pain 83:389–400, 1999.
17. Grond S, Radbruch L, Meuser T, et al. Assessment and treatment of neuropathic cancer pain following WHO guidelines. Pain 79:15–20, 1999.
18. Dellemijn P. Are opioids effective in relieving neuropathic pain? Pain 80:453–62, 1999.
19. Bruera E, MacMillan K, Hanson J. Palliative care in a cancer center: results in 1984 versus 1987. J Pain Symptom Manage 5(1):1–5, 1990.
20. Coyle N, Adelhart J, Foley KM, et al. Character of terminal illness in the advanced cancer patient: pain and other symp-

toms during the last four weeks of life. J Pain Symptom Manage 5:83–93, 1990.

21. Kalso E, Heiskanen T, Rantio M, et al. Epidural and subcutaneous morphine in the management of cancer pain: a double-blind cross-over study. Pain 67:443–9, 1996.

22. Morley JS, Watt JWG, Wells JC, et al. Methadone in pain uncontrolled by morphine. Lancet 342:1243, 1993.

23. Galer BS, Coyle N, Pasternak GW, Portenoy RK. Individual variability in the response to different opioids: report of five cases. Pain 49:87–91, 1992.

24. Ripamonti C, Bruera E. CNS adverse effects of opioids in cancer patients. Guidelines for treatment. CNS Drugs 8(1):21–37, 1997.

25. Eisenberg E, Berkey C, Carr DB, et al. Efficacy and safety of nonsteroidal antiinflammatory drugs for cancer pain: a meta-analysis. J Clin Oncol 12:2756–65, 1994.

26. Moore A, Collins S, Carroll D, McQuay H. Paracetamol with and without codeine in acute pain: a quantitative systematic review. Pain 70:193–201, 1997.

27. Ventafridda V, Tamburini M, Caraceni A, et al. A validation study of the WHO method for cancer pain relief. Cancer 59:850–6, 1987.

28. De Conno F, Ripamonti C, Sbanotto A, et al. A clinical study on the use of codeine, oxycodone, dextropropoxyphene, buprenorphine and pentazocine in cancer pain. J Pain Symptom Manage 6:423–7, 1991.

29. Radbruck L, Zech D, Grond S, et al. Pain analysis and pain therapy for lung cancer. Chirurg 65:696–701, 1994.

30. Mercadante S, Genovese G, Kargar JA, et al. Home palliative care: results in 1991 versus 1989. J Pain Symptom Manage 7:414–8, 1992.

31. Brooks DJ, Gamble W, Ahmedzai S. A regional survey of opioid use by patients receiving specialist palliative care. Palliat Med 9:229–38, 1995.

32. Freynhagen R, Zenz M, Strumpf M. WHO Step II: clinical reality or a didactic instrument? Der Schmerz 8:210–5, 1994.

33. Dhaliwal HS et al. Randomized evaluation of controlled-release codeine and placebo in chronic cancer pain. J Pain Symptom Manage 10:612–23, 1995.

34. Caraco Y, Sheller J, Wood AJJ. Pharmacogenetic determination of the effects of codeine and prediction of drug interactions. J Pharmacol Experimental Ther 278:1165–74, 1996.

35. Lurcott G. The effects of the genetic absence and inhibition of CYP2D6 on the metabolism of codeine and its derivatives, hydrocodone and oxycodone. Anesth Prog 45:154–6, 1999.

36. Lurcott G, Bertilsson L. Geographical/interracial differences in polymorphic drug oxidation. Clin Pharmacokinet Concepts 29:192–209, 1995.

37. Sindrup SH, Brosen K, Bjerring P, et al. Codeine increases pain thresholds to copper vapor laser stimuli in extensive but not poor metabolizers of sparteine. Clin Pharmacol Ther 49:686–93, 1991.

38. Cleary J, Mikus G, Somogyi Bochner F. The influence of pharmacogenetics on opioid analgesia: studies with codeine and oxycodone in the Sprague-Dawley/Dark Agouti rat model. J Pharmacol Exp Ther 271:1528–34, 1994.

39. Otton SV, Wu D, Joffe RT, et al. Inhibition by fluoxetine of cytochrome P450 2D6 activity. Clin Pharmacol Ther 53:401–9, 1993.

40. Manzey LL, Guthrie SK. Interactions of the selective serotonin reuptake inhibitors with the cytochrome P450 enzyme system: drug interactions and clinical implications. Mich Drug Lett 15:1–6, 1996.

41. Rowell FJ, Seymour RA, Rawlins MD. Pharmacokinetics of intravenous and oral dihydrocodeine and its acid metabolites. Eur J Clin Pharmacol 25:419–24, 1983.

42. Palmer RN, Eade OE, O'Shea PJ, Cuthbert MF. Incidence of unwanted effects of dihydrocodeine bitartrate in healthy volunteers. Lancet ii:620–1, 1966.

43. Barnes JN, Williams AJ, Tomson MJF, et al. Dihydrocodeine in renal failure: further evidence for an important role of the kidney in the handling of opioid drugs. BMJ 290:740–2, 1985.

44. Dayer P, Collart L, Desmeules J. The pharmacology of tramadol. Drugs 47(Suppl 1):3–7, 1994.

45. Lee CR, McTavish D, Sorkin EM. Tramadol. Drugs 46:313–40, 1993.

46. Osipova NA, Novikov GA, Beresnev VA, Loseva A. Analgesic effect of tramadol in cancer patients with chronic pain: a comparison with prolonged-action morphine sulfate. Curr Ther Res 50:812–21, 1991.

47. Tawfik MO, Elborolossy K, Nasr F. Tramadol hydrochloride in the relief of cancer pain: a double blind comparison against sustained release morphine. Pain (Suppl) 5:377, 1990.

48. Wilder-Smith CH, Schimke J, Osterwalder B, Senn HJ. Oral tramadol, a mu-opioid agonist and monoamine reuptake-blocker, and morphine for strong cancer-related pain. Ann Oncol 5:141–6, 1994.

49. Barnung SK, Treschow M, Borgbjerg FM. Respiratory depression following oral tramadol in a patient with impaired renal function. Pain 71:111–2, 1997.

50. Hennies HH, Friderichs E, Schneider J. Receptor binding, analgesic and antitussive potency of tramadol and other selected opioids. Arzneimittelforschung 38:877–80, 1988.

51. Grond S, Radbruch L, Meuser T, et al. High-dose tramadol in comparison to low-dose morphine for cancer pain relief. J Pain Symptom Manage 18:174–9, 1999.

52. Sindrup S, Andersen G, Madsen C, et al. Tramadol relieves pain and allodynia in polyneuropathy: a randomised, double-blind, controlled trial. Pain 83:85–90, 1999.

53. Harati Y, Gooch C, Swenson M, et al. Double-blind randomized trial of tramadol for the treatment of pain of diabetic neuropathy. Neurology 50:1842–6, 1998.

54. Ebert B, Thorkildsen C, Andersen S, et al. Opioid analgesics as noncompetitive N-methyl-D-aspartate (NMDA) antagonists. Biochem Pharmacol 56(5):553–9, 1998.

55. Beaver WT. Analgesic efficacy of dextropropoxyphene and dextropropoxyphene-containing combinations: a review. Hum Toxicol 3(Suppl):191–220, 1984.

56. Mercadante S, Salvaggio L, Dardanoni G, et al. Dextropropoxyphene vs morphine in opioid-naive cancer patients with pain. J Pain Symptom Manage 15:76–81, 1998.

57. Goldberg RJ, Mor V, Wiemann M, et al. Analgesic use in terrninal cancer patients: report from the National Hospice Study. J Chronic Disease 39:37–45, 1986.

58. Walsh TD, Saunders CM. Oral morphine for relief of chronic pain from cancer. N Engl J Med 305:1417, 1981.

59. Boerner V, Abbott S, Roe RL. The metabolism of morphine and heroin in man. Drug Metab Rev 4:39–73, 1975.

60. Sawe J, Dahlstrom B, Rane A. Steady-state kinetics and analgesic effect of oral morphine in cancer patients. Eur J Clin Pharmacol 24:537–42, 1983.

61. Gourlay GK, Cherry DA, Cousin MJ. A comparative study of the efficacy and pharmacokinetics of oral methadone and morphine in the treatment of severe pain in patients with cancer. Pain 25:297–312, 1986.

62. Kaiko RF, Wallenstein SL, Rogers AG, et al. Clinical analgesic studies and sources of variation in analgesic responses to morphine. In: Foley KM, Inturrisi CE, eds. Advances in pain research and therapy. New York: Raven Press, 1986:13–23.

63. Inturrisi CE. Management of cancer pain. Pharmacology and principles of management. Cancer 63:2308–20, 1989.

64. Sawe J, Svensson JO, Rane A. Morphine metabolism in cancer patients on increasing oral doses-no evidence for autoinduction or dose-dependence. Br J Clin Pharmacol 16:85–93, 1983.

65. Brunk SF, Delle M. Morphine metabolism in man. Clin Pharmacol Ther 16:51–7, 1974.

66. Hanks GW, Aherne GW, Hoskin PJ, et al. Explanation for potency of repeated oral doses of morphine? Lancet 2:732–735, 1987.

67. Kaiko RF. Age and morphine analgesia in cancer patients with postoperative pain. Clin Pharmacol Ther 28:823–6, 1980.

68. Ventafridda V, Saita L, Barletta L, et al. Clinical observations on controlled release morphine in cancer pain. J Pain Symptom Manage 4(3):124–9, 1989.

69. Dahlstrom B, Paakow L. Quantitative determination of morphine in biological samples by gas-liquid chromatography and electron capture detection. J Pharm Pharmacol 27:172–76, 1975.

70. Osborne R, Ioes S, Slevin M. Morphine intoxication in renal failure: the role of morphine-6-glucuronide. BMJ 292:1548–9, 1986.

71. Glare PA, Walsh TD. Clinical pharmacokinetics of morphine. Rev Ther Drug Monitoring 13:1–23, 1991.

72. Labella FS, Pinsky C, Havlicek V. Morphine derivates with diminished opiate receptor potency enhanced central excitatory activity. Brain Res 174:263–71, 1979.

73. Glare PA, Walsh TD, Pippenger CE. Normorphine, a neurotoxic metabolite? Lancet 335:725–6, 1990.

74. Zaw Tun N, Bruera E. Active metabolites of morphine. J Palliat Care 8:48–50, 1992.

75. Faura CC, Collins SL, Moore RA, McQuay HJ. Systemic review of factors affecting the ratios of morphine and its major metabolites. Pain 74:43–53, 1998.

76. Tiseo PJ, Thaler HT, Lapin J, et al. Morphine-6-glucuronide concentrations and opioid-related side effects: a survey in cancer patients. Pain 61:47–54, 1995.

77. Portenoy RK, Foley KM, Stulman J, et al. Plasma morphine and morphine-6-glucuronide during chronic morphine therapy for cancer pain: plasma profiles, steady state concentrations and the consequences of renal failure. Pain 47:13–9, 1991.

78. Wolff T, Samuelsson H, Hedner T. Concentrations of morphine and morphine metabolites in CSF and plasma during continuous subcutaneous morphine administration in cancer pain patients. Pain 68:209–16, 1996.

79. Finn JW, Walsh TD, MacDonald N, et al. Placebo-blinded study of morphine sulphate sustained-release tablets and immediate-release morphine sulphate solution in outpatients with chronic pain due to advanced cancer. J Clin Oncol 11:967–72, 1993.

80. Gourlay GK, Cherry DA, Onley MM, et al. Pharmacokinetics and pharmacodynamics of twenty-four-hourly Kapanol compared to twelve-hourly MS Contin in the treatment of severe cancer pain. Pain 69(3):295–302, 1997.

81. Smith K, Broomhead A, Kerr R, et al. Comparison of a once-a-day sustained-release morphine formulation with standard oral morphine treatment for cancer pain. J Pain Symptom Manage 14(2):63–73, 1997.

82. Ventafridda V, Ripamonti C, Bianchi M, et al. A randomized study on oral administration of morphine and methadone in the treatment of cancer pain. J Pain Symptom Manage 1:203–7, 1986.

83. Mercandante S, Casuccio A, Agnello A, et al. Morphine versus methadone in the pain treatment of advanced-cancer patients followed up at home. J Clin Oncol 16(11):3656–61, 1998.

84. Miller MG, McCarthy N, O'Boyle CA, Kearney M. Continuous subcutaneous infusion of morphine vs hydromorphone: a controlled trial. J Pain Symptom Manage 18(1):9–15, 1999.

85. Coda BA, O'Sullivan B, Donaldson G, et al. Comparative efficacy of patient-controlled administration of morphine, hydromorphone, or sufentanil for the treatment of oral mucositis pain following bone marrow transplantation. Pain 72(3):333–46, 1997.

86. Lo Russo P, Berman B, Silberstain P, et al. Comparison of controlled-release oxycodone (OxyContin) tablets to controlled-release morphine (MS Contin) in patients with cancer pain. American Pain Society Fifteenth Annual Scientific Meeting, Washington, DC, November 14–17, 1996 (Abstract 675).

87. Bruera E, Belzile M, Pituskin E, et al. Randomized, double-blind, cross-over trial comparing safety and efficacy of oral controlled-release oxycodone with controlled-release morphine in patients with cancer pain. J Clin Oncol 16:3222–9, 1998.

88. Kalso E, Vainio A. Morphine and oxycodone hydrochloride in the management of cancer pain. Clin Pharmacol Ther 47:639–46, 1990.

89. Heiskanen T, Kalso E. Controlled-release oxycodone and morphine in cancer related pain. Pain 73:37–45, 1997.

90. Du Pen S, Du Pen A. Intraspinal analgesic therapy in palliative care: evolving perspective. In: Portenoy RK, Bruera E, eds. Topics in palliative care, vol. 4. New York: Oxford University Press, 2000:12:217–35.

91. Ripamonti C, Bruera E. Current status of patient-controlled analgesia in cancer patients. Oncology 11(3):373–84, 1997.

92. Nahata M, Miser A, Reuning R. Analgesic plasma concentrations of morphine in children with terminal malignancy receiving a continuous subcutaneous infusion of morphine to control severe pain. Pain 18:109, 1984.

93. Waldmann C, Eason J, Rambohul E. Serum morphine levels: a comparison between continuous subcutaneous and intravenous infusion in postoperative patients. Anaesth Analg 39:768, 1984.

94. Coyle N, Mauskop A, Maggard J, Foley K. Continuous subcutaneous infusion of opiates in cancer patients with pain. Oncol Nurs Forum 13:53–7, 1986.

95. Ventafridda V, Spoldi E, Caraceni A, et al. The importance of subcutaneous morphine administration for cancer control. Pain Clin 1:47–55, 1986.

96. Bruera E, Brenneis C, Michaud M, et al. Use of the subcutaneous route for administration of narcotics in patients with cancer pain. Cancer 62:407–11, 1988.

97. Kaiko RF. Controversy in the management of chronic cancer pain: therapeutic equivalents of IM and PO morphine. J Pain Symptom Manage 1:42–6, 1986.

98. Drexel H, Dzien A, Spiegel RW, et al. Treatment of severe cancer pain by low-dose continuous subcutaneous morphine. Pain 36:169–76, 1989.

99. McDonald P, Graham P, Clayton M, et al. Regular subcutaneous bolus morphine via an indwelling cannula for pain from advanced cancer. Palliat Med 5:323–9, 1991.

100. Cole L, Hanning CD. Review of the rectal use of opioids. J Pain Symptom Manage 5(2):118–26, 1990.

101. De Boer AG, De Leede LG, Breimer DD. Drug absorption by sublingual and rectal route. Br J Anaesth 56:69–82, 1984.

102. Hojsted J, Rubeck K, Peterson H. Comparative bioavailability of a morphine suppository given rectally and in a colostomy. Eur J Clin Pharmacol 39:49–50, 1990.

103. Bruera E, Faisinger R, Spachinsky K, et al. Clinical efficacy and safety of a novel controlled-release morphine suppository and subcutaneous morphine in cancer pain: a randomized evaluation. J Clin Oncol 13:1520–7, 1995.

104. Babul N, Provencher L, Laberge F, et al. Comparative efficacy and safety of controlled-release morphine suppositories and tablets in cancer pain. J Clin Pharmacol 38:74–81, 1998.

105. De Conno F, Ripamonti C, Saita L, et al. Role of rectal route in treating cancer pain: a randomized cross-over clinical trial of oral vs rectal morphine administration in opioid-

106. naive cancer patients with pain. J Clin Oncol 13:1004–8, 1995.

106. Bruera E, Belzile M, Neumann CM, et al. Twice-daily versus once-daily morphine sulphate controlled-release suppositories for the treatment of cancer pain. A randomized controlled trial. Support Care Cancer 7:280–3, 1999.

107. Krames E. Intrathecal infusional therapies for intractable pain: patient management guidelines. J Pain Symptom Manage 8:36–46, 1993.

108. Ohlsson L, Rydberg T, Eden T, et al. Cancer pain relief by continuous administration of epidural morphine in a hospital setting and a home. Pain 48:349–54, 1992.

109. Arner S, Rawal N, Gustafsson L. Chemical experience of long-term treatment with epidural and intrathecal infusional therapies for intractable pain: patient management guidelines. J Pain Symptom Manage 8:36–46, 1993.

110. Zech DFJ, Grond S, Lynch J, et al. Validation of the World Health Organization guidelines for cancer pain relief: a 10-year prospective study. Pain 63:65–76, 1995.

111. Vainio A, Tigerstedt I. Opioid treatment for radiating cancer pain: oral administration vs epidural techniques. Acta Anaesthesiol Scand 32:179–80, 1988.

112. Fainsinger R, Schoeller T, Bruera E. Methadone in the management of cancer pain: a review. Pain 52:137–47, 1993.

113. Ripamonti C, Zecca E, Bruera E. An update on the clinical use of methadone for cancer pain. Pain 70:109–15, 1997.

114. Mercadante S, Casuccio A, Agnello A, Barresi L. Methadone response in advanced cancer patients with pain followed at home. J Pain Symptom Manage 18:188–92, 1999.

115. Wheeler WL, Dickerson ED. Clinical application of methadone. Am J Hospice Palliat Care 17(3):1–8, 2000.

116. Bruera E, Pereira J, Watanabe S, et al. Opioid rotation in patients with cancer pain. A retrospective comparison of dose ratios between methadone, hydromorphone, and morphine. Cancer 78:852–7, 1996.

117. Ripamonti C, Groff L, Brunelli C, et al. Switching from morphine to oral methadone in treating cancer pain: what is the equianalgesic dose ratio? J Clin Oncol 16(10):3216–21, 1998.

118. Davis MP, Walsh D. Methadone for relief of cancer pain: a review of pharmacokinetics, pharmacodynamics, drug interactions and protocol of administration. Support Care Cancer 9:73–83, 2001.

119. Gorman AL et al. The d- and l-isomers of methadone bind to the non-competitive site on the N-methyl-D-aspartate receptor in rat forebrain and spinal cord. Neurosci Lett 223:5–8, 1997.

120. Egbert B, Andersen S, Krogsgaard-Larsen P. Ketobemidone, methadone and pethidine are non-competitive N-methyl-D-aspartate (NMDA) antagonists in the rat cortex and spinal cord. Neurosci Lett 187:165–8, 1995.

121. Gagnon B, Bruera E. Differences in the ratios of morphine to methadone in patients with neuropathic pain versus non-neuropathic pain. J Pain Symptom Manage 18:120–5, 1999.

122. Makin MK, O'Donnell V, Skinner JM, Ellershaw JE. Methadone in the management of cancer related neuropathic pain: report of five cases. Pain Clinic 4:275–9, 1998.

123. Fitzgibbon DR, Ready LB. Intravenous high-dose methadone administered by patient controlled analgesia and continuous infusion for the treatment of cancer pain refractory to high-dose morphine. Pain 73:259–61, 1997.

124. Manfredi PL, Borsook D, Chandler SW, Payne R. Intravenous methadone for cancer pain unrelieved by morphine and hydromorphone: clinical observations. Pain 70:99–101, 1997.

125. Morley JS, Makin MK. The use of methadone in cancer pain poorly responsive to other opioids. Pain Rev 5:51–8, 1998.

126. Crews JC, Sweeney NJ, Denson DD. Clinical efficacy of methadone in patients refractory to other mu-opioid receeotor agonist analgesics for management of terminal cancer pain. Cancer 72:2266–72, 1993.

127. Santiago-Palma J, Khojainova N, Kornick C, et al. Intravenous methadone in the management of chronic cancer pain. Safe and effective starting doses when substituting methadone for fentanyl. Cancer 92:1919–25, 2001.

128. Daeninck PJ, Bruera E. Reduction in constipation and laxative requirements following opioid rotation to methadone: a report of four cases. J Pain Symptom Manage 18:303–9, 1999.

129. Mercadante S, Sapio M, Serretta R. Treatment of pain in chronic bowel subobstruction with self-administration of methadone. Support Care Cancer 5:1–3, 1997.

130. Mancini I, Hanson J, Neumann CM, Bruera E. Opioid type and other clinical predictors of laxative dose in advanced cancer patients. Palliat Med 3:49–56, 2000.

131. Gardner-Nix LS. Oral methadone for managing chronic non-malignant pain. J Pain Symptom Manage 11:321–3, 1996.

132. De Conno F, Groff L, Brunelli C, et al. Clinical experience with oral methadone administration in the treatment of pain in 196 advanced cancer patients. J Clin Oncol 14:2836–42, 1996.

133. Mercadante S, Sapio M, Serretta R, Caligara M. Patient-controlled analgesia with oral methadone in cancer pain. Ann Oncol 7:613–7, 1996.

134. Sawe J, Hansen J, Ginman C, et al. Patient-controlled dose regimen of methadone for chronic cancer pain. Br Med J 282:771–3, 1981.

135. Herrlin K, Segerdahl M, Gustafsson LL, Kalso E. Methadone, ciprofloxacin and adverse drug reactions. Lancet 356:2069–70, 2000.

136. Tarumi Y, Pereira J, Watanabe S. Methadone and fluconazole: respiratory depression by drug interaction. J Pain Symptom Manage 23:148–53, 2002.

137. Ripamonti C, Zecca E, Brunelli C, et al. Rectal methadone in cancer patients with pain. A preliminary clinical and pharmacokinetic study. Ann Oncol 6:841–3, 1995.

138. Bruera E, Watanabe S, Faisinger RL, et al. Custom-made capsules and suppositories of methadone for patients on high- dose opioids for cancer pain. Pain 62:141–6, 1995.

139. Bruera E, Faisinger R, Moore M, et al. Local toxicity with subcutaneous methadone. Experience of two centers. Pain 45:141–143, 1991.

140. Mathew P, Storey P. Subcutaneous methadone in terminally ill patients: manageable local toxicity. J Pain Symptom Manage 18:49–52, 1999.

141. Inturrisi CE, Colburn WA, Kaiko RF, et al. Pharmacokinetics and pharmacodynamics of methadone in patients with chronic pain. Clin Pharmacol Ther 41:392–401, 1987.

142. Shir Y, Yehuda DB, Palliact A. Prolonged continuous epidural methadone analgesic in the treatment of back and pelvic pain due to multiple myeloma. Pain Clin 1:255–9, 1987.

143. Jacobson L, Chabal C, Brody MC, et al. Intrathecal methadone: a dose-response study and comparison with intrathecal morphine 0,5 mg. Pain 41:147–8, 1990.

144. Levy MH. Pharmacological treatment of cancer pain. N Engl J Med 335(15):1124–32, 1996.

145. Lawlor PG, Turner K, Hanson J, et al. Dose ratio between morphine and methadone in patients with cancer pain: a retrospective study. Cancer 82:1167–73, 1998.

146. Mercadante S, Casuccio A, Calderone L. Rapid switching from morphine to methadone in cancer patients with poor response to morphine. J Clin Oncol 17(10):3307–12, 1999.

147. Mercadante S, Casuccio A, Fulfaro F, et al. Switching from morphine to methadone to improve analgesia and tolerability in cancer patients: a prospective study. J Clin Oncol 19:2898–904, 2001.

148. Anderson R, Saiers JH, Abram S, Schlicht C. Accuracy in equianalgesic dosing: conversion dilemmas. J Pain Symptom Manage 21:397–406, 2001.

149. Hagen NA, Wasylenko E. Methadone: outpatient titration and monitoring strategies in cancer patients. J Pain Symptom Manage 18:369–75, 1999.

150. Babul N, Drake AC. Putative role of hydromorphone metabolites in myoclonus. Pain 51:260–1, 1992.

151. Hagen NA, Babul N. Comparative clinical efficacy and safety of a novel controlled-release oxycodone formulation and controlled-release hydromorphone in the treatment of cancer pain. Cancer 79:1428–37, 1997.

152. Lawlor PG, Turner K, Hanson, J, et al. Dose ratio between morphine and hydromorphone in patients with cancer pain: a retrospective study. Pain 72:79–85, 1997.

153. Dunbar PJ, Chapman CR, Buckley FP, Gavrin JR. Clinical analgesic equivalence for morphine and hydromorphone with prolonged PCA. Pain 68:265–70, 1996.

154. Agency for Health Care Policy Research. Management of Cancer Pain. Clinical Practice Guidelines, Rockville, MD: U.S. Department of Health and Human Services. AHCPR Publications N. 94-0592, March 1994:52.

155. Ripamonti C, De Conno F, Groff L, et al. Equianalgesic dose/ratio between methadone and other opioid agonists in cancer pain: comparison of two clinical experiences. Ann Oncol 9:79–83, 1998.

156. Moulin DE, Kreeft JH, Murray PN, Bouquillon AI. Comparison of continuous subcutaneous and intravenous

hydromorphone infusions for management of cancer pain. Lancet 337:465–8, 1991.

157. Chaplin SR et al. Morphine and hydromorphone epidural analgesia. Anesthesiology 77:1090–4, 1992.

158. Katcher J, Walsh D. Opioid-induced itching: morphine sulfate and hydromorphone hydrochloride. J Pain Symptom Manage 17:70–2, 1999.

159. Chen ZR, Irvine RJ, Somogyi AA, Bochner F. Mu receptor binding of some commonly used opioids and their metabolites. Life Sci 48:2165–71, 1991.

160. Kantor TG, Hopper M, Laska E. Adverse effects of commonly ordered oral narcotics. J Clin Pharmacol 21:1–8, 1981.

161. Heiskanen T, Olkkola KT, Kalso E. Effects of blocking CYP2D6 on the pharmacokinetics and pharmacodynamics of oxycodone. Clin Pharmacol Ther 64:603–11, 1998.

162. Leow K, Smith M, Williams B, Cramond T. Single-dose and steady-state pharmacokinetics and pharmacodynamics of oxycodone in patients with cancer. Clin Pharmacol Ther 52:487–95, 1992.

163. Leow KP, Cramond T, Smith MT. Pharmacokinetics and pharmacodynamics of oxycodone when given intravenously and rectally to adult patients with cancer pain. Anesth Analg 80:296–302, 1995.

164. Leow KP, Smith MT, Watt JA, et al. Comparative pharmacokinetics in humans after administration of intravenous, oral and rectal oxycodone. Drug Monit 14:479–84, 1992.

165. Poyhia R, Olkkola KT, Seppala T, Kalso E. The pharmacokinetics of oxycodone after intravenous injection in adults. Br J Clin Pharmacol 32:516–8, 1991.

166. Poyhia R, Seppala T, Olkkola KT, Kalso E. The pharmacokinetics and metabolism of oxycodone after intramuscular and oral administration to healthy subjects. Br J Clin Pharmacol 33:617–21, 1992.

167. Beaver WT, Wallenstein SL, Rogers A, Houde RW. Analgesic studies of codeine and oxycodone in patients with cancer II: comparison of intramuscular oxycodone with intramuscular morphine and codeine. J Pharmacol Exp Ther 207:101–8, 1978.

168. Kaiko R, Benziger D, Fitzmartin R, et al. Pharmacokinetic-pharmacodynamic relationships of controlled-release oxycodone. Clin Pharmacol Ther 59:52–61, 1996.

169. Weinstein SC, Gaylord JC. Determination of oxycodone in plasma and identification of a major metabolite. J Pharmacol Sci 68:527–8, 1979.

170. Leow KP, Smith M. The antinociceptive potencies of oxycodone, noroxycodone, and morphine after intracerebroventricular administration in rats. Life Sci 54:1229–36, 1994.

171. Watson CP, Babul N. Efficacy of oxycodone in neuropathic pain. A randomized trial in postherpetic neuralgia. Neurology 50:1837–41, 1998.

172. Kaplan R, Parris W, Citron M, et al. Comparison of controlled-release and immediate release oxycodone tablets in patients with cancer pain. J Clin Oncol 16:3230–37, 1998.

173. Parris WC-V, Johnson B, Croghan MK, et al. The use of controlled-release oxycodone for the treatment of chronic cancer pain: a randomized, double-blind study. J Pain Symptom Manage 16:205–11, 1998.

174. Kaiko RF. The use of controlled release opioids. In: Parris WCW, ed. Cancer pain management: principles and practice. Boston: Butterworth-Heinemann, 1997:69–90.

175. Zhukovsky DS, Walsh D, Doona M. The relative potency between high dose oral oxycodone and intravenous morphine: a case illustration. J Pain Symptom Manage 18:53–5, 1999.

176. Gagnon B, Bielech M, Watanabe S, et al. The use of intermittent subcutaneous injections of oxycodone for opioid rotation in patients with cancer pain. Support Care Cancer 7:265–70, 1999.

177. Beaver WT, Wallenstein SL, Rogers A, Houde RW. Analgesic studies of codeine and oxycodone in patients with cancer. I. Comparison of oral with intramuscular codeine and of oral with intramuscular oxycodone. J Pharmacol Exper Ther 207:92–100, 1978.

178. Maddocks I, Somogyi A, Abbott F, et al. Attenuation of morphine-induced delirium in palliative care by substitution with infusion of oxycodone. J Pain Symptom Manage 12:182–9, 1996.

179. Ahmedzai S, Brooks D. Transdermal fentanyl versus sustained-release oral morphine in cancer pain: preference, efficacy, and quality of life. J Pain Symptom Manage 13:254–61, 1997.

180. Donner B, Zenz M, Strumpf M, Raber M. Long-term treatment of cancer pain with transdermal fentanyl. J Pain Symptom Manage 15:168–75, 1998.

181. Donner B, Zenz M, Tryba M, Strumpf M. Transdermal fentanyl in cancer pain: conversion from sustained release morphine to fentanyl TTS-a multicenter study. Pain 64:527–34, 1996.

182. Korte W, Morant R. Transdermal fentanyl in uncontrolled cancer pain: titration on a day-to-day basis as a procedure for safe and effective dose finding a pilot study in 20 patients. Support Care Cancer 2:123–7, 1994.

183. Korte W, de Stoutz N, Morant R. Day-to-day titration to initiate transdermal fentanyl in patients with cancer pain: short-and long-term experiences in a prospective study on 39 patients. J Pain Symptom Manage 11:139–46, 1996.

184. Maves TJ, Barcellos WA. Management of cancer pain with transdermal fentanyl: Phase IV trial, University of Iowa. J Pain Symptom Manage 7:S58–S62, 1992.

185. Zech DFJ, Grond S, Lynch J, et al. Transdermal fentanyl and initial dose-finding with patient-controlled analgesia in cancer pain. A pilot study with 20 terminally ill cancer patients. Pain 50:293–301, 1992.

186. Grond S, Zech D, Lehmann KA, et al. Transdermal fentanyl in the long-term treatment of cancer pain: a prospective study of 50 patients with advanced cancer of the gastrointestinal tract or the head and neck region. Pain 69:191–8, 1997.

187. Zech D, Lehmann KA. Transdermal fentanyl in combination with initial intravenous dose titration by patient-controlled analgesia. Anticancer Drugs 6(Suppl 3):44–9, 1995.

188. Payne R, Mathias SD, Pasta DJ, et al. Quality of life and cancer pain: satisfaction and side effects with transdermal fentanyl versus oral morphine. J Clin Oncol 16:1588–93, 1998.

189. Megens A, Artois K, et al. Comparison of the analgesic and intestinal effects of fentanyl and morphine in rats. J Pain Symptom Manage 15:253–8, 1998.

190. Zenz M, Donner B, Strumpf M. Withdrawal symptoms during therapy with transdermal fentanyl (fentanyl TTS)? J Pain Symptom Pain Manage 9:54–5, 1994.

191. Higgs C, Vella-Brincat J. Withdrawal with transdermal fentanyl. J Pain Symptom Manage 10:4–5, 1995.

192. Davies A, Bond C. Transdermal fentanyl and the opioid withdrawal syndrome. Palliat Med 10:348, 1996.

193. Hunt R. Transdermal fentanyl and the opioid withdrawal syndrome. Palliat Med 10:347–8, 1996.

194. Streisand JB, Varvel JR, Stanski DR, et al. Absorption and bioavailability of oral and transmucosal fentanyl citrate. Anesthesiology 75:223–9, 1991.

195. Fine PG, Marcus M, De Boer AJ, et al. An open label study of oral transmucosal fentanyl citrate (OTFC) for the treatment of breakthrough cancer pain. Pain 45:149, 1991.

196. Streisand JB, Busch MA, Egan TD, et al. Dose proportionality and pharmacokinetics of oral transmucosal fentanyl citrate. Anesthesiology 88:305–9, 1998.

197. Christie JM, Simmonds M, Patt R, et al. Dose titration: a multicenter study of oral transmucosal fentanyl citrate for the treatment of breakthrough pain in cancer patients using transdermal fentanyl for persistent pain. J Clin Oncol 16:3238–45, 1998.

198. Farrar JT, Clearly J, Rauck R, et al. Oral transmucosal fentanyl citrate: randomized, double-blinded, placebo-controlled trial for treatment of breakthrough pain in cancer patients. J Natl Cancer Inst 90(8):611–6, 1998.

199. Portenoy RK, Payne R, Coluzzi P, et al. Oral transmucosal fentanyl citrate (OTFC) for the treatment of breakthrough pain in cancer patients: a controlled dose titration study. Pain 79:303–12, 1999.

200. Lipman AG. New and alternative noninvasive opioid dosage forms and routes of administration. Supportive Oncology Updates 3(1):1–8, 2000.

201. Inturrisi CE, Max MB, Foley KM, et al. The pharmacokinetics of heroin in patients with chronic pain. N Engl J Med 210:1213–7, 1984.

202. Kaiko RF, Wallenstein SL, Rogers AG, et al. Analgesic and mood effects of heroin and morphine in cancer patients with postoperative pain. N Engl J Med 304:1501–5, 1981.

203. Leon WB, Morrison JD, Dundee JW, et al. Studies of drugs given before anaesthesia. The natural and semisynthetic opiates. Br J Anaesth 41:57–63, 1969.

204. Wheatley RG, Somerville ID, Jones JG. The effect of diamorphine administered epidurally or with a patient-controlled analgesia system on long-term postoperative oxygenation. Eur J Anaesthesiol 6:64–6, 1989.

205. Fisher AP, Simpson D, Hanna M. A role for epidural opioid in opioid-insensitive pain? Pain Clinic 1:233–4, 1987.

206. De Castro J, Meynadier J, Zenz M. Regional opioid analgesia. Dordrecht: Kluwer Academic, 1991.

207. Lewis JW. Pharmacological profile of buprenorphine and its clinical use in cancer pain. In: Foley KM, Inturrisi CE, eds. Advances in pain research and therapy, vol. 8: Opioid analgesics in the management of clinical pain. New York: Raven Press, 1986:267–70.

208. Jasinski DR, Pevnick JS, Griffith JD. Human pharmacology and abuse potential of the analgesic buprenorphine. Arch Gen Psychiatry 35:501–16, 1978.

209. De Conno F, Ripamonti C, Sbanotto A, Barletta L. A clinical note on sublingual buprenorphine. J Palliat Care 9(3):44–6, 1993.

210. Gal T. Naloxone reversal of buprenorphine-induced respiratory depression. Clin Pharmacol Ther 45:66–71, 1989.

211. Tive L, Ginsberg K, Pick CG, Pasternak GW. K3 receptors and levorphanol analgesia. Neuropharmacology 9:851–6, 1992.

212. Dixon R. Pharmacokinetics of levorphanol. In: Foley KM, Inturrisi CE, eds. Advances in pain research and therapy, vol. 8: Opioid analgesics in the management of clinical pain. New York: Raven Press, 1986:217.

213. Wallenstein SL, Rogers AG, Kaiko RF, Houde RW. Clinical analgesic studies of levorphanol in acute and chronic cancer pain: assay methodology. In: Foley KM, Inturrisi CE, eds. Advances in pain research and therapy, vol. 8: opioid analgesics in the management of clinical pain. New York: Raven Press, 1986:211–6.

214. Minotti V, Patoia L, Roila F, et al. Double-blind evaluation of analgesic efficacy of orally administered diclofenac, nefopam and acetylsalicylic acid plus codeina in chronic cancer pain. Pain 36:177–9, 1989.

215. Crain SM, Shen K-F. Antagonists of excitatory opioid receptor functions enhance morphine's analgesic potency and attenuate opioid tolerance/dependence liability. Pain 84:121–31, 2000.

216. Levine JD, Gordon NC, Taiwo YO, Coderre TJ. Potentiation of pentazocine analgesia by low-dose naloxone. J Clin Invest 82:1574–7, 1988.

217. Gan TJ, Ginsberg B, Glass PSA, et al. Opioid-sparing effects of a low-dose infusion of naloxone in patient-administered morphine sulphate. Anesthesiology 87:1075–81, 1997.

218. O'Brien CP. A range of research-based pharmacotherapies for addiction. Science 278:66–70, 1997.

219. Shen K-F, Crain SM. Ultra-low doses of naltrexone or etorphine increase morphine's antinociceptive potency and attenuate tolerance/dependence in mice. Brain Res 757:176–90, 1997.

220. Joshi GP, Duffy J, Chehade J, et al. Effects of prophylactic nalmefene on the incidence of morphine-related side effects in patients receiving intravenous patient-controlled analgesia. Anesthesiology 90:1007–11, 1999.

221. Ross FB, Smith MT. The intrinsic antinociceptive effects of oxycodone appear to be kappa opioid receptor mediated. Pain 73:151–7, 1997.

222. Ross FB, Wallis SC, Smith MT. Co-administration of sub-antinociceptive doses of oxycodone and morphine produces marked antinociceptive synergy with reduced CNS side-effects in rats. Pain 84:421–8, 2000.

223. McQuay HJ, Carroll D, Jadad AR, et al. Dextromethorphan for the treatment of neuropathic pain: a double-blind randomised controlled crossover trial with integral n-of-1 design. Pain 59:127–33, 1994.

224. Mercadante S, Casuccio A, Genovese G. Ineffectiveness of dextromethorphan in cancer pain. J Pain Symptom Manage 16:317–22, 1998.

225. Nelson KA, Park KM, Robinovitz E, et al. High-dose dextromethorphan versus placebo in painful diabetic neuropathy and postherpetic neuralgia. Neurology 48:1212–8, 1997.

226. Mao J, Price DD, Caruso F, Mayer DJ. Oral administration of dextromethorphan prevents the development of morphine tolerance and dependence in rats. Pain 67:361–8, 1996.

227. Grass S, Hoffman O, Xu X-J, Wiesenfeld-Hallin Z. N-methyl-D-aspartate receptor antagonists potentiate morphine's anti-nociceptive effect in the rat. Acta Physiol Scand 158:269–73, 1996.

228. Katz NP. MorphiDex (MS:DM) double-blind, multiple-dose studies in chronic pain patients. J Pain Symptom Manage 19:S37–S41, 2000.

229. Caruso FS. MorphiDex pharmacokinetic studies and single-dose analgesic efficacy studies in patients with postoperative pain. J Pain Symptom Manage 19:S31–S36, 2000.

230. Goldblum R. Long-term safety of Morphi-Dex. J Pain Symptom Manage 19(18):S50–S56, 2000.

231. Cherny N, Ripamonti C, Pereira J, et al. Strategies to manage the adverse effects of oral morphine: an evidenced-base report. J Clin Oncol 19:2542–54, 2001.

232. Paix A, Coleman A, Lees J, et al. Subcutaneous fentanyl and sufentanil infusion substitution for morphine intolerance in cancer pain management. Pain 63:263–9, 1995.

233. de Stoutz ND, Bruera E, Suarez-Almazor M. Opioid rotation for toxicity reduction in terminal cancer patients. J Pain Symptom Manage 10:378–84, 1995.

234. Sjogren P, Jensen N-H, Jensen T-S. Disappearance of morphine-induced hyperalgesia after discontinuation or substituting morphine with other opioid agonists. Pain 59:315–6, 1990.

235. Lawlor P, Walker P, Bruera E, Mitchell S. Severe opioid toxicity and somatization of psychological distress in a cancer patient with a background of chemical dependence. J Pain Symptom Manage 13:356–61, 1997.

236. Eisendrath SJ, Goldman B, Douglas J, et al. Meperidine-induced delirium. Am J Psychiatry 144:1062–5, 1987.

237. Steinberg RB, Gilman DE, Johnson III FET. Acute toxic delirium in a patient using transdermal fentanyl. Anesth Analg 75:1014–6, 1992.

238. Szeto HH, Inturrisi CE, Houde R, et al. Accumulation of normeperidine, an active metabolite of meperidine, in patients with renal failure or cancer. Ann Intern Med 86:738–41, 1977.

239. Kaiko RF, Foley KM, Grabinski PY, et al. Central nervous system excitatory effects of meperidine in cancer patients. Ann Neurol 13:180–5, 1983.

240. Parkinson SK, Bailey SL, Little WL, et al. Myoclonic seizure activity with chronic high-dose spinal opioid administration. Anesthesiology 72:743–45, 1990.

241. MacDonald N, Der L, Allan S, et al. Opioid hyperexcitability: the application of alternate opioid therapy. Pain 53:353–5, 1993.

242. Kloke M, Rapp M, Bosse B, Kloke O. Toxicity and/or insufficient analgesia by opioid therapy: risk factors and the impact of changing the opioid. A retrospective analysis of 273 patients observed at a single center. Support Care Cancer 8:479–86, 2000.

243. Ripamonti C, Dickerson D. Strategies for the treatment of cancer pain in the new millennium. Drugs 617:955–77, 2001.

9 Opioid side effects and management

CATHERINE SWEENEY AND EDUARDO D. BRUERA
The University of Texas M. D. Anderson Cancer Center

Introduction

The majority of cancer patients (approximately 80%) develop pain before they die (1). Pain in cancer patients is often underdiagnosed, and inadequate treatment with opioid analgesics is well documented (2–4). Many factors influence pain management in this patient group. Inappropriate and suboptimal education of physicians and other health care professionals has been identified as the major barrier to adequate opioid use (5,6). In developing countries, a further issue is reduced availability of opioids because of financial limitations and government regulations.

As a result of a major educational effort by a number of organizations, including the World Health Organization, the International Association for the Study of Pain, and the American Society of Clinical Oncology, opioid use has improved significantly in developed countries during the last 15 years (7). The results of such efforts have been quite variable (8). In many regions of the world, however, progress has been made, with opioids being used in higher doses and at earlier stages in palliative care (9). Cancer patients, who now have earlier exposure to opioids and generally have treatment with higher dosages, are better managed than in the past. This highly desirable increase in the use of opioids, combined with increased vigilance, has resulted in increased detection of several side effects, most notably neurotoxicity. With this increase in opioid use and the improvement in identification of adverse effects, management strategies for dealing with these unwanted effects have been developed and augmented.

Opioid side effects

Many opioid side effects have long been recognized. However, others have been more clearly identified over the past 10 to 20 years, and the clinical implications of yet others, such as effects on the immune and endocrine systems, are as yet not clear. Table 9.1 summarizes both well-known and more recently identified opioid side effects. This chapter discusses both traditional and emerging opioid side effects and their management.

Sedation

Sedation is a common adverse effect when patients initially receive opioid analgesics or after a significant increase in dose (10–14). In opioid-naive healthy volunteers, clinical doses of buprenorphine cause alterations in reaction time, muscle coordination, attention, and short-term memory (15,16). However, cancer patients receiving stable opioid doses do not develop significant impairment in psychomotor performance (11), reaction times to auditory stimuli (17), postural stability (18), or driving

Table 9.1. *Opioid side effects*

Traditional view:
- Sedation
- Nausea and vomiting
- Constipation
- Respiratory depression
- Less commonly; pruritus, anaphylaxis, sweating, urinary retention

Emerging view:
- Non-cardiogenic pulmonary edema
- Opioid-induced neurotoxicity
  severe sedation
  cognitive failure
  hallucinosis/delirium
  myoclonus/grand mal seizures
  hyperalgesia/allodynia
- Immune system effects
- Endocrine function effects (hypopituitarism, hypogonadism)

ability (12). Opioid-dependent individuals on methadone maintenance therapy appear to have normal cognitive function and reaction time (19–22). The effects of opioid administration on cognitive performance and psychomotor skills, such as driving ability, is further discussed and recommendations are made later in this chapter. In some patients with severe pain, somnolence during the first days of treatment or after an increase in dose may simply reflect increased comfort after days of pain-induced insomnia rather than true somnolence.

There are many other possible causes of sedation in patients who are taking opioid medication. Figure 9.1 summarizes the contributors to sedation in cancer patients. Accumulation of active metabolites of opioids causes sedation and may occur quite rapidly in a number of situations. It is more likely to occur in patients on high doses of opioids and in those with renal insufficiency. Renal impairment developing as a result of administration of nonsteroidal anti-inflammatory drugs (NSAIDs) or some antihypertensives may also cause buildup of active opioid metabolites (23,24). Other medication that has centrally acting sedative effects may add to sedation if used with opioids; examples include hypnotics, tricyclic antidepressants, and centrally acting antiemetics. Consideration of the use of hypnotics is particularly important in cancer patients because they are frequently prescribed to this population for significant periods of time (25,26). Alcohol may have a similar sedative enhancing effect. It is important to consider that rapidly progressing sedation may be the result of other complica-

tions, including metabolic alterations such as hypercalcemia or hyponatremia, sepsis, or progressive brain metastases (25).

Management

Patients with sedation should be carefully assessed for potential causes of their somnolence. Underlying factors such as those in Fig. 9.1 should be addressed where possible. In cancer patients who present with sedation related to opioid use, administration of naloxone is not indicated in the absence of signs of respiratory depression. Naloxone use can precipitate an unnecessary opioid withdrawal syndrome and severe pain (27).

When somnolence is encountered in the presence of residual pain, it is necessary to reexamine the possibility that previously unsuspected anxiety, depression, or other unresolved psychological distress is augmenting the patient's expression of pain, and that the opioid dose is excessive in relation to the nociceptive component of the pain. Somatization of psychosocial suffering has been identified as an independent predictor of cancer pain control in cancer patients (28). In these cases, the opioid dose should be reduced, and other symptoms should be appropriately treated.

In patients where there is persistent sedation at opioid doses necessary to achieve pain control, adjuvant opioid-sparing measures should be considered; these may allow reduction in the opioid dose. These include the use of NSAIDs, bisphosphonates, and corticosteroids. Neuropathic pain may be treated with tricyclic antidepressants or anticon-

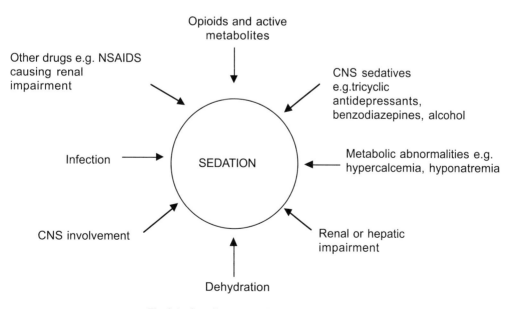

Fig. 9.1. Contributors to sedation in cancer patients.

vulsants. Non-pharmacological measures, such as radiation therapy or nerve blocks, may also be useful.

Finally, a trial of psychostimulants may be useful in patients who are sedated at opioid doses needed for adequate pain control. Psychostimulants have multiple effects as adjuvant drugs in pain management. They potentiate opioid-induced analgesia, counteract opioid-related sedation and cognitive dysfunction, and allow an escalation of opioid dose in patients with pain syndromes that are difficult to treat (29).

Dextroamphetamine has been found to antagonize opioid-induced sedation in a single-dose study involving postsurgical patients (30). Controlled clinical trials show conflicting results. A number of investigators have found that the use of methylphenidate resulted in a significant improvement in the visual analog scale for drowsiness and confusion (4,31,32). Wilwerding et al. (33) were unable to demonstrate a statistically significant benefit for methylphenidate in reducing opioid-induced drowsiness; however, a trend toward decreased drowsiness after methylphenidate was observed.

Methylphenidate significantly improved cognitive function (measured by finger-tapping speed, arithmetic, digit memitory, memory and visual memory) in patients being treated with high dose of opioids. Fernandez et al. (34) reported an uncontrolled trial involving 19 cognitively impaired patients with AIDS-related complex who demonstrated improvement in neuropsychological tests when treated with methylphenidate and dextroamphetamine.

Psychostimulants can produce adverse effects such as hallucinations, delirium, or psychosis (which can be treated with haloperidol or discontinuation of the drug). Amphetamine derivatives have other adverse effects such as decreased appetite, and tolerance to their effects can develop.

Before prescribing psychostimulants, a careful medical history must be taken to exclude any psychiatric disorder. This is important, as stimulants are contraindicated in patients with a history of hallucinations, delirium, or paranoid disorders. They are also relatively contraindicated in those with a history of substance abuse or hypertension.

In clinical practice, the usual starting doses of psychostimulants are methylphenidate 10 mg/day, dextroamphetamine 2.5 mg/day, or pemoline 20 mg/day. The drug dose can be increased if no adverse effects are observed. The therapeutic effect is evident within 2 days of treatment. Morning and noon administration is advised so as not to disturb sleep (35).

Donepezil is a reversible centrally selective acetylcholinesterase inhibitor and is used for the management of cognitive failure related to cortical dementia. A recent series of case reports and anecdotal experience from our group suggests that it may reduce sedation in patients receiving opioids (36). Randomized controlled trials are needed to better characterize this potential effect.

Nausea and vomiting

Opioid analgesia can cause nausea and vomiting in patients after initiation or increase in dose. This usually responds well to antiemetics and disappears spontaneously within the first 3 or 4 days of treatment (37,38). Some patients, particularly those receiving high doses of opioids, experience chronic and severe nausea. This may be accompanied by abdominal pain, constipation, and gas distention of the large bowel and occasionally of the small bowel. As with other symptoms in cancer patients, there are often many potential causes of nausea and vomiting, and in many patients the etiology is multifactorial. Figure 9.2 summarizes the main contributors to nausea in cancer patients.

Opioids cause chronic nausea by a number of mechanisms, including stimulation of the chemoreceptor trigger zone in the area postrema of the medulla, stimulation of the vomiting center, vertigo because of stimulation of the eighth cranial nerve, gastroparesis, and constipation. Chronic nausea has been associated with accumulation of active morphine metabolites such as morphine-6-glucuronide (M-6-G) (39). The frequency of nausea and vomiting is comparatively higher in ambulatory patients than in those confined to bed. This suggests that these drugs also act by altering the sensitivity of the vestibular center.

Management

Those exposed to opioids for the first time, or those who undergo a significant dose increase, should have universal access to antiemetics. Opioid-induced nausea and vomiting are probably most likely to be effectively treated with prokinetic agents such as metoclopramide (40–42). However, there have been no randomized controlled trials comparing different agents in the management of opioid-induced emesis. Drugs with central nervous system (CNS) effects can also be helpful, for example, because the vestibular center has a high concentration of muscarinic cholinergic (43) and histamine H_1-receptors (44); the use of anticholinergic and antihistaminic drugs may be beneficial in the specific cases of nausea related to movement. Antiemetic agents that act centrally on the CNS have the potential to cause trouble-

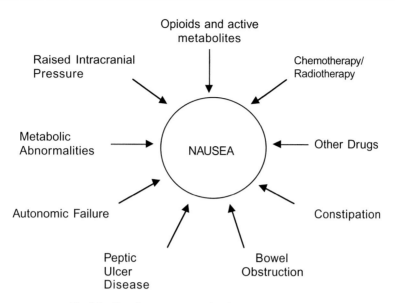

Fig. 9.2. Contributors to nausea in advanced cancer patients.

some side effects such as sedation, which can add to opioid toxicity in some patients. In patients who do not initially respond to antiemetics, the addition of corticosteroids can dramatically improve the effects of prokinetic drugs (44); the mechanism of this effect of corticosteroids is not well understood.

The etiology of nausea and vomiting in an individual cancer patient is often multifactorial, and underlying causes should, if possible, be identified and corrected. Constipation, which frequently coexists in these patients, should be treated, metabolic abnormalities corrected, and other medications that might contribute should be discontinued.

Constipation

Constipation occurs in approximately 90% of patients treated with opioids (46). Clinical observations suggest that constipation caused by opioids is a dose-related phenomenon with wide interindividual variability. Tolerance to this symptom develops slowly, and many patients require laxative therapy for as long as they take opioids.

There is recent evidence of differences between individual opioids in their constipation-inducing potential. Hunt et al. (47) performed a crossover trial of equianalgesic doses of subcutaneous fentanyl and morphine in 23 hospice cancer patients and found that patients had more frequent bowel movements while on fentanyl. Measures for nausea, delirium, and cognitive function showed no differences between the two drugs. In a retrospective study of 49 patients, the amount of laxatives needed to

achieve at least one bowel movement every 3 days was compared to the median equivalent daily dose of parenteral morphine for each opioid. Laxative doses for methadone were significantly lower than for morphine and hydromorphone. Abdominal involvement, female gender, and older age also resulted in greater need for laxatives (48). Further studies are needed in this area to look prospectively at which opioids have more favorable side effect profiles with respect to constipation.

Opioids cause constipation by affecting the intestine by one of three mechanisms: reduction in motility, reduction in secretion (pancreatic, biliary, electrolyte, and fluid), and increase in intestinal fluid absorption and blood flow (49–51).

Exogenous opioid administration extends the transit time and desiccates the intraluminal content. There is some evidence that morphine stimulates mucosal sensory receptors, which in turn activate a reflex arc to further increase fluid absorption (52).

Many factors can contribute to constipation in cancer patients. Figure 9.3 summarizes the main causes in this population. Constipation may result in a number of clinical presentations and complications that are not normally associated with absence of bowel movements; these are summarized in Table 9.2.

Management

Patients who are starting opioid medication should be advised of the likelihood of constipation developing and should be prescribed laxatives concomitantly and the dose titrated to effect. Even patients with poor oral intake

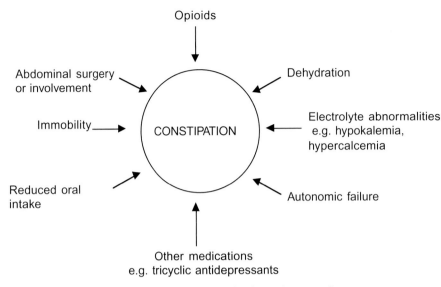

Fig. 9.3. Causes of constipation in advanced cancer patients.

should be advised that constipation may occur and of the advisability of laxative use.

All patients taking opioids should be assessed for constipation because of its prevalence in this group. Assessment of constipation has been found to be insufficient even in patients at high risk for constipation in a palliative care center; in addition, the location of patients (home or hospital) did not predict the degree of constipation on admission (53). Assessment includes at least a history of the frequency and difficulty of defecation and symptoms attributed to constipation, and a physical and rectal examination. Occasionally, an abdominal x-ray study may be required if the history is unclear (54–56). The use of a radiological constipation score may be necessary for adequate diagnosis in some patients, particularly those with cognitive failure. On a plain abdominal x-ray study, the abdomen is divided into four quadrants. Each quadrant is assessed for constipation score: 0 = no stool, 1 = stool occupying < 50% of the lumen, 2 = stool occupying > 50% of the lumen, 3 = stool completely occupying the whole lumen of the colon. The total score of all quadrants is calculated and will range from 0 to 12. A score of 7/12 or greater indicates severe constipation and requires immediate treatment (53,54,56).

In addition to opioid therapy, the majority of cancer patients also have at least one or two more of the precipitating factors described in Fig. 9.3. Therefore, the management of constipation in these patients will frequently require a multimodal approach. Management can be divided into general and therapeutic approaches. General interventions involve elimination of medical factors that may be contributing to constipation (for example, treatment of electrolyte abnormalities, discontinuation of all non-essential constipating drugs), increase in fluid intake and fiber consumption, and, if possible, the availability of comfort, privacy, and convenience during defecation. Increased fiber intake may not be desirable in patients who have poor caloric intake or are cachectic, as it may result in early satiety and prevent the ingestion of more nutritious foods.

Therapeutic interventions involve the use of laxatives, rectal suppositories, enemas, and manual disimpaction. Oral laxatives include bulk agents, osmotic agents, contact cathartics, lubricants, prokinetic drugs, and oral naloxone.

Bulk agents such as cellulose and psyllium seeds are used as a fiber supplement to increase stool bulk. They

Table 9.2. *Clinical presentations and complications of constipation*

Clinical presentations
• Abdominal pain
• Distention
• Anorexia
• Nausea and vomiting
• Urinary retention
• Increased liver or retroperitoneal pain
• Confusion
• Diarrhea

Complications of untreated constipation
• Fecal impaction
• Rectal tears, fissures, and hemorrhoids
• Bowel obstruction
• Intestinal perforation
• Inadequate absorption of oral medication

typically work after 2 to 4 days of regular use. They may cause distention, bloating, and abdominal pain and are unsuitable for patients with advanced cancer, as they require adequate oral fluid intake and may result in satiety, which can result in reduced oral intake of nutritious food. They are of doubtful effectiveness in severe constipation.

Saline laxatives such as magnesium and sodium salts act as osmotically active particles and draw fluid into the intestinal lumen resulting in a semiliquid stool that has a reduced transit time. They usually work in 3 to 6 hours; long-term use should be avoided, as the action is not physiological. Sodium salts in particular should be avoided in patients with cardiac failure or renal insufficiency, as they can lead to water and sodium retention. Lactulose and sorbitol also act as osmotic laxatives; they are not absorbed by the bowel and cause water retention in the lumen. Their onset of action is usually 24 to 48 hours. They may cause flatulence and their sweet taste is nauseating for some patients.

Contact cathartics (senna, cascara, danthron, phenophthalein, bisacodyl, docusates, and castor oil) are the most commonly administered laxatives for opioid-induced constipation. These drugs act by increasing peristalsis by way of a stimulatory effect on the myenteric plexus and reducing absorption of water and electrolytes from the bowel lumen (57). Onset of action varies between individual agents in this group, castor oil 2 to 6 hours, docusate 24 to 72 hours, and the others in the region of 6 to 10 hours. Short-term use is safe; however, overuse can cause dehydration and long-term ingestion may result in dependence on laxatives for bowel function. However, this is certainly not a contraindication to therapy for advanced cancer patients (58).

Lubricant laxatives (mineral oils) soften the stool and lubricate the stool surface. They usually work in 6 to 8 hours but are not recommended for chronic laxation in the cancer population, as long-term use is associated with perianal irritation, malabsorption of fat-soluble proteins, and potential for lipoid pneumonia (58).

Prokinetic agents such as metoclopramide and domperidone could be considered for constipation that has not responded to conventional measures. A continuous infusion of metoclopramide has been used to treat severe narcotic bowel obstruction (59).

Two types of opioid antagonists have been shown to have a beneficial effect on opioid-induced constipation. Oral naloxone, a μ-opioid antagonist, can reverse opioid-induced constipation (60,61). It has been shown that the oral administration of naloxone at a daily dose of 20% or more of the prevailing 24-hour morphine dose can pro-

vide a clinical laxative effect without antagonizing opioid analgesia (62). Some patients in this study, however, experienced opioid withdrawal. In a more recent prospective study, oral naloxone was shown to improve symptoms of opioid-induced constipation and reduce laxative use in chronic pain patients. Opioid withdrawal symptoms were seen in 4 of 22 patients (moderate side effects of yawning, sweating, and shivering were of short duration). One patient withdrew from the study because of opioid withdrawal; the other three continued without problems after a slight reduction in dose. In this study oral naloxone was started and titrated individually between 3×3 mg to 3×12 mg/day, depending on laxation and withdrawal symptoms (63).

Methylnaltrexone is a peripheral opioid receptor antagonist. Intravenous methylnaltrexone has also been shown to induce laxation in a double-blind, placebo-controlled trial of 21 patients in a methadone maintenance program who had methadone-induced constipation. No opioid withdrawal was observed, and no significant adverse effects were reported (64). A follow-up study using oral methylnaltrexone showed dose-related laxation in 12 patients on a methadone maintenance program, again with no withdrawal and no adverse effects (65).

Combined laxative treatment is not universally effective; 40% of advanced cancer patients also require the use of enemas and/or rectal manipulation (46). For most cancer patients, the use of enemas and rectal suppositories is limited to the acute, short-term management of more severe episodes of constipation. Some patients who cannot tolerate oral laxatives may be able to use long-term rectal laxatives or enemas effectively (58).

Suppositories may be inert or active. Inert suppositories usually contain glycerine and draw fluid into the rectum, acting as a stimulus for defecation. Active suppositories contain a cathartic. Where suppositories are ineffective, enemas can be used. Microenemas are useful, as their small fluid volume makes them less distressing for the patient. Docusate and bisacodyl are also available in enema form. Sodium phosphate enemas may cause fluid and electrolyte imbalances, particularly in dehydrated patients. Soap and water enemas can cause fluid overload and may irritate the rectal mucosa.

Another approach in patients with severe refractory constipation is to consider opioid rotation to methadone, which appears to be less constipating than other opioids (48). Opioid rotation is dealt with in more detail later in this chapter (see Management of opioid-induced neurotoxicity).

Other novel approaches have been described, including use of fresh bakers yeast or NSAIDs. A small preliminary study of cancer patients who initiated opioid therapy and concurrently commenced fresh bakers yeast showed it had an effect on prevention of constipation in the short term (66). Ketorolac infusion has also been shown, in a small study, to relieve opioid bowel syndrome, probably in part by its morphine sparing effect, but also possibly by a prostaglandin inhibitory effect (67). Prostaglandins inhibit intestinal motility; this has been shown to be reversed by indomethacin (68,69).

Respiratory depression

Respiratory depression as a side effect of opioid use is dose dependent. Different receptor mechanisms are responsible for opioid-induced analgesia and respiratory depression. Opioids have a direct effect on the pontine and bulbar brainstem respiratory centers, reducing respiratory drive (70). Respiratory depression generally occurs after short-term administration of high doses of opioids in opioid-naive individuals. In cancer patients who are on long-term opioid treatment, tolerance develops to the respiratory depressant effects with repeated administration of the drugs (71). Respiratory depression will not occur in the absence of other concurrent side effects, such as sedation. Patients who ignore sedation and continue to take regular opioid medication may develop respiratory depression. In renal impairment, the buildup of renally excreted morphine metabolites, such as M-6-G, can lead to respiratory depression (72). Another area where there is risk of respiratory depression in patients on long- term opioids is after the rotation from another opioid to methadone; problems with dose ratios and reduced cross tolerance result in a significant risk of respiratory depression (73,74). Pain is an effective antagonist to the respiratory depressant effects of opioids. Abolition of pain by cervical cordotomy and neurolytic blocks in patients on opioid medication has resulted in respiratory depression (75,76).

Management
In patients with respiratory depression, the opioid involved should be reduced or temporarily discontinued and treatment changed to a different opioid if necessary. Naloxone should be administered immediately in a diluted solution in small increments to avoid withdrawal symptoms. It is usually possible to start with 0.1mg every 3 to 5 minutes until reversal of the symptoms occur. The patient should be monitored as naloxone has an elimination half-life of 30 minutes, and respiratory depression may recur when the effect of the naloxone becomes attenuated by its elimination. Repeat administration or a continuous intravenous or subcutaneous infusion may be required.

Pruritis

Some side effects vary with route of administration of the opioid; pruritis, nausea and vomiting, respiratory depression, and urinary retention are more common with neuraxial (epidural and intrathecal) administration (77). Pruritis is uncommon after systemic administration of opioids, but has been reported to occur in 8.5% and 46% of patients receiving epidural and intrathecal opioids, respectively (78). The etiology is unknown but may be related to histamine release or a central effect.

Management
In the management of patients with pruritis associated with neuraxial administration of opioids, a variety of medications have shown potential, but none is universally effective. Epidural administration of droperidol (79), butorphanol (80), and naloxone (81) have each shown benefit, as has intravenous prophylactic ondansetron (82). Antihistamines, intravenous propofol, low-dose intravenous naloxone (83), and transnasal butorphanol (84) have also been used with success. Change of opioid from morphine to hydromorphone has also been reported to be effective (85,86).

Urinary retention

Urinary retention, like pruritis, is also more common with neuraxial administration of opioids (77). It is more likely to occur in opioid-naive patients and in the first days of treatment with opioids. Low-dose intravenous naloxone may be useful, but care must be taken not to induce withdrawal; alternatively, a program of intermittent catheterization can be used but is rarely needed.

Non-cardiogenic pulmonary edema

This side effect of opioid use was first described by Osler over 100 years ago (87). It has been well documented with street use of narcotics and in cases of opioid overdosage. It has also been reported after the administration of naloxone (88). In recent years, with use of high doses of opioids for management of cancer pain, this phenomenon has been described in cancer patients (89). Cancer patients who develop this problem generally have had a large increase in their opioid dose for pain relief in the previous days. In cancer patients with a non-intensive management approach, there is a high mortality associated with opioid-induced non-cardiogenic pulmonary edema, whereas in drug addicts the incidence has been described as less than 1% (87). There are several hypotheses for the mechanism of this phenomenon, including increased capillary permeability, immune complex deposition in the lung, endothelial damage from hypoxia, and an effect of opioids in an area of the brainstem, which may control capillary permeability (89).

Management

The apparent relationship between recent large increases in opioid dose and the development of non-cardiogenic pulmonary edema indicates that it should be anticipated in patients who have required massive dose increases of their opioids. Approximately 15% of patients receiving parenteral opioids require rapid increases in daily dose (90). In these patients, consideration should be given to the use of adjuvant analgesic measures with other pharmacologic and nonpharmacologic agents to try to prevent the need for rapid dose escalation. Opioid rotation may be helpful in reducing dose increases because of incomplete cross-tolerance between different opioids (91). Other potential precipitating factors, such as excessive hydration, oxygen therapy, or corticosteroids, should be limited in these patients.

Opioid-induced neurotoxicity

Opioid-induced neurotoxicity (OIN) is a recently recognized syndrome of neuropsychiatric consequences of opioid administration (92). The features of OIN include cognitive impairment, severe sedation, hallucinosis, delirium, myoclonus, seizures, hyperalgesia, and allodynia. Patients exhibiting some or all of these features are suffering from opioid-induced neurotoxicity. OIN is most often seen in patients receiving high doses of opioid analgesics for prolonged periods, often in association with psychoactive medications. Fluid depletion and renal failure are also often present. Risk factors for OIN are summarized in Table 9.3.

Sedation, cognitive failure, hallucinosis, and delirium

Sedation has been described earlier in this chapter; in cases of OIN, it is often seen in association with other features of OIN such as cognitive failure and may be a feature of delirium.

Cognitive failure is often seen in patients with advanced cancer (93), and although it has multiple causes,

Table 9.3. *Risk factors for opioid-induced neurotoxicity*

High opioid dose
Prolonged opioid exposure
Preexisting borderline cognition/delirium
Dehydration
Renal failure
Opioids with mixed agonist/antagonist activity (e.g., pentazocine, butorphanol, and nalbuphine)
Other psychoactive drugs

opioid treatment plays a major role (93–96). Figure 9.4 outlines the main causes of cognitive failure and delirium in cancer patients. Changes in cognition can be seen in patients who have recently had a significant increase in opioid dose; however, these usually subside within approximately 1 week of being maintained on the opioid (12,96,97). Cognitive dysfunction can be more severe in patients receiving higher doses or opioids having agonist/antagonist activity compared with pure agonists, in patients receiving other psychoactive medications, and in patients having borderline cognitive impairment before treatment. The impairment is usually a slowing of the cognitive abilities rather than an increase in the number of errors or major lapses in judgment (98,99).

In cancer patients on long-term opioid treatment, other factors related to the cancer also influence the level of cognitive functioning, and the picture at present is not entirely clear. Advanced cancer patients on stable doses of oral morphine have been compared to advanced cancer patients not on opioids and to healthy age-matched controls. Cancer patients performed less well than healthy controls on all assessments, and those on morphine had poorer grammatical reasoning, alertness, and cognitive function than both other groups (100). In another study that attempted to separate the impact of performance status, pain, and oral opioids on neuropsychological functioning in cancer patients, the use of long-term oral opioids did not affect any of the neuropsychological tests used. The control group consisted of cancer patients with Karnofsky Performance Status A (able to carry on normal activity and work with no special care needed) who had no pain and received no opioid medication. Those with lower performance status had slower continuous reaction times, and pain was possibly responsible for more deterioration in serial addition task than opioid treatment (101).

In an observational study involving only patients with cancer pain receiving opioids, the majority had mental status impairment, with only 23% (8 of 35) retaining full cognitive function (96). In a series of articles studying cognition and reaction time in cancer patients treated for

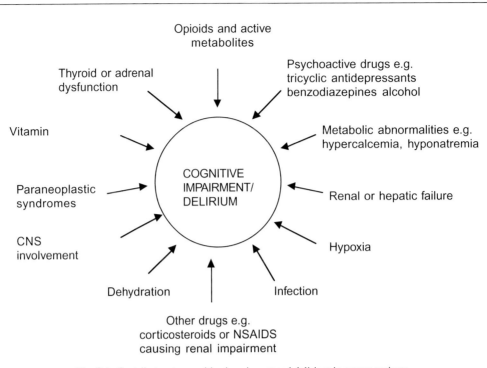

Fig. 9.4. Contributors to cognitive impairment and delirium in cancer patients.

pain, those on opioid analgesics had significant retardation in reaction time when compared to healthy controls (14,17) and cancer patients not on opioids (13).

Driving ability is an area where impairment of alertness and cognitive function has major implications. In patients with advanced cancer, the presence of malignancy itself aggravates cognitive impairment. The effects of cancer and opioid medication on driving ability have been looked at in a few studies. Cancer patients on regular morphine undergoing a series of psychologic and neurologic tests for assessment of driving ability were compared to those not on opioids. No significant difference was noted in driving ability, but there was a slight and selective effect on functions related to driving in the patients on long-term morphine therapy (12). Overall, this study suggests that cancer patients, both those receiving and not receiving opioids, have significant impairment in driving ability as compared to healthy controls. A pilot study has looked at predriver evaluation and simulator driving evaluation in patients with non-malignant pain using stable chronic opioid analgesic therapy and compared them to cerebrally compromised patients who had the same evaluations and subsequent behind wheel driving tests. The comprehensive off-road driving evaluation used measures that have been shown to be sensitive in predicting on-road driving performance. The study generally supported the notion that chronic opioid analgesic therapy did not significantly

impair the perception, cognition, coordination, and behavior measured in off-road tests, but the authors commented that methodological problems may limit the generalizability of results and recommended further research (102).

In general, patients should be advised to refrain from driving, operating machines, and performing tasks that require significant concentration and psychomotor skills for 3 to 4 days after initiation of opioid therapy and after significant increases (30%–50%) in their daily dose of opioid. In cases of doubt about driving ability in patients receiving opioids, an appropriate approach would be to ask the patient to take a driving test with the local driving authority or a skilled occupational therapist.

Hallucinations have been described in patients receiving opioid analgesia (103–107). Most of the reports have described visual hallucinations. However, tactile hallucinations have been suggested to occur more frequently (108). Occasionally, patients may have hallucinations without obvious cognitive failure (104), and their fear of having psychiatric illness may cause reluctance to reveal the situation to caregivers. In some cases, an abrupt change in the patient's mood (anxiety or depression) may be the only sign of the development of organic hallucinosis (109).

During recent years, a number of authors have documented that delirium is one of the most frequent neuropsychiatric complications in patients with advanced cancer (97,110,111). Approximately 80% of cancer patients may have delirium near death (111,112). In a recent prospective series of 131 patients with advanced cancer consecutively admitted to a tertiary palliative care unit, delirium was present in 42% on admission and developed in 45% of the remaining patients. Delirium was present in 88% of patients who died, and patients with delirium had poorer survival rates than controls (111). Patients with delirium present with combinations of cognitive failure, fluctuating levels of consciousness, changes in the sleep-wake cycle, and variable severity of psychomotor agitation, hallucinations, delusions, and other perception abnormalities (113). There are a number of possible clinical presentations of delirium; it may present with hyperactive, agitated, hyperalert features, or as a hypoactive withdrawn state. Often, mixed features of hyperactivity and hypoactivity coexist (108). Non-agitated delirium is frequently underdiagnosed (114).

Myoclonus and seizures

High doses of morphine have been found to induce myoclonus in animals and humans. The term *myoclonus* is applied to a sudden, brief, shock-like involuntary movement caused by active muscular contractions. It may involve a whole muscle or may be limited to a small number of muscle fibers (115). It has been described as being a type of tonic-clonic seizure, representing a continuum of neural effects (116,117). On the other hand, it may represent a pre-epileptiform phenomenon that, if left untreated, may progress to tonic-clonic seizures. In animals, morphine, hydromorphone, and fentanyl have been found to be capable of causing agitation, myoclonus, hyperalgesia, and seizures when administered systemically or intrathecally (118). In humans, myoclonus has been described after the administration of morphine (105,119–121), hydromorphone (122,123), meperidine (124–126), fentanyl and its derivatives (127–129), and diamorphine (130). Studies have shown that high concentrations of these opioids and their metabolites in cerebrospinal fluid may cause myoclonus (131–133). Renal impairment is a cause of metabolite accumulation in patients with myoclonus (119,127,134). In a small prospective trial, 12 of 19 patients treated with oral or parenteral morphine developed myoclonus, and one patient developed hyperalgesia (120). The frequency of patients developing myoclonus was not linked to the plasma concentration of morphine but was associated with the concomitant use of antidepressants, antipsychotics, and NSAIDS. Myoclonus was less likely to occur in patients on steroids.

Grand mal seizures may be more likely in patients who have other risk factors such as a history of seizures, brain metastases, or other metabolic abnormalities.

Hyperalgesia and allodynia

Hyperalgesia and allodynia are two of the most distressing presentations of opioid toxicity. Hyperalgesia is an exaggerated nociceptive response to noxious stimuli, whereas allodynia is an exaggerated nociceptive response to innocuous stimuli (135). Hyperalgesia and allodynia have been observed after high doses of morphine (both parenteral and intrathecal) in humans (106,120). Sjogren et al. (121,136) have described this toxicity well. They reported that eight patients demonstrated hyperalgesia and myoclonus after receiving high doses of intravenous morphine and described another series of four patients who developed hyperalgesia during systemic morphine administration. Hyperalgesia can have two presentations, one as exaggerated nociceptive response, for example, to cutaneous stimulation such as a pinprick, the second as a worsening of the underlying pain syndrome. The latter type of hyperalgesia has also been described clinically as the development of paradoxical pain (137). This is of clinical relevance, as clinicians may misinterpret this phenomenon by not recognizing it as a neurotoxic adverse effect and respond by further increasing the opioid dose in an attempt to control the pain. It is important to consider the possibility of OIN in patients who suffer a sudden aggravation of pain or cutaneous hyperalgesia.

A number of compounds have been identified as being involved in the mechanism of allodynia in animal studies, including morphine, morphine-3-glucuronide (M-3-G), normorphine, and hydromorphone. All are capable of causing allodynia in rats after intrathecal administration (138,139).

Management of opioid-induced neurotoxicity

As is the case with many symptoms in advanced cancer patients, sedation, cognitive impairment, hallucinations, and delirium with agitation or withdrawal have several potential underlying causes. In a previously mentioned prospective study of delirium in advanced cancer patients, a median (range) of three (range, 1–6) precipitating factors was identified for each episode of delirium (111). In individuals presenting with possible opioid side effects or toxicity, a detailed assessment is necessary to identify treatable causes. This includes a history (and collateral history if the patient is confused) with particular attention to medications and history of alcohol or substance abuse, a physical examination, and assessment of mental status. When any of the features of OIN are present blood tests to look at complete blood count, electrolytes, renal function, hepatic function, and calcium should be undertaken along with urinalysis, and a possible chest x-ray study if sepsis is considered. Identified possible contributing factors should be treated as appropriate. As approximately 80% of patients have delirium near death, in delirious patients where the illness trajectory suggests that death is imminent and further treatment is not planned, it is not appropriate to assess the patient in this degree of detail.

Management of sedation has been described earlier. Impaired cognitive function may also respond to a similar management strategy with treatment of underlying contributors, opioid dose reduction where possible, and a trial of psychostimulants in selected patients. Care must be taken to exclude a history of psychiatric disorders, in particular hallucinations, delirium, or paranoid ideation, as these can be precipitated or exacerbated by the use of psychostimulants.

Hallucinations, agitation or withdrawal in a patient treated with opioids should alert the clinician to the possibility of opioid toxicity. A high index of suspicion is needed in these cases. Simple and reliable instruments, such as the Mini-Mental Status Examination (140) or the Memorial Delirium Assessment Scale (141) are available for the screening, monitoring, and diagnosis of delirium in advanced cancer patients. After careful assessment and management, Lawlor et al. (111) reported an overall delirium reversibility rate of 49%. They clearly identified opioid and non-opioid psychoactive medications as precipitating factors independently associated with delirium reversibility.

Several strategies have been proposed and successfully used in the management of OIN. Table 9.4 summarizes these approaches.

Opioid rotation

It is well documented that several of the opioids as well as their active metabolites, can cause effects considered part of the syndrome of OIN. Morphine has three active metabolites: M-3-G, M-6-G, and normorphine. Morphine and its metabolites have all been shown to cause central excitation that is mediated by receptors, which seem to be distinct from the receptors involved in analgesia (132). In animal models M-3-G has been shown to antagonize the analgesic effects of morphine and M-6-G and to induce hyperalgesia, myoclonus, and convulsions (132,142). Normorphone can

Table 9.4. *Approaches to management of acute episodes of opioid-induced neurotoxicity*

Hydration
Opioid rotation
Opioid dose reduction or discontinuation
Stop other contributing drugs (e.g., hypnotics, nonsteroidal anti-inflammatory drugs)
Circadian modulation
Symptomatic treatment with haloperidol or other medications

also cause significant hyperexcitability (143). A recent analysis in patients on long-term morphine treatment indicates that elevated concentrations of M-3-G in plasma, as well as plasma and cerebrospinal fluid M-3-G/M-6-G ratios, may have a pathological role in the development of hyperalgesia, allodynia, and/or myoclonus (144). Morphine, hydromorphone, and fentanyl are capable of causing agitation, myoclonus, hyperalgesia, and tonic-clonic seizures in animals when administered systemically or intrathecally (117,118,145,146).

If neurotoxicity is thought to be secondary to accumulation of the parent opioid or its active metabolites, a change of opioid has been shown to be effective in reversing the symptoms. Several studies have shown that opioid rotation is a safe and effective method for reducing neurotoxicity and at the same time retaining analgesia (107,121,122,124,131,136,147–154). Although these studies are small and uncontrolled, all patients had evidence of OIN and all were observed to have significant improvement after the opioid rotation. Differences in analgesic or adverse effects after opioid rotation are thought to be the result of a number of mechanisms, including receptor activity, asymmetry in cross-tolerance among different opioids, different opioid efficacies, and accumulation of toxic metabolites (155). A retrospective review of the prevalence of OIN has shown a dramatic decrease in agitated delirium after the institution of hydration and opioid rotation (156). These results justify the use of opioid rotation in the management of OIN and should be the focus of future randomized controlled trials.

The ideal alternative opioid has not as yet been determined. In those patients who develop OIN while on morphine, a trial of hydromorphone or oxycodone is usually effective. The reverse (hydromorphone or oxycodone to morphine) is also effective.

If OIN develops after rotation among the first-line agonists, a second-line opioid such as methadone or parenteral fentanyl may be used. Methadone has the advantage of extremely low cost and no known active metabolites but the disadvantage of a long and variable half-life and poorly defined equianalgesic dose as compared to morphine or hydromorphone (157–159). Recent research suggests the benefit of methadone in *N*-methyl-D-aspartate receptor antagonism (159–161). Methadone is commonly administered orally or rectally with good absorption. Cross-tolerance appears to be less than with other opioids; equianalgesic doses are relatively lower in patients previously exposed to high doses of opioid agonists as compared with patients previously exposed to low doses (163–165). Rotation to methadone can be safely achieved over 3 to 4 days, gradually increasing the dose while decreasing the offending opioid by similar proportions (159). However, rotation to methadone should only be attempted by experienced specialists because of the problem with poorly defined equianalgesic ratios. Management of patients on methadone once the rotation has been completed is not different from other opioid agonists (166).

Dose reduction or discontinuation

Reduction in dosage or discontinuation of opioids have been shown in several reports to reverse OIN (106,119,167,168). This intervention is clear proof that opioids are causative agents in the neurotoxicity syndrome. The use of adjuvant opioid-sparing treatments has been mentioned earlier in this chapter. However, reduction or discontinuation of opioids is rarely possible in patients with advanced cancer pain syndromes. Aggressive opioid rotation may result in lower doses being used in individual patients, as well as programs as a whole (151,169), and this can contribute to a lower overall incidence of OIN in a palliative care program (151,156,169).

Circadian modulation

Pain and its perception vary from patient to patient, and some studies demonstrate that the pain intensity can change according to the time of day. A circadian pattern of pain can be demonstrated in patients whose pain is caused by a variety of different diseases (170), and animal experiments have shown that reactions to induced pain also follow circadian rhythmicity (171). Evidence of circadian cycling in patients with advanced cancer pain has only recently been observed. A prospective study measuring the temporal variation of pain in cancer patients found the peak pain consistently occurred in the late afternoon at 1800 hours (172). This has been supported by our group and others who found the peak use

of rescue opioids occurred between 1800 and 2200 hours, whereas the lowest doses were given between 0200 and 0600 hours (158,173–177). Further prospective studies should evaluate whether pain management regimens targeted to the circadian variation in pain intensity might reduce overall opioid requirements and the consequent development of OIN or tolerance without jeopardizing effective analgesia. Opioids with a short and predictable half-life, such as fentanyl and its derivatives, might be ideally suited to such studies.

Hydration

The active metabolites of opioid agonists are water soluble and are likely to accumulate in patients with renal failure or volume depletion. Ensuring patients receive adequate hydration, either orally or parenterally will decrease the severity and duration of OIN. In the advanced cancer patient, hydration is most easily administered either intravenously or subcutaneously (178). If the decision is made not to hydrate a terminally ill patient who is receiving opioid analgesics, it is likely that active opioid metabolites will accumulate as the patient becomes progressively volume contracted and urine output decreases. Under these conditions, patients will require careful reduction in opioid dose and ongoing assessment for signs of OIN. Should the latter develop, opioid rotation may be required.

Renal failure in patients with advanced cancer has been associated with an increase in the serum levels of M-3-G and M-6-G. These patients also developed signs of OIN (179). Although volume status was not noted, the accumulation of toxic metabolites in association with renal failure emphasizes the importance of proper hydration to prevent OIN.

In at least one study, the introduction of a policy of hydration resulted in a dramatic and significant decrease in agitated delirium (156). Unfortunately, no determinations of serum levels of opioids or metabolites were made before or after the establishment of hydration. Most effects of OIN resolve within 3 to 5 days of introduction of opioid rotation and hydration.

Other medications

Administration of naloxone may be useful in cases of massive acute opioid overdose (92). In cancer patients who have been on long-term opioid therapy for ongoing cancer pain, however, naloxone can precipitate severe pain aggravation, opioid withdrawal syndrome, or toxic-clonic seizures and, thus, should be used only in exceptional circumstances and with extreme caution (27).

Hyperactive delirium caused by opioid therapy is best treated symptomatically with haloperidol to control symptoms until other measures such as hydration and opioid rotation start to have effect (23,180,181). However, it can be difficult to determine whether the cause of delirium is opioid induced or pain related. Increased agitation is often interpreted by families and staff as increased pain, and if the cause is opioid related increasing opioid medication may result in significant aggravation of delirium and agitation (182). In most patients' hallucinations, delusions or agitation will respond rapidly to haloperidol either given orally or subcutaneously. If this is not effective, a more sedating alternative such as chlorpromazine may be needed. In a very small number of patients whose symptoms cannot be controlled using the above measures, a continuous subcutaneous infusion of midazolam may be required, usually 25 to 50 mg in a total volume of 50 ml dextrose 5% starting at 1 ml/hour and titrating until there is control of symptoms. This treatment results in significant sedation.

An array of other medications such as baclofen, barbiturates, clonazepam and other benzodiazepines, and clonidine have all been used to manage various symptoms of OIN (120,168,183–185). Few controlled trials have studied the role of these drugs, and the effectiveness reported by different groups are sometimes contradictory, as in the cases of baclofen (119,167) and diazepam (106). In addition, most of these drugs can cause various forms of neurotoxicity, and recent evidence suggests benzodiazepines may antagonize opioid analgesia (186). Although other medications may improve OIN symptoms, they do not address the underlying cause.

Prevention of OIN

Prevention and early recognition and treatment of OIN can lead to better quality of life for patients with advanced cancer. Strategies have been developed to ensure good pain control in cancer patients and at the same time to minimize the risk of OIN. Prevention is best achieved by individual assessment of risk factors in each patient and by prevention of opioid dose escalation. The main risk factors for OIN are summarized in Table 9.3. These factors should be identified and if possible managed rapidly for the prevention of OIN.

Prevention of dose escalation
Table 9.5 summarizes the main risk factors for opioid dose escalation in cancer patients. Some of them, such as neuropathic pain, tolerance, and incidental pain, are inde-

Table 9.5. *Risk factors for opioid dose escalation in cancer patients*

Neuropathic pain
Incidental pain
Tolerance
Somatization
Substance abuse

pendent predictors of poor pain control. In the following paragraphs, the two most frequently unrecognized reasons for dose escalation, psychological distress, and somatization and substance abuse, are addressed.

Psychological distress and somatization Patients with advanced cancer have a variety of ways of coping with their diagnosis and disease. Often, the perception of pain or other symptoms may be accentuated by the emotional state or by psychological distress in the patient. This condition of psychological distress, also known as somatization, can lead to excessive somatic complaints, which may have no identifiable etiologic or organic basis or may be grossly in excess of expectations based on clinical findings (187–189). Depression is closely related to somatization (190,191) and may be the most common cause. Somatization has been associated with neurological (192) and cardiovascular diseases (193), but few studies document an association in cancer patients (194–196). In one series, 28% of cancer patients referred for psychiatric evaluation were found to have evidence of somatization (197). The psychiatric diagnoses of these patients included depression, anxiety, and atypical somatiform disorder. Because perception of cancer pain is affected by multiple factors including psychosocial and emotional stressors (198,199), patients who somatize will have a tendency to express pain intensity as higher and derive little benefit (but often toxicity) from pharmacologic treatment of their pain. In addition to a history of affective disorder, previous somatization associated with stressors (e.g., back pain, headache) and the presence of high intensity for multiple symptoms simultaneously are all signs that are suggestive of somatization. Because of the absence of a "gold standard," the diagnosis of somatization is made based on a number of repeated observations and after extensive discussion with the patient and family.

Psychological distress (somatization) has been identified as an independent risk factor for poor pain management in studies evaluating a staging system for cancer pain (28,200–202). These patients are often seen as "suffering" by primary care physicians as well as specialists, who in escalating opioid analgesics often precipitate OIN (153,203,204). In such situations, unidimensional pain assessment ("Pain is what the patient calls pain and has the intensity the patient reports") is not useful, and multidimensional assessment and treatment strategies must be used (153,203,204). Acknowledgment of the existing underlying pain syndrome and physician support are important but psychological and spiritual counseling can alleviate some of the emotional suffering with a subsequent decrease in pain perception and opioid requirements (204,205). Obtaining a detailed psychosocial history from the patient, family members, and/or primary physician can help in identifying maladaptive coping mechanisms and, with careful multidimensional pain assessment, may allow for pain analgesia without OIN (204,206).

Substance abuse In a similar vein, cancer patients who have a past or active history of substance abuse present a special pain control problem. Their history of abuse reflects maladaptive coping strategies, which invariably leads to excessive expression of symptoms. This often is misinterpreted as nociception, leading to an escalation of opioids and OIN (153,203,207). Recent studies have found that approximately 4%–9% of North Americans have some form of alcohol dependence (208,209). The incidence of addictive disorders in the United States (and likely similar in developed countries) ranges from 3%–16% (210,211). It has been well documented that persons with one addictive disorder are at increased risk for other forms of substance abuse (210,212). The rates of substance abuse may be higher in medical settings, especially as abusive behavior often leads to medical diseases (213). The rates of addiction in cancer patients may also be higher, as alcohol use and abuse can play an etiologic role in several types of malignant disease (e.g., head and neck, esophageal, hepatocellular carcinoma). Patients with newly diagnosed lung cancer were questioned with respect to psychiatric symptomatology and substance abuse, 46% of whom had abused alcohol sometime in their lives, and 13% were currently abusing alcohol (214). In 200 patients admitted to a tertiary palliative care program, the prevalence of alcoholism was 27% (215). Opioid abuse and misuse are more likely to be seen in cancer patients with a history of drug or alcohol abuse (216,217), and substance abuse has been identified as an independent risk factor for poor pain management (28,200–202).

Screening for substance abuse is an important first step in the prevention of escalation of opioids and subsequent development of OIN. The CAGE questionnaire (218) has a sensitivity >85% to diagnose alcohol dependence (208)

and can be done as part of the routine history taking. A positive response to two of the four questions (cut down, annoyed by criticism, experiencing guilt, eye-opener drink in the morning) is indicative of alcohol dependence and may also indicate abuse of other substances (209). Patients should be questioned about their lifelong alcohol intake, as addictive behavior may indicate maladaptive coping strategies that are seldom if ever changed throughout life. Also, it is important to inquire about the desired effects of any substances abused, which can bring out valuable information about co-morbid psychiatric or behavioral problems (e.g., anxiety, somatization, depression, personality disorders) or unrelieved symptoms that the patient may find particularly noxious (217).

As indicated previously, multidimensional assessment and treatment strategies can be effective in identifying the maladaptive coping ("coping chemically") of these patients. A retrospective study found that after the institution of routine alcohol screening (using the CAGE questionnaire) and multidimensional assessment, patients could be identified as alcoholics and their pain treatments adapted accordingly. Alcoholic patients had higher doses of opioids on admission, but maximal dose of opioid and pain intensity during inpatient treatment was not significantly different from non-alcoholics (215). This is in contrast with earlier studies, which found that alcoholics not treated with a multidisciplinary strategy had significantly worse prognosis and pain management problems (216,218). Such treatment strategies can alert the physician to the potential risk of rapid escalation of opioids in substance abusers and help in the prevention of OIN (153,203,204).

Overall management
Cancer patients receiving opioids for pain likely will always be at some risk for the development of OIN. Prevention and early recognition and treatment of OIN will reduce morbidity in these patients. Strategies for prevention of OIN are summarized in Table 9.6. Physicians treating these patients should become familiar with the components of the syndrome to ensure early diagnosis. When faced with a patient exhibiting any or all components of OIN, the physician should ask why the individual is toxic. Is it the presence of one or several risk factors, multiple drug treatments, opioid dose escalation, or are the patient's toxic symptoms due to another reversible cause such as infection or metabolic abnormalities? Use of a multidisciplinary assessment and treatment approach will motivate the health care team to have a high index of suspicion and ensure that the same standard of care is provided to all patients. Should symptoms of OIN develop,

Table 9.6. *Prevention of further episodes of opioid-induced neurotoxicity (OIN)*

Identify and manage risk factors for OIN (Tables 9.3, 9.4)
Identify reasons for opioid dose escalation (Table 9.5)
Carefully monitor for early signs of OIN (included in Table 9.1)
Educate patient and family about risk factors and early signs of OIN
Educate primary care physician about risk factors and early signs of OIN

rapid identification can lead to swift treatment and reversal of toxicity. Once a patient has had an episode of OIN, the risk for subsequent episodes rises. Increased vigilance of this subgroup of patients should be undertaken, and should toxicity recur, treatment using opioid rotation, hydration, and so on should commence immediately. The authors have found that patients with several risk factors for OIN may require multiple opioid rotations, and the intervals between rotations decrease as the patient approaches death. Further preventative strategies, such as psychological counseling for addiction or somatization, should be instituted early, as these advanced cancer patients have short life spans and toxicity has major implications for the quality of their remaining life.

Immune system effects

There is substantial evidence to support the theory that opioids have an effect on host defense and are associated with the pathogenesis of infection among intravenous drug users (220). Morphine in vivo has been shown to suppress a variety of immune responses that involve the major cell types in the immune system including natural killer cells, T cells, B cells, macrophages, and polymorphonuclear leukocytes (PMNs) (221). There is evidence that some of this effect is by direct depression of macrophage and PMN function, but it also appears that there may be an indirect effect on the immune system, possibly through an in vivo neural-immune circuit through which morphine acts to depress the function of all cells in the immune system (221).

The importance of these findings for cancer patients, especially those with advanced cancer and short life expectancy receiving opioid analgesia, is as yet unknown. It is possible that some of the immune changes ascribed to chemotherapy and advanced cancer may be in part opioid related in some patients. At present opioid use is not contraindicated in immunosuppressed patients. Knowing whether individual opioids have different effects in these patient populations might help identify better therapies for various groups of patients.

Endocrine effects of opioids

Opioid administration is known to be associated with endocrine abnormalities. Opioid administration has been shown to inhibit adrenocorticotropic hormone (ACTH) (222) and cortisol levels, and naloxone stimulates the release of ACTH (223–225). Opioids have also been shown to inhibit vasopressin and oxytocin release at posterior pituitary level, to elevate insulin and glucagon, and inhibit somatostatin (226).

A study of 73 patients receiving long-term intrathecal opioid administration for intractable nonmalignant pain showed hypogonadotrophic hypogonadism in a large majority of patients. In addition, 15% were shown to have developed hypocorticism, and approximately the same percentage had developed growth hormone deficiency. A control group of patients with a comparable pain syndrome but not treated with opioids was used (227).

Further studies are needed to look at the effect of opioid use on endocrine function in cancer patients as the possibility exists that some of the symptoms we now ascribe to cancer may be at least in part related to endocrine dysfunction secondary to opioid administration. Most endocrine abnormalities are relatively easy to diagnose with blood tests. If some of the symptoms we currently associate with the presence of cancer such as profound fatigue, reduced libido, and loss of muscle mass are related to endocrine changes, hormonal supplementation may offer treatment options in patients with these problems.

Conclusion

Opioid side effects are relatively frequent but minor in severity. When appropriately diagnosed and managed, these side effects are rarely a cause for drug discontinuation. Increased opioid use has resulted in more frequent observation of opioid induced toxicity. The main challenges are to make an early and appropriate diagnosis in patients with multiple other possible causes for neuropsychiatric changes. This syndrome can be effectively controlled with simple measures. The potentially important effects of opioids on the immune and endocrine systems in cancer patients require further research.

References

1. Portenoy RK. Cancer pain. Epidemiology and syndromes. Cancer 63(11 Suppl):2298–307, 1989.
2. World Health Organization. Cancer pain relief and palliative care. Technical Series 804. Geneva: World Health Organization, 1990.

3. Cleeland CS, Gronin R, Hatfield AK, et al. Pain and its treatment in outpatients with metastatic cancer. N Engl J Med 330:592–6, 1994.

4. Bruera E, Brenneis C, Michaud M, MacDonald RN. Influence of the pain and symptom control team (PSCT) on the patterns of treatment of pain and other symptoms in a cancer center. J Pain Symptom Manage 4(3):112–16, 1989.

5. Von Roenn JH, Cleeland CS, Gonin R, et al. Physician attitudes and practice in cancer pain management. A survey from the Eastern Cooperative Oncology Group. Ann Intern Med 119(2):121–26, 1993.

6. Cherny NJ, Ho MN, Bookbinder M, et al. Cancer pain: knowledge and attitudes of physicians at a cancer center [abstract]. Proc Am Soc Clin Oncol 12:434, 1994.

7. World Health Organization. Cancer pain relief, 2nd ed. Geneva: World Health Organization, 1996.

8. Zenz M, Willweber-Strumpf A. Opiophobia and cancer pain in Europe. Lancet 341:1075–6, 1993.

9. Bruera E, Macmillan K, Hanson J, MacDonald RN. Palliative care in a cancer center: results in 1984 versus 1987. J Pain Symptom Manage 5(1):1–5, 1990.

10. Sjogren P, Banning AM, Christensen CB, Pedersen O. Continuous reaction time after single dose, long-term oral and epidural opioid administration. Eur J Anaesthesiol 11(2):95–100, 1994.

11. Bruera E, Macmillan K, Hanson J, MacDonald RN. The cognitive effects of the administration of narcotic analgesics in patients with cancer pain. Pain 39(1):13–6, 1989.

12. Vainio A, Ollila J, Matikainen E, et al. Driving ability in cancer patients receiving long-term morphine analgesia. Lancet 346(8976):667–70, 1995.

13. Banning A, Sjogren P, Kaiser F. Reaction time in cancer patients receiving peripherally-acting analgesics alone or in combination with opioids. Acta Anaesthesiol Scand 36(5):480–2, 1992.

14. Banning A, Sjogren P. Cerebral effects of long-term oral opioids in cancer patients measured by continuous reaction time. Clin J Pain 6(2):91–5, 1995.

15. Saarialho-Kere U, Mattila MJ, Paloheimo M, Seppala T. Psychomotor, respiratory and neuroendocrinological effects of buprenorphine and amitriptyline in healthy volunteers. Eur J Clin Pharmacol 33(2):139–46, 1987.

16. MacDonald FC, Gough KJ, Nicoll RA, Dow RJ. Psychomotor effects of ketorolac in comparison with buprenorphine and diclofenac. Br J Clin Pharmacol 27(4):453–9, 1989.

17. Sjogren P, Banning A. Pain, sedation and reaction time during long-term treatment of cancer patients with oral and epidural opioids. Pain 39(1):5–11, 1989.

18. Sjogren P, Banning AM, Larsen TK, et al. Postural stability during long-term treatment of cancer patients with epidural opioids. Acta Anaesthesiol Scand 34(5):410–12, 1990.

19. Gordon N. Reaction times of methadone treated ex-heroin addicts. Psychopharmacologia 16:337–44, 1976.

20. Lombardo WK, Lombardo B, Goldstein A. Cognitive functioning under moderate and low dosage methadone maintenance. Intl J Addictions 11(3):389–401, 1976.

21. Rothenberg S, Schottenfeld S, Meyer RE, et al. Performance differences between addicts and non-addicts. Psychopharmacology 52:299–307, 1977.

22. Joo S. Methadone substitution and driver ability: research findings and conclusions from a discussion of experts. J Traffic Med 22:101–3, 1994.

23. Fainsinger RL, Miller MJ, Bruera E. Morphine intoxication during acute reversible renal insufficiency. J Palliat Care 8(2):52–3, 1992.

24. Fainsinger R, Schoeller T, Boiskin M, Bruera E. Cognitive failure and coma after renal failure in a patient receiving captopril and hydromorphone. J Palliat Care 9(1):53–5, 1993.

25. Bruera E, Chadwick S, Weinlick A, MacDonald N. Delirium and severe sedation in patients with terminal cancer. Cancer Treat Rep 71(7–8):787–8, 1987.

26. Bruera E, Fainsinger RL, Schoeller T, Ripamonti C. Rapid discontinuation of hypnotics in terminal cancer patients: a prospective study. Ann Oncol 7(8):855–6, 1996.

27. Manfredi PL, Ribeiro S, Chandler SW, Payne R. Inappropriate use of naloxone in cancer patients with pain. J Pain Symptom Manage 11(2):131–4, 1996.

28. Bruera E, Schoeller T, Wenk R, et al. A prospective multicenter assessment of the Edmonton staging system for cancer pain. J Pain Symptom Manage 10(5):348–55, 1995.

29. Bruera E, Watanabe S. Psychostimulants as adjuvant analgesics. J Pain Symptom Manage 9(6):412–15, 1994.

30. Forrest WH Jr, Brown BW Jr, Brown CR, et al. Dextroamphetamine with morphine for the treatment of postoperative pain. N Engl J Med 296(13):712–15, 1977.

31. Bruera E, Brenneis C, Chadwick S, et al. Methylphenidate associated with narcotics for the treatment of cancer pain. Cancer Treat Rep 71(1):67–70, 1987.

32. Bruera E, Fainsinger R, MacEachern T, Hanson J. The use of methylphenidate in patients with incident cancer pain receiving regular opiates. A preliminary report. Pain 50(1):75–7, 1992.

33. Wilwerding MB, Loprinzi CL, Mailliard JA, et al. A randomized, crossover evaluation of methylphenidate in cancer patients receiving strong narcotics. Support Care Cancer 3(2):135–8, 1995.

34. Fernandez F, Adams F, Levy JK, et al. Cognitive impairment due to AIDS-related complex and its response to psychostimulants. Psychosomatics 29(1):38–46, 1988.

35. Wilens TE, Biederman J. The stimulants. Psychiatr Clin North Am 15(1):191–222, 1992.

36. Slatkin NE, Rhiner M, Maluso Bolton T. Donepezil in the treatment of opioid-induced sedation: report of six cases. J Pain Symptom Manage 21(5):425–38, 2001.

37. Allan SG. Nausea and vomiting. In: Doyle D, Hanks GW, MacDonald N, eds. Oxford: Oxford Medical Press, 1993:282–90.

38. Clarke RS. Nausea and vomiting. Br J Anaesth 56(1):19–27, 1984.

39. Hagen NA, Foley KM, Cerbone DJ, et al. Chronic nausea and morphine-6-glucuronide. J Pain Symptom Manage 6(3):125–8, 1991.

40. Bruera E, Seifert L, Watanabe S, et al. Chronic nausea in advanced cancer patients: a retrospective assessment of a

metoclopramide-based antiemetic regimen [see comments].
J Pain Symptom Manage 11(3):147–53, 1996.

41. Bruera ED, MacEachern TJ, Spachynski KA, et al.
Comparison of the efficacy, safety, and pharmacokinetics of
controlled release and immediate release metoclopramide
for the management of chronic nausea in patients with
advanced cancer [published erratum appears in Cancer
75(7):1733, 1995]. Cancer 74(12):3204–11, 1994.

42. Bruera E, Belzile M, Neumann C, et al. A double-blind,
crossover study of controlled-release metoclopramide and
placebo for the chronic nausea and dyspepsia of advanced
cancer. J Pain Symptom Manage 19(6):427–35, 2000.

43. Wamsley JK, Lewis MS, Young WS III, Kuhar MJ.
Autoradiographic localization of muscarinic cholinergic
receptors in rat brainstem. J Neurosci 1(2):176–91, 1981.

44. Palacios JM, Wamsley JK, Kuhar MJ. The distribution of
histamine H1-receptors in the rat brain: an autoradiographic study. Neuroscience 6(1):15–37, 1981.

45. Bruera ED, Roca E, Cedaro L, et al. Improved control of
chemotherapy-induced emesis by the addition of dexamethasone to metoclopramide in patients resistant to metoclopramide. Cancer Treat Rep 67(4):381–3, 1983.

46. Twycross RG, Lack SA. Control of alimentary symptoms in
far advanced cancer. London: Churchill Livingstone,
1986:166–207.

47. Hunt R, Fazekas B, Thorne D, Brooksbank M. A comparison of subcutaneous morphine and fentanyl in hospice cancer patients. J Pain Symptom Manage 18(2):111–19, 1999.

48. Mancini I, Hanson J, Neumann C, Bruera E. Opioid type
and other clinical predictors of laxative dose in advanced
cancer patients. a retrospective study. J Palliat Med
3(1):49–56, 2000.

49. De Luca A, Coupar IM. Insights into opioid action in the
intestinal tract. Pharmacol Ther 69(2):103–15, 1996.

50. Portenoy RK. Constipation in the cancer patient: causes
and management. Med Clin North Am 71(2):303–11, 1987.

51. Manara L, Bianchetti A. The central and peripheral influences of opioids on gastrointestinal propulsion. Annu Rev
Pharmacol Toxicol 25:249–73, 1985.

52. Brown NJ, Coupar IM, Rumsey RD. The effect of acute and
chronic administration of morphine and morphine withdrawal
on intestinal transit time in the rat. J Pharm Pharmacol
40(12):844–8, 1988.

53. Bruera E, Suarez-Almazor M, Velasco A, et al. The assessment of constipation in terminal cancer patients admitted to
a palliative care unit: a retrospective review. J Pain
Symptom Manage 9(8):515–19, 1994.

54. Starreveld JS, Pols MA, Van Wijk HJ, et al. The plain
abdominal radiograph in the assessment of constipation.
Gastroenterology 28(7):335–8, 1990.

55. Smith RG, Lewis S. The relationship between digital rectal
examination and abdominal radiographs in elderly patients.
Age Ageing 19(2):142–3, 1990.

56. McKay LF, Smith RG, Eastwood MA, et al. An investigation of colonic function in the elderly. Age Ageing
12(2):105–10.

57. Hardcastle JD, Wilkins JL. The action of sennosides and
related compounds on human colon and rectum. Gut
11(12):1038–42, 1970.

58. Mancini IL, Bruera E. Constipation in advanced cancer
patients. Support Care Cancer 6(356):364, 1998.

59. Bruera E, Brenneis C, Michaud M, MacDonald N.
Continuous SC infusion of metoclopramide for treatment of
narcotic bowel syndrome [letter]. Cancer Treat Rep
71(11):1121–2, 1987.

60. Kreek MJ, Schaefer RA, Hahn EF, Fishman J. Naloxone, a
specific opioid antagonist, reverses chronic idiopathic constipation. Lancet 1(8319):261–2, 1983.

61. Culpepper-Morgan JA, Inturrisi CE, Portenoy RK, et al.
Treatment of opioid-induced constipation with oral naloxone: a pilot study. Clin Pharmacol Ther 52(1):90–5, 1992.

62. Sykes NP. An investigation of the ability of oral naloxone to
correct opioid-related constipation in patients with
advanced cancer. Palliat Med 10(2):135–44, 1996.

63. Meissner W, Schmidt U, Hartmann M, et al. Oral naloxone
reverses opioid-associated constipation. Pain 84(1):105–9,
2000.

64. Yuan CS, Foss JF, O'Connor M, et al. Methylnaltrexone for
reversal of constipation due to chronic methadone use: a
randomized controlled trial. JAMA 283(3):367–72, 2000.

65. Yuan CS, Foss JF. Oral methylnaltrexone for opioid-
induced constipation [letter]. JAMA 284(11):1383–4, 2000.

66. Wenk R, Bertolino M, Ochoa J, et al. Laxative effects of
fresh baker's yeast [letter]. J Pain Symptom Manage
19(3):163–4, 2000.

67. Joishy SK, Walsh D. The opioid-sparing effects of intravenous ketorolac as an adjuvant analgesic in cancer pain:
application in bone metastases and the opioid bowel syndrome. J Pain Symptom Manage 16(5):334–9, 1998.

68. Frantzides CT, Lianos EA, Wittmann D, et al.
Prostaglandins and modulation of small bowel myoelectric
activity. Am J Physiol 262(3 Pt 1):G488–G497, 1992.

69. Thor P, Konturek JW, Konturek SJ, Anderson JH. Role of
prostaglandins in control of intestinal motility. Am J
Physiol 248(3 Pt 1):G353–G359, 1985.

70. Florez J, McCarthy LE, Borison HL. A comparative study
in the cat of the respiratory effects of morphine injected
intravenously and into the cerebrospinal fluid. J Pharmacol
Exp Ther 163(2):448–55, 1968.

71. Walsh TD. Opiates and respiratory function in advanced
cancer. Recent Results Cancer Res 89:115–17, 1984.

72. Osborne RJ, Joel SP, Slevin ML. Morphine intoxication in
renal failure: the role of morphine-6-glucuronide. Br Med J
(Clin Res Ed) 292(6535):1548–9, 1986.

73. Hunt G, Bruera E. Respiratory depression in a patient
receiving oral methadone for cancer pain. J Pain Symptom
Manage 10(5):401–4, 1995.

74. Oneschuk D, Bruera E. Respiratory depression during
methadone rotation in a patient with advanced cancer. J
Palliat Care 16(2):50–4, 2000.

75. Hanks GW, Twycross RG, Lloyd JW. Unexpected complication of successful nerve block. Morphine induced respi-

ratory depression precipitated by removal of severe pain. Anaesthesia 36(1):37–9, 1981.

76. Wells CJ, Lipton S, Lahuerta J. Respiratory depression after percutaneous cervical anterolateral cordotomy in patients on slow-release oral morphine [letter]. Lancet 1(8379):739, 1984.

77. Cousins MJ, Mather LE. Intrathecal and epidural administration of opioids. Anesthesiology 61(3):276–310, 1984.

78. Ballantyne JC, Loach AB, Carr DB. Itching after epidural and spinal opiates. Pain 33(2):149–60, 1988.

79. Horta ML, Ramos L, Goncalves ZR. The inhibition of epidural morphine-induced pruritus by epidural droperidol. Anesth Analg 90(3):638–41, 2000.

80. Gunter JB, McAuliffe J, Gregg T, et al. Continuous epidural butorphanol relieves pruritus associated with epidural morphine infusions in children. Paediatr Anaesth 10(2):167–72, 2000.

81. Choi JH, Lee J, Choi JH, Bishop MJ. Epidural naloxone reduces pruritus and nausea without affecting analgesia by epidural morphine in bupivacaine. Can J Anaesth 47(1):33–7, 2000.

82. Yeh HM, Chen LK, Lin CJ, et al. Prophylactic intravenous ondansetron reduces the incidence of intrathecal morphine-induced pruritus in patients undergoing cesarean delivery. Anesth Analg 91(1):172–5, 2000.

83. Saiah M, Borgeat A, Wilder-Smith OH, et al. Epidural-morphine-induced pruritus. propofol versus naloxone. Anesth Analg 78(6):1110–13, 1994.

84. Dunteman E, Karanikolas M, Filos KS. Transnasal butorphanol for the treatment of opioid-induced pruritus unresponsive to antihistamines. J Pain Symptom Manage 12(4):255–60, 1996.

85. Katcher J, Walsh D. Opioid-induced itching: morphine sulfate and hydromorphone hydrochloride. J Pain Symptom Manage 17(1):70–2, 1999.

86. Chaplan SR, Duncan SR, Brodsky JB, Brose WG. Morphine and hydromorphone epidural analgesia. A prospective, randomized comparison. Anesthesiology 77(6):1090–4, 1992.

87. Cooper A, White D, Matthay R. Drug-induced pulmonary disease. Am Rev Respir Dis 133:488–505, 1986.

88. Taff RH. Pulmonary edema following naloxone administration in a patient without heart disease. Anesthesiology 59(6):576–7, 1983.

89. Bruera E, Miller MJ. Non-cardiogenic pulmonary edema after narcotic treatment for cancer pain [see comments]. Pain 39(3):297–300, 1989.

90. Bruera E, Brenneis C, Michaud M, et al. Use of the subcutaneous route for the administration of narcotics in patients with cancer pain. Cancer 62(2):407–11, 1988.

91. Foley K. The treatment of cancer pain. N Engl J Med 313(84):93, 1985.

92. Bruera E, Pereira J. Acute neuropsychiatric findings in a patient receiving fentanyl for cancer pain. Pain 69(1–2):199–201, 1997.

93. Bruera E, Miller L, McCallion J, et al. Cognitive failure in patients with terminal cancer. a prospective study. J Pain Symptom Manage 7(4):192–5, 1992.

94. Stiefel F, Fainsinger R, Bruera E. Acute confusional states in patients with advanced cancer. J Pain Symptom Manage 7(2):94–8, 1992.

95. Fainsinger R, Young C. Cognitive failure in a terminally ill patient. J Pain Symptom Manage 6(8):492–4, 1991.

96. Leipzig RM, Goodman H, Gray G, et al. Reversible, narcotic-associated mental status impairment in patients with metastatic cancer. Pharmacology 35(1):47–54, 1987.

97. Breitbart W, Bruera E, Chochinov H, Lynch M. Neuropsychiatric syndromes and psychological symptoms in patients with advanced cancer. J Pain Symptom Manage 10(2):131–41, 1995.

98. Zacny JP, Lichtor JL, Thapar P, et al. Comparing the subjective, psychomotor and physiological effects of intravenous butorphanol and morphine in healthy volunteers. J Pharmacol Exp Ther 270(2):579–88, 1994.

99. Zacny JP, Lichtor JL, Flemming D, et al. A dose-response analysis of the subjective, psychomotor and physiological effects of intravenous morphine in healthy volunteers. J Pharmacol Exp Ther 268(1):1–9, 1994.

100. Clemons M, Regnard C, Appleton T. Alertness, cognition and morphine in patients with advanced cancer. Cancer Treat Rev 22(6):451–68, 1996.

101. Sjogren P, Olsen AK, Thomsen AB, Dalberg J. Neuropsychological performance in cancer patients: the role of oral opioids, pain and performance status. Pain 86(3):237–45, 2000.

102. Galski T, Williams JB, Ehle HT. Effects of opioids on driving ability. J Pain Symptom Manage 19(3):200–8, 2000.

103. Crawford RD, Baskoff JD. Fentanyl-associated delirium in man. Anesthesiology 53(2):168–9, 1980.

104. Bruera E, Schoeller T, Montejo G. Organic hallucinosis in patients receiving high doses of opiates for cancer pain. Pain 48(3):397–9, 1992.

105. Poyhia R, Vainio A, Kalso E. A review of oxycodone's clinical pharmacokinetics and pharmacodynamics. J Pain Symptom Manage 8(2):63–7, 1993.

106. De Conno F, Caraceni A, Martini C, et al. Hyperalgesia and myoclonus with intrathecal infusion of high-dose morphine. Pain 47(3):337–9, 1991.

107. Paix A, Coleman A, Lees J, et al. Subcutaneous fentanyl and sufentanil infusion substitution for morphine intolerance in cancer pain management. Pain 63(2):263–9, 1995.

108. Lawlor P, Gagnon B, Mancini IL, et al. Phenomenology of delirium and its subtypes in advanced cancer patients: a prospective study [abstract]. J Palliat Care 14(3):106, 1998.

109. Lowe GR. The phenomenology of hallucinations as an aid to differential diagnosis. Br J Psychiatry 123(577):621–33, 1973.

110. Stiefel F, Holland J. Delirium in cancer patients. Int Psychogeriatr 3(2):333–6, 1991.

111. Lawlor PG, Gagnon B, Mancini IL, et al. Occurrence, causes, and outcome of delirium in patients with advanced cancer: a prospective study. Arch Intern Med 160(6):786–94, 2000.

112. Massie MJ, Holland J, Glass E. Delirium in terminally ill cancer patients. Am J Psychiatry 140(8):1048–50, 1983.

113. Lipowski ZJ. Update on delirium. Psychiatr Clin North Am 15(2):335–46, 1992.

114. Bruera E, Miller MJ, Macmillan K, Kuehn N. Neuropsychological effects of methylphenidate in patients

receiving a continuous infusion of narcotics for cancer pain. Pain 48(2):163–6, 1992.

115. Nunez Olarthe JM. Opioid-induced myoclonus. Eur J Palliat Care 2:146–50, 1996.

116. Marsden CD. The nosology and pathophysiology of myoclonus. In: Marsden CD, Fahn S, eds. Movement disorders. London: Butterworth, 1982:196–248.

117. Sagratella S. Enkephalinase inhibition and hippocampal excitatory effects of exogenous and endogenous opioids. Prog Neuropsychopharmacol Biol Psychiatry 18(6):965–78, 1994.

118. Shohami E, Evron S. Intrathecal morphine induces myoclonic seizures in the rat. Acta Pharmacol Toxicol (Copenh) 56(1):50–4, 1985.

119. Sjogren P, Dragsted L, Christensen CB. Myoclonic spasms during treatment with high doses of intravenous morphine in renal failure. Acta Anaesthesiol Scand 37(8):780–2, 1993.

120. Potter JM, Reid DB, Shaw RJ, et al. Myoclonus associated with treatment with high doses of morphine: the role of supplemental drugs [see comments]. BMJ 299(6692):150–3, 1989.

121. Sjogren P, Jonsson T, Jensen NH, et al. Hyperalgesia and myoclonus in terminal cancer patients treated with continuous intravenous morphine. Pain 55(1):93–7, 1993.

122. MacDonald N, Der L, Allan S, Champion P. Opioid hyperexcitability: the application of alternate opioid therapy. Pain 53(3):353–5, 1993.

123. Babul N, Darke AC. Putative role of hydromorphone metabolites in myoclonus [letter] [published erratum appears in Pain 52(1):123, 1993] [comment]. Pain 51(2):260–1, 1992.

124. Kaiko RF, Foley KM, Grabinski PY, et al. Central nervous system excitatory effects of meperidine in cancer patients. Ann Neurol 13(2):180–5, 1983.

125. Hochman MS. Meperidine-associated myoclonus and seizures in long-term hemodialysis patients [letter]. Ann Neurol 14(5):593, 1983.

126. Danziger LH, Martin SJ, Blum RA. Central nervous system toxicity associated with meperidine use in hepatic disease. Pharmacotherapy 14(2):235–8, 1994.

127. Rao TL, Mummaneni N, El Etr AA. Convulsions: an unusual response to intravenous fentanyl administration. Anesth Analg 61(12):1020–1, 1982.

128. Benthuysen JL, Smith NT, Sanford TJ, et al. Physiology of alfentanil-induced rigidity. Anesthesiology 64(4):440–6, 1986.

129. Bowdle TA, Rooke GA. Postoperative myoclonus and rigidity after anesthesia with opioids. Anesth Analg 78(4):783–6, 1994.

130. Cartwright PD, Hesse C, Jackson AO. Myoclonic spasms following intrathecal diamorphine. J Pain Symptom Manage 8(7):492–5, 1993.

131. Szeto HH, Inturrisi CE, Houde R, et al. Accumulation of normeperidine, an active metabolite of meperidine, in patients with renal failure of cancer. Ann Intern Med 86(6):738–41, 1977.

132. Labella FS, Pinsky C, Havlicek V. Morphine derivatives with diminished opiate receptor potency show enhanced central excitatory activity. Brain Res 174(2):263–71, 1979.

133. Hagen N, Thirlwell MP, Dhaliwal HS, et al. Steady-state pharmacokinetics of hydromorphone and hydromorphone-3-

glucuronide in cancer patients after immediate and controlled-release hydromorphone. J Clin Pharmacol 35(1):37–44, 1995.

134. Babul N, Darke AC, Hagen N. Hydromorphone metabolite accumulation in renal failure [letter]. J Pain Symptom Manage 10(3):184–6, 1995.

135. International Association for the Study of Pain. Classification of chronic pain. Descriptions of chronic pain syndromes and definitions of pain terms. Pain 3:S1–226, 1986.

136. Sjogren P, Jensen NH, Jensen TS. Disappearance of morphine-induced hyperalgesia after discontinuing or substituting morphine with other opioid agonists. Pain 59(2):313–6, 1994.

137. Stillman MJ, Moulin DE, Foley K. Paradoxical pain following high-dose spinal morphine. Pain 4:S389, 1987.

138. Yaksh TL, Harty GJ. Pharmacology of the allodynia in rats evoked by high dose intrathecal morphine. J Pharmacol Exp Ther 244(2):501–7, 1988.

139. Yaksh TL, Harty GJ, Onofrio BM. High dose of spinal morphine produce a nonopiate receptor-mediated hyperesthesia: clinical and theoretic implications. Anesthesiology 64(5):590–7, 1986.

140. Folstein MF, Folstein SE, McHugh PR. "Mini-mental state." A practical method for grading the cognitive state of patients for the clinician. J Psychiatr Res 12(3):189–98, 1975.

141. Breitbart W, Rosenfeld B, Roth A, et al. The Memorial Delirium Assessment Scale. J Pain Symptom Manage 13(3):128–37, 1997.

142. Smith MT, Watt JA, Cramond T. Morphine-3-glucuronide—a potent antagonist of morphine analgesia. Life Sci 47(6):579–85, 1990.

143. Glare PA, Walsh TD, Pippenger CE. Normorphine, a neurotoxic metabolite? [letter]. Lancet 335(8691):725–6, 1990.

144. Sjogren P, Thunedborg LP, Christrup L, et al. Is development of hyperalgesia, allodynia and myoclonus related to morphine metabolism during long-term administration? Six case histories. Acta Anaesthesiol Scand 42(9):1070–5, 1998.

145. Mao J, Price DD, Mayer DJ. Thermal hyperalgesia in association with the development of morphine tolerance in rats: roles of excitatory amino acid receptors and protein kinase C. J Neurosci 14(4):2301–12, 1994.

146. Borgbjerg FM, Frigast C. Segmental effects on motor function following different intrathecal receptor agonists and antagonists in rabbits. Acta Anaesthesiol Scand 41(5):586–94, 1997.

147. Moss JH. Anileridine-induced delirium. J Pain Symptom Manage 10(4):318–20, 1995.

148. Eisendrath SJ, Goldman B, Douglas J, et al. Meperidine-induced delirium. Am J Psychiatry 144(8):1062–5, 1987.

149. Parkinson SK, Bailey SL, Little WL, Mueller JB. Myoclonic seizure activity with chronic high-dose spinal opioid administration. Anesthesiology 72(4):743–5, 1990.

150. Steinberg RB, Gilman DE, Johnson F III. Acute toxic delirium in a patient using transdermal fentanyl [see comments]. Anesth Analg 75(6):1014–16, 1992.

151. de Stoutz ND, Bruera E, Suarez-Almazor M. Opioid rotation for toxicity reduction in terminal cancer patients. J Pain Symptom Manage 10(5):378–84, 1995.

152. Maddocks I, Somogyi A, Abbott F, et al. Attenuation of morphine-induced delirium in palliative care by substitu-

tion with infusion of oxycodone. J Pain Symptom Manage 12(3):182–9, 1996.

153. Lawlor P, Walker P, Bruera E, Mitchell S. Severe opioid toxicity and somatization of psychosocial distress in a cancer patient with a background of chemical dependence. J Pain Symptom Manage 13(6):356–61, 1997.

154. Hagen N, Swanson R. Strychnine-like multifocal myoclonus and seizures in extremely high-dose opioid administration: treatment strategies [see comments]. J Pain Symptom Manage 14(1):51–8, 1997.

155. Mercadante S. Opioid rotation for cancer pain: rationale and clinical aspects. Cancer 86(9):1856–66, 1999.

156. Bruera E, Franco JJ, Maltoni M, et al. Changing pattern of agitated impaired mental status in patients with advanced cancer: association with cognitive monitoring, hydration, and opioid rotation. J Pain Symptom Manage 10(4):287–91, 1995.

157. Fainsinger R, Schoeller T, Bruera E. Methadone in the management of cancer pain: a review. Pain 52(2):137–47, 1993.

158. Bruera E, Pereira J, Watanabe S, et al. Opioid rotation in patients with cancer pain. A retrospective comparison of dose ratios between methadone, hydromorphone, and morphine. Cancer 78(4):852–7, 1996.

159. Ripamonti C, Zecca E, Bruera E. An update on the clinical use of methadone for cancer pain. Pain 70(2–3):109–15, 1997.

160. Choi DW, Viseskul V. Opioids and non-opioid enantiomers selectively attenuate N-methyl-D-aspartate neurotoxicity on cortical neurons. Eur J Pharmacol 155(1–2):27–35, 1988.

161. Krug M, Matthies R, Wagner M, Brodemann R. Non-opioid antitussives and methadone differentially influence hippocampal long-term potentiation in freely moving rats. Eur J Pharmacol 231(3):355–61, 1993.

162. Ebert B, Andersen S, Krogsgaard-Larsen P. Ketobemidone, methadone and pethidine are non-competitive N-methyl-D-aspartate (NMDA) antagonists in the rat cortex and spinal cord. Neurosci Lett 187(3):165–8, 1995.

163. Bruera E, Sloan P, Mount B, et al. A randomized, double-blind, double-dummy, crossover trial comparing the safety and efficacy of oral sustained-release hydromorphone with immediate-release hydromorphone in patients with cancer pain. Canadian Palliative Care Clinical Trials Group. J Clin Oncol 14(5):1713–17, 1996.

164. Lawlor P, Turner K, Hanson J, Bruera E. Dose ratio between morphine and hydromorphone in patients with cancer pain: a retrospective study. Pain 72(1–2):79–85, 1997.

165. Ripamonti C, De Conno F, Groff L, et al. Equianalgesic dose/ratio between methadone and other opioid agonists in cancer pain: comparison of two clinical experiences. Ann Oncol 9(1):79–83, 1998.

166. De Conno F, Groff L, Brunelli C, et al. Clinical experience with oral methadone administration in the treatment of pain in 196 advanced cancer patients. J Clin Oncol 14(10):2836–42, 1996.

167. Krames ES, Gershow J, Glassberg A, et al. Continuous infusion of spinally administered narcotics for the relief of pain due to malignant disorders. Cancer 56(3):696–702, 1985.

168. Eisele JH, Grigsby EJ, Dea G. Clonazepan treatment of myoclonic contractions associated with high-dose opioids: case report. Pain 49:231–2, 1992.

169. Fainsinger RL, Louie K, Belzile M, et al. Decreased opioid doses used on a palliative care unit. J Palliat Care 12(4):6–9, 1996.

170. Labrecque G, Vanier MC. Biological rhythms in pain and in the effects of opioid analgesics. Pharmacol Ther 68(1):129–47, 1995.

171. Frederickson RC, Burgis V, Edwards JD. Hyperalgesia induced by naloxone follows diurnal rhythm in responsivity to painful stimuli. Science 198(4318):756–8, 1977.

172. Sittl R, Kamp HD, Knoll R. Zirkadiane rhythmik des Schmerzempfindens bei tumorpatienten. Nevenheilkunde 9:22–4, 1990.

173. Wilder-Smith CH, Wilder-Smith OH. Smolensky MH, et al. (eds.) Diurnal patterns of pain in cancer patients during treatment with long-acting opioid analgesics. Proceedings of the Fifth International Conf on Biological Rhythms and Medication, Amelia Island, Florida, 1992.

174. Canier MC, Labrecque G, Lepage-Savary D, et al. (eds.) Temporal changes in the hydromorphone analgesia in cancer patients. Proceedings of the Fifth International Conf on Biological Rhythms and Medication, Amelia Island, FL, 1992.

175. Citron ML, Kalra JM, Seltzer VL, et al. Patient-controlled analgesia for cancer pain: a long-term study of inpatient and outpatient use. Cancer Invest 10(5):335–41, 1992.

176. Bruera E, Macmillan K, Kuehn N, Miller MJ. Circadian distribution of extra doses of narcotic analgesics in patients with cancer pain: a preliminary report. Pain 49(3):311–14, 1992.

177. Bruera E, Fainsinger R, Spachynski K, et al. Clinical efficacy and safety of a novel controlled-release morphine suppository and subcutaneous morphine in cancer pain: a randomized evaluation. J Clin Oncol 13(6):1520–7, 1995.

178. Fainsinger RL, MacEachern T, Miller MJ, et al. The use of hypodermoclysis for rehydration in terminally ill cancer patients. J Pain Symptom Manage 9(5):298–302, 1994.

179. Ashby M, Fleming B, Wood M, Somogyi A. Plasma morphine and glucuronide (M3G and M6G) concentrations in hospice inpatients. J Pain Symptom Manage 14(3):157–67, 1997.

180. Breitbart W, Marotta R, Platt MM, et al. A double-blind trial of haloperidol, chlorpromazine, and lorazepam in the treatment of delirium in hospitalized AIDS patients. Am J Psychiatry 153(2):231–7, 1996.

181. Settle EC Jr, Ayd FJ Jr. Haloperidol: a quarter century of experience. J Clin Psychiatry 44(12):440–8, 1983.

182. Coyle N, Breitbart W, Weaver S, Portenoy R. Delirium as a contributing factor to "crescendo" pain: three case reports. J Pain Symptom Manage 9(1):44–7, 1994.

183. Fromm GH. Baclofen as an adjuvant analgesic. J Pain Symptom Manage 9(8):500–9, 1994.

184. Luo L, Puke MJ, Wiesenfeld-Hallin Z. The effects of intrathecal morphine and clonidine on the prevention and reversal of spinal cord hyperexcitability following sciatic nerve section in the rat. Pain 58(2):245–52, 1994.

185. Waldman HJ. Centrally-acting skeletal muscle relaxants and associated drugs. J Pain Symptom Manage 9(7):434–41, 1994.

186. Gear RW, Miaskowski C, Heller PH, et al. Benzodiazepine mediated antagonism of opioid analgesia. Pain 71(1):25–9, 1997.

187. Lipowski ZJ. Somatization: the concept and its clinical application. Am J Psychiatry 145(11):1358–68, 1988.

188. Massie MJ. Somatoform disorder and cancer. In: Holland JC, Rowlands JH, eds. Handbook of psychooncology. Oxford: Oxford University Press, 1989:317–19.

189. Wickramasekera IE. Somatization. Concepts, data, and predictions from the high risk model of threat perception. J Nerv Ment Dis 183(1):15–23, 1995.

190. Katon W. Depression: relationship to somatization and chronic medical illness. J Clin Psychiatry 45(3 Pt 2):4–12, 1984.

191. Katon W, Kleinman A, Rosen G. Depression and somatization: a review. Part II. Am J Med 72(2):241–7, 1982.

192. Marsden CD. Hysteria—a neurologist's view. Psychol Med 16(2):277–88, 1986.

193. Bass C, Wade C, Hand D, Jackson G. Patients with angina with normal and near normal coronary arteries: clinical and psychosocial state 12 months after angiography. BMJ 287(6404):1505–8, 1983.

194. Fobair P, Hoppe RT, Bloom J, et al. Psychosocial problems among survivors of Hodgkin's disease. J Clin Oncol 4(5):805–14, 1986.

195. Devlen J, Maguire P, Phillips P, Crowther D. Psychological problems associated with diagnosis and treatment of lymphomas. II: prospective study. BMJ 295(6604):955–7, 1987.

196. Loge JH, Abrahamsen AF, Ekeberg O, et al. Psychological distress after cancer cure: a survey of 459 Hodgkin's disease survivors. Br J Cancer 76(6):791–6, 1997.

197. Chaturvedi SK, Hopwood P. Maguire P. Non-organic somatic symptoms in cancer. Eur J Cancer 29A(7):1006–8, 1993.

198. Cherny NI, Coyle N, Foley KM. Suffering in the advanced cancer patient: a definition and taxonomy. J Palliat Care 10(2):57–70, 1994.

199. Breitbart W. Cancer pain management guidelines: implications for psychooncology. Psychooncology 3:103–8, 1994.

200. Bruera E, Watanabe S. New developments in the assessment of pain in cancer patients. Support Care Cancer 2(5):312–18, 1994.

201. Bruera E, Macmillan K, Hanson J, MacDonald RN. The Edmonton staging system for cancer pain: preliminary report. Pain 37(2):203–9, 1989.

202. Vigano A, Watanabe S, Bruera E. Methylphenidate for the management of somatization in terminal cancer patients. J Pain Symptom Manage 10(2):167–70, 1995.

203. Watanabe S, Carmody D, Bruera E. Successful multidimensional intervention in a patient with intractable neuropathic cancer pain. J Palliat Care 13(2):52–4, 1997.

204. Robinson K, Bruera E. The management of pain in patients with advanced cancer: the importance of multidimensional assessments. J Palliat Care 11(4):51–3, 1995.

205. Dalton JA, Feuerstein M. Fear, alexithymia and cancer pain. Pain 38(2):159–70, 1989.

206. Turk DC, Sist TC, Okifuji A, et al. Adaptation to metastatic cancer pain, regional/local cancer pain and non-cancer pain: role of psychological and behavioral factors. Pain 74(2–3):247–56, 1998.

207. Chapman CR, Gavrin J. Suffering and its relationship to pain. J Palliat Care 9(2):5–13, 1993.

208. Poulin C, Webster I, Single E. Alcohol disorders in Canada as indicated by the CAGE questionnaire. Canadian Med Assoc J 157(11):1529–35, 1997.

209. O'Connor PG, Schottenfeld RS. Patients with alcohol problems. N Engl J Med 338(9):592–602, 1998.

210. Regier DA, Myers JK, Kramer M, et al. The NIMH Epidemiologic Catchment Area program. Historical context, major objectives, and study population characteristics. Arch Gen Psychiatry 41(10):934–41, 1984.

211. Savage SR. Long-term opioid therapy: assessment of consequences and risks. J Pain Symptom Manage 11(5):274–86, 1996.

212. Lehman WE, Barrett ME, Simpson DD. Alcohol use by heroin addicts 12 years after drug abuse treatment. J Stud Alcohol 51(3):233–44, 1990.

213. Moore RD, Bone LR, Geller G, et al. Prevalence, detection, and treatment of alcoholism in hospitalized patients. JAMA 261(3):403–7, 1989.

214. Ginsburg ML, Quirt C, Ginsburg AD, MacKillop WJ. Psychiatric illness and psychosocial concerns of patients with newly diagnosed lung cancer. Canadian Med Assoc J 152(5):701–8, 1995.

215. Bruera E, Moyano J, Seifert L, et al. The frequency of alcoholism among patients with pain due to terminal cancer. J Pain Symptom Manage 10(8):599–603, 1995.

216. McCorquodale S, De Faye B, Bruera E. Pain control in an alcoholic cancer patient. J Pain Symptom Manage 8(3):177–80, 1993.

217. Passik SD, Portenoy RK, Ricketts PL. Substance abuse issues in cancer patients. Part 2: Evaluation and treatment. Oncology 12(5):729–34, 1998.

218. Ewing JA. Detecting alcoholism. The CAGE questionnaire. JAMA 252(14):1905–7, 1984.

219. Bruera E, MacDonald S. Audit methods: the Edmonton Symptom Assessment System. In: Higginson Irene, ed. Clinical audit in palliative care. Oxford: Radcliffe Medical Press, 1993:61–77.

220. Risdahl JM, Khanna KV, Peterson PK, Molitor TW. Opiates and infection. J Neuroimmunol 83(1–2):4–18, 1998.

221. Eisenstein TK, Hilburger ME. Opioid modulation of immune responses: effects on phagocyte and lymphoid cell populations. J Neuroimmunol 83(1–2):36–44, 1998.

222. Grossman A, Besser GM. Opiates control ACTH through a noradrenergic mechanism. Clin Endocrinol 17(3):287–90, 1982.

223. Volavka J, Bauman J, Pevnick J, et al. Short-term hormonal effects of naloxone in man. Psychoneuroendocrinology 5(3):225–34, 1980.

224. Morley JE, Baranetsky NG, Wingert TD, et al. Endocrine effects of naloxone-induced opiate receptor blockade. J Clin Endocrinol Metab 50(2):251–7, 1980.

225. Allolio B, Winkelmann W, Hipp FX, et al. Effects of a met-enkephalin analog on adrenocorticotropin (ACTH), growth hormone, and prolactin in patients with ACTH hypersecretion. J Clin Endocrinol Metab 55(1):1–7, 1982.

226. Pfeiffer A, Herz A. Endocrine actions of opioids. Horm Metab Res 16(8):386–97, 1984.

227. Abs R, Verhelst J, Maeyaert J, et al. Endocrine consequences of long-term intrathecal administration of opioids. J Clin Endocrinol Metab 85(6):2215–22, 2000.

10 Nonopioid analgesics

BURKHARD HINZ, HANNS ULRICH ZEILHOFER, AND KAY BRUNE
Friedrich Alexander University Erlangen-Nuremberg

History of antipyretic analgesics

Fever was the cardinal symptom of disease in the hippocratic medicine. It was assumed to result from an imbalance of body fluids. Therefore, it was the aim of Hippocratic medicine to correct the balances of fluids by either bloodletting, purgation, sweating, or, above all, administering drugs that normalized body temperature. The leading compound in the 18th and 19th centuries for that purpose was quinine, which became scarce in continental Europe during and after the Napoleonic wars as a result of the continental blockade. The emerging synthetic chemistry and drug industry concentrated on producing chemical analogs of quinine and its derivative quinoline as substitutes of the natural products. Moreover, pharmaceutical chemists attempted to isolate substances with similar antipyretic activity from other plants. The results of these efforts were the three prototypes of antipyretic non-opioid analgesic drugs still in use. On the basis of the work of Piria in Italy, Kolbe synthesized salicylic acid as an antipyretic agent in 1859. In 1897, salicylic acid was acetylated by Hoffmann to form aspirin. In 1882, Knorr and Filehne in Erlangen synthesized and tested the non-acidic agent phenazone (antipyrine), which proved to be effective in the clinic. Phenazone was the first pure synthetic drug worldwide. Its introduction as an antipyretic and later as an analgesic led to the discovery of various phenazone derivatives that are still used every year in ton quantities. Almost at the same time, Cahn and Hepp in Strasbourg found that acetanilide may also reduce fever. Acetanilide was introduced as antifebrin, but was later replaced by phenacetin and finally by paracetamol (acetaminophen), which is believed to be safer.

For more than 100 years, the mode of action of these compounds was poorly understood. With the emergence of scientific medicine, many puzzling results were obtained. Experimental and clinical findings within the last 30 years have added important insights into the mode of action of antipyretic analgesics. Consequently, a coherent pharmacological explanation of their effects and major side effects may now be given. It started with the pioneering discovery by Vane, who showed that aspirin and related drugs suppress the production of prostaglandins (1,2). This simple monocausal explanation, however, could not reconcile all experimental findings (3–6). For example, salicylic acid and paracetamol cause no inhibition of prostaglandin synthesis in the inflamed tissue at pharmacologically meaningful concentrations.

Mode of action of antipyretic analgesics

Impact of biodistribution on pharmacological effects of antipyretic analgesics

After the discovery that aspirin-like drugs may exert their pharmacological action by suppressing the synthesis of prostaglandins, we wondered why aspirin and its pharmacological relatives, the (acidic) nonsteroidal anti-inflammatory drugs (NSAIDs) exerted anti-inflammatory activity and analgesic effects, but the non-acidic drugs phenazone and paracetamol were analgesic only (7). We speculated that all acidic anti-inflammatory analgesics, which are highly bound to plasma proteins and show a similar degree of acidity (pK_A values between 3.5 and 5.5), should lead to a specific drug distribution within the body of humans or animals (Fig. 10.1). High concentrations of these compounds are reached in blood, liver, spleen, and bone marrow (as a result of high protein binding and an open endothelial layer of the vasculature), but also in body compartments with acidic extracellular

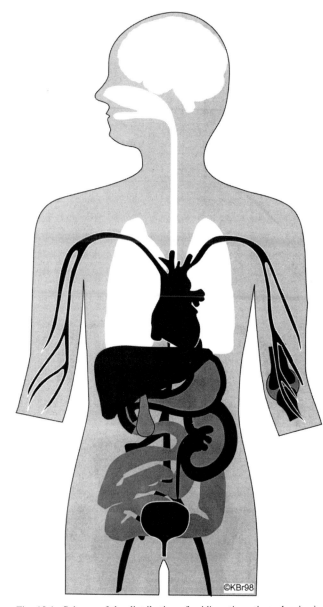

Fig. 10.1. Scheme of the distribution of acidic antipyretic analgesics in the human body (transposition of the data from animal experiments to human conditions). Dark areas indicate high concentrations of acidic antipyretic analgesics: stomach and upper wall of the gastrointestinal tract, blood, liver, bone marrow, spleen (not shown), inflamed tissue (e.g., joints) as well as the kidney (cortex > medulla). Some acidic antipyretic analgesics are excreted in part unchanged in urine and achieve high concentration in this body fluid. Others encounter entero-hepatic circulation and are found in high concentrations as conjugates in the bile.

pH values (8). The latter type of compartments includes the inflamed tissue, the wall of the upper gastrointestinal tract, and the collecting ducts of the kidneys. By contrast, paracetamol and phenazone, compounds with almost neutral pK_A values and a scarce binding to plasma proteins, should distribute homogeneously and quickly

throughout the body because of their ability to easily penetrate barriers such as the blood-brain barrier (9). It is obvious that the degree of inhibition of prostaglandin synthesis resulting from inhibition of the responsible enzymes (cyclooxygenases, Fig. 10.2) depends on the potency of the drug and its local concentration.

Impact of biodistribution on side effects of antipyretic analgesics

High drug concentrations resulting from the accumulation of NSAIDs should lead to an almost complete inhibition of cyclooxygenases in some body compartments (e.g., the inflamed tissue, blood, stomach wall, and kidney), whereas equal distribution throughout the body might lead to some inhibition throughout. These observations and contentions did explain the fact that only the acidic, antipyretic analgesics (NSAIDs) are anti-inflammatory and cause acute side effects in the gastrointestinal tract (ulcerations), the blood (inhibition of platelet aggregation), and the kidney (fluid and potassium retention), whereas the non-acidic drugs paracetamol and phenazone, as well as their derivatives, are devoid of both anti-inflammatory activity and gastric and (acute) renal toxicity. Finally, chronic inflammation of the upper respiratory tract (e.g., asthma, nasal polyps) leads to the accumulation of inflammatory prostaglandin-producing cells in the respiratory mucosa. Inhibition of cyclo-oxygenases shifts part of the metabolism of the prostaglandin precursor arachidonic acid to the production of leukotrienes, which may induce pseudoallergic reactions (i.e., aspirin asthma). Patients with allergy compose a well-defined risk group (10) and should receive antipyretic analgesics, particularly acidic NSAIDs, only under the control of a physician.

Cyclooxygenase isoforms

The enzyme cyclooxygenase (COX) catalyzes the first step of the synthesis of prostanoids by converting arachidonic acid and molecular oxygen into prostaglandin H_2, which is the common substrate for specific prostaglandin synthases. The enzyme is bifunctional, with fatty-acid COX activity (catalyzing the conversion of arachidonic acid to prostaglandin G_2) and prostaglandin hydroperoxidase activity (catalyzing the conversion of prostaglandin G_2 to prostaglandin H_2). In the early 1990s, COX was demonstrated to exist as two distinct isoforms, which are encoded by different genes, but share a 60% identity in their amino acid sequence (11–13). COX-1 is constitu-

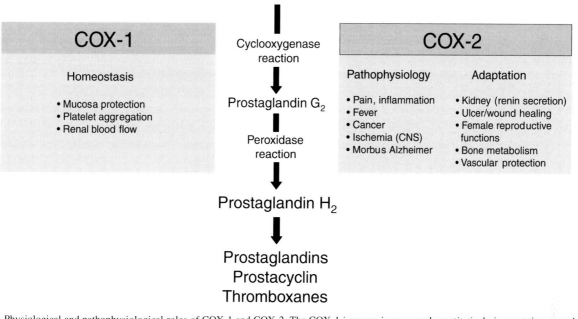

Fig. 10.2. Physiological and pathophysiological roles of COX-1 and COX-2. The COX-1 isozyme is expressed constitutively in most tissues and fulfills housekeeping functions by producing prostaglandins. The COX-2 isoform is an inducible enzyme, which becomes expressed in inflammatory cells (e.g., macrophages, synoviocytes) after exposure to endotoxin, mitogens, or proinflammatory cytokines. COX-2 has been implicated in the pathophysiology of various inflammatory and mitogenic disorders. However, in some tissues (e.g., genital tract, bone, kidney, endothelial cells), COX-2 is already significantly expressed even in the absence of inflammation and appears to fulfill various physiological functions.

tively expressed as a "housekeeping" enzyme in most tissues and mediates physiological responses (e.g., cytoprotection of the stomach, platelet function). On the other hand, COX-2, which is encoded by an immediate-early gene, can be upregulated by various proinflammatory agents, including endotoxin, cytokines, and mitogens. COX-2 expressed by cells that are involved in inflammation (e.g., macrophages, monocytes, synoviocytes) has emerged as the isoform that is primarily responsible for the synthesis of the prostanoids involved in pathological processes such as acute and chronic inflammatory states. COX-2-derived prostaglandins may cause inflammation by virtue of their chemotactic and edema-promoting actions.

The expression of the COX-2 enzyme is regulated by a broad spectrum of other mediators involved in inflammation. Glucocorticoids and anti-inflammatory cytokines (interleukin-4 [IL-4], IL-10, IL-13) have been reported to inhibit the expression of the COX-2 isoenzyme (12,14,15). Moreover, evidence is emerging to suggest that products of the COX-2 pathway may exert feedback regulatory actions on the expression of its biosynthesizing enzyme. Accordingly, a recent study using the rat model of carrageenan-induced inflammation (16) has shown that prostaglandins produced by COX-2 at sites of

inflammation may potentiate COX-2 expression via a positive feedback loop. Similar findings were reported by Hinz et al., who showed that prostaglandin E_2 may upregulate COX-2 messenger RNA expression in murine macrophages (17) and human blood monocytes (18) via an adenylyl cyclase/cyclic adenosine monophosphate-dependent mechanism.

NSAIDs interfere with the enzymatic activity of COX-2. However, all conventional NSAIDs inhibit both COX-1 and COX-2 at therapeutic doses, although they vary in their relative potencies against the two isoenzymes (19). Whereas many of the side effects of NSAIDs (e.g., gastrointestinal ulceration and bleeding, platelet dysfunctions) are due to a suppression of COX-1-derived prostanoids, inhibition of COX-2-derived prostanoids facilitates the anti-inflammatory, analgesic, and antipyretic effects of NSAIDs. Thus, the hypothesis that specific inhibition of COX-2 might have therapeutic actions similar to those of NSAIDs, but without causing the unwanted side effects, was the rationale for the development of specific inhibitors of the COX-2 enzyme as a new class of anti-inflammatory and analgesic agents with improved gastrointestinal tolerability.

Unfortunately, the simple concept of COX-2 being an exclusively proinflammatory and inducible enzyme cannot be held any longer. COX-2 has also been shown to be expressed under basal conditions in organs as the ovary, uterus, brain, spinal cord, kidney, cartilage, bone, and even gut, suggesting that this isozyme may play a more complex physiological role than formerly expected (20,21). In the rat kidney, COX-2 is expressed constitutively, particularly in the macula densa, the site of regulation of glomerular blood flow and renin release (22). Upregulation of COX-2 expression in the macula densa has been observed after salt restriction (22). Studies in humans indicate that COX-2 is present in the glomerular podocytes and in the vasculature of the kidney (23,24). COX-2 expression has also been observed in the uterine epithelium at different times during early pregnancy (25). Here, COX-2 may be involved in the implantation of the ovum, in the angiogenesis needed for the establishment of the placenta, and in the induction of labor (26). Furthermore, recent findings suggest that COX-2 may be involved in ovulation as female COX-2 knock-out mice are infertile (27). An overview about regulation, functions, and distribution of the COX isozymes is given in Fig. 10.2.

Mechansims of hyperalgesia

Recent findings shed light on the molecular basis of sensitization to painful stimuli. It has been shown that prostaglandins regulate the sensitivity of so-called polymodal nociceptors. These receptors are present in almost all tissues throughout the body. A significant portion of these nociceptors cannot be easily activated by physiological stimuli, such as (mild) pressure or (some) increase of temperature (28,29). However, after tissue trauma and the release of prostaglandins, "silent" polymodal nociceptors become responsive (30). They change their characteristics and become excitable to pressure, temperature changes, and tissue acidosis. This process results in a phenomenon called hyperalgesia—in some instances allodynia. Moreover, it has been demonstrated that prostaglandin E_2 and other inflammatory mediators facilitate the activation of tetrodotoxin (TTX)-resistant Na^+ channels in dorsal root ganglion neurons (31–33). A certain type of TTX-resistant Na^+ channels has recently been cloned (34) that appears to be selectively expressed in small and medium-sized dorsal root ganglion neurons. Compelling evidence indicates that these small dorsal root ganglion neurons are the somata which give rise to thinly and unmyelinated C and $A\delta$ nerve fibers, the latter conducting nociceptive stimuli. Modulation of these Na^+ channels involves activation of the adenylyl cyclase enzyme and increases in cyclic adenosine monophosphate (AMP), possibly leading to protein kinase A-dependent phosphorylation of the channels. On the basis

of this mechanism, prostaglandins produced during inflammatory states may significantly increase the excitability of nociceptive nerve fibers, thereby contributing to the activation of "sleeping" nociceptors. It appears reasonable that at least a part of the peripheral antinociceptive action of acidic antipyretic analgesics arises from prevention of this sensitization. Figure 10.3 (35) summarizes mechanisms underlying the activation and sensitization of the nociceptive primary afferent terminal.

Apart from sensitizing peripheral nociceptors, prostaglandins may also act in the central nervous system to produce hyperalgesia in the spinal cord dorsal horn (30). Some of these central forms of hyperalgesia seem to be reversed by inhibition of prostaglandin synthesis. The role of COX in the central nervous system is not yet entirely clear. However, it has been shown that COX-2 expression is induced in the hippocampus during epileptiform activity (36). It appears likely that COX-2 expression is increased via NMDA receptor activation and a calcium-dependent mechanism in the central nervous system. COX-2 is expressed constitutively in the spinal cord and becomes upregulated briefly after damage of (e.g., a paw [limb] trauma in the corresponding sensory segments of the spinal cord) (37). There is compelling evidence that activity-dependent increases in COX-2 mRNA demonstrated in the spinal cord might facilitate transmission of the nociceptive input (37). Furthermore, in a recent study Smith et al. (38) reported that the specific COX-2 inhibitor celecoxib suppressed inflammation-induced prostaglandin levels in cerebrospinal fluid, whereas the selective COX-1 inhibitor SC-560 was inactive in this respect. Thus, apart from generating prostaglandins in the periphery, COX-2 probably mediates a neurological component of inflammatory pain in the central nervous system. Moreover, it has been shown that the non-acidic antipyretic analgesics of the phenazone type exert their analgesic effects predominantly in the spinal cord that is easily accessible to these compounds resulting from physicochemical characteristics that allow fast passage through the blood-brain barrier (30). In agreement with this finding, we have recently shown that paracetamol reduces nociception-induced prostaglandin production in the spinal cord by an as yet unknown mechanism (39).

Several lines of evidence suggest that the analgesic action of antipyretic analgesics in the spinal cord might be not only due to reduced prostaglandin levels but also to an increase of other arachidonic acid metabolites (40). Production of 12-HPETEs appears to be a mediator of opioid-induced analgesia in the midbrain (Fig. 10.4) and these recent findings may provide a molecular basis for

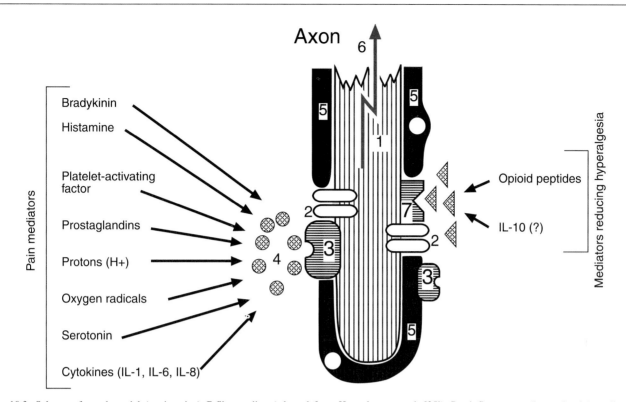

Fig. 10.3. Scheme of a polymodal (nociceptive) C-fiber ending (adapted from Heppelmann et al. [35]). Pro-inflammatory (hyperalgesic) mediators increase the sensitivity of a nociceptive C-fiber ending by either increasing the availability of receptor-coupled ion channels or causing the Schwann cells to contract. In addition, recent data suggest that cytokines may cause nociceptors to develop new μ receptors. 1 = axon, C-fiber ending; 2 = sodium channel; 3 = receptors of pain mediators (e.g., prostaglandin receptor, EP-3); 4 = pain mediators; 5 = Schwann cells covering the C-fiber ending; 6 = propagation of depolarization; 7 = receptors of antinociceptive mediators (e.g., μ receptor).

the purported clinical potentiation of opioid action by antipyretic analgesics (41).

Antipyretic analgesics for the treatment of cancer pain

Cancer pain reflects syndromes with a complex etiology involving soft tissue injury or mechanical distortion (tumor expansion in viscera, bone/fascia), lytic processes (e.g., in tumor erosion of the bone or skin), release of neurohumors that activate small afferents, and nerve injury secondary to tumor compression, activation of immune processes, or iatrogenic events such as nerve section for tumor removal (e.g., in postmastectomy pain or radiation injury). The potent inhibitory effect of antipyretic analgesics on pain secondary to bony invasion clearly reflects the important role of prostaglandins in mediating the pain secondary to the lytic processes of tumor invasion. Antipyretic analgesics are the first line of implementation according to the sequence staged scheme of World Health Organization (WHO) for cancer pain. With progressive incrementation in the pain state, their

use is supplemented by the addition of opioid drugs. By virtue of their combined analgesic and anti-inflammatory actions, acidic antipyretic analgesics have been shown to be especially effective in the treatment of moderate to severe pain resulting from bone metastases, mechanical distention of the periosteum, mechanical compression of muscles and tendons (e.g., associated with sarcoma), mechanical distention of the pleura or peritoneum (e.g., associated with intrathoracic or intra-abdominal tumors), and inflammation and stiffness of joints or muscles due to anticancer therapy (42). Non-acidic antipyretic analgesics possess a similar analgesic potency, although they lack anti-inflammatory activity. Remarkably, it is impossible to predict which antipyretic analgesic is best tolerated by a particular cancer pain patient. Moreover, neither the minimal effective analgesic dose nor the toxic dose is known for the individual patient with cancer pain and may be higher or lower than the recommended dose range of the respective antipyretic analgesic (43). However, the pharmacokinetic differences of antipyretic analgesics (Table 10.1) and their profile of adverse effects have some bearing on their optimal clinical use.

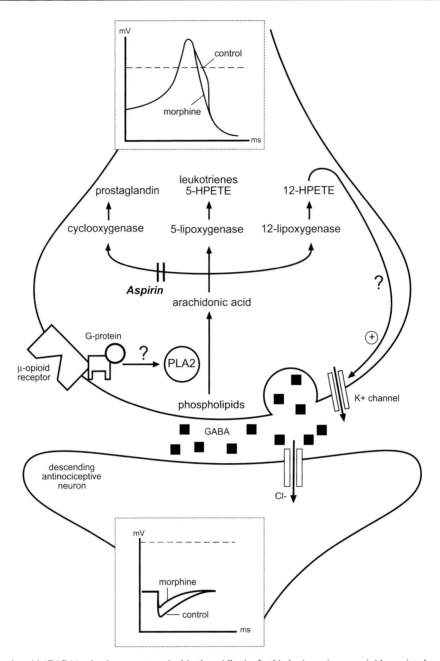

Fig. 10.4. A γ-aminobutyric acid (GABA)-releasing nerve terminal in the midbrain. In this brain region, μ-opioid agonists located at presynaptic termi-nals of inhibitory GABAergic interneurons activate phospholipase A$_2$ (PLA$_2$) via a so far unknown mechanism. This in turn increases intracellular levels of arachidonic acid, which is metabolized by COX, 5-lipoxygenase, and 12-lipoxygenase. Products of the 12-lipoxygenase pathway include 12-hydroper-oxyeicosatetraenoic acid (12-HPETE), which activates presynaptic potassium conductance and decreases the duration of the action potential. Shortening the action potential reduces GABA release into the synaptic cleft, possibly reducing its inhibitory effects on descending "antinociceptive" neurons. The presynaptic action of opioids causes the inhibitory postsynaptic potentials to become smaller. COX inhibitors, such as aspirin, may facilitate the action of opioids by shunting the arachidonic acid metabolism toward the 12-lipoxygenase pathway, thereby increasing the production of 12-HPETE (adapted from Vaughan et al. [40] and Williams et al. [41]).

Acidic antipyretic analgesics

Based on the finding that aspirin at high doses (>3 g/day) not only inhibits fever and pain but also interferes with inflammation, Winter, in the United States, developed an assay to search for drugs with a similar profile of activity (44,45). Within the past 40 years, hundreds of those com-pounds were discovered. Amazingly, all that survived the test of experimental pharmacology and clinical trials turned out to be acids with a high degree of lipophilic-hydrophilic polarity, similar pK_A values, and a high degree of plasma protein binding in vivo (for review on chemical and pharmacological properties of acidic antipyretic analgesics, see references 46,47). Suggestions for indications, including treatment of cancer pain, are listed in Table 10.1.

Apart from aspirin, all these compounds differ in potency. The dose necessary to achieve a certain degree of effect ranges from a few milligrams (e.g., lornoxicam) to about 1 g (e.g., salicylic acid). They may also differ in their pharmacokinetic characteristics, including the speed of absorption (time to peak, t_{max}), which may also depend on the galenic formulation used, the maximal plasma concentrations (c_{max}), the elimination half-life ($t_{1/2}$), and the oral bioavailability. Interestingly, all widely used drugs lack a relevant degree of so-called COX-2 selectivity. This is surprising, as they have all been selected on the basis of high anti-inflammatory potency and low gastrotoxicity

(which is believed to depend on COX-1 inhibition). The key characteristics of the most important NSAIDs are compiled in Table 10.2 (most data are from references 45, 47, and 48). This table includes aspirin, which differs in many respects from the other NSAIDs, and because of its historical and actual importance, is discussed in detail later. Apart from aspirin, the drugs can be categorized in four groups: 1) NSAIDs with low potency and short elimination half-life, 2) NSAIDs with high potency and short elimination half-life, 3) NSAIDs with intermediate potency and intermediate elimination half-life, and 4) NSAIDs with high potency and long elimination half-life.

NSAIDs with low potency and short elimination half-life

The prototype of this type of compounds is ibuprofen. Depending on its galenic formulation, fast or slow

Table 10.1. *Indications for antipyretic analgesics*

Acidic antipyretic analgesics (antiinflammatory antipyretic analgesics, NSAIDs)[a]			
Acute and chronic pain, produced by inflammation of different etiology	High dose	Middle dose	Low dose
Arthritis: chronic polyarthritis (rheumatoid arthritis), ankylosing spondilytis (Morbus Bechterew) acute gout (gout attack)	Diclofenac, indomethacin, ibuprofen, piroxicam (Phenylbutazone)[b]	Diclofenac, indomethacin, ibuprofen, piroxicam, (Phenylbutazone)[b]	No
Cancer pain (e.g., bone metastatis)	(Indomethacin[c]), diclofenac[c], ibuprofen[c], piroxicam[c]	(Indomethacin[c]), diclofenac[c], ibuprofen[c], piroxicam[c]	Aspirin[d], ibuprofen[c]
Active arthrosis (acute pain-inflammatory episodes)	No	Diclofenac, indomethacin, ibuprofen, piroxicam	Ibuprofen, ketoprofen
Myofascial pain syndromes (antipyretic analgesics are often prescribed but of limited value)	No	Diclofenac, ibuprofen, piroxicam	Ibuprofen, ketoprofen
Posttraumatic pain, swelling	No	(Indomethacin), diclofenac, ibuprofen	Aspirin[d], ibuprofen[c]
Postoperative pain, swelling	No	(Indomethacin), diclofenac, ibuprofen	Ibuprofen

Non-acidic antipyretic analgesics			
Acute pain and fever	Pyrazolinones (high dose)	Pyrazolinones (low dose)	Anilines (high dose is toxic)
Spastic pain (colics)	Yes	Yes	No
Conditions associated with high fever	Yes	Yes	No
Cancer pain	Yes	Yes	Yes
Headache, migraine	No	Yes	Yes[f]
General disturbances associated with viral infections	No	Yes[e]	Yes

[a] Dosage range of NSAIDs and example of monosubstances (but note dosage prescribed for each agent).
[b] Indicated only in gout attacks.
[c] Compare the sequence staged scheme of WHO for cancer pain.
[d] Blood coagulation and renal function must be normal.
[e] If other analgesics and antipyretics are contraindicated (e.g. gastroduodenal ulcer, blood coagulation disturbances, asthma).
[f] In particular patients.

Table 10.2. *Acidic antipyretic analgesics: Physicochemical and pharmacological data, therapeutic dosage*

Pharmakokinetic/ Chemical subclasses	pK$_A$	Binding to plasma proteins	Oral bioavailability	t$_{max}$[a]	t$^{1}/_{2}$[b]	Single dose for adults (maximal daily dose)
Low potency/short elimination half-life: Salicylates: Aspirin	3.5	50–70%	~50% dose-dependent	~15 min	~15 min	0.05–1 g[c] (~6 g)
Salicylic acid	3.0	80–95% dose-dependent	80–100%	0.5–2 hr	2.5–4.5 hr dose-dependent	0.5–1 g (6 g)
2-Arylpropionic acids: Ibuprofen	4.4	99%	100%	0.5–2 hr	2 hr	200–800 mg (2,4 g)
Anthranilic acids: Mefenamic acid	4.2	90%	70%	2–4 hr	1–2 hr	250–500 mg (1.5 g)
High potency/short elimination half-life: 2-Arylpropionic acids: Flurbiprofen	4.2	>99%	No data	1.5–3 hr	2.5–4(–8) hr	50–100 mg (200 mg)
Ketoprofen	5.3	99%	~90%	1–2 hr	2–4 hr	25–100 mg (200 mg)
Aryl-/Heteroarylacetic acids: Diclofenac	3.9	99.7%	~50% dose-dependent	1–12 hr[e] very variable	1–2 hr	25–75 mg (150 mg)
Indomethacin	4.5	99%	~100%	0.5–2 hr	2–3(–11 h)[d] very variable	(25–75 mg) (200 mg)
Oxicams: Lornoxicam	4.7	99%	~100%	0.5–2 hr	4–10 hr	4–12 mg (16 mg)
Intermediate potency/ intermediate elimination half-life: Salicylates: Diflunisal	3.3	98–99% dose-dependent	80–100%	2–3 hr	8–12 hr dose-dependent	250–500 mg (1 g)
2-Arylpropionic acids: Naproxen	4.2	99%	90–100%	2–4 hr	12–15 hr[d]	250–500 mg (1.25 g)
Arylacetic acids: 6-Methoxy-2-naphthylacetic acid (active metabolite of nabumetone)	4.2	99%	20–50%	3–6 hr	20–24 hr	0.5–1 g (1.5 g)
High potency/long elimination half-life: Oxicams: Piroxicam	5.9	99%	~100%	3–5 hr	14–160 hr[d]	20–40 mg; initial: 40 mg
Tenoxicam	5.3	99%	~100%	0.5–2 hr	25–175 hr[d]	20–40 mg; initial: 40 mg
Meloxicam	4.08	99.5%	89%	7–8 hr	20 hr[e]	7.5–15 mg

[a] Time to reach maximum plasma concentration after oral administration.
[b] Terminal half-life of elimination.
[c] Single dose for inhibition of thrombocyte aggregation: 50–100 mg; single analgesic dose: 0.5–1 g.
[d] Enterohepatic circulation.
[e] Monolithic acid-resistant tablet or similar galanic form.

absorption of ibuprofen may be achieved (50). A fast absorption of ibuprofen was observed when it was administered as a lysine salt (51). The bioavailability of ibuprofen is close to 100%, and the elimination is always fast even in patients suffering from mild or severe impairment of the liver (metabolism) or kidney function (46). Therefore, ibuprofen is used in single doses between 200 mg and 1 g. A maximum dose of 3.2 g/day (United States) or 2.4 g/day (Europe) for rheumatoid arthritis is possible. Ibuprofen (at low doses) appears particularly useful for the treatment of acute occasional inflammatory pain. At high doses it may also be used, although with less benefit, for the treatment of chronic rheumatic diseases. At high doses, this otherwise harmless compound has been shown to increase its toxicity (52). Ibuprofen is also used as the pure S-enantiomer because only this enantiomer is a (direct) COX-inhibitor. On the other hand, the R-enantiomer, composing 50% of the usual racemic mixture, is converted to the S-enantiomer in the human body (53). Therefore, it is possible but not proven that the use of the pure S-enantiomer offers any therapeutic or toxicological benefit. Other drugs of this group are salicylates and mefenamic acid. The latter does not appear to offer major advantages; on the contrary, this compound and other fenamates are rather toxic to the central nervous system at overdosage (central nervous system). The drugs of this group are particularly useful for blocking occasional mild inflammatory pain.

NSAIDs with high potency and short elimination half-life

The drugs of this group are prevailing in the therapy of rheumatic pain. The most widely used compound worldwide is diclofenac, which appears to be slightly less active on COX-1 as compared to COX-2 (54). This is taken as a reason for its relatively low incidence of gastrointestinal side effects (55). The limitations of diclofenac result from the usual galenic formulation, consisting of a monolythic acid-resistant encapsulation. This may cause retarded absorption of the active ingredient because of the retention of such monolythic formulations in the stomach for hours or even days (46). Moreover, diclofenac encounters a considerable first-pass metabolism, which causes a limited (about 50%) oral bioavailability. Consequently, a lack of therapeutic effect may require adaptation of the dosage or change of the drug. New galenic formulations (e.g., microencapsulations, salts) remedy some of these deficits. The slightly higher incidence of liver toxicity with diclofenac may result from the high degree of first-pass metabolism, but other interpretations appear feasible.

This group also contains other important drugs such as lornoxicam, flurbiprofen, and indomethacin (very potent), as well as ketoprofen and fenoprofen (less active). All of them show high oral bioavailability and good efficacy, but also a relative high risk of unwanted drug effects (55).

NSAIDs with intermediate potency and intermediate elimination half-life

The third group is intermediate in potency and speed of elimination, and contains drugs such as diflunisal and naproxen.

NSAIDs with high potency and long elimination half-life

The fourth group consists of the oxicams (meloxicam, piroxicam, and tenoxicam). These compounds owe their slow elimination to slow metabolism together with a high degree of enteropathic circulation (46,56). The long half-life (days) does not make these oxicams drugs a first choice for acute pain of (probably) short duration. Their main indication is inflammatory pain likely to persist for days (e.g., pain resulting from cancer [bone metastases] or chronic polyarthritis). The high potency and long persistence in the body may be the reason for the somewhat higher incidence of serious adverse drug effects in the gastrointestinal tract and in the kidney (55). It has been claimed that meloxicam is particularly well tolerated by the gastrointestinal tract because it inhibits predominantly the COX-2 isozyme. These results are not fully accepted. Accordingly, when tested in the human whole blood assay, the COX-2 selectivity of meloxicam is not superior to that of diclofenac (19).

Compounds of special interest

A few compounds deserve special discussion. The most popular one is aspirin. Aspirin actually comprises two active compounds: acetic acid, which is released before, during, and after absorption, and salicylic acid. Aspirin is about 100 times more potent as an inhibitor of the COX enzymes than salicylic acid, which is practically devoid of this effect at analgesic doses. The acetate released from aspirin acetylates a serin residue in the active center of COX-1 (highly effective) and COX-2 (less effective). Consequently, aspirin inactivates both COX isoforms permanently. Building on this knowledge, more bulky aspirin analogs, exclusively acetylating COX-2, are being investigated (57). With the exception of blood platelets, most cells compensate the enzyme loss as a result of acetylation by the production of new enzyme. Therefore, a single dose of aspirin blocks the platelet COX-1 and thereby thromboxane synthesis, for many days. When low doses are administered, absorbed aspirin acetylates the COX-1 isozyme of platelets passing through the capillary bed of the gastrointestinal tract, but not the COX enzyme of endothelial cells outside the gut. This is due to the rapid cleavage of aspirin leaving little if any unmetabolized aspirin after primary liver passage. These latter cells continue to release prostacyclin and maintain their antithrombotic activity. Thus, low-dose aspirin has its only indication in the prevention of thrombotic and embolic events. It may cause bleeding from existing ulcers because of its long-lasting platelet effect and topical irritation of the gastrointestinal mucosa. Aspirin may be used as a solution (effervescent) or as a (lysine) salt, allowing very fast absorption, distribution, and fast pain relief. The inevitable irritation of the gastric mucosa may be acceptable in otherwise healthy patients. It may be added that the old claims that aspirin is less toxic to the gastrointestinal tract than salicylic acid are not based on scientific evidence, but date from a letter by the father of the discoverer, Hoffmann. He found his daily dose of 10 g aspirin much more palatable than the same amount of sodium salicylate. Aspirin should not be used in pregnant women (premature bleeding, closure of ductus arteriosus) or children before puberty (Reye's syndrome).

Specific COX-2 Inhibitors

Specific COX-2 inhibitors are expected to exert anti-inflammatory and analgesic effects without causing gastric ulcerogenic effects or platelet dysfunction. By definition, a substance may be regarded as a specific COX-2 inhibitor if it causes no clinically meaningful COX-1 inhibition (i.e., suppression of platelet thromboxane formation and gastric prostaglandin synthesis) at maximal therapeutic doses. Such compounds usually reveal a more than 100-fold difference in the concentration that inhibits COX-2 versus COX-1 in respective biochemical in vitro assays (58). Among the variety of available test systems, the ex vivo whole-blood assay has emerged as the best method to estimate COX-2 selectivity in humans. This assay provides a direct indication of the ability of a test substance to inhibit the enzymatic activities of COX-1 (i.e., thromboxane formation from platelets during blood clotting) and COX-2 (i.e., prostaglandin E_2 synthesis in lipopolysaccharide-stimulated monocytes).

X-ray crystallography of the three-dimensional structures of COX-1 and COX-2 has yielded insights into how COX-2 specificity is achieved. Within the hydrophobic channel of the COX enzyme, a single amino acid difference in position 523 (isoleucin in COX-1, valin in COX-2) has been detected that is critical for the COX-2 selectivity of several drugs. Accordingly, the smaller valin molecule

in COX-2 gives access to a side pocket, which has been proposed to be the binding site of COX-2-selective substances. Consequently, the total NSAID-binding site is about 17% larger in COX-2 than in COX-1 (59). Thus, the increased NSAID-binding pocket of the COX-2 isozyme can bind bulky inhibitors more readily than the COX-1 isoform. Celecoxib (SC58635) and rofecoxib (MK-966) are novel specific COX-2 inhibitors of the diarylheterocyclic family (Fig. 10.5). The 4-methylsulfonylphenyl and 4-sulfonamoylphenyl groups of these compounds have been shown to interact with specific residues within the "side pocket" of the COX-2 isozyme (60).

Celecoxib and rofecoxib have been shown to be effective analgesics in dental pain models (61), as well as having effective anti-inflammatory and analgesic substances in patients with rheumatoid arthritis and osteoarthritis (61). Celecoxib (SC58635) was approved in December 1998 by the U.S. Food and Drug Administration. Rofecoxib became available in 1999. Celecoxib is indicated for relief of the signs and symptoms of osteoarthritis (recommended oral dose 200 mg/day administered as a single dose or 100 mg twice a day) and rheumatoid arthritis in adults (recommended oral dose 100 to 200 mg twice a day). Rofecoxib is indicated for relief of the signs and symptoms of osteoarthritis (recommended starting dose 12.5 mg once daily, maximum recommended daily dose 25 mg), for the mangement of acute pain in adults, and for the treatment of primary dysmenorrhea (recommended initial doses 50 mg once daily; use of rofecoxib for more than 5 days in the management of pain has not been studied). At therapeutic dosages, celecoxib and rofecoxib have no effect on COX-1-dependent thromboxane formation and gastric prostaglandin synthesis. The pharmacokinetic profile of celecoxib and rofecoxib is compiled in Table 10.3. In comparison with celecoxib, rofecoxib has a longer half-life and is more potent and selective in vitro. However, their pharmacokinetic characteristics (slow absorption, slow elimination) make both drugs unlikely candidates for the treatment of acute pain of short duration. Whereas the metabolism of rofecoxib is primarily mediated through cytosolic enzymes, celecoxib is metabolized predominantly via cytochrome P4502C9 (CYP2C9). Thus, significant interactions may occur when celecoxib is administered together with drugs that inhibit CYP2C9. For instance, concomitant administration of celecoxib and fluconazole may increase celecoxib plasma levels. Accordingly, celecoxib should be used at the lowest recommended dose in such patients. As NSAIDs have been reported to elevate plasma lithium levels, patients receiving specific COX-2

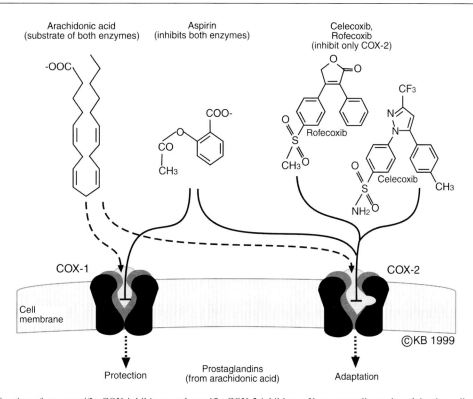

Fig. 10.5. Mode of action of non-specific COX inhibitors and specific COX-2 inhibitors. X-ray crystallography of the three-dimensional structures of COX-1 and COX-2 indicate that the total NSAID-binding site is about 17% larger in COX-2 than in COX-1. Thus, the increased NSAID-binding pocket of the COX-2 isozyme can bind bulky inhibitors more readily than the COX-1 isoform. The specific COX-2 inhibitors celecoxib and rofecoxib have been shown to interact with specific residues within the "side pocket" of the COX-2 isozyme.

inhibitors and lithium should be observed carefully for signs of lithium toxicity. Furthermore, specific COX-2 inhibitors may diminish the antihypertensive effect of angiotensin-converting enzyme inhibitors. In patients receiving warfarin, anticoagulant activity should be monitored, particularly in the first few days after initiating therapy with specific COX-2 inhibitors.

Published clinical studies support the hypothesis that specific COX-2 inhibitors may provide a significantly improved risk-benefit ratio in terms of gastrointestinal safety as compared with conventional NSAIDs. Accordingly, the use of specific COX-2 inhibitors, rather than traditional NSAIDs, should be preferred in patients

at increased risk of serious upper gastrointestinal complications. These patients include individuals older than 60 years, those with a history of peptic ulcer disease, and those taking glucocorticoids (with a high-dose NSAID) and anticoagulants. In the Vioxx Gastrointestinal Outcomes Research (VIGOR) study (62), treatment with rofecoxib at twice the approved maximal dose for long-term use resulted in significantly lower rates of clinically important upper gastrointestinal events and complicated upper gastrointestinal events than did treatment with a standard dose of naproxen. Moreover, the incidence of complicated upper gastrointestinal bleeding and bleeding from beyond the duodenum was significantly lower

Table 10.3. *Specific COX-2 inhibitors: Physicochemical and pharmacological data, therapeutic dosage*

Chemical/pharmacological class	Binding to plasma proteins	Oral bioavailability	t_{max}[a]	$t^{1/2}$[b]	Single dose (maximal daily dose) for adults
Celecoxib	94–98%	60–80%	2–4 hr	11 hr	100–200 mg (400 mg)
Rofecoxib	~98%	~100%	2–4 hr	~17 hr	12.5–25 mg (50 mg)

[a] Time to reach maximum plasma concentration after oral administration.
[b] Terminal half-life of elimination.

among patients who received rofecoxib. In the celecoxib long-term Arthritis Safety Study (CLASS) (63), incidences of symptomatic ulcers and/or ulcer complications were not significantly different in patients taking celecoxib versus NSAIDs who were also taking concomitant low-dosage aspirin, indicating that the use of low-dose aspirin may abrogate the gastrointestinal-sparing effects of celecoxib. By contrast, analysis of non-aspirin users alone demonstrated that celecoxib, at a dosage twofold to fourfold greater than the maximum therapeutic dosages, was associated with a significantly lower incidence of symptomatic ulcers and/or ulcer complications compared with NSAIDs.

The involvement of COX-2 in human renal functions is supported by clinical studies (64,65) that showed that specific COX-2 inhibitors, similar to other NSAIDs, may cause peripheral edema, hypertension, and exacerbation of preexisting hypertension by inhibiting water and salt excretion by the kidneys. Moreover, in healthy elderly volunteers, specific COX-2 inhibitors decreased renal prostacyclin production and led to a significant transient decline in urinary sodium excretion (64,65). However, although decreases in sodium excretion were comparable between NSAIDs and specific COX-2 inhibitors, only NSAIDs were shown to reduce the glomerular filtration rate in volunteers with normal renal function (64). On the basis of these data, it seems plausible to use specific COX-2 inhibitors with caution in patients with fluid retention, hypertension, and heart failure. Finally, celecoxib should not be administered in patients with allergic-type reactions to sulfonamides.

Controlled clinical trials will gain more insights into possible long-term side effects associated with the use of specific COX-2 inhibitors. Interestingly, COX-2 is induced in tissue on the edges of ulcers, and in animal studies, selective COX-2 inhibitors have been shown to retard ulcer healing (66). Thus, in patients with NSAID-associated ulcers, it will be obligatory to show whether effective ulcer healing occurs in patients switched to specific COX-2 inhibitors. Likewise, studies are required to demonstrate that COX-2 inhibitors are safe in distinct subgroups (patients with erosions or prior history of ulcer disease).

Furthermore, COX-2 localized in the endothelium has been shown to exert vasoprotective and antiatherogenic actions by virtue of its major product, prostacyclin, the latter being a potent inhibitor of platelet aggregation, activation and adhesion of leukocytes, and accumulation of cholesterol in vascular cells. Upregulation of endothelial COX-2 has been shown to be induced by laminar shear stress (67) or lysophosphatidylcholin (component of atherogenic lipoproteins) (68), suggesting that COX-2 may provide an adaptive vascular protection. As specific COX-2 inhibitors do not inhibit platelet COX-1, they might, at least in theory, unfavorably alter the thromboxane-prostacyclin balance by inhibiting COX-2-dependent synthesis of vasoprotective prostacyclin in endothelial cells. However, hitherto published clinical studies have yielded discrepant results in this regard. In the CLASS trial no difference was noted in the incidence of cardiovascular events (cerebrovascular accident, myocardial infarction, angina) between celecoxib and NSAIDs (ibuprofen, diclofenac) (63). On the other hand, in the VIGOR study, patients receiving rofecoxib had a significant fourfold increase in the incidence of myocardial infarctions, as compared with patients randomized to naproxen (62). However, as both compounds are known to cause a similar inhibition of systemic prostacyclin production without altering platelet-derived thromboxane synthesis, the apparent discrepancy of these studies in terms of cardiovascular outcome is most likely due to differences in the study protocols (e.g., eligibility criteria, study population, study duration) and the use of different NSAID comparators. Accordingly, 22% of the patients included in the CLASS trial took aspirin as a cardioprotective agent, whereas the entry criteria for the VIGOR study precluded aspirin consumption. In addition, the VIGOR study was performed on patients with rheumatoid arthritis, a condition that has been associated with an enhanced rate of cardiovascular events. By contrast, in the CLASS trial, patients were included with osteoarthritis that had not been associated with an increased risk of cardiovascular complications. As a consequence, a possible thrombogenicity of specific COX-2 inhibitors deserves further well-controlled studies.

The involvement of the COX-2 isozyme in other pathological states suggests that specific COX-2 inhibitors may have further indications in conditions such as colonic polyposis, colorectal cancer, and Alzheimer's disease (69–73). Specific COX-2 inhibitors have been shown to possess a strong chemopreventive action against colon carcinogenesis in rats, inhibiting tumors to a greater degree than conventional NSAIDs (74). With regard to the functions of the COX isozymes, Tsujii et al. (75) found that COX-2 may modulate the production of angiogenic factors by colon cancer cells, whereas COX-1 regulates angiogenesis in endothelial cells. Moreover, recent studies indicate that COX-2 overexpression is not necessarily unique to cancer of the colon but may be a common feature of other epithelial cells. Accordingly, increased COX-2 levels have been identified in lung (76,77), breast (78,79), and gastric cancers (80,81). On the basis of these data, it is conceivable that specific COX-2 inhibitors might be used as adjuvants in the treatment of tumors as well as in cancer prevention. At present, there are few data on the use of specific COX-2 inhibitors for the relief of cancer pain.

Non-acidic antipyretic analgesics

Aniline derivatives

The main representative of this group, paracetamol (acetaminophen), was discovered at the same time as aspirin. Its pharmacokinetic and pharmacodynamic data are compiled in Table 10.4. Paracetamol is a very weak (possibly indirect) inhibitor of the COX isozymes. Induction of fever is clearly blocked by paracetamol in several species. The major advantage of paracetamol lies in its relative lack of (serious) side effects if dose limits are obeyed, although serious events have been observed with low doses in a few cases (82). Paracetamol is metabolized to highly toxic nucleophilic benzoquinones, which bind covalantly to DNA and structural proteins in parenchymal cells (e.g., in liver and kidney), where these reactive intermediates are produced (for review see reference 83). The consequence is cell death and death of the whole organism resulting from liver necrosis. When detected early, overdosage can be antagonized within the first 12 hours after intake by administration of N-acetylcysteine or glutathione that regenerate detoxifying mechanisms. Paracetamol should not be given to patients with seriously impaired liver function.

The predominant indication for paracetamol is fever and mild forms of pain (e.g., pain in the context of viral infections). Many patients with recurrent headache also benefit from paracetamol and its low toxicity. Paracetamol is also used in children, but despite its somewhat lower toxicity in juvenile patients, fatalities resulting from involuntary overdosage have been reported. To what extent paracetamol acts synergistically in combination with aspirin and caffeine (84), but also causes the so-called analgesic nephropathy, is unclear (85). The mechanism appears uncertain (86). Also, claims that such combinations are more frequently abused than single-entity analgesics are supported only by (weak) epidemiological data. Paracetamol has been shown to be as effective and potent as aspirin in single-dose studies in cancer pain (87). Acetanilide and phenacetine, the precursors of paracetamol, have been banned because of their higher toxicity.

Pyrazolinone derivatives

After the discovery of phenazone 120 years ago, the drug industry tried to improve this compound in three aspects. Phenazone was chemically modified 1) to have a more potent compound, 2) to yield a water-soluble derivative to be given parenterally, and 3) to find a compound, which is eliminated faster and more reliably than phenazone in all patients. The best known results of these attempts are aminophenazone, dipyrone, and propyphenazone (Table 10.4). Aminophenazone is not in use anymore because it might lead to the formation of nitrosamines that may increase the risk of stomach cancer. The other two compounds differ from phenazone in

Table 10.4. *Non-acidic antipyretic analgesics: Physicochemical and pharmacological data, therapeutic dosage*

Chemical/pharmacological class	Binding to plasma proteins	Oral bioavailability	t_{max}[a]	$t^{1/2}$[b]	Single dose (maximal daily dose) for adults
Anilin derivatives:					
Paracetamol (acetaminophen)	5–50% dose-dependent	70–100% dose-dependent	0.5–1.5 hr	1.5–2.5 hr	0.5–1 g (4 g)
Pyrazolinone derivatives:					
Phenazone	<10%	~100% dose-dependent	0.5–2 hr	11–12 hr	0.5–1 g (4 g)
Propyphenazone	~10%	~100% dose-dependent	0.5–1.5 hr	1–2.5 hr	0.5–1 g (4 g)
Metamizol-Na[c]	<20%	–	–	–	0.5–1 g (4 g)
4-Methylaminophenazone[d]	58%	~100%	1–2 hr	2–4 hr	–
4-Aminophenazone[d]	48%	–	–	4–5.5 hr	–

[a] Time to reach maximum plasma concentration after oral administration.
[b] Terminal half-life of elimination.
[c] Noraminopyrinemethansulfonate-Na.
[d] Metabolites of metamizol.

their potency and elimination half-life (88), their water solubility (dipyrone is a water-soluble prodrug of methylaminophenazone), and their general toxicity (propyphenazone and dipyrone do not lead to the formation of nitrosamines in the acidic environment of the stomach). Phenazone, propyphenazone, and dipyrone are used in many countries worldwide (Latin America, many countries in Asia, Eastern Europe, and Central Europe) as the dominant antipyretic analgesics.

Dipyrone has been alleged to cause agranulocytosis. Although there appears to be a statistically significant link, the incidence is extremely rare (1 case per million treatment periods) (89,90). All antipyretic analgesics have also been claimed to cause Stevens-Johnson syndrome and Lyell's syndrome, as well as shock reactions. New data indicate that the incidence of these events is in the same order of magnitude as occurs with other drugs (e.g., penicillins) (91–93).

All non-acidic phenazone derivatives lack anti-inflammatory activity and are devoid of gastrointestinal and (acute) renal toxicity. In contrast to paracetamol, dipyrone is safe when given in overdosage (94). If one compares aspirin, paracetamol and, for example, propyphenazone when used for the same indication (e.g., occasional headache), it is obvious that aspirin is more dangerous than either propyphenazone or paracetamol.

References

1. Vane J. Towards a better aspirin. Nature 367:215–16, 1994.
2. Vane JR. Inhibition of prostaglandin synthesis as a mechanism of action of aspirin-like drugs. Nature New Biol 231:232–5, 1971.
3. McCormack K, Brune K. Dissociation between the antinociceptive and anti-inflammatory effects of the nonsteroidal anti-inflammatory drugs. A survey of their analgesic efficacy. Drugs 41:533–47, 1991.
4. Brune K. Spinal cord effects of antipyretic analgesics. Drugs 47(Suppl 5):21–7, 1994.
5. Hinz B, Kraus V, Pahl A, Brune K. Salicylate metabolites inhibit cyclooxygenase-2-dependent prostaglandin E_2 synthesis in murine macrophages. Biochem Biophys Res Commun 274:197–202, 2000.
6. Hinz B, Brune K, Rau T, Pahl A. Flurbiprofen enantiomers inhibit inducible nitric oxide synthase expression in RAW 264.7 macrophages. Pharm Res 18:151–6, 2001.
7. Brune K. How aspirin might work: a pharmacokinetic approach. Agents Actions 4:230–2, 1974.
8. Brune K, Glatt M, Graf P. Mechanism of action of anti-inflammatory drugs. Gen Pharmacol 7:27–33, 1976.
9. Brune K, Rainsford KD, Schweitzer A. Biodistribution of mild analgesics. Br J Clin Pharmacol 10(Suppl 2):279–84, 1980.
10. Hoigne RV, Szczeklik A. Allergic and pseudoallergic reactions associated with nonsteroidal anti-inflammatory drugs. In: Borda IT, Koff RS, eds. NSAIDs: a profile of adverse effects. Philadelphia: Hanley & Belfus, and St Louis: Mosby-Yearbook, 1992:57–184.
11. Fu JY, Masferrer JL, Seibert K, et al. The induction and suppression of prostaglandin H_2 synthase (cyclooxygenase) in human monocytes. J Biol Chem 265:16737–40, 1990.
12. Masferrer JL, Zweifel BS, Seibert S, Needleman P. Selective regulation of cellular cyclooxygenase by dexamethasone and endotoxin in mice. J Clin Invest 86:1375–9, 1990.
13. Xie W, Chipman JG, Robertson DL, et al. Expression of a mitogen-responsive gene encoding prostaglandin synthase is regulated by mRNA splicing. Proc Natl Acad Sci USA 88:2692–6, 1991.
14. Niiro H, Otsuka T, Izuhara K, et al. Regulation by interleukin-10 and interleukin-4 of cyclooxygenase-2 expression in human neutrophils. Blood 89:1621–8, 1997.
15. Onoe Y, Miyaura C, Kaminakayashiki T, et al. IL-13 and IL-4 inhibit bone resorption by suppressing cyclooxygenase-2-dependent prostaglandin synthesis in osteoblasts. J Immunol 156:758–64, 1996.
16. Nantel F, Denis D, Gordon R, et al. Distribution and regulation of cyclooxygenase-2 in carrageenan-induced inflammation. Br J Pharmacol 128:853–9, 1999.
17. Hinz B, Brune K, Pahl A. Prostaglandin E_2 up-regulates cyclooxygenase-2 expression in lipopolysaccharide-stimulated RAW 264.7 macrophages. Biochem Biophys Res Commun 272:744–8, 2000.
18. Hinz B, Brune K, Pahl A. Cyclooxygenase-2 expression in lipopolysaccharide-stimulated human monocytes is modulated by cyclic AMP, prostaglandin E_2 and nonsteroidal anti-inflammatory drugs. Biochem Biophys Res Commun 278:790–6, 2000.
19. Patrignani P, Panara MR, Sciulli MG, et al. Differential inhibition of human prostaglandin endoperoxide synthase-1 and -2 by nonsteroidal anti-inflammatory drugs. J Physiol Pharmacol 48:623–31, 1997.
20. Brune K, Zeilhofer HU, Hinz B. Cyclo-oxygenase inhibitors: new insights. In: Emery P, ed. Fast Facts—Rheumatology Highlights 1998–99, Oxford Health Press 1999:18–24.
21. Hinz B, Brune K. Cyclooxygenase-2—Ten years later. J Pharmacol Exp Ther 300:367–75, 2002
22. Harris RC, McKanna JA, Akai Y, et al. Cyclooxygenase-2 is associated with the macula densa of rat kidney and increases with salt restriction. J Clin Invest 94:2504–10, 1994.
23. Komhoff M, Grone JJ, Klein T, et al. Localization of cyclooxygenase-1 and cyclooxygenase-2 in adult and fetal human kidney: implication for renal function. Am J Physiol 272:F460–8, 1997.
24. Khan KNM, Verturini CM, Bunch RT, et al. Interspecies differences in renal localization of cyclooxygenase isoforms: implication in nonsteroidal antiinflammatory drug-related nephrotoxicity. Toxicol Pathol 27:612–20, 1998.
25. Chakraborty I, Das SK, Wang J, Dey SK. Developmental expression of the cyclo-oxygenase-1 and cyclo-oxygenase-2

genes in the peri-implantation mouse uterus and their differential regulation by the blastocyst and ovarian steroids. J Mol Endocrinol 16:107–22, 1996.

26. Gibb W, Sun M. Localization of prostaglandin H synthase type 2 protein and mRNA in term human fetal membranes and decidua. J Endocrinol 150:497–503, 1996.

27. Lim H, Paria BC, Das SK, et al. Multiple female reproductive failures in cyclooxygenase 2-deficient mice. Cell 91:197–208, 1997.

28. Schaible HG, Schmidt RF. Time course of mechanosensitivity changes in articular afferents during a developing experimental arthritis. J Neurophysiol 60:2180–95, 1988.

29. Kress M, Koltzenburg M, Reeh PW, Handwerker HO. Responsiveness and functional attributes of electrically localized terminals of cutaneous C-fibers in vivo and in vitro. J Neurophysiol 68:581–95, 1992.

30. Neugebauer V, Geisslinger G, Rümenapp P, et al. Antinociceptive effects of R(−)- and S(+)-flurbiprofen on rat spinal dorsal horn neurons rendered hyperexcitable by an acute knee joint inflammation. J Pharmacol Exp Ther 275:618–28, 1995.

31. Gold MS, Zhang L, Wrigley DL, Traub RJ. Prostaglandin E_2 modulates TTX-R I(Na) in rat colonic sensory neurons. J. Neurophysiol 88:1512–22, 2002.

32. England S, Bevan S, Docherty RJ. PGE_2 modulates the tetrodotoxin-resistant sodium current in neonatal rat dorsal root ganglion neurones via the cyclic AMP-protein kinase A cascade. J Physiol (Lond) 495:429–40, 1996.

33. Gold MS, Reichling DB, Shuster MJ, Levine JD. Hyperalgesic agents increase a tetrodotoxin-resistant Na^+ current in nociceptors. Proc Natl Acad Sci USA 93:1108–12, 1996.

34. Akopian AN, Sivilotti L, Wood JN. A tetrodotoxin-resistant voltage-gated sodium channel expressed by sensory neurons. Nature 379:257–62, 1996.

35. Heppelmann B, Messlinger K, Neiss WF, Schmidt RF. Ultrastructural three-dimensional reconstruction of group III and group IV, sensory nerve endings ("free nerve endings") in the knee joint capsule of the cat: evidence for multiple receptive sites. J Comp Neurol 292:103–11, 1990.

36. Yamagata K, Andreasson KI, Kaufmann WE, et al. Expression of a mitogen-inducible cyclooxygenase in brain neurons: regulation by synaptic activity and glucocorticoids. Neuron 11:371–86, 1993.

37. Beiche F, Scheuerer S, Brune K, et al. Upregulation of cyclooxygenase-2 mRNA in the rat spinal cord following peripheral inflammation. FEBS Lett 390:165–9, 1996.

38. Smith CJ, Zhang Y, Koboldt CM, et al. Pharmacological analysis of cyclooxygenase-1 in inflammation. Proc Natl Acad Sci USA 95:13313–18, 1998.

39. Muth-Selbach US, Tegeder I, Brune K, Geisslinger G. Acetaminophen inhibits spinal prostaglandin E_2 release after peripheral noxious stimulation. Anesthesiology 91:231–9, 1999.

40. Vaughan CW, Ingram SL, Connor MA, Christie MJ. How opioids inhibit GABA-mediated neurotransmission. Nature 390:611–14, 1997.

41. Williams JT. The painless synergism of aspirin and opium. Nature 390:557, 1997.

42. Bonica JJ. Cancer pain. In: Bonica JJ, ed. The management of pain. Philadelphia: Lea & Febiger, 1990:400–60.

43. Portenoy RK. Cancer pain management. Semin Oncol 20(Suppl 1):19–35, 1993.

44. Winter CA, Risley EA, Nuss GW. Carrageenin-induced edema in hind paw of the rat as an assay for anti-inflammatory drugs. Proc Soc Exp Biol 111:544–52, 1962.

45. Otterness IG, Bliven ML. Laboratory models for testing nonsteroidal anti-inflammatory drugs. In: Lombardino J, ed. Nonsteroidal anti-inflammatory drugs. New York: John Wiley & Sons, 1985:111–252.

46. Brune K, Lanz R. Pharmacokinetics of non-steroidal anti-inflammatory drugs. In: Bonta IL, Bray MA, Parnham MJ, eds. Handbook of inflammation, vol. 5. The Pharmacology of inflammation, 1985:413–49.

47. Hinz B, Dorn CP, Shen TY, Brune K. Anti-inflammatory—antirheumatic drugs. In: Ullmann's encyclopedia of industrial chemistry, 6th ed. Weinheim: Wiley-VCH, 2000 Electronic Release.

48. Herzfeldt CD, Kümmel R. Dissociation constants, solubilities and dissolution rates of some selected nonsteroidal anti-inflammatories. Drug Dev Ind Pharm 9:767–93, 1983.

49. Verbeck RK, Blackburn JL, Loewen GR. Clinical pharmacokinetics of non-steroidal anti-inflammatory drugs. Clin Pharmacokinet 8:297–331, 1983.

50. Laska EM, Sunshine A, Marrero I, et al. The correlation between blood levels of ibuprofen and clinical analgesic response. JAMA 40:1–7, 1986.

51. Geisslinger G, Menzel S, Wissel K, Brune K. Single dose pharmacokinetics of different formulations of ibuprofen and aspirin. Drug Invest 5:238–42, 1993.

52. Kaufman DW, Kelly JP, Sheehan JE, et al. Nonsteroidal anti-inflammatory drug use in relation to major upper gastrointestinal bleeding. Clin Pharmacol Ther 53:485–94, 1993.

53. Rudy AC, Knight PM, Brater DC, Hall SD. Stereoselective metabolism of ibuprofen in humans: administration of R-, S- and racemic ibuprofen. J Pharmacol Exp Ther 259:1133–9, 1991.

54. Tegeder I, Lotsch J, Krebs S, et al. Comparison of inhibitory effects of meloxicam and diclofenac on human thromboxane biosynthesis after single doses and at steady state. Clin Pharmacol Ther 65:533–44, 1999.

55. Henry D, Lim LL, Garcia Rodriguez LA, et al. Variability in risk of gastrointestinal complications with individual nonsteroidal anti-inflammatory drugs: results of a collaborative meta-analysis. Br Med J 312:1563–6, 1996.

56. Schmid J, Buisch U, Heinzel G, et al. Meloxicam: pharmacokinetics and metabolic pattern after intravenous infusion and oral administration to healthy subjects. Drug Metab Dispos 23:1206–13, 1995.

57. Kalgutkar AS, Crews BC, Rowlinson SW, et al. Aspirin-like molecules that covalently inactivate cyclooxygenase-2. Science 280:1268–70, 1998.

58. Lipsky PE. The clinical potential of cyclooxygenase-2-specific inhibitors. Am J Med 106:51S–7S, 1999.

59. Luong C, Miller A, Barnett J, et al. Flexibility of the NSAID binding site in the structure of human cyclooxygenase-2. Nature Struct Biol 3:927–33, 1996.

60. Kurumbail RG, Stevens AM, Gierse JK, et al. Structural basis for selective inhibition of cyclooxygenase-2 by anti-inflammatory agents. Nature 384:644–8, 1996.

61. Lane NE. Pain management in osteoarthritis: the role of COX-2 inhibitors. J Rheumatol 24(Suppl 49):20–4, 1997.

62. Bombardier C, Laine L, Reicin A, et al. Comparison of upper gastrointestinal toxicity of rofecoxib and naproxen in patients with rheumatoid arthritis. VIGOR Study Group. N Engl J Med 343:1520–8, 2000.

63. Silverstein FE, Faich G, Goldstein JL, et al. Gastrointestinal toxicity with celecoxib vs nonsteroidal anti-inflammatory drugs for osteoarthritis and rheumatoid arthritis: the CLASS study: a randomized controlled trial. Celecoxib Long-term Arthritis Safety Study. JAMA 284:1247–55, 2000.

64. Catella-Lawson F, McAdam B, Morrison BW, et al. Effects of specific inhibition of cyclooxygenase-2 on sodium balance, hemodynamics, and vasoactive eicosanoids. J Pharmacol Exp Ther 289:735–41, 1999.

65. McAdam BF, Catella-Lawson F, Mardini IA, et al. Systemic biosynthesis of prostacyclin by cyclooxygenase (COX)-2: the human pharmacology of a selective inhibitor of COX-2. Proc Natl Acad Sci USA 96:272–7, 1999.

66. Schmassmann A, Peskar BM, Stettler C, et al. Effects of inhibition of prostaglandin endoperoxide synthase-2 in chronic gastro-intestinal ulcer models in rats. Br J Pharmacol 123:795–804, 1998.

67. Topper JN, Cai J, Falb D, Gimbrone MA. Identification of vascular endothelial genes differentially responsive to fluid mechanical stimuli: cyclooxygenase-2, manganese superoxide dismutase, and endothelial cell nitric oxide synthase are selectively up-regulated by steady laminar shear stress. Proc Natl Acad Sci USA 93:10417–22, 1996.

68. Zembowicz A, Jones SL, Wu KK. Induction of cyclooxygenase-2 in human umbilical vein endothelial cells by lysophosphatidylcholine. J Clin Invest 96:1688–92, 1995.

69. Kune GA, Kune S, Watson LF. Colorectal cancer risk, chronic illnesses, operations, and medications: case control results from the Melbourne Colorectal Cancer Study. Cancer Res 48:4399–404, 1988.

70. Thun MJ, Namboodiri MM, Heath CW. Aspirin use and reduced risk of fatal colon cancer. N Engl J Med 325:1593–6, 1991.

71. Giardiello FM, Hamilton SR, Krush AJ, et al. Treatment of colonic and rectal adenomas with sulindac in familial adenomatous polyposis. N Engl J Med 328:1313–16, 1993.

72. Oshima M, Dinchuk JE, Kargman SL, et al. Suppression of intestinal polyposis in Apc^{δ716} knockout mice by inhibition of cyclooxygenase 2 (COX-2). Cell 87:803–9, 1996.

73. Tocco G, Freire-Moar J, Schreiber SS, et al. Maturational regulation and regional induction of cyclooxygenase-2 in rat brain: implications for Alzheimer's disease. Exp Neurol 144:339–49, 1997.

74. Kawamori T, Rao CV, Seibert K, Reddy BS. Chemopreventive activity of celecoxib, a specific cyclooxygenase-2 inhibitor, against colon carcinogenesis. Cancer Res 58:409–12, 1998.

75. Tsujii M, Kawano S, Tsuji S, et al. Cyclooxygenase regulates angiogenesis induced by colon cancer cells. Cell 93:705–16, 1998.

76. Hida T, Yatabe Y, Achiwa H, et al. Increased expression of cyclooxygenase 2 occurs frequently in human lung cancers, specifically in adenocarcinomas. Cancer Res 58:3761–4, 1998.

77. Wolff H, Saukkonen K, Anttila S, et al. Expression of cyclooxygenase-2 in human lung carcinoma. Cancer Res 58:4997–5001, 1998.

78. Hwang D, Scollard D, Byrne J, Levine E. Expression of cyclooxygenase-1 and cyclooxygenase-2 in human breast cancer. J Natl Cancer Inst 90:455–60, 1998.

79. Parrett ML, Harris RE, Joarder FS, et al. Cyclooxygenase-2 gene expression in human breast cancer. Int J Oncol 10:503–7, 1997.

80. Sakamoto C. Roles of COX-1 and COX-2 in gastrointestinal pathophysiology. J Gastroenterol 33:618–24, 1998.

81. Ristimäki A, Honkanen N, Jänkälä H, et al. Expression of cyclooxygenase-2 in human gastric carcinoma. Cancer Res 57:1276–80, 1997.

82. Bridger S, Henderson K, Glucksman E, et al. Deaths from low dose paracetamol poisoning. Am Med J 316:1724–5, 1998.

83. Seeff LB, Cuccherini BA, Zimmerman HJ, et al. Paracetamol hepatotoxicity in alcoholics. Ann Intern Med 104:399–404, 1986.

84. Laska EM, Sunshine A, Mueller F, et al. Caffeine as an analgesic adjuvant. JAMA 251:1711–18, 1984.

85. Elseviers MM, De Broe ME. Combination analgesic involvement in the pathogenesis of analgesic nephropathy: the European perspective. Am J Kidney Dis 28 (Suppl 1):48–55, 1996.

86. Porter GA. Paracetamol/aspirin mixtures: experimental data. Am J Kidney Dis 28(Suppl 1):30–3, 1996.

87. Beaver WT. Nonsteroidal antiinflammatory analgesics in cancer pain. In: Foley KM, ed. Advances in pain research and therapy. New York: Raven Press, 1990:109–31.

88. Levy M, Zylber-Katz E, Rosenkranz B. Clinical pharmacokinetcs of dipyrone and its metabolites. Clin Pharmacokinet 28:216–34, 1995.

89. Kaufman DW, Kelly JP, Levy M, Shapiro S. The drug etiology of agranulocytosis an aplastic anemia. Monographs in epidemiology and biostatistics 18. Oxford: Oxford University Press, 1991.

90. The International Agranulocytosis and Aplastic Anemia Study: risks of agranulocytosis and aplastic anemia: a first report of their relation to drug use with special reference to analgesics. JAMA 256:1749–57, 1986.

91. Roujeau JC, Kelly JP, Naldi L, et al. Drug etiology of Stevens-Johnson syndrome and toxic epidemal necrolysis,

first results from an international case-control study. N Engl J Med 333:1600–9, 1995.

92. Mockenhaupt M, Schlingmann J, Schroeder W, Schoepf E. Evaluation of non-steroidal anti-inflammatory drugs (NSAIDs) and muscle relaxants as risk factors for Stevens-Johnson syndrome (SJS) and toxic epidermal necrolysis (TEN). Pharmacoepidemiology and Drug Safety 5:116, 1996.

93. The International Collaborative Study of Severe Anaphylaxis. Epidemiology 9:141–6, 1998.

94. Wolhoff H, Altrogge G, Pola W, Sistovaris N. Metamizol—akute Überdosierung in suizidaler Absicht. Dtsch Med Wochenschr 108:1761–4, 1983.

11 Adjuvant analgesic drugs

RUSSELL K. PORTENOY
Albert Einstein College of Medicine

GERMAINE ROWE
Staten Island University Hospital

Introduction

The term *adjuvant analgesic* can be applied to any drug that has a primary indication other than pain, but is analgesic in some painful conditions. This term is often used synonymously with the term *co-analgesic* when it refers to a drug that is administered with another analgesic, usually an opioid. In the cancer population, this combination is usually administered to enhance pain relief when a syndrome is poorly responsive to the opioid, or to allow opioid dose reduction when opioid-related side effects are problematic. The adjuvant analgesics also may be considered a subset of a larger group of adjuvant drugs some of which are specifically co-administered with analgesics to treat side effects.

Rapid advances in basic and clinical pharmacology have dramatically expanded the role of the adjuvant analgesics. For this reason, the term *adjuvant* is actually a misnomer in many settings. Many of these drugs are used alone, as primary analgesics, when pain is likely to be responsive. This is particularly true in populations with chronic non-malignant pain. Given this expanding use, it is important to understand both the pharmacology of these drugs and their therapeutic role in the management of cancer pain.

General considerations

The effective use of an adjuvant analgesic depends on systematic assessment of the patient. This assessment clarifies the nature of the pain, infers pain pathophysiology, identifies a specific pain syndrome, and allows an understanding of the pain as one of potentially numerous problems that may undermine quality of life. Over time, repeated assessments must track changes in pain, side effects, or any of the broader quality of life concerns may impel a shift in therapeutic strategy.

Positioning therapy

Although the individual patient can benefit dramatically from the addition of an adjuvant analgesic, extensive experience in the cancer population indicates that these drugs are, as a group, less reliable analgesics than the opioids. For this reason, there is a general consensus that patients who experience moderate or severe cancer pain usually should be offered a trial of an opioid drug as the primary analgesic. It should be recognized, however, that the data that justify this impression are actually minimal, and it is certainly possible that some syndromes could be more readily addressed by early and aggressive use of adjuvant analgesics. For example, many experienced clinicians perceive that paroxysmal lancinating neuropathic pain (e.g., the intense stabbing ear pain that may be associated with recurrent head and neck cancer) is often poorly responsive to opioids, but potentially very responsive to selected adjuvant drugs, such as those in the anticonvulsant class. These patients might be offered a trial of an anticonvulsant first or promptly after initiation of an opioid regimen that fails to control the pain.

Given the potential for additive toxicity when opioid dose changes are combined with changes in other drug therapies, it usually is best to optimize the opioid regimen before initiating a trial of an adjuvant analgesic. Although some clinicians attempt to improve patient response by initiating both an opioid and an adjuvant analgesic concurrently, this approach requires careful monitoring and presumably carries additional risk. Should significant toxicity occur, both drugs must be discontinued, and there would be no certainty about which was the offending agent. Usually, only a few days are required to identify an opioid dose that appears to provide the best balance between efficacy and side effects.

The use of an adjuvant analgesic as a means to improve pain control after an opioid regimen has been shown to be inadequate alone must be understood in relation to the other options that exist in this situation (Table 11.1). In the absence of data from comparative clinical trials, the decision to use an adjuvant analgesic drug instead of an alternative therapy, such as a trial of spinally administered opioids or a nerve block, is usually a matter of clinical judgment.

Knowledge, skills, and expectations

To select and properly administer an adjuvant analgesic, the clinician must be familiar with the drug's approved indications, unapproved indications accepted in medical practice, likely side effects and potential serious adverse effects, usual time-action relationship, pharmacokinetics, and specific dosing guidelines for pain. Few of the adjuvant analgesics have been studied in cancer patients, and the information used to develop dosing guidelines is usually extrapolated from other patient populations. Given the medical co-morbidities that are common among cancer patients, it is usually best to begin cautiously by incorporating low initial doses and gradual dose escalation. This approach may reduce early side effects, allow acclimation to the drug, and identify dose-dependent analgesic effects that can be explored to optimize the balance between pain relief and adverse effects. The use of low initial doses and slow dose titration also may delay the onset of analgesia, however, and patients must be forewarned of this possibility.

There is great variability in the response to all adjuvant analgesics. Although there are likely to be characteristics of the patient or the pain that systematically alter response, the outcomes achieved by any individual patient

Table 11.1. *Therapeutic options when pain is poorly responsive to an opioid therapy*

Approach	Therapeutic options
Pharmacologic techniques	Use of an adjuvant analgesic to enhance analgesia and reduce systemic opioid requirement
	Use of spinal opioids
	Identify an opioid with a more favorable therapeutic index (opioid rotation)
	Improve tolerability through more aggressive side effect management
Nonpharmacologic techniques	Anesthetic, surgical, rehabilitative, psychologic, neurostimulatory, and complementary approaches

are yet unpredictable. There is remarkable intraindividual variability even to different drugs within the same class. This variability implies the potential utility of sequential trials in identifying the most effective therapy. The process of sequential drug trials, like the use of low initial doses and dose titration, should be explained to the patient at the start of therapy to enhance adherence and reduce the distress that may occur as treatments fail.

The use of adjuvant analgesics implies the endorsement of polypharmacy in selected patients. If a drug is added to an existing regimen and yields demonstrable benefit without cumulative side effects that otherwise impair function or quality of life, there is ample justification for continuing. This assessment must be informed by the overall goals of care. Additional pain relief at the price of some mental clouding may not be acceptable for patients whose goals include restoration of function, but may be completely appropriate for those who seek comfort as the major goal.

Clinical use of the adjuvant analgesics

The term *adjuvant analgesic* can now be applied to a large number of specific drugs in diverse classes (Table 11.2) (1). A useful clinical classification distinguishes those drug classes that may be considered multipurpose analgesics from those with more specific indications. These distinctions are derived from the nature of the supporting evidence for analgesic effects and current clinical practice. Future studies will undoubtedly provide a better empirical basis of the selection of drugs for varied pain problems.

Multipurpose analgesics

A large number of clinical trials in diverse patient populations offer evidence that some drug classes produce nonspecific analgesic effects that potentially could be relevant to pain syndromes of any type. This description clearly applies to the corticosteroids, antidepressants, and alpha-2-adrenergic agonists. In the cancer population, however, only the corticosteroids have been used as multipurpose analgesics in practice. The effectiveness of the opioids as first-line analgesics has relegated the use of the antidepressants and adrenergic agonists to those syndromes that are relatively less responsive to opioid therapy, specifically the neuropathic pain syndromes.

Corticosteroids

In the cancer population, the corticosteroids have been shown to improve pain, appetite, nausea, malaise, and

Table 11.2. *Adjuvant analgesics*

Class	Examples
Antidepressants	
Tricyclic antidepressants	Amitriptyline
	Desipramine
"Newer" antidepressants	SSRIs, SNRIs; others
	e.g., Paroxetine
	Venlafaxine
	Nefazodone
	Trazodone
	Maprotiline
Anticonvulsants	Gabapentin
	Carbamazepine
	Phenytoin
	Valproate
	Clonazepam
	Topiramate
	Lamotrigine
Oral local anesthetics	Mexiletine
	Tocainide
Alpha-2 adrenergic agonists	Clonidine
	Tizanidine
NMDA receptor antagonists	Dextromethorphan
	Ketamine
	Amantadine
Corticosteroids	Dexamethasone
	Prednisone
Topical agents	Capsaicin
	Local anesthetics
	NSAIDs
Neuroleptics	Pimozide
Miscellaneous drugs for neuropathic pain	Baclofen
	Calcitonin
Drugs for bone pain	Bisphosphonates
	Calcitonin
	Gallium nitrate
	Strontium-89
	Samarium-153
Drugs for bowel obstruction	Scopolamine
	Glycopyrrolate
	Octreotide

Abbreviations: SSRI, selective serotonin reuptake inhibitor; SNRI, selective norepinephrine reuptake inhibitor; NMDA, *N*-methyl-D-aspartate; NSAID, nonsteroidal anti-inflammatory drug.

overall quality of life (2–4). Based on extensive clinical experience, the accepted pain-related indications are refractory neuropathic pain, bone pain, pain associated with capsular expansion or duct obstruction, pain from bowel obstruction, pain caused by lymphedema, and headache caused by increased intracranial pressure. Current data are inadequate to evaluate drug-selective differences, dose-response relationships, predictors of efficacy, or the durability of favorable effects.

The analgesic effects of corticosteroids presumably result from a variety of mechanisms. Mass effect from an expanding neoplasm could be lessened by reduction of peritumoral edema, and anti-inflammatory effects could inhibit the release of compounds that sensitize or activate primary afferent nerves. Corticosteroids may have a direct salutary effect on abnormal discharges produced by injured nerves, and positive mood effects could have indirect benefits.

The risk of adverse effects associated with corticosteroid therapy increases with both the dose and duration of use. Long-term administration for pain usually is considered only for patients with advanced disease, whose limited life expectancy and overriding need for symptom control justify the risk. One large survey observed that the most common side effect is oral candidiasis (5). Potential serious adverse effects include increased risk of infection, myopathy, diabetes, fluid overload (ranging from peripheral edema to congestive heart failure), cushingoid habitus, increased risk of skin breakdown, and neuropsychiatric syndromes (ranging from mild dysphoria or mental clouding to severe anxiety or depression, or even psychosis). Patients who receive corticosteroids must be carefully monitored for these potential toxicities.

The typical low-dose approach to corticosteroid therapy involves treatment with prednisone, 5 to 10 mg, or dexamethasone, 1 to 2 mg, once or twice daily. Treatment is continued as long as potential benefits appear to outweigh adverse effects. If pain is not controlled, dose escalation should be considered. Clinical observations strongly suggest that there is a dose-response relationship for many of the pain syndromes that are the target of this therapy. Dose escalation also is associated with increasing risk of adverse effects, and the risks and benefits must be weighed carefully in each case. A therapeutic trial of a much higher dose may be appropriate, particularly if the disease is far advanced and the patient is perceived to be at the end of life.

In the setting of rapidly worsening, severe pain (sometimes called "crescendo" pain), which usually is related to neoplastic injury to nerve or bone, or to duct obstruction, a trial of a high steroid dose should be considered. Typically, an opioid is tried first, but an alternative approach is needed when quick escalation of the opioid dose does not control the pain and yields somnolence or other side effects. In this setting, the steroid regimen may begin with dexamethasone at a relatively high dose (20 to 100 mg intravenously), which is then followed by a similarly high divided daily dose (e.g., 4 mg to 24 mg orally in four divided doses). This dose is gradually tapered over weeks as an alternative analgesic approach is implemented, such as radiation therapy or neural blockade. There is extensive experience in the use of this approach (specifically, dexamethasone 100 mg intravenously, followed by 24 mg every 6 hours) in the treatment of spinal cord compression, and the risks appear to be small (6,7).

Drugs used for neuropathic pain

Numerous drugs may be considered for the management of neuropathic pain. As noted, the corticosteroids are often considered in the setting of advanced disease. Drugs in a variety of other classes also may be helpful. As noted, some of these classes, specifically the antidepressants and the alpha-2-adrenergic agonists, are actually best considered multipurpose analgesics; but in the cancer population, they are typically used for neuropathic pain that has been shown to be relatively poorly responsive to an opioid.

During the past few years, the anticonvulsant gabapentin has become a commonly selected first-line adjuvant analgesic for neuropathic pain. The evidence of efficacy in controlled clinical trials (8,9), a relatively favorable side effect profile, and the lack of hepatic metabolism and known drug-drug interactions has encouraged the early use of this drug for neuropathic pain of all types. Favorable effects and good tolerability also have been demonstrated in a series of patients with cancer-related neuropathic pain (10).

Other than gabapentin, there is no one specific drug conventionally selected for an early trial in cancer-related neuropathic pain. At the present time, drug selection might be guided by the likelihood of side effects, by cost or convenience, or by the desire to concurrently treat another symptom targeted by the drug. In most cases, drug selection is by trial and error. Typically, the more familiar classes of drugs, specifically the antidepressants and the anticonvulsants (other than gabapentin), are tried first. Given the long history of effective treatment of lancinating neuropathic pain with anticonvulsants, there is also a tendency to select one of these drugs first for pain with this type of phenomenology. Again, however, this decision making is not informed by comparative clinical trials, but rather by tradition and clinical experience.

Antidepressants

The analgesic efficacy of antidepressant drugs has been established in many disorders (11). Most studies have evaluated the tricyclic antidepressants (TCAs). Both the tertiary amine TCAs (including amitriptyline, doxepin, imipramine, and clomipramine) and the secondary amine compounds (including desipramine and nortriptyline) have analgesic effects. The supporting evidence is best for amitriptyline and desipramine (12,13).

There are few controlled trials of the selective serotonin reuptake inhibitors (SSRIs), the selective norepinephrine reuptake inhibitors, and other atypical antidepressants such as maprotiline, venlafaxine, and nefazodone (11). The limited evidence favors analgesic effects for paroxetine and venlafaxine (14,15), and there are mixed reports on others, including fluoxetine, citalopram, and trazodone. Isolated cases suggest that other drugs, such as mirtazepine and buproprion, are also potentially analgesic, and though it is reasonable to highlight those drugs that have been studied, it is likely that others may be analgesic in some patients.

The analgesia produced by antidepressant drugs is believed to be attributable to their actions on endogenous monoaminergic pain modulating systems, particularly those that use norepinephrine or serotonin. Although positive mood effects or improved sleep may be beneficial, they are not required for analgesic efficacy. There is also evidence that the tricyclic drugs may increase plasma morphine concentration through a pharmacokinetic interaction (16).

When used for neuropathic pain, the available evidence suggests that the antidepressant drugs, at least the tricyclic antidepressants, can relieve both continuous and paroxysmal neuropathic components (12,13). As noted, however, anticonvulsant medications still tend to be tried first if the predominating component of the pain is lancinating.

Amitriptyline is the best studied of the analgesic TCAs. If evidence of analgesic efficacy were the only criterion for selection, a trial of this drug would be justified in most cases. The side effect liability of amitriptyline is relatively high, however, and includes somnolence, anticholinergic effects (e.g., dry mouth, constipation, blurred vision, urinary retention), and cardiovascular effects (most commonly hypotension). Patients who are unable to tolerate amitriptyline or are predisposed to its side effects should be considered for a trial of an alternative drug. Given the potential for side effects, many clinicians begin with a trial of a secondary amine drug, specifically desipramine or nortriptyline, in medically frail patients. If a patient cannot tolerate a secondary TCA, or is so predisposed to adverse effects that the safest approach is justified, therapy can be initiated with one of the analgesic SSRIs or related drugs. For example, patients with advanced illness and those with severe heart disease, symptomatic prostatic hypertrophy, neurogenic bladder, preexisting organic brain syndrome, or narrow-angle glaucoma are appropriate for an initial trial of a non-TCA drug for pain.

The initial doses of a TCA should be low, generally 10 mg at night in the elderly and the medically frail, and 25 mg at night in others. The dose should be increased every few days by the size of the starting dose. Analgesic effects usually occur within 4 to 7 days after achieving an effective daily dose, which typically falls in the range of 50 to 150 mg for amitriptyline and desipramine. The available data suggest a dose-response relationship for analgesia, and if neither analgesia nor intolerable side effects occur as doses are increased, a trial of higher doses may be indicated. A willingness to increase the dose is also important if major depression is present and treatment for depressed mood is a goal of therapy.

Dosing data for the non-tricyclic antidepressants is limited. Nonetheless, it is likely that a dose-response relationship for analgesic effects exists for all these drugs. Accordingly, a trial of paroxetine can be slowly titrated from 10 or 20 mg/day at the start to 60 or 80 mg/day in an effort to identify analgesic effects.

Although there are no data relating a specific plasma drug concentration to analgesia, measurement of plasma drug concentration, if available, can help guide therapy. In the United States, plasma concentrations may be obtained commercially for all of the tricyclic antidepressants. If adherence to therapy is good, a relatively low concentration (compared to the reference antidepressant range) suggests poor absorption or rapid metabolism of the drug. In the absence of side effects, this finding warrants further dose escalation regardless of the administered dose. Conversely, dose escalation usually is not pursued if the concentration approaches or exceeds the upper limit of the antidepressant range. It also is prudent to obtain an electrocardiogram as higher doses are administered.

If therapy with an antidepressant is not successful, the dose should be tapered before treatment is stopped. This reduces the risk of withdrawal phenomena such as insomnia or mood change. A poor result with one antidepressant also does not predict failure with another.

Anticonvulsants and related drugs

As noted, it is common practice to select gabapentin as one of the early therapies for cancer-related neuropathic pain. Treatment usually starts with a low dose, 100 to 300 mg/day, and the dose is gradually titrated upward. In clinical practice, the effective dose range is very broad. Some patients respond to 300 mg/day in divided doses, whereas others do not reach a maximal response until the dose is increased to 6000 mg/day, and sometimes higher. In the absence of treatment-limiting side effects, dose escalation should continue until analgesic effects are maximized (i.e., a higher dose does not improve analgesia further). The maximum dose that was studied in the controlled trials was 3600 mg/day. In most cases, dose titration can be performed at intervals of just a few days.

Many anticonvulsant drugs other than gabapentin have been evaluated as treatments for neuropathic pains (17,18). Although there is almost no published experience in the treatment of cancer-related pain, the efficacy of these drugs in diverse types of neuropathic pain suggests their utility for the medically ill. Some of these drugs have been used for decades, including carbamazepine, phenytoin, divalproex, and clonazepam. The use of carbamazepine in the cancer population is limited by its potential to produce bone marrow suppression, particularly leukopenia. Clonazepam, a benzodiazepine, may be useful if pain is complicated by anxiety or insomnia.

There are more limited data supporting the analgesic efficacy of newer anticonvulsants, including lamotrigine, topiramate, tiagabine, and oxcarbazepine. In the United States, zonisamide and levtiracetam are also commercially available and may be considered in refractory cases. There is particularly good evidence that lamotrigine is analgesic (18), and clinical experience with topiramate also has been favorable. Felbamate is analgesic but should be considered only in extreme cases because of its recently recognized potential for life-threatening aplastic anemia.

All anticonvulsants are administered according to the dosing schedules typically used for seizures. Plasma concentrations of carbamazepine, phenytoin, and valproate can be monitored to ensure that maximum anticonvulsant doses have been reached if pain relief does not occur with routine dose escalation. Like other adjuvant analgesics, sequential trials may be necessary to identify the most useful agent.

The gamma-aminobutyric acid agonist, baclofen, which is marketed for spasticity and not seizures, is often discussed with the anticonvulsants because of its established analgesic efficacy in lancinating neuropathic pain (19). A long clinical experience with this drug suggests that it may be useful in all types of neuropathic pain. The therapeutic dose varies widely, ranging from 30 mg/day to more than 200 mg/day. Gradual dose escalation from a low initial dose optimizes the likelihood of benefit. Because abrupt discontinuation of this drug has been associated with seizures, tapering of the dose is necessary in the event of a poor response.

Local anesthetics

Systemic local anesthetic drugs are analgesic in neuropathic pains and other pain syndromes (20–22). There is limited published evidence of effectiveness for cancer-related neuropathic pain (23–25). In most cases, however, chronic therapy is accomplished using oral local anesthetic drugs. Oral formulations of mexiletine, tocainide, and flecainide have established analgesic efficacy (26,27) and may be valuable in the treatment of any type of neuropathic pain. Given the limited experience in the medically ill, however, these drugs usually are considered after treatment trials with anticonvulsants and antidepressants have proved ineffective. In the United States, mexiletine has been the preferred oral local anesthetic, a view that may be justified by a relatively better therapeutic index for serious cardiac and neurologic toxicity.

Treatment with mexiletine typically is started at 150 mg once or twice per day. This low initial dose will reduce the likelihood of adverse effects and allow exploration of the dose-response relationship for pain. Gradual dose escalation should proceed until favorable effects occur, side effects become troublesome, or the usual maximal daily dose of 900 mg to 1200 mg is reached. The electrocardiogram should be monitored at higher doses, and plasma mexiletine plasma concentrations can be obtained to guide dosing in the higher range. Gastrointestinal toxicity (usually nausea) and central nervous system side effects (usually dizziness) often are treatment-limiting. Patients with a history of heart disease (either myocardial dysfunction or arrhythmia) may be at increased risk of serious adverse effects, and should undergo an appropriate cardiac evaluation before oral local anesthetic therapy is initiated.

Local anesthetic infusions also may play a therapeutic role. In rare cases, long-term subcutaneous lidocaine infusion has been used to manage refractory neuropathic pain (24). Usually, however, brief intravenous infusions are tried in the hope of achieving rapid relief, which can sometimes continue for a prolonged period. These brief infusions may be used to manage acute flares of pain (20,21) or pain with a "crescendo" pattern. Because prolonged pain relief sometimes can follow a brief infusion, a brief infusion may be considered in any patient with refractory neuropathic pain as well. There also are limited data suggesting that the response to a brief lidocaine infusion predicts the analgesic efficacy of mexiletine therapy (28).

Published reports have focused on the use of lidocaine, which has been administered in a dose range of 2 to 5 mg/kg over 20 to 30 minutes (20–23). This dose range has not been systematically evaluated in the medically ill, and safety considerations may warrant a lower initial dose. There are clear concentration-dependent effects,

and the most reasonable approach may involve repeated brief infusions in gradually escalating doses.

Alpha-2-adrenergic agonists

The alpha-2-adrenergic agonists have established analgesic efficacy in a variety of pain syndromes (29–31). Like the antidepressants, these drugs may be considered multipurpose analgesics but generally are considered for neuropathic pain refractory to opioids in the cancer population. In the United States, tizanidine and clonidine are used for pain. Clonidine is approved for epidural use and has been shown to have better efficacy for neuropathic than nociceptive pain by this route (31).

Given limited experience in the medically ill and the likelihood that a relatively small minority of patients will experience a strong analgesic response (29), the adrenergic agonists also are best considered after trials with other drugs have failed. Tizanidine is less hypotensive than clonidine and should be considered first for a systemic trial. The analgesic dose range of tizanidine appears to be between 4 mg/day and 40 mg/day; higher doses may be tried if effects are inadequate and the drug is tolerated. A clonidine trial can be implemented by either the oral or the transdermal route, and the effective dose range appears to between 0.2 mg/day and 0.6 mg/day for most patients. Higher doses may be tried but are often poorly tolerated because of somnolence, dry mouth, and dizziness.

NMDA receptor antagonists

The N-methyl-D-aspartate (NMDA) receptor complex is involved with the development of both neuropathic pain and opioid tolerance (32). NMDA-receptor antagonists are undergoing intensive investigation as potential analgesics and coanalgesics for this reason. Three NMDA antagonists are commercially available in the United States: the dissociative anesthetic ketamine, the antitussive dextromethorphan, and the antiviral amantadine. All of these drugs are now considered for refractory neuropathic pain.

There are both controlled trials and case reports that establish the analgesic efficacy of intravenous and oral ketamine (33–36). The side effect liability of this drug is relatively high, however, and includes disturbing nightmares, confusion, and periods of dissociation. These effects can occur even at the subanesthetic doses used to treat pain. This possibility suggests that ketamine should be used cautiously and generally should be tried only after other interventions have failed. The doses reported to be useful have ranged 0.1 to 1.5 mg/kg per hour, administered via continuous intravenous or subcutaneous infusion. When administered orally, the injectable formulation is used, and the starting dose is usually 10 to 25 mg/day. Doses are escalated gradually. Some clinicians recommend concurrent administration of a benzodiazepine to reduce the risk of side effects.

Dextromethorphan has also been shown to be analgesic in a controlled trial (37). At the present time, the drug may be administered using a commercially available antitussive that contains neither alcohol nor guaifenesin. The starting dose can be as high as 120 to 240 mg/day in three to four divided doses. This dose should be increased gradually. Doses higher than 1 g have been administered safely, at least for the short term.

A single dose controlled trial of amantadine demonstrated that this drug can have analgesic effects in cancer-related neuropathic pain (38). Additional experience with chronic administration is needed to determine whether the drug can play a role in medically ill patients with opioid-refractory pain.

Neuroleptics

Pimozide may be analgesic in patients with lancinating or paroxysmal pains (39), but side effects are common, and the drug is seldom used. The data supporting the use of other neuroleptics, such as fluphenazine and haloperidol, are very meager. Given the potential for side effects, the use of these drugs is best limited to the treatment of delirium. Methotrimeprazine, a phenothiazine neuroleptic, has established analgesic effects but is no longer commercially available in the United States.

Benzodiazepines

As described previously, the anticonvulsant clonazepam often is used to treat neuropathic pains. A survey of cancer patients with neuropathic pains suggested that alprazolam may also have analgesic effects (40). Although there is no evidence that other benzodiazepines are analgesic, patients with cancer pain also commonly experience anxiety and muscle spasms, phenomena that may exacerbate the intensity of pain and respond well to diazepam or other drugs in this class. The salutary effects of the benzodiazepines, therefore, may relate to a variety of effects, and it may be impossible to determine the degree to which psychotropic or primary analgesic actions contribute to this outcome. The potential for somnolence and cognitive impairment must be monitored carefully during treatment.

Other systemic drugs for neuropathic pain

Several controlled trials have suggested that calcitonin might be effective in diverse types of neuropathic pain

(41,42). Although the mechanism is not understood and confirmation in additional trials is warranted, the convenience and low side effect profile associated with the commercially available intranasal formulation justifies a trial in patients with difficult neuropathic pain syndromes. Dose-response has not been examined and duration of effect have not been examined. Based solely on anecdotal observations, it may be reasonable to begin with a single 200 IU intranasal dose and, if not effective, increase the dose several times before concluding that the treatment is ineffective.

Neuropathic pain associated with focal autonomic changes suggests the diagnosis of complex regional pain syndrome (formerly known as reflex sympathetic dystrophy or causalgia) (43). This pattern signals an increased likelihood that sympathetic nervous function is involved in the pathophysiology of the pain. In this situation, a variety of drugs have been tried, including calcium channel blockers such as verapamil, beta blockers such as propranolol, and alpha-adrenergic blockers such as prazocin and phenoxybenzamine. None of these drugs is supported by data from controlled clinical trials, and their use in the medically ill is uncommon.

Topical analgesics

Topical analgesic therapies may particularly benefit medically ill patients with chronic pain by providing pain relief that complements a systemic analgesic regimen without the risk of additional side effects. Topical therapies include local anesthetics, nonsteroidal anti-inflammatory drugs (NSAIDs), and capsaicin (44).

Recently, a patch that allows cutaneous application of concentrated lidocaine was approved for use in patients with postherpetic neuralgia (45). This formulation appears to be well accepted by patients and is now considered for a trial in patients with all types of neuropathic pain. This patch, which provides a soft protective cover and presumably increases the contact time between the anesthetic and the skin, may increase the utility of the topical anesthetics for pain management. The patch has been approved with instructions to apply it 12 hours per day; many patients find it useful if worn continuously.

Cutaneous anesthesia can be produced by topical application of local anesthetics, including a commercially available 1:1 mixture of lidocaine and prilocaine (known as an eutectic mixture of local anesthetics [EMLA])(46) and high-concentration lidocaine (47). Although this phenomenon may offer a theoretical advantage, there is no evidence that cutaneous anesthesia is prerequisite to analgesia. The lidocaine patch, for example, does not produce reliable anesthesia in the area applied. If an anesthetic cream or gel is considered for a trial, therefore, it is reasonable to begin with a lower concentration (e.g., lidocaine 5% cream) and then proceed to the more costly EMLA or compounded high-concentration cream if this is ineffective. Dosing frequency and method for creams and gels are empiric. If possible, these formulations should be applied under an occlusive dressing, which increases skin penetration and could theoretically augment analgesic efficacy.

Theoretically, topical local anesthetics should be preferred in the treatment of neuropathic pains that are peripherally generated, particularly those that are associated with allodynia. In practice, however, the relative safety of the approach suggests that a trial of the lidocaine patch or an anesthetic cream may be considered for all types of neuropathic pain.

There is substantial evidence that topical NSAIDs can be effective for soft tissue pain and perhaps joint pain (48). A trial of a compounded formulation containing diclofenac, ketoprofen, or another NSAID is reasonable when pain in the medically ill is related to chronic soft tissue injury. Although these drugs are likely to be safe, there is little support for a trial of their efficacy for neuropathic pain.

Patients with neuropathic pain caused by peripheral nerve injury also can be considered for a trial of topical capsaicin. Capsaicin depletes peptides such as substance P in primary afferent nociceptors. Although efficacy in neuropathic pain has been suggested in both open-label and controlled studies (49–51), anecdotal experience has been mixed. A therapeutic trial of the high-concentration formulation (0.075%) is reasonable in patients with neuropathic pains presumed to have a strong peripheral input. An adequate trial is generally believed to require four applications daily for 1 month. Burning that occurs on application may remit over time or be managed by some patients using an oral or topical analgesic. Sometimes, a switch to a lower concentration formulation (0.05%) is helpful. Topical capsaicin has also been demonstrated to have efficacy in painful arthropathy (52) and mucositis pain (53).

Other drugs have been compounded into topical formulations and are now being applied in an empirical fashion. These include ketamine, amitriptyline, or other antidepressants, varied anticonvulsants, and a variety of alternative anesthetics. To date, there is no scientific support for the efficacy of these formulations. Nonetheless, some experienced clinicians perceive benefit from mixtures and offer trials to patients with challenging neuro-

pathic pains. The cost of this therapy, the low risk of toxicity, and the lack of proven efficacy must be balanced against these anecdotal reports of benefit on a case-by-case basis.

Drugs used for bone pain

Radiation therapy is usually considered when bone pain is focal and poorly controlled with an opioid, or is associated with impending fracture. Symptomatic relief also may be provided using an opioid, or an opioid combined with an NSAID or corticosteroid. These drugs are appropriate for multifocal bone pain as well, as are several other adjuvant analgesics. These include bisphosphonate compounds (54,55), calcitonin (56,57), gallium nitrate (58), and bone-seeking radionuclides (59,60).

There have been no comparative trials of these adjuvant analgesics for bone pain, and the selection of one over another is usually based on convenience, patient preference, and several clinical indicators. Based on the abundance of supporting evidence, the benefit to nonpainful skeletal comorbidities (such as fracture rate), and convenience, the bisphosphonates are generally preferred as the first-line approach. There is strong evidence that certain bisphosphonates, including pamidronate and clodronate, can be analgesic. Pamidronate is available in the United States and usually is administered via brief infusion at a dose of 60 mg. Doses are typically repeated every other week, and two or three doses are needed to determine efficacy.

There is strong evidence that treatment with oral clodronate can be analgesic in patients with painful bone metastases (61). In the United States, two other oral bisphosphonates are commercially available, alendronate and risendronate. Although these drugs have not been adequately studied for this indication, it is likely that they can be effective and should be considered for patients who are unable to be treated with pamidronate. Failure to respond to one of these drugs should not exclude a trial with pamidronate.

Data supporting the use of calcitonin and gallium nitrate are very limited. Evidence is much better for the bone-seeking radiopharmaceuticals, strontium-89, and samarium-153. These drugs should be considered for patients with refractory multifocal pain caused by osteoblastic lesions or lesions with an osteoblastic component. Samarium-153 allows imaging with bone scintigraphy during treatment for bone pain. Patients who receive these drugs should have life expectancies greater than 3 months, adequate bone marrow reserve, and no further planned therapy with myelosuppressive chemotherapy. Patients with a platelet count below 60,000 or a white blood cell count below 2400 generally should not be treated. The onset of effect is often slow (2 weeks or longer), and peak effects may not be attained for more than 1 month. Some patients experience a flare of pain before analgesic effects occur. The chief adverse effect is bone marrow suppression, with thrombocytopenia that may be irreversible.

Drugs used for the pain of bowel obstruction

Patients with malignant bowel obstruction may benefit from aggressive pharmacotherapy to control pain and other symptoms, including distention, nausea, and vomiting (62,63). This treatment is particularly important if the patient is not a candidate for surgical decompression. Anecdotal reports suggest that anticholinergic drugs, the somatostatin analog octreotide, and corticosteroids may be useful adjuvant analgesics in this setting. The optimal use of these drugs may minimize the number of patients who must be considered for chronic drainage using nasogastric or percutaneous catheters.

Anticholinergic drugs presumably reduce intestinal motility and intraluminal secretions (64,65). Scopolamine (hydrobromide and butylbromide), atropine, and glycopyrrolate have been used effectively for symptom control. Scopolamine butylbromide and glycopyrrolate have lesser penetration through the blood-brain barrier and, therefore, may be less likely to produce central nervous system toxicity.

Patients with refractory pain from bowel obstruction may also be considered for a trial of the somatostatin analog octreotide (66). This drug inhibits the secretion of gastric, pancreatic, and intestinal secretions and reduces gastrointestinal motility.

Patients with bowel obstruction may benefit from corticosteroid therapy (67,68). No information exists concerning the most effective drug, dose, or dosing regimen. Like the many other pain-related indications for these drugs, bowel obstruction is managed empirically by offering an initial trial, usually with a loading dose, then continuing treatment in patients who respond for as long as needed. One case series, for example, described the use of dexamethasone in a dose range of 8 to 60 mg/day (67).

Conclusion

There have been extraordinary advances in analgesic pharmacology during the past few decades. Drugs that have been commercialized for diverse purposes have been discovered to be analgesic. Although the opioid analgesics continue to be the mainstay therapy for moderate to severe cancer pain, the availability of these other drugs provides a means to achieve better pain control when poor opioid responsiveness is encountered. In some cases, the effectiveness of these therapies suggests that they should be positioned early in the treatment strategy.

References

1. Portenoy RK. Adjuvant analgesics in pain management. In: Doyle D, Hanks GW, MacDonald N, eds. Oxford textbook of palliative medicine, 2nd ed. Oxford: Oxford University Press, 1998:361–90.
2. Bruera E, Roca E, Cedaro L, et al. Action of oral methylprednisolone in terminal cancer patients: a prospective randomized double-blind study. Cancer Treat Rep 69:751–4, 1985.
3. Della Cuna GR, Pellegrini A, Piazzi M. Effect of methylprednisolone sodium succinate on quality of life in preterminal cancer patients: a placebo-controlled, multicenter study. The Methylprednisolone Preterminal Cancer Study Group. Eur J Cancer Clin Oncol 25:1817–21, 1989.
4. Tannock I, Gospodarowicz M, Meakin W, et al. Treatment of metastatic prostatic cancer with low-dose prednisone: evaluation of pain and quality of life as pragmatic indices of response. J Clin Oncol 7:590–7, 1989.
5. Hanks GW, Trueman T, Twycross RG. Corticosteroids in terminal cancerùa prospective analysis of current practice. Postgrad Med J 59:702–6, 1983.
6. Greenberg HS, Kim J, Posner JB. Epidural spinal cord compression from metastatic tumor: results with a new treatment protocol. Ann Neurol 8:361–6, 1980.
7. Breitbart W, Stiefel F, Kornblith AB, Pannulo S. Neuropsychiatric disturbance in cancer patients with epidural spinal cord compression receiving high dose corticosteroids: a prospective comparison study. Psychooncology 2:233–45, 1993.
8. Backonja M, Beydoun A, Edwards KR, et al. Gabapentin for the symptomatic treatment of painful neuropathy in patients with diabetic mellitus: a randomized controlled trial. JAMA 280:1831–36, 1998.
9. Rowbotham M, Harden N, Stacey B, et al. Gabapentin for the treatment of postherpetic neuralgia: a randomized controlled trial. JAMA 280:1837–42, 1998.
10. Caraceni A, Zecca E, Martini C, De Conno F. Gabapentin as an adjuvant to opioid analgesia for neuropathic cancer pain J Pain Symptom Manage 17:441–5, 1999.
11. Monks R, Merskey H. Psychotropic drugs. In: Wall PD, Melzack R, eds., Textbook of pain, 4th ed. New York: Churchill Livingstone, 1999:1155–86.
12. Kishore-Kumar R, Max MB, Schafer SC, et al. Desipramine relieves postherpetic neuralgia. Clin Pharmacol Ther 47:305–12, 1990.

13. Max MB, Lynch SA, Muir J, et al. Effects of desipramine, amitriptyline, and fluoxetine on pain in diabetic neuropathy. N Engl J Med 326:1250–6, 1992.

14. Goldenberg DL, Schmid C, Ruthazer R, et al. A randomized double-blind crossover trial of fluoxetine and amitriptyline in the treatment of fibromyalgia. Arthritis Rheum 39:1852–9, 1996.

15. Sindrup SH, Gram LF, Brosen K, et al. The selective serotonin reuptake inhibitor paroxetine is effective in the treatment of diabetic neuropathy symptoms. Pain 42:135–44, 1990.

16. Ventafridda V, Bianchi M, Ripamonti C, et al. Studies on the effects of antidepressant drugs on the antinociceptive action of morphine and on plasma morphine in rat and man. Pain 43(2):155–62, 1990.

17. Tremont-Lukats IW, Megeff C, Backonja MM. Anticonvulsants for neuropathic pain syndromes: mechanisms of action and place in therapy. Drugs 60:1029–52, 2000.

18. Vestergaard K, Andersen G, Gottrup H, et al. Lamotrigine for central poststroke pain: a randomized controlled trial. Neurology 56:184–90, 2001.

19. Fromm GH, Terrence CF, Chattha AS. Baclofen in the treatment of trigeminal neuralgia: double-blind study and long-term follow-up. Ann Neurol 15:240–4, 1984.

20. Galer BS, Miller KV, Rowbotham MC. Response to intravenous lidocaine infusion differs based on clinical diagnosis and site of nervous system injury. Neurology 43:1233–5, 1993.

21. Rowbotham MC, Reisner-Keller LA, Fields HL. Both intravenous lidocaine and morphine reduce the pain of postherpetic neuralgia. Neurology 41:1024–8, 1991.

22. Kastrup J, Petersen P, Dejgard A, et al. Intravenous lidocaine infusion—a new treatment for chronic painful diabetic neuropathy. Pain 28:69–75, 1987.

23. Elleman K, Sjogren P, Banning A, et al. Trial of intravenous lidocaine on painful neuropathy in cancer patients. Clin J Pain 5:291–4, 1989.

24. Brose WG, Cousins MJ. Subcutaneous lidocaine for treatment of neuropathic cancer pain. Pain 45:145–8, 1991.

25. Chong SF, Bretscher ME, Mailliard JA, et al. Pilot study evaluation local anesthetics administered systemically for treatment of pain in patients with advanced cancer. J Pain Symptom Manage 13:112–7, 1997.

26. Dejgard A, Petersen P, Kastrup J. Mexiletine for treatment of chronic painful diabetic neuropathy. Lancet 1:9–11, 1988.

27. Lindstrom P, Lindblom U. The analgesic effect of tocainide in trigeminal neuralgia. Pain 28:45–50, 1987.

28. Galer BS, Harle J, Rowbotham MC. Response to intravenous lidocaine infusion predicts subsequent response to oral mexiletine: a prospective study. J Pain Symptom Manage 12:161–7, 1996.

29. Byas-Smith MG, Max MB, Muir J, Kingman A. Transdermal clonidine compared to placebo in painful diabetic neuropathy using a two-stage "enriched enrollment" design. Pain 60:267–74, 1995.

30. Fogelholm R, Murros K. Tizanidine in chronic tension-type headache: a placebo-controlled, double-blind cross-over study. Headache 32:509–13, 1992.

31. Eisenach JC, DuPen S, Dubois M, et al. Epidural clonidine analgesia for intractable cancer pain. The Epidural Clonidine Study Group. Pain 61:391–400, 1995.

32. Price DD, Mayer DJ, Mao J, Caruso FS. NMDA-receptor antagonists and opioid receptor interactions as related to analgesia and tolerance. J Pain Symptom Manage 19:S7–S11, 2000.

33. Mathisen LC, Skjelbred P, Skoglund LA, et al. Effect of ketamine, an NMDA receptor inhibitor, in acute and chronic orofacial pain. Pain 61:215–20, 1995.

34. Cherry DA, Plummer JL, Gourlay GK, et al. Ketamine as an adjunct to morphine in the treatment of pain. Pain 62:119–21, 1995.

35. Persson J, Axelsson G, Hallin RG, et al. Beneficial effects of ketamine in a chronic pain state with allodynia, possibly due to central sensitization. Pain 60:217–22, 1995.

36. Nikolajsen L, Hansen PO, Jensen TS: Oral ketamine therapy in the treatment of postamputation stump pain. Acta Anaesthesiol Scand 41:427–9, 1997.

37. Nelson KA, Park KM, Robinovitz E, et al. High-dose oral dextromethorphan versus placebo in painful diabetic neuropathy and postherpetic neuralgia. Neurology 48:1212–18, 1997.

38. Pud D, Eisenberg E, Spitzer A, et al. The NMDA receptor antagonist amantadine reduces surgical neuropathic pain in cancer patients: a double-blind, randomized, placebo-controlled trial. Pain 75:349–54, 1998.

39. Lechin F, van der Dijs B, Lechin ME, et al. Pimozide therapy for trigeminal neuralgia. Arch Neurol 46:960–3, 1989.

40. Fernandez F, Adams F, Holmes VF. Analgesic effect of alprazolam in patients with chronic, organic pain of malignant origin. J Clin Psychopharmacol 7:167–9, 1987.

41. Gobelet C, Waldburger M, Meier JL. The effect of adding calcitonin to physical treatment on reflex sympathetic dystrophy. Pain 48:171–5, 1992.

42. Jaeger H, Maier C. Calcitonin in phantom limb pain: a double-blind study. Pain 48:21–7, 1992.

43. Galer BS, Schwartz L, Allen RJ. Complex regional pain syndromes Type I: reflex sympathetic dystrophy and Type II: causalgia. In: Loeser JD, Butler SH, Chapman CR, Turk DC, eds. Bonica's management of pain. Philadelphia: Lippincott, 2001:388–411.

44. Rowbotham MC. Topical analgesic agents. In: Fields HL, Liebeskind JC, eds. Pharmacological approaches to the treatment of chronic pain: new concepts and critical issues. Seattle: IASP Press, 1994:211–29.

45. Galer BS, Rowbotham MC, Perander J, Friedman E. Topical lidocaine patch relieves postherpetic neuralgia more effectively than a vehicle topical patch: results of an enriched enrollment study. Pain 80:533–8, 1999.

46. Ehrenstrom Reiz GM, Reiz SL. EMLA—a eutectic mixture of local anaesthetics for topical anaesthesia. Acta Anaesthesiol Scand 26:596–8, 1982.

47. Rowbotham MC, Davies PS, Fields HL. Topical lidocaine gel relieves postherpetic neuralgia. Ann Neurol 37:246–53, 1995.

48. Vaile JH, Davis P. Topical NSAIDs for musculoskeletal conditions. A review of the literature. Drugs 56:783–99, 1998.

49. Watson CP, Evans RJ, Watt VR. Post-herpetic neuralgia and topical capsaicin. Pain 33:333–40, 1988.

50. Tandan R, Lewis GA, Krusinski PB, et al. Topical capsaicin in painful diabetic neuropathy. Controlled study with long-term follow-up. Diabetes Care 15:8–14, 1992.

51. Ellison N, Loprinzi CL, Kugler J, et al. Phase III placebo-controlled trial of capsaicin cream in the management of surgical neuropathic pain in cancer patients. J Clin Oncol 15:2974–80, 1997.

52. Towheed TE, Hochberg MC. A systematic review of randomized controlled trials of pharmacological therapy in osteoarthritis of the knee, with an emphasis on trial methodology. Semin Arthritis Rheum 26:755–70, 1997.

53. Berger A, Henderson M, Nadoolman W, et al. Oral capsaicin provides temporary relief for oral mucositis pain secondary to chemotherapy/radiation therapy [published erratum appears in J Pain Symptom Manage 11(5):331, 1996] J Pain Symptom Manage 10:243–8, 1995.

54. Mannix K, Ahmedzai SH, Anderson H, et al. Using bisphosphonates to control the pain of bone metastases: evidence-based guidelines for palliative care. Palliat Med 14:455–61, 2000.

55. Hortobagyi GN, Theriault RL, Porter L, et al. Efficacy of pamidronate in reducing skeletal complications in patients with breast cancer and lytic bone metastases. N Engl J Med 335:1785–91, 1996.

56. Mystakidou K, Befon S, Hondros K, et al. Continuous subcutaneous administration of high-dose salmon calcitonin in bone metastasis: pain control and beta-endorphin plasma levels. J Pain Symptom Manage 18:323–30, 1999.

57. Roth A, Kolaric K. Analgesic activity of calcitonin in patients with painful osteolytic metastases of breast cancer. Results of a controlled randomized study. Oncology 43:283–7, 1986.

58. Warrell RP Jr, Lovett D, Dilmanian FA, et al. Low-dose gallium nitrate for prevention of osteolysis in myeloma: results of a pilot randomized study. J Clin Oncol 11:2443–50, 1993.

59. Porter AT, McEwan AJ, Powe JE, et al. Results of a randomized phase-III trial to evaluate the efficacy of strontium-89 adjuvant to local field external beam irradiation in the management of endocrine resistant metastatic prostate cancer. Int J Radiat Oncol Biol Phys 25:805–13, 1993.

60. Serafini AN, Houston SJ, Resche I, et al. Palliation of pain associated with metastatic bone cancer using samarium-153 lexidronam: a double-blind placebo-controlled clinical trial. J Clin Oncol 16:1574–81, 1998.

61. Heidenreich A, Hofmann R, Engelmann, UHL. The use of bisphosphonate for the palliative treatment of painful bone metastasis due to hormone refractory prostate cancer. J Urol 165:136–40, 2001.

62. Ripamonti C. Management of bowel obstruction in advanced cancer patients. J Pain Symptom Manage 9:193–200, 1994.

63. Baines M, Oliver DJ, Carter RL. Medical management of intestinal obstruction in patients with advanced malignant disease. A clinical and pathological study. Lancet 2:990–3, 1985.

64. Ripamonti C, Mercadante S, Groff L, et al. Role of octreotide, scopolamine butylbromide, and hydration in symptom control of patients with inoperable bowel obstruction and nasogastric tubes: a prospective randomized trial. J Pain Symptom Manage 19:23–34, 2000.

65. Muir JC, von Gunten CF. Antisecretory agents in gastrointestinal obstruction. Clin Geriatr Med 16:327–34, 2000.

66. Mercadante S, Spoldi E, Caraceni A, et al. Octreotide in relieving gastrointestinal symptoms due to bowel obstruction. Palliat Med 7:295–9, 1993.

67. Fainsinger RL, Spachynski K, Hanson J, et al. Symptom control in terminally ill patients with malignant bowel obstruction (MBO). J Pain Symptom Manage 9:12–18, 1994.

68. Philip J, Lickiss N, Grant PT, Hacker NF. Corticosteroids in the management of bowel obstruction on a gynecological oncology unit. Gynecol Oncol 74:68–73, 1999.

SECTION IV NONPHARMACOLOGICAL APPROACHES

12 Anesthesiological procedures

SUELLEN M. WALKER AND MICHAEL J. COUSINS
Royal North Shore Hospital, Australia

Introduction

Improvements in the understanding of the pathophysiology of pain, increased availability of pharmacological agents, adoption of different modes of drug administration, and development of comprehensive multidisciplinary care have all contributed to increasing the number of patients with effective control of cancer pain. The Guidelines for Cancer Pain Relief established by the World Health Organization (1) have been useful in emphasizing the effectiveness of oral morphine as a mainstay of cancer pain treatment. Although the analgesic "ladder" drew attention to the importance of using opioids of increasing potency and adding adjuvant therapies as necessary (2), the strategy today is to tailor the ingredients of a multimodal oral regimen to each patient's requirements at a particular stage of the disease. However, 10%–20% of patients will require more intensive measures to control pain, particularly in the terminal phases of their illness. Treatment options include primary therapies such as radiotherapy, chemotherapy, and surgery to reduce pain in specific cases; parenteral or spinal administration of analgesic agents; neurolytic blocks; and surgical neuroablative procedures. In a prospective study of 2118 patients with cancer pain managed according to WHO Guidelines, anesthetic nerve blocks were performed in 8% of patients, neurolytic nerve blocks in 3%, and spinal analgesic administration (epidural and intrathecal) in 3% of patients (2). The true incidence of patients requiring interventional analgesic techniques remains unknown, as the size of the group from which patients in reported series are selected is unknown, and inclusion criteria for spinal therapies or nerve blocks vary in different centers according to local experience, expertise, and referral patterns. Invasive procedures should be considered in patients whose pain is uncontrolled by other means, or if high-dose oral therapies are associated with unacceptable side effects (3,4). There is a growing consensus that intraspinal opioid therapy, which has the advantages of reversibility and a more favorable risk to benefit ratio, may be warranted before irreversible neuroablative approaches (5,6).

Peripheral neural blockade

Local anesthetic agents

Local anesthetic agents have a long history of use for anesthesia and analgesia because of their ability to reversibly inhibit increases in sodium channel permeability and impair axonal conduction. Local anesthetics may be administered at multiple sites along the neuraxis, and the effects and potential complications will vary according to the route used.

Local anesthetics have significant systemic toxic effects if an excessive dose is given or the dose is inadvertently injected intravascularly (e.g., during epidural injection). The relative toxicity of different agents varies and is also influenced by the rate of injection and rapidity with which a particular plasma concentration is achieved. Central nervous system symptoms range from light-headedness and perioral numbness at low plasma concentrations to visual and auditory disturbances, muscular twitching, loss of consciousness, convulsions, coma, and respiratory arrest at high concentrations (7,8). Cardiovascular toxicity relates to effects of local anesthetics on the electrophysiology of cardiac muscle with resultant arrhythmias, depression of cardiac muscle contractility, and a biphasic action on peripheral vasculature (vasodilataion at high concentrations). Preparations containing S-bupivacaine rather than the racemic mixture are associated with reduced cardiac toxicity, as is the newer agent ropivacaine (marketed as a solution containing only the S-isomer) (7). In a crossover trial of intrathecal bupivacaine and ropivacaine in one patient with cancer pain, no differences were seen in pain intensity, level of sensory disturbances, motor weakness, or required number of rescue boluses (9). Further long-term studies are required.

Systemic absorption of lower non-toxic doses of local anesthetics may contribute to an analgesic effect, as additional effects of lignocaine on the N-methyl-D-aspartate (NMDA) and neurokinin-1 receptor have been identified (10). These factors must be considered in the interpretation of diagnostic blocks, or may be used for a therapeutic effect. Systemically administered local anesthetic, such as subcutaneous infusion of lignocaine, has been shown to improve management of refractory neuropathic pain in patients with cancer (11).

Peripheral local anesthetic blockade

Neural blockade can have diagnostic, prognostic, and therapeutic roles in cancer therapy. Before neuroablative procedures are carried out, local anesthetic blocks can allow the patient to experience the sensation of numbness, as some patients will prefer the pain to the complete loss of sensation (12). However, a good response to a local anesthetic block is not always prognostic of a long-term favorable response to an ablative surgical or neurolytic procedure (4,12).

Subcutaneous infiltration of local anesthetic provides localized analgesia and anesthesia, but the duration of action is limited, and injection (particularly of adrenaline-containing solutions) is painful. Peripheral nerve blocks may be useful in managing acute pain exacerbations (e.g., fractured femur), but single blocks have little to offer the longer term care of patients with cancer pain. Prolongation of peripheral local anesthetic actions can be achieved with continuous infusion via catheters (e.g., plexus or epidural catheters). Future development of local anesthetic preparations, such as microspheres or slow-release suspension formulations, may allow a more prolonged effect after single injections.

Catheter techniques Percutaneous catheters can be sited near peripheral nerves to allow repeated administration or infusion of local anesthetic and prolonged sensory blockade. Complications may relate to effects of the local anesthetic (incorrect dosage or accumulation of local anesthetic may lead to systemic toxicity) or to technical complications of the catheter technique (trauma, subsequent infection, hematoma formation, dislodgement of the catheter, mechanical failure of the infusion device). Case reports of the use of brachial plexus, psoas, sheath, femoral, and sciatic nerve sheath catheters described benefit for periods of days or weeks in patients with cancer pain (13–15). Evaluation of long-term benefits and complications requires further studies.

Local anesthetic preparations Bupivacaine has been formulated in a number of slow-release preparations that have the potential to enhance the efficacy and safety of local anesthetic block. Delayed release and uptake of the local anesthetic results in lower peak plasma levels in animal studies (16,17), and therefore the risk of systemic toxicity is reduced. In addition, a prolonged local anesthetic effect and sensory block (17,18) may be achieved after wound infiltration or peripheral nerve blockade, which would reduce the need for catheter insertion and ongoing infusions. The duration of sensory block varies with the nature of the formulation. Formulations being investigated include liposomal vesicles (19) and microspheres of varying composition (20,21). Dexamethasone in the suspending solution of the microspheres prolongs the block by up to 5 times, but the mechanism is unclear (22,23). At this time, human toxicity studies after peripheral nerve blockade with such preparations are incomplete (24). In one case report of epidural administration for cancer pain management, analgesia was prolonged from 4 hours with a plain bupivacaine solution to 11 hours with a liposomal preparation, which is of little additional benefit in a patient with ongoing pain (25). The main application of these preparations may be in the management of acute and postoperative pain rather than chronic cancer pain.

Butyl aminobenzoate is an amino-ester local anesthetic with low water solubility, but when formulated as a suspension with polysorbate (BAB suspension) and/or polyethylene glycol (butamben), there is slow and prolonged release of the drug (26). BAB suspension also has an apparent selectivity for A-delta and C fibers, with minimal motor blockade and sparing of bowel and bladder function following epidural administration (27,28). This may relate in part to confinement of the suspension within the epidural space, as the permeability of the dura for BAB suspension is much lower than other anaesthetics such as lignocaine and bupivacaine (29). Prolonged analgesia has been observed after peripheral nerve blocks (30) and repeated epidural administration (31) of butamben suspension in animal models. Analgesia has been provided for weeks to months in patients with cancer pain by a series of epidural injections of 10% (27,28) or 5% (32) butamben suspension. A total of 48 of 67 cancer patients were successfully treated with 5% butamben epidural and/or peripheral nerve blocks, with a 74% mean reduction in opioid requirements, and a median duration of pain relief of 12 weeks (range 1–96 weeks) (32).

Neurolytic blocks

Neurolytic blocks may be suitable for patients who have limited life expectancy, well-localized pain that has been difficult to control with other measures (4,33,34), and disease that is unresponsive to further definitive antitumor therapy (35). Careful evaluation of the patient is essential and includes determination of the risk-benefit ratio for each patient. Relief of intractable pain and reduction in analgesic requirements occurs after successful blocks (36) and may be a sufficient advantage for some patients to accept potential side effects and complications.

Neurolytic agents such as phenol and alcohol produce demyelination and degeneration. Phenol has local anesthetic as well as neurolytic effects, resulting in painless injection, but the block produced by phenol tends to be less profound and of shorter duration than alcohol (34).

Peripheral neurolytic block Neurolytic block of peripheral nerves has limited application. The current agents (alcohol, phenol, glycerol) are non-selective for sensory nerves, and there is a lack of efficacy data from controlled studies for most peripheral sites of injection. Disadvantages of peripheral neurolytic blocks relate to:

1. Failure due to overlapping sensory innervation
2. Potential for motor deficit and unintended damage to adjacent tissues
3. Impermanence resulting from nerve regeneration
4. Development of neuralgia and deafferentation pain. Neuropathic pain is reported to develop in 14%–30% of patients after peripheral neurolytic blocks (34).

Percutaneous glycerol injection into the trigeminal ganglion has a clinical role in the management of refractory tic douloureux. High initial success rates have been reported (75%–90%) (34), and there appears to be a low incidence of corneal anaesthesia and anaesthesia dolorosa. Maxillary and mandibular nerve blocks have been used to control pain resulting from tumor-invading structures innervated by these branches of the trigeminal nerve (34). Initial pain relief has been reported in 86% of patients (37), but recurrence of pain occurs in up to 30% of patients.

Neurolytic thoracic paravertebral block was beneficial in a small number of patients with cancer pain restricted to a few thoracic dermatomes, but repeated blocks were required and the benefit was often of short duration (38).

Subarachnoid neurolytic block The aim of intrathecal neurolytic blocks is to produce a chemical posterior rhizotomy and interrupt pain pathways from the affected area. To avoid indiscriminate neural injury, extreme attention must be paid to the technical aspects of these procedures (patient selection, injection site, volume and concentration of injectate, patient position) (34,39).

Results of neurolytic blocks are difficult to assess because of the subjective nature of patient response and also differences in type of tumor, and sites and doses of alcohol injected. Review of large series suggested 60% good relief, 21% fair relief, and 18% poor relief (34,40). Patt and Reddy (39) reported 56 intrathecal neurolytic blocks in 37 patients with excellent to good relief in 73%, fair in 13%, poor in 11%, and unavailable in 3%. Duration of pain relief varies with mean duration between 2 weeks and 3 months.

Complication rates range from 1% to 14% (34). The action of neurolytic substances on other nerve fibers may result in motor paresis, loss of sphincter function, impairment of touch and proprioception, and dysesthesias. The efficacy of neurolytic blocks is reduced in the presence of previous radiation or inflammation in the region of nerve roots. Deafferentation or neuropathic pain may not be improved, or may be exacerbated by neurolytic blocks. Nerve regeneration, an incomplete block, or progression of disease beyond the area innervated by the nerves initially blocked may result in recurrent pain that requires a repeat neurolytic block (33,35) or alternative therapy.

Sympathetic plexus blockade

The role of the sympathetic nervous system in a range of pain states, including neuropathic and visceral pain, is being increasingly recognized. The peripheral sympathetic nervous system begins as efferent preganglionic fibers in the intermediolateral column of the spinal cord, passing out in the ventral roots from T1–L2 to form the sympathetic chain at the side of the vertebral bodies. The preganglionic fibers pass a variable distance to reach ganglia in the chain, and postganglionic fibers are widely distributed. The sympathetic chain also receives afferent visceral fibers that conduct pain from the head, neck and upper extremity (cervicothoracic or stellate ganglion), abdominal viscera (celiac plexus), lower limbs and lower abdominal viscera (lumbar sympathetic ganglia), pelvic organs (hypogastric plexus), and perineum (ganglion impar) (41). Because the sympathetic ganglia are separated from somatic nerves (except in the thoracic region), it is possible to achieve selective blockade of sympathetic fibers at these sites without effects on motor or cutaneous sensory function. Neurolytic blocks of the sympathetic plexus can be effective in controlling visceral cancer pain (42). Details of the techniques for sympathetic blockade are found elsewhere (41).

Celiac plexus block

The efficacy of neurolytic celiac plexus block (NCPB) for upper abdominal pain associated with cancer is supported by a meta-analysis of published series (43). Studies included predominantly patients with pancreatic cancer (63%), and blocks were performed with 50 to 150 ml of 50%–100% alcohol. Good to excellent pain relief was reported in 89% of patients in the first 2 weeks. Partial to complete relief was maintained in 90% of patients at 3 months, and until death in 70%–90% of patients (43). Significant early analgesia and reduction in analgesic consumption has been shown in patients undergoing NCPB compared to patients treated with pharmacological therapy (44,45). Although long-term results did not differ between the groups in one study (44), NCPB prevented the deterioration in quality of life seen in patients treated with NSAID and morphine alone (45). Minor complications of NCPB include local pain (96% of patients), diarrhea (44% of patients), and hypotension (38% of patients) (43). Major complications are rare but may have a significant impact on quality of life (e.g., paraplegia, superior mesenteric venous thrombosis) (46), and non-neurological (pneumothorax, shoulder or chest pain, hematuria) complications have been reported in 1% of patients. Addition of radiographical contrast to the neurolytic solution and performance of the block under fluoroscopic or computerized tomography guidance is recommended to increase the safety and efficacy of the block (47).

As an alternative to celiac plexus block, the splanchnic nerves can be blocked dorsally at the anterolateral margins of the T11–12 vertebral body. Needles should closely hug the vertebral body to reduce the risk of pneumothorax. Generally, lesser volumes of neurolytic agent are required to produce blockade at this level, and 3 to 5 ml of 10% phenol bilaterally has been recommended (48). A prospective randomized study in 61 patients with pancreatic cancer pain compared three posterior percutaneous celiac plexus block techniques: transaortic celiac plexus block with 30 ml absolute alcohol, classic retrocrural block with 15 ml absolute alcohol, and bilateral splanchnic nerve block with 7 ml absolute alcohol each side (49). No statistically significant differences were found among the three techniques in terms of either

immediate or up-to-death results, and similar rates of minor complications were seen, except for orthostatic hypotension, which occurred less with the transaortic procedure. However, splanchnic nerve block may have advantages when there is anatomical distortion in the region of the celiac plexus that limits the local spread of the neurolytic solution (50). Using a single needle anterior approach, long-lasting pain relief was obtained when contrast containing neurolytic solution was seen (on computed tomography scanning) to spread to all four quadrants of the celiac area. If spread of the neurolytic solution was restricted to one or two quadrants as a result of regional infiltration or compression by tumor, long-lasting pain relief was not achieved (50). NCPB is effective in a higher percentage of patients if performed early after pain onset, when the pain is still only or mainly of celiac type (49), and if the tumor is localized to the head of the pancreas rather than the tail (51). As disease progresses, other sources of pain may develop such as somatic pain from peritoneal involvement (52), and the probability of patients remaining completely pain free diminishes with increased survival time (49). In cases of advanced cancer, improved results have been reported with administration of local anesthetic through an indwelling celiac catheter (53), or alternative techniques such as epidural administration (54) may be required to provide more generalized analgesia.

Visceral pain may be a significant component of pain associated with advanced stage carcinomas of the pelvis. Afferent fibers innervating pelvic organs travel in sympathetic nerves that can be blocked at the level of the fifth lumbar/first sacral vertebrae (superior hypogastric plexus) (34,55). Of 227 patients with gynecological, colorectal, or genitourinary cancer, 79% had a positive response to a diagnostic local anesthetic block and proceeded to percutaneous neurolytic superior hypogastric plexus block. Reductions in pain and opioid requirements were maintained during 3 months of follow-up care in 72% of patients. Patients with extensive retroperitoneal disease were less likely to respond, presumably because of inadequate spread of neurolytic solution (56).

Central neural blockade and spinal drug administration

Spinal administration may be used as a general term that encompasses delivery of drug to a potential space outside the dura (*epidural* administration) or delivery directly into the cerebrospinal fluid (*intrathecal* or subarachnoid administration). Further details of the techniques of epidural and intrathecal injection are available in texts (57). Spinal drug delivery should be considered in appropriately selected patients when severe cancer pain cannot be controlled with systemic drugs because of inadequate effect or dose-limiting side effects (58–60). Ongoing outpatient management of refractory cancer pain is possible with implanted catheters and pumps for spinal drug delivery (61,62). The site of drug delivery (epidural, intrathecal, or intracerebroventricular) and choice of system (tunneled catheter, fully implanted system, internal or external infusion device) depend on the site and nature of the pain, expected duration of therapy, local expertise in invasive techniques, availability of ongoing outpatient care, cost, and perceived risk-benefit ratio for each patient.

Spinal opioids

Demonstration of spinally mediated opioid analgesia in animal studies by Yaksh and Rudy in 1976 (63) was followed relatively rapidly by case reports of administration of spinal opioids to patients with refractory cancer pain (64,65). Cousins and Mather (66) reviewed the pharmacology and initial clinical use of spinal opioids in 1984. Spinal opioids are increasingly used for cancer pain management, as the lower doses required often result in a decrease in systemic side effects, and long-term delivery systems (epidural and intrathecal) have been developed. In a retrospective survey (67) of patients receiving intrathecal morphine for cancer and non-cancer pain, the mean percent relief was 61%.

Pharmacokinetics of spinal opioids

Pharmacokinetic models for epidural and intrathecal opioids have been described (66) but are predominantly based on acute bolus administration rather than chronic infusion. A close relationship exists between lipid solubility and both onset and duration of analgesia (66,68). The duration of analgesia is inversely related to the lipid solubility of the agent, but is also influenced by the rate of dissociation from receptors (62). Morphine is relatively hydrophilic, and high cerebrospinal fluid (CSF) concentrations are achieved after *intrathecal* administration. Morphine diffuses slowly from CSF to opioid receptors, nonspecific binding sites, and clearance sites (arachnoid granulations), resulting in a long duration of analgesia and greater migration to the brain, with the potential for delayed respiratory depression in opioid-naive patients. Uptake into the systemic circulation occurs to a minor degree (66). Spinal administration of morphine offers more benefit in terms of dose sparing between spinal and systemic routes than other opioids (60).

The kinetics of *epidural* injection are further complicated by factors of dural penetration, fat deposition, and systemic absorption (69,70). After epidural injection of morphine, only a low concentration of the more lipid soluble, non-ionized moiety will be present in solution and therefore peak CSF concentration and central distribution of morphine is obtained slowly (cervical CSF concentrations peak between 1 and 3 hours) (70,71). The larger doses of opioid required for epidural administration result in high plasma levels of morphine initially (66,70), but the duration of analgesia follows CSF, rather than plasma, opioid concentrations. Hydromorphone has similar CSF and blood kinetics to morphine, but a faster onset of analgesia that may relate to an initial supraspinal effect (71). Epidural methadone has been administered for cancer pain management (72), but dose requirements and adverse effects tend to be greater than with morphine (73). Phenylpiperidine derivatives (meperidine, fentanyl, alfentanil, lofentanil) are highly lipid soluble and have a rapid onset of analgesia after epidural dosing that coincides with an early peak drug concentration in CSF (74,75). As lipid solubility increases, a greater proportion of epidurally administered drug reaches the systemic circulation. Plasma concentrations of alfentanil, which has high-lipid solubility, are similar after epidural and intravenous administration; therefore, epidural administration offers little clinical advantage (76) Epidural meperidine has potential advantages because of its combined opioid and local anesthetic action (77); however, long-term administration may be complicated by central excitatory effects (78).

Pharmacodynamics and efficacy of spinal opioids

Opioid receptors are found throughout the spinal gray matter but are most prominent in the substantia gelatinosa, and are predominantly of the mu subtype (70% mu, 20% delta, and 10% kappa) (79). Opioids act at presynaptic sites to reduce primary afferent transmitter release and, at postsynaptic sites, produce hyperpolarization via activation of potassium channels to inhibit dorsal horn neurons. When systemic opioids fail to provide adequate analgesia or are associated with excessive side effects (clouding of consciousness, nausea, vomiting), optimization of opioid delivery to receptors by spinal administration may result in enhanced analgesia (4), and the associated reduction in systemic opioid concentrations may minimize side effects.

Determining the relative efficacy of different routes of administration is difficult in the absence of dose equivalence data. In an animal model, spinal morphine was more effective than systemic morphine in inhibiting evoked dorsal horn neuronal responses after spinal nerve ligation in rats (80). This may suggest that the spinal route is more efficacious than the systemic route. Alternatively, an improved effect may be due to a relatively higher dose being administered spinally, as fewer dose-limiting side effects are seen when compared to systemic administration (80). Many clinical trials report improvement in pain with conversion from oral to spinally administered opioids, but often the preceding opioid doses and attempts at optimization of opioid type and dose are not reported. In a double-blind, crossover study of nine patients with cancer pain, both epidural and subcutaneous administration of morphine were comparable in terms of efficacy and acceptability for the patient, and both treatments provided better pain relief with less adverse effects then prestudy oral morphine (81). In a series of 92 patients with cancer pain, 19 patients required subcutaneous opioid because of efficacy or uncontrolled side effects. However, 13 of these patients subsequently progressed to intrathecal morphine, supplemented in some cases by clonidine, calcitonin, or bupivacaine, and achieved improvements in pain relief (82).

Conversion from systemic to spinal routes of opioid administration requires selection of an approximately equianalgesic dosage, which is then titrated according to effect. The epidural starting dose is generally 10% and the intrathecal dose 1% of the 24-hour intravenous morphine requirement; however, conversion rates need to be individually determined (81). A conversion tool has been suggested that further adjusts the initial dose according to the severity of pain (visual analog scale [VAS] score), previous systemic opioid requirements, presence of neuropathic pain, and the age of the patient (83). As the spinal dose is titrated against the analgesic response, preexisting systemic opioid is gradually tapered to prevent withdrawal effects. One suggested regimen is an initial reduction by 50% of the calculated 24-hour systemic opioid dose, followed by further 20% reductions daily (6), with concomitant titration up of the spinal dose.

If an inadequate response is achieved with one opioid, an improvement may be achieved by rotation to a different opioid. Changing from epidural morphine to buprenorphine improved analgesia in 32% of patients and reduced side effects, and changing from buprenorphine to morphine improved analgesia in a further 46% of patients (84). Improvement in drug-related complications was found when epidural morphine therapy was changed to buprenorphine or methadone (85). Intrathecal

DADL (D-Ala2-D-Leu5) enkephalin, a moderately selective delta receptor agonist, has been used to provided analgesia in patients tolerant to morphine (86). Sufentanil has a high intrinsic efficacy necessitating lower fractional receptor occupancy (87) and may be more effective in the presence of tolerance to other opioids (88), but its use is currently limited by cost (89).

Evidence for the safety and efficacy of spinally administered opioids, alone and in combination with other analgesic agents, is emerging. Details of duration of treatment, analgesic agents and doses, outcome, and complication rates in large series are outlined in Table 12.1. At this stage, it remains difficult to clearly define the role of epidural and intrathecal opioid therapy from the published studies. Criteria for treatment success vary among authors: 1. The nature of pain (i.e., nociceptive or neuropathic) may not be well defined, 2. Selection criteria vary, 3. The stage of illness at which patients are referred for more aggressive pain management differs among institutions, and 4. Assessment of outcome and duration of follow-up care are variable. Confirmation of reduced side effects, improved efficacy, and risk-benefit advantages of spinal therapies compared with systemic treatment requires further controlled trials (90).

Side effects of spinally administered opioids
Side effects of spinally administered opioids include the following:

1. Respiratory depression, resulting from cephalad migration of hydrophilic morphine, has been reported after bolus spinal administration in opioid naive patients. In many series of patients with cancer pain who previously received opioids by other routes, respiratory depression after spinal opioids has not been seen (84,91–96). Respiratory depression may rarely occur in these patients if doses are escalated rapidly, complications such as liver failure supervene (97,98), or if intrathecal pump refills are inadvertently injected subcutaneously or directly into the catheter via a side port (98). An infusion of naloxone reverses respiratory depression, without reversal of analgesia.
2. Nausea and vomiting after epidural morphine has been observed 6 hours after administration, which coincides with other evidence of rostral spread of morphine in CSF to intracerebral structures (99). Short-term epidural use of lipid-soluble opioids such as meperidine, fentanyl, and sufentanil (100–102) may be associated with the lowest incidence of nausea and vomiting, but comparison between different

Table 12.1. *Spinal therapy in cancer pain management*

Year (Ref)	Site/type of catheter	Number	Medication	Duration	Outcome	Complication: Minor	Complication: Major
1983 (93)	Epidural: percutaneous catheter and external filter	105 patients (215 catheters)	Morphine (90 patients) 4–30 mg/day (mean: 12.6 mg/day) Buprenorphine (12 patients) 0.6–2.1 mg/day (mean: 1.1 mg/day) Bupivacaine 0.25% (6 patients) 5–10 ml/day	7–283 days (mean: 65 days)	• 67% satisfactory with epidural opioid alone	• 15 catheter tips cultured – 5/15 *Staphylococcus albus* positive but no clinical infection	• sepsis – one case (?other focus – catheter colonized with St. *aureus* – no CNS infection)
(1985) (96)	Epidural: catheter tunneled to anterior abdominal wall	15 patients (22 catheters)	Morphine 4–45 mg/day (mean: 14.6 mg/day)	5–280 days (mean: 89.6 days)	• ceased oral opioid 53% • reduced oral opioid 47% • returned home 87%	• dislodged (7/22) 32% • pain on injection (4/22) 18%	
1986 (84)	Epidural: catheter tunneled to anterior abdominal wall	89 patients (113 catheters) 61 patients (92 catheters)	Morphine (4–60 mg/day (mean: 17 mg) Buprenorphine 0.3–4.5 mg/day (mean: 1.3 mg)	7–397 days (mean: 49 days) 7–262 days (mean: 53 days)	• 45% patients satisfactory analgesia • 67% patients satisfactory analgesia	• pain on injection 14% • 46% side effects with morphine (changing to buprenorphine improved 32%) • 20% s/effects with buprenorphine (changing to morphine improved 46%)	
1990 (247)	Epidural tunneled percutaneous	350 patients				• superficial infection 8.6%	• epidural abscess 4.3% • deep track infection 2.3% • treat with antibiotics and catheter removal, no surgery; catheter replaced in 15/19 patients
1991 (103)	Epidural: tunneled catheter	16 patients (18 catheters)	Morphine 2–360mg/day (mean: 79.4 mg/day) Morphine + bupivacaine 0.125%	5–965 days (mean: 31.5 days)	• relief with morphine alone (6/16) 37% • relief with morphine and bupivacaine (10/16) 63%	• dislodged (8/18) 44% • superficial infection (1/18) 5% • pain on injection (4/16) 25%	• epidural haematoma—one case (prostate cancer with DIC, bone metastases)
1991 (72)	Epidural: percutaneous	70 patients	Methadone 12–32 mg/day (mean: 18.6 mg/day)	3–140 days (mean: 27 days)	• good pain control (56/70) 80%	• technical failure requiring new catheter: dislodge, pain on injection, local infection, occlusion— 47 catheters	

(continued)

Table 12.1. *Spinal therapy in cancer pain management (continued)*

Year (Ref)	Site/type of catheter	Number	Medication	Duration	Outcome	Complication: Minor	Complication: Major
1991 (246)	Epidural percutaneous 78%; SC portal 22%	225 patients	Morphine 13.4 +/− 6.9 mg/day (mean: 5–80 mg/day)	47.3 days 47.4 (7–420)	• satisfactory analgesia 59%	• dislodged 7% • occlusion 3.5% • leakage 2.2% • superficial infection 4%	• epidural haematoma 0.8% (2 patients)
1992 (118)	Epidural: tunneled catheter + filter + external infusion pump	15 patients	Morphine 12–290 mg/day (mean: 92 mg/day)	4–325 days (mean: 60.4 days)	• initial VAS 7–9 – reduced to VAS 4 or less • improved sleep	• kink in catheter 2% • bacterial contamination of 0.6% reservoirs; epidural filters culture negative; no clinical infections	
1987 (94)	Epidural: catheter tunnelled and subcutaneous Dacron cuff	52 patients (58 catheters)	Morphine 1–375 mg/day (mean: 58.3 mg/day Buprenorphine: 1 patient	4–306 days (mean: 61 days)	• oral opioid reduced • activity increased • reduced hospital admission	• pain on injection (2/58) 3% • infections 0%	
1988 (134)	Epidural: catheter tunneled and subcutaneous Dacron cuff	28 patients	Bupivacaine 0.125%–0.5% Mean dose: 480 mg/day (0.25%) 960 mg/day (0.375%) 1400 mg/day (0.5%)		• LA added as opioid alone inadequate in these 28 of total 213 patients)	• decrease BP >20% in 3/28 patients in first 24 hours only • no toxicity even with maximum dose 1800 mg/day for 16 days	• epidural infection—one case
1998 (230)	Epidural 79% percutaneous 21% SC portal	91 patients 137 catheters	Morphine (108 caths) Sufentanil (24 caths) Bupivacaine (135 caths) Clonidine (39 caths)	total 4326 days range: 1–457 days	• >50% decrease in oral or parenteral opioids in 76% of patients with neuropathic pain and 73% with neuropathic pain	• dislodged catheter (all percutaneous) 9% • leakage 4% • superficial infection 43%	• 11 epidural abscess 12% all treated with IV antibiotic + 4 surgical decompression – 9 recovered, 3 treated conserva-tively and died from infection • 1 meningitis • 1 paravertebral abscess
1994 (224)	Epidural: percuta-neous catheter (41 tunneled for short distance – no difference in complication) Epidural: tunneled catheter and subcutaneous portal	149 patients (198 catheters) (52 catheters)	Morphine Sufentanil (15 patients) Clonidine (6 patients) Bupivacaine (doses not reported)			• dislodged 21% • leakage 14% • occlusion 12% • pain on injection 6% • infection 13.6% (5.9/1000 catheter days) • dislodged 0% • leakage 5% • occlusion 2% • pain on injection 2.5% • infection 13.6% (2.8/1000 catheter days)	• meningitis—one case catheter removed • edidural abscess—one case 70 days after port • unexplained neurological symptoms after 133 days in one patient; ?abscess on MRI, infiltration only at operation

Year (Ref)	Technique	Patients	Drug/dose	Duration	Outcome	Complications	Other
1991 (227)	Epidural: tunneled catheter and subcutaneous poral	7 patients	Morphine 6–120 mg/day	7–180 days (mean: 60 days)	all good to excellent pain control	• occluded – 2 catherers • superficial infection – 1	
1988 (91)	Epidural: tunneled catheter (subcutaneous portal 2/69 centers) (external infusion 6/69) intrathecal: tunneled catheter	750 patients 18 patients	Morphine 6–480 mg/day (mean: 46.2 mg/day) Morphine 0.4–50 mg/day (mean: 9.6 mg/day)	3–450 days (mean: 124 days) 3–90 days (mean: 47 days)	18 patients proceeded to intrathecal catheters as inadequate response	• dislodged • catheter occlusion • fibrosis • pain on injection • superficial infection (incidence not reported)	• meningitis—one patients with agranulcytosis
1991 (223)	Epidural: tunneled catheter and subcutaneous portal Intrathecal: tunneled catheter and subcutaneous portal	284 patients 17 patients	Morphine min: 0.5–200 mg/day max: 1–3072 mg/day Morphine minimum: 0.5–5 mg/day (mean: 1.6 mg/day) maximum: 2–130 mg/day (mean: 21 mg/day)	1–1215 days (mean: 96 days) 6–961 days (mean: 147 days)		• leakage 2.1% • occlusion 10.9% • pain on injection 12% (required resiting to intrathecal in 7 patients) • superficial infection 8.1%	• meningitis—one case with intrathecal catheter, no sequelae
1985 (97)	Epidural (3/53) Intrathecal (49/52) • tunneled	52 patients	Morphine in 7% dextrose 1–10 mg/day (mean: 2.5 mg/day)	30–420 days (mean: 125 days)	• 81% good or excellent pain relief • improved activity 67%	• superficial infection (2/52) 4%	• respiratory depression (1/52) • meningitis (1/52)
1991 (209)	Intrathecal: tunneled catheter and external filter	52 patients	Morphine 1–210 mg/day (0.2–7.5 mg/ml) Bupivacaine 1–318 mg/day (0.2–5 mg/ml)	1–305 days (mean: 23 days)	• adequate analgesia 3.8% • good 23.1% • very good 59.6% • excellent 13.5% • improved sleep and activity • decreased total opioid requirement	• motor/BP/sphincter side effects with bupivacaine >60–70 mg/day • paraesthesia in all patients with bupivacaine>3 mg/hr	• clonus–5 patients also had cerebral metastases (morphine: 2,18,24,48. 60 mg/day)
1993 (133)	Intrathecal: percutaneous tunneled	51 patients	Morphine 34 patients Morphine + bupivacaine 17 patients	3140 total days	• morphine alone satisfactory in 34 • 10 improved significantly with combination; 4 moderate • 3 no benefit with addition of bupivacaine	• dislodgment 8% • disconnection 17% • CSF leak 6% • headache 10%	
1994 (221)	Intrathecal: tunneled percutaneous catheter and external infusion pump	15 patients (life expectancy <2 months bedridden)	Morphine 2–10 mg/day (mean: 5.4 mg/day) + bupivacaine, 0.25% 5 ml/day (12.5 mg) to 0.5% 5 ml/day (25 mg)	8–25 days (mean: 15.7 days)	• good pain relief 86% of patients	• dislodged catheter 6% • motor weakness 12%	• no neurologic sequelae or meningitis

(continued)

Table 12.1. *Spinal therapy in cancer pain management (continued)*

Year (Ref)	Site/type of catheter	Number	Medication	Duration	Outcome	Complication: Minor	Complication: Major
1994 (132)	Intrathecal: tunneled catheter, filter and external infusion	53 patients	Morphine 0.5–72 mg/day (mean: 8 mg/day) + bupivacaine 9–250 mg/day (mean: 56 mg/day)		• reduction in VAS • decreased oral analgesic and sedatives • sleep improved • no treatment failures	• urinary detention (bup>30 mg/day) 33% • paraesthesia (bup>45 mg/day) 41% • impaired gait (bup>45 mg/day) 33%	
1995 (232)	Intrathecal: • tunneled and external filter (prospective review for complications)	200 patients	Morphine, buprenorphine, fentanyl, bupivacaine	1–575 days (median 33 days; total 14,485 days)		• perfect function 93% • skin breakdown at insertion site 2% • PDPH 15.5% • CSF leak 3.5% • pain on injection 4.5% (bolus injection only) • dislodgment 5.5% • occlusion 1% • cather leak 1.5% • superficial infection 0.5%	• epidural haematoma 0.5% (trauma to unknown epidural tumour: paralysis right leg) • 2 patients paraplegia >1 week after insertion ?progression of intraspinal tumor • epidural abscess 0% • meningitis 0.5%
1994 (82)	Intrathecal: • subcutaneous port – bolus 10 patients; infusion 23 patients	33 patients	Morphine <10 mg/day: 10 patients 10–50 mg/day: 13 patients >50 mg/day: 1 pt • add calcitonin (4 pts); bupivacaine (1 pt); clonidine (10 pts)	<90 days: 21 patients > 90 days: 12 patients	• 25 good until death: 7 difficult to control in terminal phase; insufficient pain relief in 1	• CSF leaf 9% • obstruction 12%	• meningitis 3 patients (9%) all accidental disconnections in external tubing
1997 (248)	Intrathecal: • percutaneous 10 patients • subcutaneous port 40 patients	50 patients	Morphine Initial: 2.5 mg/day (0.4–8.3) Final: 9.2 mg/day (1–94) Average: 5.4 mg/day (1–23)	7–584 days (mean: 142 days)	• all at least moderate relief which allowed discontinuation of oral or parenteral opioid	• CSF leak 12% (temporary percutaneous catheter)	• no respiratory depression • no clinically detectable infections

Year (ref)	Method	Patients	Drug/dose	Duration	Outcome	Complications
1995 (233)	Intrathecal catheter • 21 DuPen externalized catheters • 60 catheter and implanted pump	72 patients 81 catheters	Morphine (99% of patients) Bupivacaine (12%) Clonidine (9%)	median 56 days (1–1830 days) total: 9090 catheter days		• pocket infection 5.5% • tunnel infection 1.3% • meningitis 2.8% • infection rate 0.77 per 1000 catheter days (1.6 with DuPen and 0.64 with implanted pump) • respiratory depression – 2 cases – inadvertent subcutaneous injection during refill; escalation of oral opioid and liver failure
1984 (98)	Epidural: implanted pump Intrathecal: implanted group	8 patients 6 patients	Morphine 2–50 mg/day Morphine 0.5–75 mg/day	42–390 days (mean: 180 days)	• poor respone after 2 months therapy (early failure due to intraspinal tumor in 4/6 patients) • 3 patients required neurolysis after 6 mo	• dislodged catheter (2/14) 14%
1985 (95)	Epidural: implanted pump Intrathecal: implanted pump	5 patients (4 required subsequent intrathecal) 11 patients	Morphine Initial: 4.4–9.0 mg/day (mean: 6.5 mg/day) Final: 0.8–48 mg/day (mean: 20.7 mg/day) Initial: 1.7–7.6 mg/day (mean: 3.3 mg/d) Final: 4.5–56 mg/day (mean: 32.3 mg/day)	30–540 days (mean: 176 days)	• good to excellent pain relief (15/16) 94% • improved quality of life	• dislodged catheter 19% • obstructed catheter 6% • myoclonic spasms – 2 morphine 21 and 37 mg/day

Abbreviations: CNS, central nervous systems; DIC, disseminated intravascular coagulation; LA, local anesthetic; BP, blood pressure; SC, subcutaneous; MRI, magnetic resonance imaging; CSF, cerebrospinal fluid; VAS, visual analog scale; PDPH, post-dural puncture headache.

agents is still inadequate. The incidence of nausea and vomiting seems to be less with repeated epidural dosing and is low in patients who require long-term spinal opioid therapy (62).

3. Pruritus occurs in up to 24% of patients after acute administration of spinal morphine but diminishes with chronic administration (84,93,95).

4. Urinary retention is usually self-limiting with chronic administration (84,93–96,98).

5. Hyperalgesia may develop with chronic high doses of spinal morphine (103,104). High concentrations of intrathecal morphine and associated hyperalgesia have been investigated in rats. This effect is non-opiate receptor mediated (105), as it is exaggerated rather than reversed by naltrexone, and may relate to high levels of the metabolite morphine-3-glucuronide, or to enhanced NMDA receptor activation (62).

6. Endocrine abnormalities have been noted after prolonged intrathecal administration of opioids (106,107). The majority of patients have been found to develop hypogonadotropic hypogonadism, with reduced levels of testosterone in men, reduced estradiol and progesterone in women, and reduced luteinizing hormone in both men and women. The associated reduced libido improved in most patients after administration of gonadal steroids. A smaller proportion of patients (15%) developed growth hormone deficiency or central hypocorticism (106).

Intracerebroventricular opioids

Opioids can be delivered supraspinally via intracerebroventricular (ICV) catheters and have an analgesic effect that is thought to be mediated by activation of descending inhibitory pathways that project to the spinal cord. Recently, the antinociceptive effect of ICV morphine has been shown to be mediated in part through release of serotonin (5-hydroxytryptamine [5HT]) in the spinal cord, activation of $5HT_3$ receptors and subsequent release of the inhibitory neurotransmitter gamma-amino butyric acid (GABA) (108). Comparative data of epidural, subarachnoid, and ICV opioids in patients with cancer pain suggest similar efficacy, with 58%–75% of patients achieving excellent pain relief (61). ICV morphine has been shown to improve analgesia in cancer patients whose pain was uncontrolled by other measures (109–115) (Table 12.2). After ICV injection, high concentrations of morphine are achieved in ventricular CSF (115). Analgesia occurs within 10 minutes, reaches a maximum between 6 and 10 hours, and persists for 12 to 48 hours (113,116). Symptoms and side effects after

injection may include nausea and vomiting, diaphoresis, sedation, and confusion (117). A suggested initial intraventricular dose is one tenth of the intrathecal dose (5). Daily doses range from 0.15 to 2 mg initially (depending on previous requirements for oral opioid), tend to increase slowly (115), and may reach as high as 15 mg/day (109).

Patients with pain uncontrolled by less invasive measures, obstruction to circulation of CSF making lumbar intrathecal therapy ineffective, or local factors precluding foreign body implantation in the thoracic and lumbar region may be suited to ICV catheters (4,5,117). Pain in any site can be controlled by ICV opioids, but intractable pain in the head and neck region has been suggested as a specific indication for this route of therapy (97,113).

Combinations of spinal analgesic agents

In some patients with advanced cancer, pain may not be adequately controlled by opioids, either by systemic or regional administration. Management of pain resistant to spinal opioids requires thorough reevaluation. Disease progression, development of new pain types (e.g., bone pain resulting from pathological fracture, neuropathic pain resulting from compression of peripheral nerves or the spinal cord) and malfunction of the spinal delivery system must all be considered. Opioids alone are most effective for the management of continuous somatic pain, whereas neuropathic pain, visceral pain, and intermittent or incident pain tend to be less responsive (85,103,118,119), and control may be improved by use a combination of analgesic drugs. For example, delivering a spinal opioid with a local anesthetic improves the control of incident (i.e., movement-related) pain (120,121), whereas the addition of clonidine to an opioid enhances the control of neuropathic pain (122). Evidence from controlled trials for the efficacy of spinal analgesic combination therapy has been recently reviewed (123). Currently, there is insufficient evidence to determine the indications or comparative benefits for the large number of possible combinations of spinal analgesic agents.

Interest in the development of combination spinal analgesic therapy has focused on the following aims:

1. Improvement in analgesic efficacy. When two drugs are administered together their effects may be (a) antagonistic if the combination's effect is less than the sum of the effects produced by each agent alone; (b) additive if their combined effect equals the sum of the effects produced by each agent alone; or (c) synergistic

Table 12.2. *Intracerebroventricular therapy in cancer pain management*

Year (Ref)	Catheter	Number	Medication	Duration	Outcome	Complication: Minor	Complication: Major
1985 (97)	Intraventricular	18 patients	Morphine 0.12–2 mg/day (mean: 0.66 mg/day)	12–230 days (mean: 66 days)	• 89% good or excellent pain relief • 56% improved activity	• superficial infection (1/18) 5%	• respiratory depression (1/18) • visual hallucinations and behavior changes (1/18)
1986 (117)	Intraventricular: Broviac	2 patients	Morphine 0.5–24 mg/day		• excellent relief	• tachycardia, perspiration and burning pain in face and limbs 2–15 min after injection	
1987 (114)	Intraventricular: Ommaya reservoir	20 patients	Morphine 4–60 mg/day (mean: 20.5 mg/day)	3–150 days (mean: 100 days)	• initial adequate relief 80% • ongoing relief 55% • cordotomy as progress of disease 10%	• transient diaphoresis after injection 35% • obstructed and replaced reservoir 5% • leaking reservoir 5%	• meningitis (1/20) – reservoir not removed, treated with intra-ventricular antibiotics
1993 (109)	Intraventricular: Ommaya or Cordis reservoir	52 patients	Morphine 0.15–20 mg/day (mean: 3.1 mg/day)	1–525 days 65% patients died within 3 months		• dislodged ventricular catheter 2% • blocked catheter 6% • colonized reservoir 4%	• meningitis (1/52) – intra-ventricular antibiotics, reservoir not removed

if the effect of the combination exceeds the sum of the effects produced by each agent alone. Preclinical studies have identified a number of synergistic interactions with intrathecal co-administration of different compounds (124), but few clinical studies have been performed to rigorously characterize whether various combinations have additive or synergistic interactions (125). Clinically the distinction between the latter two types of interaction is less important than confirming that analgesia is improved when the combination is compared to a single agent, with no increase in side effects.

2. Reduction in side effects. The limited efficacy of single agents may result in dose escalation and dose-limiting side effects (e.g., neostigmine). The combination of two agents with the common desired endpoint of analgesia but with different side effect profiles may enhance the therapeutic ratio of the therapy.

3. Reduction in the development of opioid tolerance. Tolerance to opioid analgesia refers to a decline in analgesic effect during ongoing drug administration and the need to escalate opioid dose to maintain the same effect. Combination of a non-opioid analgesic with an opioid may reduce the development of tolerance indirectly by reducing the opioid requirement. Van Dongen et al. (126) reported a diminished progression of intrathecal morphine dose during intrathecal co-administration of morphine and bupivacaine when compared to intrathecal morphine alone. Alternatively, some analgesic agents may directly affect the development of tolerance. With respect to the latter mechanism, opioid tolerance in part involves excitatory amino acids that provoke central sensitization and hyperalgesia (127). Manipulations that inhibit NMDA receptor activation, calcium influx, or the intracellular consequences of NMDA receptor activation (128,129) may forestall tolerance and dependence. Therefore in addition to a combined analgesic effect, infusion of an NMDA antagonist with an opioid may reduce opioid tolerance and dose escalation during chronic administration.

Spinal local anesthetic
In patients with cancer pain inadequately controlled by opioid alone, safe and effective management has been demonstrated with addition of local anesthetic to the epidural or intrathecal infusion (83,103,130–133). Bupivacaine is the agent most frequently used, as it has a long duration of action and exhibits little tachyphylaxis (8,130). Local anesthetics can provide intense segmental

analgesia and anesthesia, but high doses are associated with side effects. Reductions in blood pressure resulting from sympathetic fiber blockade are often seen in the first 24 hours of treatment (130,134), but after this initial stabilization, postural hypotension is rarely a significant problem. Bowel and bladder dysfunction may occur with epidural bupivacaine concentrations greater than 0.15% or intrathecal doses greater than 30 mg/day (130). Motor weakness has been shown to occur with epidural bupivacaine concentrations greater than 0.35% (130) and with intrathecal doses greater than 45 mg/day (132). After acute bolus administration, bupivacaine toxicity is seen at serum concentrations of 1 to 2 μg/ml; but in a group receiving chronic epidural bupivacaine, serum concentrations were frequently 4 to 5 μg/ml without symptoms of central nervous system toxicity (130). The majority of patients can remain active and be managed at home with appropriate family and nursing support (135). The side effects associated with high doses of local anesthetic may be acceptable to some patients with otherwise intractable pain, or those who are bedridden in the terminal phases of their illness (135).

Prolonged use of intrathecal combinations of morphine and bupivacaine has been reported in case series of patients with cancer pain (131) with two series reporting adequate pain control until death in 105 patients (132,136). In 51 patients with cancer pain, 17 proceeded from morphine only to a morphine/bupivacaine spinal infusion mixture. Pain control subsequently improved in 10 patients, with only moderate improvement in 4 patients; 11 patients required continuation of oral morphine supplementation (133). In these case series, bupivacaine was added when pain control was inadequate with opioid alone. Interpretation of this data is hampered by lack of randomization, variable inclusion criteria (particularly type of pain), and variable definitions of satisfactory pain relief. Two prospective studies have shown improvement in analgesia with bupivacaine and morphine combinations compared to opioid alone, although there was neither blinding nor randomization in one study (137) and incomplete blinding in the other (126). In both studies, pain intensity at the time of entry varied among patients, and infusions were titrated to effect in individual patients.

Non-opioid spinal analgesic agents
Both presynaptic and postsynaptic effects at the primary afferent synapse in the dorsal horn can modulate pain transmission, and analgesic agents either enhance endogenous inhibitory mechanisms or reduce excitatory

transmission. Several classes of receptors are found on the terminals of the primary afferents, where they are coupled to voltage-gated calcium channels and reduce transmitter release. Receptors located on the soma of second-order neuron are coupled to potassium channels, and activation leads to hyperpolarization of the projection neuron. If a receptor subtype is present both presynaptically and postsynaptically the joint inhibition of transmitter release and hyperpolarization of the second-order neuron yields potent and selective blockade (124). Nociception may also be modulated by agents that block or reduce excitation. Antagonists of the postsynaptic NMDA receptor or agents that alter the intracellular consequences of NMDA receptor activation, have analgesic actions by reducing excitatory nociceptive transmission.

As pain presents as an event with several pharmacologically and functionally distinct components, analgesia may be improved by use of a combination of analgesic agents acting at different receptor sites (124). Analgesic efficacy, side effects, and systemic and local toxicity of potential spinal analgesics must be carefully evaluated before clinical use. Much of the current data relating to non-opioid spinal analgesics is based on case reports or short-term administration, and it is difficult to determine the most appropriate long-term regimen. The requirements for neurotoxicological evaluation of agents before spinal administration in routine clinical practice have been outlined (138). A systematic progression from initial animal studies (behavioral testing of efficacy and side effects, evaluation of effects on spinal cord blood flow, and histopathological examination after acute and chronic administration) followed by carefully conducted and standardized clinical evaluations is required. There is limited or conflicting data relating to the neurotoxicity of many agents under current investigation (139). In relation to combination therapy, additional tests are required to ensure physical and chemical stability of the drug solutions and preservatives, as well as compatibility with the range of infusion devices now available (140).

Clonidine   The analgesic activity of alpha-2-adrenergic agonists, such as clonidine, is mediated through presynaptic and postsynaptic alpha-2 receptors localized in the superficial layers of the spinal dorsal horn (124,141). Reduction of pain intensity after epidural clonidine correlates with its concentrations in the CSF, but not in serum (142), and much lower bolus doses of clonidine are needed to produce potent and long-lasting analgesia through the intrathecal route than via the epidural or systemic routes (143). Clonidine has potential advantages as a spinal analgesic agent.

1. Analgesia is produced by a different mechanism (144); therefore clonidine may be effective in individuals tolerant to morphine (145). Alpha-2 agonists significantly shift the opioid dose-response curve to the left when they are co-administered intrathecally (144), and have a synergistic analgesic action (146). Addition of clonidine to intrathecal infusions of morphine (147) and hydromorphone (148) has successfully controlled previously intractable cancer pain. Continuous epidural infusions of morphine and clonidine have been effectively managed with patients at home (149).

2. Clonidine may be more effective for neuropathic pain (121,150). In a double-blind, crossover study 85 patients with intractable cancer pain received epidural clonidine or placebo in addition to ongoing epidural morphine. Epidural clonidine (30 μg/hr) resulted in successful analgesia in 45% of patients (placebo 21%), particularly in patients with neuropathic pain (56% vs. 5%) (121).

3. The side effect profile of clonidine differs from opioids. Clonidine has a hypotensive action that is counteracted at larger doses by a direct peripheral vasoconstrictive effect (151,152). Rebound hypertension may occur with sudden cessation of spinally administered clonidine (121). Marked bradycardia has been reported (153), but only minor reductions in heart rate not requiring treatment have been seen in many series (103,121,151,152,154). Sedation is usually transient (103,149,151), but may persist for up to 6 hours with larger bolus doses (149,152). Clonidine does not produce respiratory depression (151,154), and nausea was less marked with the combination of epidural clonidine and morphine compared to morphine alone (121).

GABA (gamma-amino butyric acid) agonists   Activation of GABA-A receptors results in an increase in inhibitory chloride conductance. Midazolam binds to the benzodiazepine site of the GABA-A receptor complex and increases the amplitude and duration of GABA-induced synaptic current (155). Intrathecal midazolam has antinociceptive effects (156–158) and displays additive or synergistic interactions with opioids (157,159). Synergistic analgesia has also been shown between spinally administered midazolam and glutamate receptor antagonists acting at the NMDA receptor or the AMPA receptor. Analgesia was achieved at lower doses when the agents were combined, and this was associated with a reduction in untoward behavioral changes and motor disturbances seen at doses required for single agent analgesia (160). Improvements in control of severe cancer pain by the addition of intrathecal midazolam to intrathecal opioid and/or local anesthetic have been reported in isolated cases (161,162).

Studies of the neurotoxicity of spinally administered midazolam have yielded conflicting results. Histological studies with light microscopy have failed to show any increase in neurotoxic effects over control animals after acute (163) or chronic administration (164–166). However, evaluation that included electron microscopy has found signs of neurotoxicity in rat (167) and rabbit models (168). The role of midazolam, the preservative-containing solution, and the pH of the solution in the long-term safety of intrathecal administration require further evaluation.

Baclofen is an agonist at GABA-B receptors. In animal models, baclofen has been shown to elicit dose-dependent analgesia (144). Clinically, spinal subarachnoid administration of baclofen has been used to manage spasticity (62,169), but analgesic effects have not been extensively studied.

NMDA antagonists   Systemic non-competitive NMDA receptor antagonists (dextromethorphan, dextrorphan, ketamine, and MK-801) reduce excitatory nociceptive transmission in the spinal cord. When delivered as a sole agent spinally, ketamine has no acute effect on tail flick latency (170), but has been shown to reduce allodynia in rat models of neuropathic pain (171,172). In clinical practice, spinally administered ketamine has limitations for use as a sole agent, both in terms of efficacy and dose-limiting side effects (173–175) and therefore may be better suited to combination therapy. Both animal (170,176) and clinical studies (177) have shown potentiation of opioid analgesia by an NMDA-receptor antagonist. In addition, intrathecally co-infused NMDA antagonists attenuate morphine tolerance in animal models (178–180). These data suggest that a combination of NMDA antagonist and opioid may have advantages for long-term infusions in clinical practice.

In patients with terminal cancer pain, addition of once daily *epidural* ketamine 0.2 mg/kg to the regimen of twice daily epidural morphine administration resulted in improved analgesia when compared to a control group (who received a third daily bolus of epidural morphine 2 mg). Two other parts in this study found a benefit with addition of neostigmine 100 µg, but no benefit with epidural midazolam 500 µg (181). A blinded crossover trial of twice daily bolus doses of *intrathecal* morphine with or without addition of ketamine 1 mg has also been conducted in patients with terminal cancer pain. Addition of ketamine reduced the dose requirements for both intrathecal morphine and breakthrough analgesia, but there was no statistical difference in the incidence of side effects, possibly because of the small number of patients studied (182). Preservative-free ketamine appears not to cause neurotoxicity (183,184), but further studies are required to establish long-term safety.

Neuronal calcium channel blocker   Neuronal (N-type) voltage-gated calcium channel antagonists (VGCC) reduce presynaptic transmitter release and have potential roles as analgesic agents (185–187). Intrathecal administration of ziconotide (SNX 111, a synthetic omega-conopeptide) produces antinociception in animal models of acute (185,186,188) and persistent pain (189). In clinical studies, intrathecal ziconotide has been shown to reduce postoperative daily patient-controlled analgesia (morphine) consumption (190) and has improved control of chronic neuropathic pain (191). However, many patients experience dose-limiting side effects (dizziness, nystagmus, ataxia, and sedation) (190,192). Therefore, combination therapy that allows the use of smaller doses has potential benefits. In an animal model, acute intrathecal co-administration of ziconitide and morphine produced an additive analgesic effect acutely that was sustained with chronic intrathecal infusion. Although there was no cross-tolerance with morphine, co-administration of ziconotide with morphine did not prevent or reverse opioid tolerance (193). The clinical efficacy of ziconotide and other newly developed N-type VGCC blockers is currently being investigated.

Neostigmine   A high density of muscarinic cholinergic receptors is found in the spinal dorsal horn, and intrathecal administration of muscarinic agonists results in behavioral analgesia (194,195). Neostigmine inhibits acetylcholinesterase and reduces the breakdown of acetylcholine. In clinical trials, intrathecal neostigmine produces dose-related analgesia, with the therapeutic dose lying between 50 and 500 µg (196). Two patients with metastatic abdominal cancer achieved relief of pain for approximately 20 hours after single intrathecal injections of neostigmine (100 and 200 µg, respectively) (197). However, side effects of nausea, vomiting, urinary retention, motor weakness, and decreased deep tendon reflexes are common at high doses (144–146). Therefore interest is now focused on potential benefits of low doses of neostigmine co-administered with other intrathecal analgesics. Synergistic analgesic interactions have been shown between neostigmine and morphine (200–202), and also neostigmine and clonidine (194,200,201). In a controlled trial conducted in patients with terminal cancer pain, addition of a bolus of epidural neostigmine (100 µg) to epidural morphine increased the duration of analgesia (181). An additive analgesic effect has been reported between intrathecal neostigmine and epidural clonidine in a volunteer study (203), but this combination has not been investigated for the management of cancer pain.

Somatostatin Somatostatinergic pain-inhibiting mechanisms have been identified. Epidural or intrathecal somatostatin resulted in "excellent" or "good" pain relief in six of eight patients with terminal cancer and intractable pain unrelieved by large doses of opioids (204). However, all patients required escalating doses of somatostatin during treatment (mean duration 11.3 days; dose range 250–3000 µg daily infusion). The clinical role of spinal somatostatin is limited, as it decreases spinal cord blood flow, may augment postsynaptic effects of glutamate leading to local neuronal injury, and has been found to have deleterious morphological effects on the spinal cord in mice, rats, and cats (205). In addition, somatostatin is unsuitable for prolonged infusion as it is a relatively unstable peptide, and the stable analog octreotide (somatostatin-14) may be more clinically useful (206). Intrathecal treatment with octreotide (5–20 µg/hr for 13–90 days) has been used in patients with cancer pain unrelieved by oral opioids. Pain scores were reduced, and supplemental oral opioid use also decreased (207).

Adenosine Adenosine agonists acting at the A1 receptor in the superficial layers of the spinal dorsal horn produce analgesia. Multiple potential analgesic mechanisms include presynaptic reduction in transmitter release, postsynaptic effects, inhibitory actions that suppress spinal NMDA-mediated responses in sensitized pain states, release of neurotransmitters such as norepinephrine, and interactions with opioids (208–210). Adenosine-receptor agonists produce antinociception in animal models of acute pain (211) and reduce hyperalgesia and allodynia in inflammatory (209) and nerve injury (212) models. In clinical case reports, intravenous infusion of adenosine (213) and intrathecal injection of adenosine (214) and its agonist R-PIA (215) have been shown to reduce allodynia and hyperalgesia in patients with neuropathic pain. No behavioral or histological evidence of neurotoxicity has been found in animal studies (216), and preliminary efficacy and safety studies have been conducted in adult volunteers (217,218). Spinal adenosine potentiates morphine in an additive manner,

and a combination of spinal morphine with inhibitors of endogenous adenosine metabolism or reuptake produced a complete reversal of allodynia in a nerve injury model (208). The role of adenosine in combination spinal therapy for the management of cancer pain requires further evaluation.

Spinal delivery systems

The choice of epidural or intrathecal administration, and the type of spinal delivery system, requires consideration of many factors:

1. The patient's life expectancy and required duration of therapy
2. The site, type, and expected progression of the tumor
3. Patient and social factors if systems requiring daily injections or home treatment are used
4. Varying availability of ongoing care and expertise with invasive techniques among geographic regions.
5. Drug and dose requirements in regard to the choice between epidural and intrathecal therapy
6. Cost and risk-benefit ratios

Epidural catheters have potential advantages, as segmental delivery of local anesthetic can be achieved in patients with severe neuropathic pain (e.g., tumor invading the brachial plexus). The dura also offers a potential barrier to infection. However, catheter dislodgement and the development of epidural fibrosis that limits drug delivery to the epidural space are potential disadvantages. As intrathecal catheters deliver drug directly into the CSF, lower doses are required and this route may be preferable for long-term therapy. Nitescu et al. (219) compared sequential epidural and intrathecal administration of morphine-bupivacaine in 25 patients with advanced cancer pain. Lower volumes and doses were required for the intrathecal route, with a mean dose ratio of one seventh of the epidural dose being effective intrathecally. Pain relief was reported as poor at the end of the epidural treatment and improved on commencement of intrathecal therapy. This is likely to reflect mechanical factors such as catheter tip fibrosis affecting drug delivery with prolonged epidural catheterization.

The method of drug delivery via catheters is also variable. In the short term, percutaneous catheters may be used. Temporary percutaneous catheters are often used for epidural or intrathecal drug trials to ensure that the patient's pain responds to spinal therapy without excessive side effects before proceeding to implantation of more invasive systems. Low cost and ease of insertion of percutaneous catheters may make this simple delivery system sufficient if the patient is expected to live only 1 to 2 weeks (5,220,221). Tunneled catheters with external filters or cuffs have a lower incidence of infection and dislodgement than percutaneous catheters (93,94,134,136,222–224). Fully implanted epidural or intrathecal catheters may be connected to subcutaneous patient-activated reservoirs (225) that deliver a fixed volume of drug, or subcutaneous portals that can be accessed by percutaneous injection (223,226,227) to deliver intermittent boluses or external infusions. No difference in pain scores or neuropsychological function was found when intermittent bolus administration of morphine was compared with continuous infusion (226), but greater dose escalation was seen in the continuous infusion group. Advantages of infusion techniques are more evident when using combination therapies. Bolus doses of local anesthetic may result in motor weakness and hemodynamic instability (60), and many nonopioid analgesics have a shorter duration of action than spinally administered morphine.

Implanted infusion pumps are being used increasingly and have several advantages: 1. Continuous infusion of analgesics is possible; 2. The reservoir requires only intermittent accessing and refilling; and 3. Patients are not hampered by external pumps or the requirement for frequent injections. Implanted pump systems are most suited to low volume intrathecal rather than epidural infusions to avoid too frequent refilling of the reservoir (volume 18–50 ml). The choice between programmable pumps and constant delivery pumps (228) is influenced by the nature and stability of the patient's pain pattern, access to specialized centers, life expectancy, and cost. Disadvantages of implanted pumps include the greater complexity of insertion and the current limited life span of 3 to 5 years for pump batteries in programmable models. In patients with a life expectancy of longer than 3 months, implanted pumps become cost effective (5,6), and are likely to have fewer catheter-related problems and lower infection rates.

Spinal delivery systems can also be used during acute exacerbations of pain or subsequent surgery. Intrathecal pumps have been accessed to deliver subarachnoid local anesthetic and provide surgical anesthesia in patients requiring urological procedures or operative procedures on lower limbs, or to deliver local anesthetic for brief periods of severe exacerbation of pain (98,229). Care must be taken to aspirate concentrated drug solutions from intrathecal catheters before injection, and physicians familiar with the use of these systems should access the pump in an aseptic manner.

Complications of spinal delivery systems

Infection. Complications related to infection vary in severity and incidence, and may be more likely in diabetic, immunosuppressed, or debilitated terminal patients. Possible routes of contamination include hematogenous spread from a distant infectious process, contamination of the injectate, and colonization of percutaneous catheters (230). Colonization of percutaneous catheters by skin flora can be reduced by minimizing the frequency of changes of drug syringe/cassette (230), using antimicrobial filters (231), careful exit site care with secure fixation of the catheter (232), and monitoring for any sign of infection (60).

The highest incidence of superficial infections (i.e., involving the catheter site, but not resulting in epidural abscess or meningitis) is seen with percutaneous catheters. Tunneling catheters for a short distance does not appear to improve infection rates (224), but use of a long subcutaneous tunnel and a fibrous cuff or external filter is associated with fewer superficial infections (93,94,118). Implanted systems with a subcutaneous portal have a lower incidence of catheter-related problems, with reported infection rates of 8%–12% (223,224). If treated early, superficial infections can be limited to the subcutaneous tissues and are not associated with epidural abscess formation or meningitis. Catheter removal may not be mandatory. The relative benefits and risks for individual patients need to be assessed, as there is currently insufficient information to support specific guidelines (233).

Central nervous system infection is a serious potential complication of spinal therapy. Symptoms of epidural abscess include increasing pain, new onset of back pain, and development of motor and sensory deficits (230). The incidence of epidural abscess and/or meningitis in patients with spinal delivery systems varies in different series from 0%–16% (230,233) (Table 12.1). The true incidence of infectious complications is difficult to determine, as cases are often reported in isolation (234), the number of patients undergoing invasive treatments is unknown and continues to change, and the type of delivery system varies. In one series, implanted pumps with intrathecal catheters had a lower incidence of infection (0.64 infections per 1000 catheter-days) compared with externalized DuPen catheters (1.6 infections per 1000 catheter-days). By multivariate Cox regression, only duration of surgery of at least 100 minutes was significantly associated with infection (233). The incidence of infection also varies in different units depending on the selection of patients, experience with the technique, and level of follow-up care (235). Centers with large numbers of patients tend to have lower incidences of infection (233). Patients with suspected spinal epidural abscess require prompt neurological evaluation, investigation with computed tomography or magnetic resonance imaging, and aggressive management, which usually includes removal of the system. In some cases intrathecal reservoirs and catheters have been retained (233) and used to sample CSF and administer intrathecal antibiotics (236).

Epidural fibrosis. Formation of a sheath of fibrous tissue around chronically implanted epidural catheters has been shown in postmortem studies (237). Pain on injection occurs in up to 12% of patients with long-term epidural catheters (84,91,94,103,223,224) resulting from fibrosis around the catheter tip, and can be managed by replacing the epidural catheter or converting to an intrathecal catheter. Delivery of opioid to its site of action can be reduced by epidural fibrosis (91) and lead to a recurrence of pain. Factors limiting fibrosis formation include morphine solutions without additives, a pH of approximately 5, and the use of silicone or polyurethane epidural catheters (60). Spinal cord compression by precipitation of the sodium hydroxide solute within bupivacaine around an epidural catheter tip has been reported (238) after 11 months of therapy in a patient with cancer pain.

Neurotoxicity and neurological complications. In experimental animals with chronically implanted catheters, mild deformation and local demyelination have been reported to occur where catheters contact the spinal cord. The same changes were seen in animals given saline or opioids (239). These findings indicate the need for caution in the site of placement of spinal catheters. However, the potential roles of insertion trauma, catheter material, analgesic solution, drug preservatives, and treatment duration are difficult to delineate in the evaluation of therapy-induced damage (240). No significant postmortem neurotoxic effects were seen in 10 cancer patients treated with morphine or morphine and bupivacaine intrathecal infusions via polyamide lumbar catheters for a mean of 98 days (range 8–452 days) (241). Neurological deficits may relate to the underlying disease process with infiltration or compression by malignant tissue, effects of previous radiotherapy and antineoplastic drugs, or infection (242). Even in the absence of spinal catheterization, compression of the spinal cord or cauda equina results in clinical symptoms of back pain, sensory disturbances, incontinence, and motor weakness, which may progress to paralysis in about 5% of cancer patients with progressive disease (243).

The known presence of epidural or spinal metastases presents a dilemma. Neurological complications may occur in these patients as a result of tumor progression, vertebral collapse, or obstruction of vascular supply, but may also be precipitated by trauma from spinal catheterization with bleeding or CSF leakage. Epidural and spinal metastases are often associated with severe pain, and in such cases, spinal administration may be a necessary last resort (232), providing patients are adequately informed of potential risks. In one series of 57 cancer patients with refractory pain, epidural metastases were found in 40 patients and spinal stenosis in 33 patients (244). During the period of intrathecal treatment, patients with confirmed epidural metastases and total spinal canal stenosis needed significantly higher daily doses of opioid and bupivacaine, and had higher rates of radicular pain at injection and poor distribution of analgesia. The presence of epidural metastasis affected catheter insertion complications (multiple attempts to achieve dural puncture, aspiration of bloody CSF, difficulty advancing catheter) and complications of intrathecal pain treatment only when it was associated with spinal stenosis. Unexpected paraparesis within 48 hours after dural puncture and intrathecal catheterization occurred in 5 of 201 patients (2.5%) (244). Loss of CSF below the level of a subarachnoid block may trigger collapse of the tumor against the spinal cord ("spinal coning") or exacerbate epidural venous engorgement. Some authors suggest that spinal catheters should be carefully placed cephalad to known metastases to minimize direct trauma and to improve efficacy, as tumor progression may result in obstruction of CSF circulation (94,110,220,245) and hinder diffusion of drugs. Ongoing chemotherapy or radiotherapy is not necessarily a contraindication to the placement of a spinal catheter (4).

Epidural hematoma. Epidural hematoma formation is a rare but potentially serious complication of spinal therapies (103,232,246), as it may result in spinal cord compression and paraplegia if not recognized. The presence of a coagulopathy (e.g., as a result of liver function abnormalities or administration of anticoagulants) significantly increases the risk of epidural hematoma formation after epidural or intrathecal injection.

Mechanical problems. Mechanical problems such as catheter obstruction and dislodgement must be excluded if pain rapidly increases in patients during spinal therapy. The incidence of catheter dislodgement is highest for percutaneous epidural catheters (up to 40%) (96,103,220,224) and reduced by use of a subcutaneous portal (223,224) or an implanted intrathecal system. Mechanical failure of implanted infusion devices may occur and result in loss of analgesia and withdrawal effects. Newer programmable implanted models require battery replacement but have an expected life span of 3 to 5 years.

Conclusion

Invasive pain management procedures should be considered if patients with cancer pain are not achieving adequate pain relief, or are experiencing dose-limiting side effects, despite a range of systemic therapies for pain and symptom management. Such measures are necessary in a minority of patients with cancer, but have the potential to significantly improve the patient's quality of life. Neurolytic procedures, such as celiac plexus block in patients with upper abdominal cancer, improve pain control and reduce requirements for other analgesic medication. The development of improved catheters and pump systems for spinal delivery has increased the potential for this route of administration of analgesic agents. This may be necessary in both the short term for patients with debilitating terminal disease, as well as in the longer term for patients with slowly progressive disease or neuropathic pain states relating to the cancer or its treatment. Improved pain control has been achieved in many cancer patients with spinal administration of opioids and local anesthetics. Based on an increased understanding of pain pathophysiology, a range of nonopioid spinal analgesics are now being investigated, and it is hoped that these agents will further increase the ability to achieve control of pain and symptoms in patients with cancer-related pain.

References

1. World Health Organization. Cancer pain relief. Geneva, 1986.
2. Zech DFJ, Grond S, Lynch J, et al. Validation of World Health Organization Guidelines for cancer pain relief: a 10-year prospective study. Pain 63:65–76, 1995.
3. Rosen SM. Procedural control of cancer pain. Semin Oncol 21:740–7, 1994.
4. Swarm RA, Cousins MJ. Anaesthetic techniques for pain control. In Doyle D, Hanks G, MacDonald N, eds. Oxford textbook of palliative medicine. Oxford: Oxford Medical Publications, 1993:204–21.
5. Gildenberg PL. Administration of narcotics in cancer pain. Stereotact Funct Neurosurg 59:1–8, 1992.
6. Krames ES. Intrathecal infusional therapies for intractable pain: patient management guidelines. J Pain Symptom Manage 8:36–46, 1993.
7. Covino BG, Wildsmith JAW. Clinical pharmacology of local anesthetic agents. In: Cousins MJ, Bridenbaugh PO, eds. Neural blockade in clinical anesthesia and pain management, 3rd ed. Philadelphia: Lippincott-Raven, 1998:97–128.
8. Tucker GT, Mather LE. Properties, absorption, and disposition of local anaesthetic agents. In: Cousins MJ, Bridenbaugh PO, eds. Neural blockade in clinical anesthesia and management of pain, 3rd ed. Philadelphia: JB Lippincott, 1998:55–95.
9. Mercadante S, Calderone L, Barresi L. Intrathecal ropivacaine in cancer pain. Reg Anaesth Pain Med 23:621, 1998.
10. Nagy I, Woolf CJ. Lignocaine selectively reduces C fibre-evoked neuronal activity in rat spinal cord in vitro by decreasing N-methyl-D-aspartate and neurokinin receptor-mediated post-synaptic depolarizations; implications for the development of novel centrally acting analgesics. Pain 64:59–70, 1996.
11. Brose WB, Cousins MJ. Subcutaneous lidocaine for treatment of neuropathic cancer pain. Pain 45:145–8, 1991.
12. Loeser JD. Neurosurgical approaches in palliative care. In: Doyle D, Hanks G, MacDonald N, eds. Oxford textbook of palliative medicine. Oxford: Oxford Medical Publications, 1993:221–9.
13. Fischer HBJ, Peters TM, Fleming IM, Else TA. Peripheral nerve catheterization in the management of terminal cancer pain. Reg Anesth 21:482–5, 1996.
14. Sato S, Yamashita S, Iwai M, et al. Continuous interscalene block for cancer pain. Reg Anesth 19:73–75, 1994.
15. Douglas I, Bush D. The use of patient-controlled boluses of local anaesthetic via a psoas sheath catheter in the management of malignant pain. Pain 82:105–7, 1999.
16. Boogaerts J, Declercq A, Lafont N, et al. Toxicity of bupivacaine encapsulated into liposomes and injected intravenously: comparison with plain solutions. Anesth Analg 76:553–5; 1993.
17. Grant GJ, Vermeulen K, Langerman L, et al. Prolonged analgesia with liposomal bupivacaine in a mouse model. Reg Anesth 19:264–9, 1994.
18. Masters DB, Berde CB, Dutta SK, et al. Prolonged regional nerve blockade by controlled release of local anesthetic from a biodegradable polymer matrix. Anesthesiology 79:340–6, 1993.
19. Grant GJ, Barenholz Y, Piskoun B, et al. DRV liposomal bupivacaine: preparation, characterization, and in vivo evaluation in mice. Pharm Res 18:336–43, 2001.
20. Kohane DS, Lipp M, Kinney RC, et al. Sciatic nerve blockade with lipid-protein-sugar particles containing bupivacaine. Pharm Res 17:1243–9, 2000.
21. Estebe JP, Le Corre P, Du Plessis L, et al. The pharmacokinetics and pharmacodynamics of bupivacaine-loaded microspheres on a brachial plexus block model in sheep. Anesth Analg 93:447–55, 2001.
22. Castillo J, Curley J, Hotz J, et al. Glucocoticoids prolong rat sciatic nerve blockade in vivo from bupivacaine microspheres. Anesthesiology 85:1157–66, 1996.
23. Drager C, Benziger D, Gao F, Berde CB. Prolonged intercostal nerve blockade in sheep using controlled-release of bupivacaine and dexamethasone from polymer microspheres. Anesthesiology 89:969–79, 1998.
24. Malinovsky JM, Benhamou D, Alafandy M, et al. Neurotoxicological assessment after intracistrenal injection

of liposomal bupivacaine in rabbits. Anesth Analg 85:1331–6, 1997.

25. Lafont ND, Legros FJ, Boogaerts JG. Use of liposome-associated bupivacaine in a cancer pain syndrome. Anaesthesia 51:578–9, 1996.

26. Grouls RJE, Ackerman EW, Machielsen EJA, Korsten HHM. Butyl-p-aminobenzoate. Preparation, characterization and quality control of a suspension injection for epidural analgesia. Pharm Weekly [Sci] 13:13–7, 1991.

27. Korsten HHM, Ackerman EW, Grouls RJE, et al. Long-lasting epidural sensory blockade by n-butyl-p-aminobenzoate in the terminally ill intractable cancer pain patient. Anesthesiology 75:950–60, 1991.

28. Shulman M. Treatment of cancer pain with epidural butyl-amino-benzoate suspension. Reg Anesth 12:1–4, 1987.

29. Grouls R, Korsten E, Ackerman E, et al. Diffusion of n-butyl-p-aminobenzoate (BAB), lidocaine and bupivacaine through the human dura-arachnoid mater in vitro. Eur J Pharm Sci 12:125–31, 2000.

30. McCarthy RJ, Kerns JM, Nath HA, et al. The antinociceptive and histologic effect of sciatic nerve blocks with 5% butamben suspension in rats. Anesth Analg 94:711–6, 2002.

31. Mitchell VA, White DM, Cousins MJ. The long-term effect of epidural administration of butamben suspension on nerve injury-induced allodynia in rats. Anesth Analg 89:989–94, 1999.

32. Shulman M, Lubenow TR, Nath HA, et al. Nerve blocks with 5% butamben suspension for the treatment of chronic pain syndromes. Reg Anesth Pain Med 23:395–401, 1998.

33. Coles PG, Thompson GE. The role of neurolytic blocks in the treatment of cancer pain. Int Anesth Clin 29:93–104, 1991.

34. Patt RB, Cousins MJ. Techniques for neurolytic neural blockade. In: Cousins MJ, Bridenbaugh PO, eds. Neural blockade in clinical anesthesia and pain management, 3rd ed. Philadelphia: Lippincott-Raven, 1998:1007–61.

35. Lamer TJ. Treatment of cancer-related pain: when orally administered medications fail. Mayo Clin Proc 69:473–80, 1994.

36. Boys L, Peat SJ, Hanna MH, Burn K. Audit of neural blockade for palliative care patients in an acute unit. Palliat Med 7:205–11, 1993.

37. Hakanson S. Trigeminal neuralgia treated by the injection of glycerol into the trigeminal cistern. Neurosurgery 9:638–46, 1981.

38. Antila H, Kirvela O. Neurolytic thoracic paravertebral block in cancer pain. Acta Anaesthesiol Scand 42:581–5, 1998.

39. Patt RB, Reddy S. Spinal neurolysis for cancer pain: indications and recent results. Ann Acad Med Singapore 23:216–20, 1994.

40. Drechsel U. Treatment of cancer pain with neurolytic agents. Recent Results Cancer Res 89:137–47, 1984.

41. Breivik H, Cousins MJ, Lofstrom JB. Sympathetic neural blockade of the upper and lower extremity. In Cousins, MJ, Bridenbaugh PO, eds. Neural blockade in clinical anesthe-

sia and pain Management, 3rd ed. Philadelphia: Lippincott-Raven, 1998:411–47.

42. de Leon-Casasola OA. Critical evaluation of chemical neurolysis of the sympathetic axis for cancer pain. Cancer Control 7:142–8, 2000.

43. Eisenberg E, Carr DB, Chalmers TC. Neurolytic celiac plexus block for treatment of cancer pain: a meta-analysis. Anesth Analg 80:290–5, 1995.

44. Polati E, Finco G, Gottin L, et al. Prospective randomized double-blind trial of neurolytic celiac plexus block in patients with pancreatic cancer. Br J Surg 85:199–201, 1998.

45. Kawamata M, Ishitani K, Ishikawa K, et al. Comparison between celiac plexus block and morphine treatment on quality of life in patients with pancreatic cancer pain. Pain 64:597–602, 1996.

46. Fitzgibbon DR, Schmiedl UP, Sinanan MN. Computed tomography-guided neurolytic celiac plexus block with alcohol complicated by superior mesenteric venous thrombosis. Pain 92:307–10, 2001.

47. Ischia S, Polati E, Finco G, et al. 1998 Labat Lecture: the role of the neurolytic celiac plexus block in pancreatic cancer pain management: do we have the answers? Reg Anesth Pain Med 23:611–4, 1998.

48. Boas RA. Sympathetic blocks in clinical practice. Int Anesthesiol Clinics 16:149, 1978.

49. Ischia S, Ischia A, Polati E, Finco G. Three posterior percutaneous celiac plexus block techniques. A prospective randomized study in 61 patients with pancreatic cancer pain. Anesthesiology 76:534–40, 1992.

50. De Cicco M, Matovic M, Bortolussi R, et al. Celiac plexus block: injectate spread and pain relief in patients with regional anatomic distortions. Anesthesiology 94:561–5, 2001.

51. Rykowski JJ, Hilgier M. Efficacy of neurolytic celiac plexus block in varying locations of pancreatic cancer: influence on cancer pain. Anesthesiology 92:347–54, 2000.

52. Mercadante S, Nicosia F. Celiac plexus block: a reappraisal. Reg Anesth Pain Med 23:37–48, 1998.

53. Vranken JH, Zuurmond WW, de Lange JJ. Increasing the efficacy of a celiac plexus block in patients with severe cancer pain. J Pain Symptom Manage 22:966–77, 2001.

54. Shulman M, Harris JE, Lubenow TR, et al. Comparison of epidural butamben to celiac plexus neurolytic block for the treatment of the pain of pancreatic cancer. Clin J Pain 16:304–9, 2000.

55. Yeo SN, Chong JL. A case report on the treatment of intractable anal pain from metastatic carcinoma of the cervix. Ann Acad Med Singapore 30:632–5, 2001.

56. Plancarte R, de Leon-Casasola OA, El-Helaly M, et al. Neurolytic superior hypogastric plexus block for chronic pelvic pain associated with cancer. Reg Anesth 22:562–8, 1997.

57. Cousins MJ, Veering BT. Epidural neural blockade. In: Cousins MJ, Bridenbaugh PO, eds. Neural blockade in clinical anesthesia and pain management, 3rd ed. Philadelphia: Lippincott-Raven, 1998:243–322.

58. Ferrante FM, Bedder M, Caplan RA, et al. Practice guidelines for cancer pain management. Anesthesiology 84:1243, 1996.

59. Scott DA, Beilby DS, McClymont C. Postoperative analgesia using epidural infusions of fentanyl with bupivacaine: a prospective analysis of 1014 patients. Anesthesiology 83:727–37, 1995.

60. Mercadante S. Problems of long-term spinal opioid treatment in advanced cancer patients. Pain 79:1–13, 1999.

61. Ballantyne JC, Carr DB, Berkey CS, et al. Comparative efficacy of epidural, subarachnoid, and intracerebroventricular opioids in patients with pain due to cancer. Reg Anesth 21:542–56, 1996.

62. Carr DB, Cousins MJ. Spinal route of analgesia: opioids and future options. In: Cousins MJ, Bridenbaugh PO, eds. Neural blockade in clinical anesthesia and pain management, 3rd ed. Philadelphia: Lippincott-Raven, 1998:915–83.

63. Yaksh TL, Rudy TA. Analgesia mediated by a direct spinal action of narcotics. Science 192:1357–8, 1976.

64. Wang JK, Nauss LE, Thomas JE. Pain relief by intrathecally applied morphine in man. Anesthesiology 50:149–51, 1979.

65. Cousins MJ, Mather LE, Glynn CJ, et al. Selective spinal analgesia. Lancet 1(8126):1141–2, 1979.

66. Cousins MJ, Mather LE. Intrathecal and epidural administration of opioids. Anesthesiology 61:276–310, 1984.

67. Paice JA, Penn RD, Shott S. Intraspinal morphine for chronic pain: a retrospective, multicenter study. J Pain Symptom Manage 11:71–80, 1996.

68. Max MB, Inturrisi CE, Kaiko RF, et al. Epidural and intrathecal opiates: cerebrospinal fluid and plasma profiles in patients with chronic cancer pain. Clin Pharmacol Ther 38:631–41, 1985.

69. Nordberg G, Hedner T, Mellstrand T, Dahlstrom B. Pharmacokinetic aspects of epidural morphine analgesia. Anesthesiology 58:545–51, 1983.

70. Gourlay GK, Cherry DA, Cousins MJ. Cephalad migration of morphine in CSF following lumbar epidural administratin in patients with cancer pain. Pain 23:317–26, 1985.

71. Brose WG, Tanelian DL, Brodsky JB, et al. CSF and blood pharmacokinetics of hydromorphone and morphine following lumbar epidural administration. Pain 45:11–5, 1991.

72. Shir Y, Shapira SS, Shenkman Z, et al. Continuous epidural methadone treatment for cancer pain. Clin J Pain 7:339–41, 1991.

73. Jacobsen L, Chabal C, Brody MC, et al. Intrathecal methadone and morphine for postoperative analgesia: a comparison of efficacy, duration and side-effects. Anesthesiology 70:742–6, 1989.

74. Glynn CJ, Mather LE, Cousins MJ, et al. Peridural meperidine in humans: analgesic response, pharmacokinetics and transmission into CSF. Anesthesiology 55:520–6, 1981.

75. Sjostrom S, Hartvig P, Persson P, Tamsen A. Pharmacokinetics of epidural morphine and meperidine in man. Anesthesiology 67:877, 1987.

76. Coda BA, Brown MC, Schaffer RL, et al. A pharmacokinetic approach to resolving spinal and systemic contribu-

tions to epidural alfentanil analgesia and side-effects. Pain 62:329–37, 1995.

77. Ngan Kee WD. Intrathecal pethidine: pharmacology and clinical applications. Anaesth Intens Care 26:137–46, 1998.

78. Kaiko RF, Foley KM, Grabinski PY, et al. Central nervous system excitatory effects of meperidine in cancer patients. Ann Neurol 13:180–5, 1983.

79. Dickenson AH. Where and how do opioids work. In: Gebhart GF, Hammond DL, Jensen TS, eds. Progress in pain research and management, vol 2. Proceedings of the 7th World Congress on Pain. Seattle: IASP Publications, 1993:525–52.

80. Suzuki R, Chapman V, Dickenson AH. The effectiveness of spinal and systemic morphine on rat dorsal horn neuronal responses in the spinal nerve ligation model of neuropathic pain. Pain 80:215–28, 1999.

81. Kalso E, Heiskanen T, Rantio M, et al. Epidural and subcutaneous morphine in the management of cancer pain: a double-blind cross-over study. Pain 67:443–9, 1996.

82. Devulder J, Ghys L, Dhondt W, Rolly G. Spinal analgesia in terminal care: risk versus benefit. J Pain Symptom Manage 9:75–81, 1994.

83. DuPen SL, Williams AR. The dilemma of conversion from systemic to epidural morphine: a proposed conversion tool for treatment of cancer pain. Pain 56:113–8, 1994.

84. Carl P, Crawford ME, Ravlo O, Bach V. Long term treatment with epidural opioids. A retrospective study comprising 150 patients treated with morphine chloride and buprenorphine. Anaesthesia 41:32–8, 1986.

85. Samuelsson H, Malmberg F, Eriksson M, Hedner T. Outcomes of epidural morphine treatment in cancer pain: nine years of clinical experience. J Pain Symptom Manage 10:105–12, 1995.

86. Krames ES, Wilkie DJ, Gershow J. Intrathecal D-Ala2-D-Leu5-enkephalin (DADL) restores analgesia in a patient analgetically tolerant to intrathecal morphine sulfate. Pain 24:205–9, 1986.

87. Dirig DM, Yaksh TL. Differential right shifts in the dose-response curve for intrathecal morphine and sufentanil as a function of stimulus intensity. Pain 62:321–8, 1995.

88. de Leon-Casasola OA, Lema MJ. Epidural bupivacaine/sufentanil therapy for postoperative pain control in patients tolerant to opioid and unresponsive to epidural bupivacaine/morphine. Anesthesiology 80:303–9, 1994.

89. Manfredi PL, Chandler SW, Patt R, Payne R. High-dose epidural infusion of opioids for cancer pain: cost issues. J Pain Symptom Manage 13:118–21, 1997.

90. Bedder MD. Epidural opioid therapy for chronic nonmalignant pain: critique of current experience. J Pain Symptom Manage 11:353–6, 1996.

91. Arner S, Rawal N, Gustafsson LL. Clinical experience of longterm treatment with epidural and intrathecal opioids— a nationwide survey. Acta Anaesth Scand 32:253–9, 1988.

92. Brazenor GA. Long term intrathecal administration of morphine: a comparison of bolus injection via reservoir with continuous infusion by implanted pump. Neurosurgery 21:484–91, 1987.

93. Crawford ME, Anderses HB, Augustenborg G, et al. Pain treatment on an outpatient basis utilizing extradural opiates. A Danish multicentre study comprising 105 patients. Pain 16:41–7, 1983.

94. DuPen SL, Peterson DG, Bogosian AC, et al. A new permanent exteriorized epidural catheter for narcotic self-administration to control cancer pain. Cancer 59:986–93, 1987.

95. Krames ES, Gershow J, Glassberg A, et al. Continuous infusion of spinally administered narcotics for the relief of pain due to malignant disorders. Cancer 56:696–702, 1985.

96. Malone BT, Beye R, Walker J. Management of pain in the terminally ill by administration of epidural narcotics. Cancer 55:438–40, 1985.

97. Lazorthes Y, Veride JC, Bastide R, et al. Spinal versus intraventricular chronic opiate administration with implantable drug delivery devices for cancer pain. Appl Neurophysiol 48:234–41, 1985.

98. Coombs DW, Maurer LH, Saunders RL, Gaylor M. Outcomes and complications of continuous intraspinal narcotic analgesia for cancer pain control. J Clin Oncol 2:1414–20, 1984.

99. Bromage PR, Camporesi EM, Durant PAC, Nielsen CH. Rostral spread of epidural morphine. Anesthesiology 56:431–6, 1982.

100. Brownridge P. Epidural and intrathecal opiates for postoperative pain relief. Anaesthesia 38:74, 1983.

101. Donadoni R, Rolly G, Noorduin H, Vanden Bussche G. Epidural sufentanil for postoperative pain relief. Anaesthesia 40:634, 1985.

102. Welchew EA. The optimum concentration for epidural fentanyl. A randomised double-blind comparison with and without 1:200000 adrenaline. Anaesthesia 38:1037–41, 1983.

103. Hogan Q, Haddox JD, Abram S, et al. Epidural opiates and local anesthetics for the management of cancer pain. Pain 46:271–9, 1991.

104. De Conno F, Caraceni A, Martini C, et al. Hyperalgesia and myoclonus with intrathecal infusion of high-dose morphine. Pain 47:337–9, 1991.

105. Yaksh TL, Harty GJ, Onofrio BM. High doses of spinal morphine produce a nonopiate receptor-mediated hyperesthesia: clinical and theoretic implications. Anesthesiology 64:590–7, 1986.

106. Abs R, Verhelst J, Maeyaert J, et al. Endocrine consequences of long-term intrathecal administration of opioids. J Clin Endocrinol Metab 85:2215–22, 2000.

107. Finch PM, Roberts LJ, Price L, et al. Hypogonadism in patients treated with intrathecal morphine. Clin J Pain 16:251–4, 2000.

108. Kawamata T, Omote K, Toriyabe M, et al. Intracerebroventricular morphine produces antinociception by evoking gamma-aminobutyric acid release through activation of 5-hydroxytryptamine 3 receptors in the spinal cord. Anesthesiol 96:1175–82, 2002.

109. Cramond T, Stuart G. Intraventricular morphine for intractable pain of advanced cancer. J Pain Symptom Manage 8:465–73, 1993.

110. Leavens ME, Stratton Hill C, Cech DA, et al. Intrathecal and intraventricular morphine for pain in cancer patients: initial study. J Neurosurg 56:241–5, 1982.

111. Lenzi A Galli G, Gandolfini M, Marini G. Intraventricular morphine in paraneoplastic painful syndrome of the cervicofacial region: experience in thirty eight cases. Neurosurgery 17:6–11, 1985.

112. Lobato RD, Madrid JL, Fatela LV, et al. Analgesia elicited by low-dose intraventricular morphine in terminal cancer patients. In: Fields HL, ed. Advances in pain research and therapy, vol 9. New York: Raven Press, 1985:673–81.

113. Nurchi GN. Use of intraventricular and intrathecal morphine in intractable pain associated with cancer. Neurosurgery 15:801–3, 1984.

114. Obbens EA, Stratton Hill C, Leavens ME, et al. Intraventricular morphine administration for control of chronic cancer pain. Pain 28:61–8, 1987.

115. Smith MT, Wright AWE, Williams BE, et al. Cerebrospinal fluid and plasma concentrations of morphine, morphine-3-glucuronide, and morphine-6-glucuronide in patients before and after initiation of intracerebroventricular morphine for cancer pain management. Anesth Analg 88:109–16, 1999.

116. Sandouk P, Serrie A, Urtizberea M, et al. Morphine pharmacokinetics and pain assessment after intracerebroventricular administration in patients with terminal cancer. Clin Pharmacol Ther 49:442–8, 1991.

117. Dagi TF, Chilton J, Caputy A, Won D. Long-term intermittent percutaneous administration of epidural and intrathecal morphine for pain of malignant origin. Am Surg 52:155–8, 1986.

118. Ohlsson L, Rydberg T, Eden T, et al. Cancer pain relief by continuous administration of epidural morphine in a hospital setting and at home. Pain 48:349–53, 1992.

119. Samuelsson H, Hedner T. Pain characterization in cancer patients and the analgetic response to epidural morphine. Pain 46:3–8, 1991.

120. Scott NB, Mogensen T, Bigler D, et al. Continuous thoracic extradural 0.5% bupivacaine with or without morphine: effect on quality of blockade, lung function and the surgical stress response. Br J Anaesth 62:253–7, 1989.

121. Eisenach JC, DuPen S, Dubois M, et al. The epidural clonidine study group. Epidural clonidine analgesia for intractable cancer pain. Pain 61:391–9, 1995.

122. Siddall PJ, Molloy AR, Walker S, et al. The efficacy of intrathecal morphine and clonidine in the treatment of pain after spinal cord injury. Anesth Analg 91:1493–8, 2000.

123. Walker SM, Goudas LC, Cousins MJ, Carr DB. Combination spinal analgesic chemotherapy: a systematic review. Anesth Analg 95:674–715, 2002.

124. Yaksh TL, Malmberg AB. Interaction of spinal modulatory receptor systems. In: Fields HL, Liebeskind JC, eds. Progress in pain management and research, vol 1, Seattle: IASP Press, 1994:151–71.

125. Solomon RE, Gebhart GF. Synergistic antinociceptive interactions among drugs administered to the spinal cord. Anesth Analg 78:1164–72, 1994.

126. van Dongen RT, Crul BJ, van Egmond J. Intrathecal coadministration of bupivacaine diminishes morphine dose progression during long-term intrathecal infusion in cancer patients. Clin J Pain 15:166–72, 1999.

127. Mao J, Price DD, Mayer DJ. Mechanisms of hyperalgesia and morphine tolerance: a current view of their possible interactions. Pain 62:259–74, 1995.

128. Elliott K, Minami N, Kolesnikov YA, et al. The NMDA receptor antagonists, LY274614 and MK-801, and the nitric oxide synthase inhibitor, NG-nitro-L-arginine, attenuate analgesic tolerance to the mu-opioid morphine but not to kappa opioids. Pain 56:69–75, 1994.

129. Mayer DJ, Mao J, Price DD. The development of morphine tolerance and dependence is associated with translocation of protein kinase C. Pain 61:365–74, 1995.

130. DuPen SL, Kharasch ED, Williams A, et al. Chronic epidural bupivacaine-opioid infusion in intractable cancer pain. Pain 49:293–300, 1992.

131. Mercadante S. Intrathecal morphine and bupivacaine in advanced cancer pain patients implanted at home. J Pain Symptom Manage 9:201–7, 1994.

132. Sjoberg M, Nitescu P, Appelgren L, Curelaru I. Long-term intrathecal morphine and bupivacaine in patients with refractory cancer pain. Results from a morphine: bupivacaine dose regimen of 0.5:4.75 mg/ml. Anesthesiology 80:284–97, 1994.

133. Van Dongen RT, Crul BJ, De Bock M. Long-term intrathecal infusion of morphine and morphine/bupivacaine mixtures in the treatment of cancer pain: a retrospective analysis of 51 cases. Pain 55:119–23, 1993.

134. DuPen SL, Ramsey DH. Compounding local anesthetics and narcotics for epidural analgesia in cancer out-patients. Anesthesiology 69:A405, 1988.

135. DuPen SL, Williams AR. Management of patients receiving combined epidural morphine and bupivacaine for the treatment of cancer pain. J Pain Symptom Manage 7:125–7, 1992.

136. Sjoberg M, Appelgren L, Einarsson S, et al. Long-term intrathecal morphine and bupivacaine in "refractory" cancer pain. 1. Results from the first series of 52 patients. Acta Anaesth Scand 35:30–43, 1991.

137. Nitescu P, Dahm P, Appelgren L, Curelaru I. Continuous infusion of opioid and bupivacaine by externalized intrathecal catheters in long-term treatment of "refractory" nonmalignant pain. Clin J Pain 14:17–28, 1998.

138. Abram SE. Spinal cord toxicity of epidural and subarachnoid analgesics. Reg Anesth 21:84–8, 1996.

139. Hodgson PS, Neal JM, Pollock JE, Liu SS. The neurotoxicity of drugs given intrathecally (spinal). Anesth Analg 88:797–809, 1999.

140. Wulf H, Gleim M, Mignat C. The stability of mixtures of morphine hydrochloride, bupivacaine hydrochloride, and clonidine hydrochloride in portable pump reservoirs for the management of chronic pain syndromes. J Pain Symptom Manage 9:308–11, 1994.

141. Goudas LC. Clonidine. Curr Opin Anesth 8:455, 1995.

142. Eisenach JC, De Kock M, Klimscha W. Alpha(2)-adrenergic agonists for regional anesthesia. A clinical review of clonidine (1984–1995). Anesthesiology 85:655–74, 1996.

143. Goudas LC, Carr DB, Filos KS, et al. The spinal clonidine—opioid analgesic interaction: from laboratory animals to the postoperative ward. A literature review of preclinical and clinical evidence. Analgesia 3:277–90, 1998.

144. Yaksh TL, Reddy S. Studies in the primate on the analgetic effects associated with intrathecal actions of opiates, alpha adrenergic agonists and baclofen. Anesthesiology 54:451–67, 1981.

145. Coombs DW, Saunders RL, Lachance D, et al. Intrathecal morphine tolerance: use of intrathecal clonidine, DADLE, and intraventricular morphine. Anesthesiol 62:358–63, 1985.

146. Ossipov MH, Suarez LJ, Spaulding TC. Antinociceptive interactions between alpha-adrenergic and opiate agonists at the spinal level in rodents. Anesth Analg 68:194–200, 1989.

147. Van Essen EJ, Bovill JG, Ploeger EJ, Beerman H. Intrathecal morphine and clonidine for control of intractable cancer pain. A case report. Acta Anaesth Belg 39:109–12, 1988.

148. Coombs DW, Saunders RL, Fratkin JD, et al. Continuous intrathecal hydromorphone and clonidine for intractable cancer pain. J Neurosurg 64:890–4, 1986.

149. Eisenach JC, Rauck RL, Buzzanell C, Lysak SZ. Epidural clonidine analgesia for intractable cancer pain: phase 1. Anesthesiology 71:647–52, 1989.

150. Lee Y-W, Yaksh TL. Analysis of drug interaction between intrathecal clonidine and MK-801 in peripheral neuropathic pain rat model. Anesthesiology 82:741–8, 1995.

151. Eisenach J, Detweiler D, Hood D. Hemodynamic and analgesic actions of epidurally administered clonidine. Anesthesiology 78:277–87, 1993.

152. Filos KS, Goudas LC, Patroni O, Polyzou V. Hemodynamic and analgesic profile after intrathecal clonidine in humans. Anesthesiology 81:591–601, 1994.

153. Mendez R, Eisenach JC, Kashtan K. Epidural clonidine after cesarean section. Anesthesiology 73:848–52, 1990.

154. Eisenach JC, Lysak SZ, Viscomi CM. Epidural clonidine analgesia following surgery: phase 1. Anesthesiology 71:640–6, 1989.

155. Kohno T, Kumamoto E, Baba H, et al. Actions of midazolam on GABAergic transmission in substantia gelatinosa neurons of adult rat spinal cord slices. Anesthesiology 92:507–15, 2000.

156. Goodchild CS, Noble J. The effects of intrathecal midazolam in the rat: evidence of spinally mediated analgesia. Br J Anaesth 59:1563–70, 1987.

157. Plummer JL, Cmielewski PL, Gourlay GK, et al. Antinociceptive and motor effects of intrathecal morphine combined with intrathecal clonidine, noradrenaline, carbachol or midazolam in rats. Pain 49:145–52, 1992.

158. Hara K, Saito Y, Kirihara Y, et al. The interaction of antinociceptive effects of morphine and GABA receptor

agonists within the rat spinal cord. Anesth Analg 89:422–7, 1999.

159. Wang C, Chakrabarti MK, Whitwam JG. Synergism between the antinociceptive effects of intrathecal midazolam and fentanyl on both A delta and C somatosympathetic reflexes. Neuropharmacology 32:303–5, 1993.

160. Nishiyama T, Gyermek L, Lee C, et al. Analgesic interaction between intrathecal midazolam and glutamate receptor antagonists on thermal-induced pain in rats. Anesthesiology 91:531–7, 1999.

161. Aguilar JL, Espachs P, Roca G, et al. Difficult management of pain following sacrococcygeal chordoma: 13 months of subarachnoid infusion. Pain 59:317–320, 1994.

162. Barnes RK, Rosenfeld JV, Fennessy SS, Goodchild CS. Continuous subarachnoid infusion to control severe cancer pain in an ambulant patient. Med J Aust 161:549–51, 1994.

163. Erdine S, Yucel A, Ozyalcin S, et al. Neurotoxicity of midazolam in the rabbit. Pain 80:419–23, 1999.

164. Schoeffler P, Auroy P, Bazin JE, et al. Subarachnoid midazolam: histologic study in rats and report of its effect on chronic pain in humans. Reg Anesth 16:329–32, 1991.

165. Bahar M, Cohen ML, Grinshpoon Y, et al. An investigation of the possible neurotoxic effects of intrathecal midazolam combined with fentanyl in the rat. Eur J Anaesth 15:695–701, 1998.

166. Serrao JM, Mackenzie JM, Goodchild CS, Gent JP. Intrathecal midazolam in the rat: an investigation of possible neurotoxic effects. Eur J Anaesth 75:115–22, 1990.

167. Svensson BA, Welin M, Gordh T, Westman J. Chronic subarachnoid midazolam (Dormicum) in the rat. Morphologic evidence of spinal cord neurotoxicity. Reg Anesth 20:426–34, 1995.

168. Bozkurt P, Tunali Y, Kaya G, Okar I. Histological changes following epidural injection of midazolam in the neonatal rabbit. Paediatr Anaesth 7:385–9, 1997.

169. Coffey RJ et al. Intrathecal baclofen for intractable spasticity of spinal origin: results of a long-term multicenter study. J Neurosurg 78:226–32, 1993.

170. Joo G, Horvath G, Klimscha W, et al. The effects of ketamine and its enantiomers on the morphine- or dexmedetomidine-induced antinociception after intrathecal administration in rats. Anesthesiology 93:231–41, 2000.

171. Dickenson AH, Sullivan AF, Stanfa LC, McQuay HJ. Dextromethorphan and levorphanol on dorsal horn nociceptive neurones in the rat. Neuropharmacology 30:1303–8, 1991.

172. Mao J, Price DD, Hayes RL, et al. Intrathecal treatment with dextrorphan or ketamine potently reduces pain-related behaviours in a rat model of peripheral mononeuropathy. Brain Res 605:164–8, 1993.

173. Hawksworth C, Serpell M. Intrathecal anesthesia with ketamine. Reg Anesth Pain Med 23:283–8, 1998.

174. Kathirvel S, Sadhasivam S, Saxena A, et al. Effects of intrathecal ketamine added to bupivacaine for spinal anaesthesia. Anaesthesia 55:899–904, 2000.

175. Kawana Y, Sato H, Shimada H, et al. Epidural ketamine for postoperative pain relief after gynecologic operations: a double-blind study and comparison with epidural morphine. Anesth Analg 66:735–8, 1987.

176. Yamamoto T, Yaksh TL. Studies on the spinal interaction of morphine and the NMDA antagonist MK-801 on the hyperesthesia observed in a rat model of sciatic mononeuropathy. Neurosci Lett 135:67–70, 1992.

177. Wong CS, Liaw WJ, Tung CS, et al. Ketamine potentiates analgesic effect of morphine in postoperative epidural pain control. Reg Anesth 21:534–41, 1996.

178. Miyamoto H, Saito Y, Kirihara Y, et al. Spinal coadministration of ketamine reduces the development of tolerance to visceral as well as somatic antinociception during spinal morphine infusion. Anesth Analg 90:136–41, 2000.

179. Shimoyama N, Shimoyama M, Inturrisi CE, Elliott KJ. Ketamine attenuates and reverses morphine tolerance in rodents. Anesthesiology 85:1357–66, 1996.

180. Dunbar S, Yaksh TL. Concurrent spinal infusion of MK801 blocks spinal tolerance and dependence induced by chronic intrathecal morphine in the rat. Anesthesiology 84:1177–88, 1996.

181. Lauretti GR, Gomes JM, Reis MP, Pereira NL. Low doses of epidural ketamine or neostigmine, but not midazolam, improve morphine analgesia in epidural terminal cancer pain therapy. J Clin Anesth 11:663–8, 1999.

182. Yang CY, Wong CS, Chang JY, Ho ST. Intrathecal ketamine reduces morphine requirements in patients with terminal cancer pain. Can J Anaesth 43:379–83, 1996.

183. Borgbjerg FM, Svensson BA, Frigast C, Gordh T. Histopathology after repeated intrathecal injections of preservative-free ketamine in the rabbit: a light and electron microscopic examination. Anesth Analg 79:105–11, 1994.

184. Malinovsky J-M, Lepage J-Y, Cozian A, et al. Is ketamine or its preservative responsible for neurotoxicity in the rabbit? Anesthesiology 78:109–15, 1993.

185. Malmberg AB, Yaksh TL. Effect of continuous intrathecal infusion of omega-conopeptides, N-type calcium channel blockers, on behaviour and antinociception in the formalin and hot-plate tests in rats. Pain 60:83–90, 1995.

186. Malmberg AB, Yaksh TL. Voltage-sensitive calcium channels in spinal nociceptive processing: blockade of N- and P-type channels inhibits formalin-induced nociception. J Neurosci 14:4882–90, 1994.

187. White DM, Cousins MJ. Effect of subcutaneous administration of calcium channel blockers on nerve injury-induced hyperalgesia. Brain Res 801:50–8, 1998.

188. Wang YX, Pettus M, Gao D et al. Effects of intrathecal administration of ziconotide, a selective neuronal N-type calcium channel blocker, on mechanical allodynia and heat hyperalgesia in a rat model of postoperative pain. Pain 84:151–8, 2000.

189. Bowersox SS, Gadbois T, Singh T, et al. Selective N-type neuronal voltage-sensitive calcium channel blocker, SNX-111, produces spinal antinociception in rat models of acute, persistent and neuropathic pain. J Pharmacol Exp Ther 279:1243–9, 1996.

190. Atanassoff PG, Hartmannsgruber MW, Thrasher J, et al. Ziconotide, a new N-type calcium channel blocker, admin-

istered intrathecally for acute postoperative pain. Reg Anesth Pain Med 25:274–8, 2000.

191. Brose WG, Gutlove DP, Luther RR, et al. Use of intrathecal SNX-111, a novel N-type voltage-sensitive calcium channel blocker in the management of intractable brachial plexus avulsion pain. Clin J Pain 13:256–9, 1997.

192. Penn RD, Paice JA. Adverse effects associated with the intrathecal administration of ziconotide. Pain 85:291–6, 2000.

193. Wang YX, Gao D, Pettus M, et al. Interactions of intrathecally administered ziconotide, a selective blocker of neuronal N-type voltage-sensitive calcium channels, with morphine on nociception. Pain 84:271–81, 2000.

194. Hood DD, Eisenach JC, Tong C, et al. Cardiorespiratory and spinal cord blood flow effects of intrathecal neostigmine methylsulfate, clonidine, and their combination in sheep. Anesthesiology 82:428–35, 1995.

195. Yaksh TL, Grafe MR, Malkmus S, et al. Studies on the safety of chronically administered intrathecal neostigmine methylsulfate in rats and dogs. Anesthesiology 82:412–27, 1995.

196. Hood DD, Eisenach JC, Tuttle R. Phase I safety assessment of intrathecal neostigmine methylsulfate in humans. Anesthesiology 82:331–43, 1995.

197. Klamt JG, Dos RM, Barbieri NJ, Prado WA. Analgesic effect of subarachnoid neostigmine in two patients with cancer pain. Pain 66:389–91, 1996.

198. Lauretti GR, Hood DD, Eisenach JC, Pfeifer BL. A muticenter study of intrathecal neostigmine for analgesia following vaginal hysterectomy. Anesthesiology 89:913–8, 1998.

199. Lauretti GR, Mattos AL, Gomes JM, Pereira NL. Postoperative analgesia and antiemetic efficacy after intrathecal neostigmine in patients undergoing abdominal hysterectomy during spinal anesthesia. Reg Anesth 22:527–33, 1997.

200. Naguib M, Yaksh TL. Antinociceptive effects of spinal cholinesterase inhibition and isobolographic analysis of the interaction with mu and alpha 2 receptor systems. Anesthesiology 80:1338–48, 1994.

201. Abram SE, Winne RP. Intrathecal acetyl cholinesterase inhibitors produce analgesia that is synergistic with morphine and clonidine in rats. Anesth Analg 81:501–7, 1995.

202. Hwang JH, Hwang KS, Choi Y, et al. An analysis of drug interaction between morphine and neostigmine in rats with nerve-ligation injury. Anesth Analg 90:421–6, 2000.

203. Hood DD, Mallak KA, Eisenach JC, Tong C. Interaction between intrathecal neostigmine and epidural clonidine in human volunteers. Anesthesiology 85:315–25, 1996.

204. Mollenholt P, Rawal N, Gordh T, Olsson Y. Intrathecal and epidural somatostatin for patients with cancer—analgesic effects and postmortem neuropathologic investigations of spinal cord and nerve roots. Anesthesiology 81:534–42, 1994.

205. Yaksh TL. Spinal somatostatin for patients with cancer—risk-benefit assessment of an analgesic (editorial). Anesthesiology 81:531–3, 1994.

206. Abram SE. Continuous spinal anesthesia for cancer and chronic pain. Reg Anesth 18:406–13, 1993.

207. Penn RD, Paice JA, Kroin JS. Octreotide: a potent new nonopiate analgesic for intrathecal infusion. Pain 49:13–9, 1992.

208. Lavand'homme PM, Eisenach JC. Exogenous and endogenous adenosine enhance the spinal antiallodynic effects of morphine in a rat model of neuropathic pain. Pain 80:31–6, 1999.

209. Poon A, Sawynok J. Antinociception by adenosine analogs and inhibitors of adenosine metabolism in an inflammatory thermal hyperalgesia model in the rat. Pain 74:235–45, 1998.

210. Gomes JA, Li X, Pan HL, Eisenach JC. Intrathecal adenosine interacts with a spinal noradrenergic system to produce antinociception in nerve-injured rats. Anesthesiology 91:1072–9, 1999.

211. Sawynok J. Adenosine receptor activation and nociception. Eur J Pharmacol 347:1–11, 1998.

212. Lee YW, Yaksh TL. Pharamacology of the spinal adenosine receptor which mediates the antiallodynic action of intrathecal adenosine agonists. J Pharmacol Exp Ther 277:1642–8, 1996.

213. Sollevi A, Belfrage M, Lundeberg T, et al. Systemic adenosine infusion: a new treatment modality to alleviate neuropathic pain. Pain 61:155–8, 1995.

214. Belfrage M, Segerdahl M, Arner S, Sollevi A. The safety and efficacy of intrathecal adenosine in patients with chronic neuropathic pain. Anesth Analg 89:136–42, 1999.

215. Karlsten R, Gordh T. An A_1-selective adenosine agonist abolishes allodynia elicited by vibration and touch after intrathecal injection. Anesth Analg 80:844–7, 1995.

216. Chiari A, Yaksh TL, Myers RR, et al. Preclinical toxicity screening of intrathecal adenosine in rats and dogs. Anesthesiology 91:824–32, 1999.

217. Eisenach JC, Hood DD, Curry R. Phase I safety assessment of intrathecal injection of an American formulation of adenosine in humans. Anesthesiology 96:24–8, 2002.

218. Eisenach JC, Hood DD, Curry R. Preliminary efficacy assessment of intrathecal injection of an American formulation of adenosine in humans. Anesthesiology 96:29–34, 2002.

219. Nitescu P, Appelgren L, Linder L-E, et al. Epidural versus intrathecal morphine-bupivacaine: assessment of consecutive treatments in advanced cancer pain. J Pain Symptom Manage 5:18–26, 1990.

220. Hicks F, Simpson KH, Tosh GC. Management of spinal infusions in palliative care. Palliat Med 8:325–32, 1994.

221. Mercadante S. Intrathecal morphine and bupivacaine in advanced cancer pain patients implanted at home. J Pain Symptom Manage 9:201–7, 1994.

222. Tryba M, Zenz M, Strumpf M. Long term epidural catheters in terminally ill patients—a prospective study of complications in 129 patients. Anesthesiology 73:A784, 1990.

223. Plummer JL, Cherry DA, Cousins MJ, et al. Long-term spinal administration of morphine in cancer and non-cancer pain: a retrospective study. Pain 44:215–20, 1991.

224. De Jong PC, Kansen PJ. A comparison of epidural catheters with or without subcutaneous injection ports for treatment of cancer pain. Anesth Analg 78:94–100, 1994.

225. Poletti CE, Cohen AM, Todd DP, et al. Cancer pain relieved by long-term epidural morphine with permanent indwelling systems for self-administration. J Neurosurg 55:581–4, 1981.

226. Gourlay GK, Plummer JL, Cherry DA, et al. Comparison of intermittent bolus with continuous infusion of epidural morphine in the treatment of severe cancer pain. Pain 47:135–40, 1991.

227. Shaves M, Barnhill D, Bosscher J, et al. Indwelling epidural catheters for pain control in gynaecologic cancer patients. Obstet Gynecol 77:642–4, 1991.

228. Harbaugh RE, Coombs DW, Saunders RL, et al. Implanted continuous epidural morphine infusion system. J Neurosurg 56:803–6, 1982.

229. Coombs DW, Fine N. Spinal anesthesia using subcutaneously implanted pumps for intrathecal drug infusion. Anesth Analg 73:226–31, 1991.

230. Smitt PS, Tsafka A, Teng-van de Zande F, et al. Outcome and complications of epidural analgesia in patients with chronic cancer pain. Cancer 83:2015–22, 1998.

231. De Cicco M, Matovic M, Castellani GT, et al. Time-dependent efficacy of bacterial filters and infection risk in long-term epidural catheterization. Anesthesiology 82:765–71, 1995.

232. Nitescu P, Sjoberg M, Appelgren L, Curelaru I. Complications of intrathecal opioids and bupivacaine in the treatment of 'refractory' cancer pain. Clin J Pain 11:45–62, 1995.

233. Byers K, Axelrod P, Michael S, Rosen S. Infections complicating tunnelled intraspinal catheter systems used to treat chronic pain. Clin Infect Dis 21:403–8, 1995.

234. Van Diejen D, Driessen JJ, Kaanders JH. Spinal cord compression during chronic epidural morphine administration in a cancer patient. Anaesthesia 42:1201–3, 1987.

235. Cherry DA, Plummer JL, Gourlay GK. Letter to the editor about epidural opiates and local anesthetics for the management of cancer pain. Pain 48:469, 1992.

236. Schoeffler P, Pichard E, Ramboatiana R, et al. Bacterial meningitis due to infection of a lumbar drug release system in patients with cancer pain. Pain 25:75–7, 1986.

237. Coombs DW, Fratkin JD, Frederick AM, et al. Neuropathologic lesions and CSF morphine concentrations during chronic continuous intraspinal morphine infusion. A clinical and post mortem study. Pain 21:337–51, 1985.

238. Johnston SP, Harland MKW. Spinal cord compression from precipitation of drug solute around an epidural catheter. Br J Neurosurg 12:445–7, 1998.

239. Yaksh TL, Noueihed RY, Durant AC. Studies of the pharmacology and pathology of intrathecally administered 4-anilinipiperidine analogues and morphine in the rat and cat. Anesthesiology 64:54–66, 1986.

240. Sjoberg M, Karlsson P-A, Nordborg C, et al. Neuropathologic findings after long-term intrathecal infusion of morphine and bupivacaine for pain treatment in cancer patients. Anesthesiology 76:173–86, 1992.

241. Wagemans MF, van der Valk P, Spoedler EM, et al. Neurohistopathological findings after continuous intrathecal administration of morphine or a morphine/bupivacaine mixture in cancer pain patients. Acta Anaesthesiol Scand 41:1033–8, 1997.

242. Smitt PS, Tsafka A, van den Bent MJ, et al. Spinal epidural abscess complicating epidural analgesia in 11 cancer patients: clinical findings and magnetic resonance imaging. J Neurol 246:815–20, 1999.

243. Schiff D, Shaw EG, Cascino TL. Outcome after spinal re-irradiation for malignant epidural spinal cord compression. Ann Neurol 37:583–9, 1995.

244. Appelgren L, Nordberg C, Sjoberg M, et al. Spinal epidural metastasis: implications for spinal analgesia to treat 'refractory' cancer pain. J Pain Symptom Manage 13:25–42, 1997.

245. Cherry DA, Gourlay GK, Cousins MJ. Epidural mass associated with lack of efficacy of epidural morphine and undetectable CSF morphine concentrations. Pain 25:69–73, 1986.

246. Erdine S, Aldemir T. Long-term results of peridural morphine in 225 patients. Pain 45:155–9, 1991.

247. Du Pen SL, Peterson DG, Williams A, Bogosian AJ. Infection during chronic epidural catheterization: diagnosis and treatment. Anesthesiology 73:905–9, 1990.

248. Gestin Y, Vainio A, Pegurier AM. Long-term intrathecal infusion of morphine in the home care of patients with advanced cancer. Acta Anaesthesiol Scand 41:12–7, 1997.

13 Psychological interventions

DIANE NOVY
University of Texas-Houston Health Science Center

Introduction

Pain is a multidimensional symptom to which there are many contributors. Nociception is perceived by an individual and then expressed. Psychosocial factors such as somatization, anxiety, depression, and intrapsychic and cultural beliefs influence the perception and expression of pain. Psychological interventions are both important and helpful in the management of pain.

Currently, many comprehensive cancer treatment centers include psychological intervention as an integral part of an interdisciplinary treatment plan to address pain and pain-related problems (1). At less comprehensive cancer clinics and hospitals, there is a growing appreciation of the important interaction between biomedical and psychosocial variables. This chapter reviews assessment of the most relevant psychosocial variables and then focuses on the major psychological interventions.

Although the research literature on psychological interventions for individuals with cancer pain is relatively young, a number of different treatments have been used. The main treatments include cognitive-behavioral, psychoeducational, and supportive therapies. To maximize therapeutic effectiveness, psychological research protocols and clinical practices often combine aspects of each of these types of therapies into a "package." Depending on the specific therapeutic technique, the format may be individual, group, or family sessions. The duration of treatment ranges from brief periods, including times of crisis, to longer term periods.

Patients with cancer have many unique problems including multiple physical, psychological, and social stresses as discussed in Chapter 5. After appropriate multidimensional assessment of patients, it is essential to individually tailor psychological interventions to their particular needs.

It is not unusual to find psychological interventions conducted by persons representing a wide variety of mental health backgrounds. These include chaplains, licensed professional counselors, psychiatric nurses, psychiatrists, psychologists, and social workers. Some interdisciplinary treatment teams even have more than one type of mental health clinician (2).

Although interdisciplinary teams are becoming the standard of care for cancer-related problems, there still may be some reluctance on the part of the patient to be assessed and treated by a mental health clinician. Therefore, it is important to incorporate an explanation that pain is a sensory/physical and emotional (i.e., with affective, behavioral, and cognitive dimensions) experience. After an appropriate and sensitive explanation, initially reluctant patients typically will be more receptive to assessment and treatment that focus on biomedical and psychosocial factors (3).

Psychosocial assessment

In most cases, a mental health clinician gathers psychosocial information from a face-to-face interview with a patient and possibly from one or more family members. In addition to demographic and clinical information about a patient's background and current situation, including emotional and social support, the interview focuses on sensory/physical, affective, behavioral, and cognitive dimensions (Table 13.1). The interview may be supplemented with self-report questionnaires and with information on certain relevant issues from significant others and members of the treatment team. However, sensitivity to a patient's physical condition often makes it necessary to streamline the ideal assessment. Although a review of the array of the self-report questionnaires is beyond the scope of this chapter, the interested reader is referred to Turk and Melzack (4).

Table 13.1. *Relevant dimensions of a psychological assessment*

Dimensions	Examples
Sensory/physical	Pain intensity, effects of pain on life
Affect	Anger, anxiety, depression, frustration
Behavior	Pain interference in activity, pacing
Cognition	Maladaptive patterns of thinking and self-talk

Sensory/physical

Medical members of the treatment team usually provide other team members with initial assessment and subsequent updated biomedical information. The mental health clinician will need a basic understanding of the variable biomedical characteristics of cancer and cancer pain that differentially affects an individual's risk for psychological and behavioral morbidity. This includes an understanding of the different types of pain syndromes, as well as familiarity with the parameters of appropriate pharmacological treatment (1). Other major biomedical characteristics of cancer for the mental health clinician to consider include extent of disease (e.g., stage and aggressiveness), magnitude of medical treatment (e.g., surgery, radiotherapy, chemotherapy, invasive procedures for pain/symptom control), prognosis (e.g., favorable, guarded, dismal), and phase in the disease time line (e.g., diagnosis/pretreatment, immediately posttreatment, extended treatment, and disseminated disease or pending death) (5). It is important for the mental health clinician to integrate information about current medical status and previous treatments when assessing patients who no longer have active disease but who have indefinite periods of treatment-related pain and are at risk for psychological and behavioral morbidity.

Additional relevant biomedical information concerns the sensory/physical dimension of pain. Like the variable characteristics of cancer, sensory/physical information about pain also may come from the medical members of the team. This does not preclude the mental health clinician from seeking further clarification about the pain (e.g., ratings of average, highest, lowest, and range of pain intensity, effects of pain on life and factors that diminish and exacerbate pain). This information helps the mental health clinician understand the roles various behavioral, cognitive, emotional, environmental, and physiological stimuli have in relation to exacerbations of pain (6).

Affect

Evaluation of anger, anxiety, depression, and frustration is part of a psychosocial assessment. The similarity of presentation of some symptoms of depression and disease-related somatic complaints such as decreased activity, fatigue, loss of concentration, sleep disruption, and weight loss makes depression difficult to recognize among patients with cancer. Because of this overlap, the mental health clinician will have to listen carefully and also take in information from behavioral observations and reports of significant others.

Although the majority of patients with cancer adjust to the stresses of the disease and its symptoms without a diagnosable mood disorder (6,7), patients with pain report significantly more anxiety and depression than those without pain (8). Among those who do report negative emotions, most often these represent acute reactions to cancer, pain, or treatment. For example, cancer treatment provides many opportunities for anticipatory anxiety: the next procedure, the next check-up, the cause of new or different pain, and the possibility of relapse. In another regard, some patients have long-standing mood disturbances that are exacerbated by their illness or challenged by the treatment setting (9,10).

Although relatively few patients with cancer commit suicide, the majority of suicides reported are among patients who had severe, inadequately controlled, or poorly tolerated pain and depression (11). Therefore, standard assessment of affect also should include evaluation of suicide ideation. For purposes of treatment, it is important to determine whether thoughts of suicide are related to depression or to a desire to have control over intolerable symptoms (1).

Behavior

There are various ways that a mental health clinician can gather information about a patient's verbal and nonverbal behaviors to communicate the experience of pain. In addition to a mental health clinician's own assessment and observation of behaviors, it is useful to ask other team members and the patient's significant others for their assessments. Of particular importance are the immediate consequences of the patient's pain behavior. This needs to be assessed to determine if medical staff or significant others are reinforcing behaviors that are inappropriate or excessive. Although this is not usually the case among patients with cancer pain, pain behaviors that foster excessive dependency may be targets for psychological intervention (6). It is also important to assess the range of behaviors patients are physically capable of engaging in but restrict because of pain. A useful way to probe this variable is to ask for a rating of pain interference in activity. It also is useful to query about how a patient paces his or her activity level. It is not unusual for a patient to overdo activities during some periods, particularly when pain is diminished, and then suffer consequences of increased pain afterward. Finally, the mental health clinician will want to ask about which behavioral strategies are currently being used and how effective they are for pain management. For those patients who already use some techniques, subsequent treatment would build on the techniques that are effective and introduce new techniques as well. For patients who do not use any techniques, greater preparation will be necessary.

Cognition

In the context of cancer pain, the assessment of cognition has to do with gathering information about a patient's thoughts and beliefs about his or her disease and condition and ability to handle the associated problems, including pain. Of particular focus are maladaptive patterns of thinking that are unrealistic or distorted. Such errors in thinking have the potential to impact the maintenance and exacerbation of pain and interfere with treatment (e.g., belief that there is nothing the patient can do to reduce pain and belief that pain is inevitable and should be tolerated). In a related vein, it also is important to ask about a patient's self-talk. This pertains to internal dialogues that reflect thoughts about his or her condition or pain. Both the cognitive errors and self-talk can be assessed in the clinical interview and/or by asking the patient to self-monitor his or her pain and record any thoughts or feelings that accompany the pain (12). It also is useful to query about the use and effect of any cognitive coping strategies.

Interventions

Cognitive-behavioral techniques

The underlying postulate of cognitive-behavioral techniques is that mental and physical symptoms are partly a function of maladaptive behaviors, feelings, and thoughts (13). The purpose of the related and complementary techniques is to identify and correct behaviors, feelings, and thoughts that contribute to symptom development and symptom maintenance. A second, equally important, purpose is to enhance the adequacy of patients' cognitive and behavioral coping repertoires, as these affect intrapersonal and interpersonal responses to the patient (12). As the name implies, cognitive-behavioral techniques incorporate both behavioral and cognitive approaches to accomplish psychological change (Table 13.2). In clinical practice, different cognitive-behavioral techniques often are combined and tailored to a patient's individual needs.

Although the underlying techniques vary, the behavioral approaches described here have apparent similarities. Common to each of them are principles of operant conditioning (14) and respondent conditioning (15) that relate the techniques to pain control. Hence, a focus on

Table 13.2. *Selected cognitive behavioral techniques*

Technique	Types	Purpose
Biofeedback	EEG, EMG, conductance, skin temperature	Used to teach self-regulation of physiological responses
Hypnosis	Anesthesia, direct diminution, displacement, dissociation, sensory substitution	Used to include a state of sustained attention and concentration and openness to suggestion
Relaxation	Autogenic, mediation, progressive muscle	Used to reduce skeletal muscle tension and reactivity to pain
Imagery	Guided imagery with generalization of skills to disease or pain focus	Used to help achieve a sense of control over pain
Distraction and attention diversion		Used to change the focus from pain to non-painful sensation, positive thoughts, pleasant images, or aspects of the environment
Cognitive restructuring		Used to bring awareness and a reality check into the evaluation process
Stress inoculation		Used for help to provide sufficient knowledge, self-understanding, and coping to facilitate better ways of handling expected stressful encounters

Abbreviations: EEG, electroencephalography; EMG, electromyography.

consequences of pain behaviors and stimuli that preceded pain is the basis for grouping the techniques as behavioral. However, it is important to note that the techniques are not purely behavioral as they also share varying degrees of focus on cognitive processes.

One behavioral approach, biofeedback, refers to a collection of techniques used to teach self-regulation of physiological responses. Physiological functioning is monitored with instrumentation that can give visual and/or auditory feedback to the patient about what is happening to bodily functions that are normally unavailable to awareness. In the first phase of treatment, the patient is trained to develop an increased awareness of the specific physiological response (e.g., muscular tension, hand temperature, heart rate, or blood pressure, depending on the focus of the specific biofeedback modality used). Then the patient is taught to gain voluntary control of his or her physiological response(s) by means of feedback from various physiological systems. In the third phase, treatment involves using the newly acquired voluntary controls in the natural environment (12).

The most common types of biofeedback are electroencephalographic (EEG), electromyographic (EMG), skin conductance, and skin temperature (13). The most typical format for biofeedback training is individual sessions. In addition to mastery of relaxation of the body, biofeedback training is thought to help patients reduce sympathetically mediated and affective responses that induce, facilitate, or maintain pain. Although there are no reported randomized controlled studies of the efficacy of this approach in treating patients with cancer pain, clinical reports suggest EEG and EMG biofeedback may be useful for cancer-related pain (16,17).

Another behavioral approach, hypnosis, is a formal induction of a state of sustained attention and concentration, reduced peripheral awareness, and openness to suggestion (18). There are three basic, equally important, phases: 1) the initial conceptualization that includes the development of rapport and dealing with any of the patient's questions concerning the nature of hypnotherapy, 2) the actual training, and 3) the transfer of training or generalization (12). The format for hypnosis is individual sessions. The five major hypnotic techniques that have been used for the treatment of cancer pain are anesthesia, direct diminution, sensory substitution, displacement, and dissociation (19–22). The technique of anesthesia refers to hypnotic suggestions that render a body area numb and insensitive to pain. Direct diminution and sensory substitution change the meaning of pain so that it is less important and painful (e.g., turning down the volume; interpreting pain as coldness). Displacement suggestions change the location of the pain. Dissociation is used to separate pain from the patient's awareness. Posthypnotic suggestion and self-hypnosis are additional techniques that are used to extend pain relief (2). Although there are shortcomings in the reported outcome studies, there are some anecdotal and controlled investigations that support of the use of hypnosis to relieve cancer-related pain (23–26).

An array of relaxation techniques represents another behavioral approach. Relaxation can range from passive techniques such as meditation to the more active ones like progressive muscle relaxation (25). Most relaxation techniques adhere to a format of individual or group sessions several times a week coupled with daily home practice. Patients often are given an audiotape as an adjunct to facilitate home practice. There is considerable anecdotal evidence yet sparse collaboration by controlled randomized design research to support relaxation techniques (26–28). The two most commonly used relaxation procedures are progressive muscle relaxation and autogenic relaxation (13).

In regard to progressive relaxation, it is important to point out that this is not a single method, but a group of techniques that vary considerably in procedural detail, complexity, and length. Regretfully, although outcome studies generally support progressive relaxation, not all reviews have distinguished between the techniques (29). The abbreviated method based on Wolpe's (30) modification of Jacobson's (31) original method often is used with patients with pain. The abbreviated method consists of systematically tensing and relaxing several of 16 major muscle groups. Frequently the clinician will offer instructions and suggestions (e.g., "Smooth it out" or "Let it go further") about what the patient should do following tension release. Although progressive relaxation methods originally were developed to reduce skeletal muscle tension and secondarily diminish pain, it also is thought to help pain sufferers by reducing their reactivity to their pain (32).

In contrast to progressive relaxation, autogenic training is based on passive concentration (33). In autogenic relaxation, the patient uses self-statements and visual images to achieve relaxation. Typical exercises begin with the image and sensation of heaviness, warmth (in some instances coolness is used), and relaxation of specific muscle groups until the whole body is involved. The heaviness is directed at muscular relaxation, whereas warmth is directed at vascular dilation. The patient concentrates on his or her body sensations without trying to directly or volitionally bring about change. In addition to helping achieve a relaxed state, autogenic training is designed to strengthen independence and to give control back to the patient (34).

Imagery is a behavioral approach that is closely aligned with relaxation. It can be used in individual or group sessions. Imagery involves having patients develop a mental image associated with feelings of peacefulness and calmness or with a positive past experience. Patients are involved in the decision about the selection of the image. The inclusion of various senses enhances the vividness of the image and facilitates the imagery process and relaxation (12). Once patients appreciate the usefulness of the technique for relaxation they can generalize their imagery skills to a disease and/or pain specific focus. When patients are in a relaxed state, they can be instructed to focus on an image that symbolizes their disease or a specific symptom like pain. Patients are taught to modify their image in a therapeutic manner. They learn that by becoming involved with their image, there is little attention to focus on their discomfort. With instruction and practice, patients can use and terminate the imagery as needed. By so doing, they can experience a greater sense of control over their pain (35).

It is important to point out that the content of the image does not seem to be the important factor; rather the manner in which the imagery is presented, the involvement of the patient, and practice appear key. When appropriate, it may be possible to teach family members about imagery so they can help their loved one use the technique when needed. As with relaxation, primarily anecdotal reports support use of imagery (26,35).

In addition to the primarily behaviorally rooted techniques, cognitive-behavioral interventions also include techniques for changing cognitions derived from principles of information processing (36). Central to information processing are studies of human perception that show that before a person is aware of seeing or hearing a stimulus, the sensory inflow coming through the eyes or ears has already passed through many stages of selection, interpretation, and appraisal. During this process, a large proportion of the original inflow has been excluded (37). One of the major assumptions of cognitive approaches to pain management is that the pain experience is based partly on the appraisals and psychological significance to the individual. Negative expectation, interpretation, and anticipatory fears such as unavoidable pain, loss of control, disfigurement, and subjective perceptions of rejection are common among patients with cancer. The goal of cognitive approaches to pain management is to modify the thoughts that may be contributing to the pain problems. Specifically, cognitive techniques aim to enhance perceptions of control and resourcefulness and to reduce demoralization (12). A related goal is to teach specific cognitive coping skills to deal with pain (6). Unfortunately, no study has directly tested the effectiveness of the individual cognitive techniques; however, different combinations of the techniques have demonstrated favorable results within multicomponent treatment packages (38–40). A few of the most widely used cognitive techniques are described in the following paragraphs. The formats used for these techniques are individual or group therapy.

Distraction and attention diversion are two related cognitive techniques. The goal of these techniques is to change the focus from pain to nonpainful sensations, positive thoughts, pleasant images, or aspects of the environment (12,41). To do this, the mental health clinician teaches the patient about the role that attention plays in the reduction of pain. Specifically, the clinician guides the patient to experiment with his or her awareness and helps the patient see that he or she can only be fully aware of whatever is the focus of attention at the moment. The patient learns that he or she can shift and control the focus (12). When patients successfully use this technique, it is thought that they can fill their minds with thoughts that may actually help to lessen their distress.

Another cognitive technique is cognitive restructuring. Restructuring involves reconceptualization of the thoughts and feelings that have a negative effect on a patient's overall adjustment and his or her experience of pain. In stressful situations such as dealing with cancer and cancer-related pain, deviations in the thinking process can play a major role on a patient's overall adjustment. At the same time that the nature of the situation is being evaluated, the patient is assessing his or her resources for dealing with it. This is the "risk-resources equation," which affects a patient's response to the situation under evaluation. The processes involved in the response are automatic, involuntary, and not within awareness (37).

Under conditions of stress and depleted resources, patients may make extreme, one-sided, absolutistic, and global judgments of their situation. When the appraisals tend to be extreme and one-sided, the behavioral inclinations also tend to be extreme. For example, a person who is susceptible to fear reactions may interpret a body sensation deemed by the physician insignificant and unrelated to the disease in a catastrophic manner. A depression-prone person may interpret a brief physician follow-up appointment as a rejection and want to withdraw from treatment.

Reconceptualization of such deviations in thinking is accomplished by active collaboration between clinician and patient. Cognitive restructuring training seeks to bring awareness and a reality check into a patient's evaluation process. As this technique applies specifically to cancer pain, the mental health clinician will query about several things related to when pain was particularly severe. These include what the situation was at the time of the pain; what thoughts the patient had before, during, and after the pain episode; what things were tried to decrease pain; and what resources are available to help deal with the pain. By examining the answers to these questions, the patient and clinician can identify negative thoughts and feelings that are not based on well-grounded evidence, and the patient can learn to develop alternative ways of responding (12).

A third cognitive technique, stress inoculation training, often is used in conjunction with cognitive restructuring and behavioral techniques. This technique also is closely related to stress management and psychoeducation. As patients identify negative reactivity, training in stress inoculation and stress management helps them deal more adaptively with those situations. Because lack of preparation and surprise contribute to distressing, ineffective coping efforts, stress inoculation training bolsters a patient's preparedness and assimilatory processes. In this way, a patient can learn to pace himself or herself, as he or she learns to master stressful situations gradually. The goals of this technique are to help patients acquire sufficient knowledge, self-understanding, and coping skills to facilitate better ways of handling expected stressful encounters (42,43).

Several related steps are usually followed in stress inoculation. Among these steps, the clinician helps the patient appreciate the fact that his or her stress reflects a normal reaction to a difficult situation. The clinician also helps the patient reframe stressful reactions not as signs of weakness, but as normal, or adaptive reactions. In a related vein, the clinician helps the patient appreciate that there are not prescribed emotional stages that stressed individuals go through, nor is there a correct way to cope. In regard to cancer-related pain and stress, the clinician also helps a patient discover and appreciate the variable nature of certain features of the stress and pain, and how the patient unwittingly, unknowingly, and often inadvertently exacerbates and helps maintain the stress reactions to certain experiences. The clinician helps the patient develop gradual mastery of stress by exposure to a more manageable reconceptualization of stress. This reconceptualization acts as the basis for coping more effectively.

The patient also is taught to draw a distinction between "changeable" and "unchangeable" aspects of the stressful situations and to "fit" either problem-focused or emotion-focused coping efforts to the situation (44). Finally, the patient is taught to break down global stressors into specific short-term intermediate, and long-term coping goals (43).

After the reconceptualization phase of stress inoculation is a focus on individually tailored coping skills acquisition and rehearsal. The newly learned or refined coping skills are rehearsed in vivo. The final phase of stress inoculation training includes opportunities for the patient to apply the variety of coping skills on a graduated basis across other levels of stressors.

Several authors (45–47) have reported the benefits of stress inoculation for patients with cancer and their families. Jay and Elliott (48,49) developed an innovative videotape application of this technique for parents of children with pediatric leukemia who were undergoing bone marrow aspirations or lumbar punctures. Relative to parents who received a child-focused intervention, the parents who received stress inoculation training evidenced less anxiety and better coping skills (43).

Psychoeducation

The overall goal of education for patients with cancer and cancer-related pain is to reduce the sense of helplessness and inadequacy as a result of lack of knowledge, uncertainty, and unpredictability that seem to contribute to the distress and suffering of patients with cancer (Table 13.3). Although education may cover technical disease and treatment issues, it also may include information about pain control and medical and psychosocial issues. Examples of educational topics, although not directly related to pain per se, are body image and sexuality, diet and exercise, emotional reactions of patients and possible responses of others to cancer, goal setting, medical system, relating to caregivers, side effects of both the disease and treatment, survival, and talking with family and friends. Some formats for the delivery of the information are educational materials (e.g., audiotapes, books, videos, and various web sites), talking to other patients with cancer, and question-and-answer group sessions. Depending on the topic under discussion, different members of the treatment team or auxiliary staff may participate as the group leader. In instances when educational meetings include individuals who have had cancer, lessons learned from their personal experiences are often shared.

Table 13.3. *Other psychological interventions*

Intervention	Purpose
Psychoeducation	Used to reduce the sense of helplessness and inadequacy caused by lack of knowledge, uncertainty, and unpredictability
Supportive psychotherapy	Used to focus on the cancer and its implications, while exploring those issues from the past and present that affect adjustment

Psychoeducational interventions can be individually tailored to a specific patient or tailored to groups of patients with similar needs. In regard to groups, a few general guidelines exist in the literature. A short-term, structured, psychoeducational group intervention is the recommended model for newly diagnosed and/or patients with good prognosis. The focus for these individuals is leaning how to live with cancer and cancer-related pain. Ongoing weekly group support educational programs are recommended for patients with advanced metastatic disease. The foci of these groups are daily coping, pain management, and issues related to death and dying (50).

Given that the effectiveness of psychoeducation often is evaluated along with other types of psychological interventions, it is difficult to assess the specific impact of psychoeducation. Overall, the combined intervention packages, including increased knowledge from psychoeducation, appear to be helpful to patients (51). Unexpected survival benefits were found among subjects in studies with an educational component (52,53). Authors of these studies speculated that the survival benefit resulted from changes patients made in their health habits and coping styles and in improving communication with their doctors and better adhering to treatment (54). In clinical practice, because patients are aware of the potential benefits of education, it is not unusual for them to specifically request these services.

Supportive psychotherapy

In contrast to the didactic cognitive-behavioral and psychoeducational interventions, supportive psychotherapy is more "patient-centered." Supportive psychotherapy as described in this chapter is an integration of crisis intervention and psychodynamic principles that are modified for patients with cancer. The goals of treatment include maintaining a primary focus on the cancer and its implications while exploring those issues from the past and

present that affect overall adjustment to illness (55) (Table 13.3).

Feelings and fears about the illness and its outcome, including pain, are important topics to patients. Patients often consider these topics to be too burdensome or difficult to discuss with family and friends. Hence, the mental health clinician is an ideal person with whom to explore feelings that otherwise would be unexpressed. Within a supportive psychotherapy context, the clinician can assure the patient that most of the fears are not unique to his or her particular situation; rather they are common to others in similar situations (55). Supportive psychotherapy can be used alone and in conjunction with the other interventions discussed. Depending on the needs of the patient, the format may be individual, group, or family sessions.

Aspects of the supportive psychotherapeutic framework will vary with the exigencies of the illness. The utmost challenge lies in adapting a structure to the illness reality, even as the illness changes, without sacrificing the uniqueness of the therapeutic interaction. The uniqueness of the interaction requires flexibility in the duration, location, and scheduling of individual psychotherapy sessions according to a patient's needs. In cases involving a group format, flexibility also must be allowed.

There has been some research on the positive impact of supportive group psychotherapy for patients with cancer. Among the positive effects, three studies demonstrated a survival benefit (53,54,56). These studies had a few key components in common that may have contributed significantly to their overall effectiveness. In each study the patients were provided a supportive, stable, and consistent environment (57).

One of the life-extending studies, a randomized prospective trial conducted over a 10-year period by Spiegel and associates (56), examined the effects of weekly support groups for patients with metastatic breast cancer. Because the support groups from Spiegel's study serve as a clear example of the intervention under review, a full description follows. The supportive groups were relatively unstructured and were designed to encourage direct discussion about living with cancer. The goal was to provide an environment in which patients could talk about their fears and concerns regarding the disease and its progression. Group members decided the topics they wished to discuss. For example, issues discussed included concerns about their doctors and medical treatment, the effects of the illness on their families, fears about dying and death, and ways to live fully in the time that was left. Because the patients were all in a similar situation, they were able to discuss these issues without undue concern about the impact it might have on others. In addition, they had the opportunity to share what they had learned from living with a life-threatening illness and help others who struggled with the same issues. By doing this they enhanced their own sense of competence and value. From this therapeutic environment, patients had social support, a sense of belonging, and the opportunity to express their thoughts and feelings about living with cancer. Such an environment was thought to improve patients' coping capabilities and enhance social support, both within the group and outside it (11, 23).

The potential benefits of supportive psychotherapy for cancer pain sufferers have enabled it to become one of the most utilized psychological interventions. Among its uses is in the management of the suicidal cancer patient. In this circumstance, it is particularly important for the clinician to maintain a supportive therapeutic relationship with a crisis intervention framework. Further, it is helpful if the clinician conveys the attitude that much can be done to improve the quality, if not the quantity, of life even if the prognosis is poor. This includes actively treating specific symptoms (e.g., pain, nausea, insomnia, anxiety, and depression). The supportive method also involves giving back a sense of control by helping the patient to focus on that which can still be controlled and involving family and friends (11).

Conclusions and future directions

After careful psychosocial assessment, an array of complementary psychological interventions can be individually tailored to help patients with cancer and cancer-related pain. There is a growing body of evidence to support the use of multicomponent psychological treatments. Although more and better studies are needed to fully support treatments for cancer pain, there are an impressive number of controlled randomized studies to support the effectiveness of combinations of the treatments on emotional well-being (5). Other issues for future work include testing the efficacy of individual components of current multicomponent interventions. Research along these lines could lead to interventions that are briefer and more economical and could help to identify the mechanisms responsible for the therapeutic effects of the treatments.

Finally, it is important to emphasize that the psychological interventions discussed in this chapter are best thought of as part of an integrated treatment plan by an interdisciplinary team. Management of pain and other

specific symptoms requires a team approach, enlisting expertise from a wide variety of clinical groups (1,58–60). The challenge of addressing both the biomedical and psychosocial issues involved in pain is to develop rational and effective management strategies. Therapies directed primarily at psychosocial variables have a profound impact on nociception, and somatic therapies directed at nociception have beneficial effects on the psychosocial aspects of pain (1).

References

1. Breitbart W, Payne DK. Pain. In: Holland JC, ed. Psycho-oncology. New York: Oxford University Press, 1998:450–67.
2. Cleeland CS, Tearnan BH. Behavioral control of pain. In: Holzman AD, Turk DC, eds. Pain management: a handbook of psychological treatment approaches. New York: Pergamon Press, 1986:193–212.
3. Turk DC, Fernandez E. On the putative uniqueness of cancer: do psychological principles apply? Behav Res Ther 28:1–3, 1990.
4. Turk DC, Melzack R, eds. Handbook of pain assessment, 2nd ed. New York: Guilford Press, 2002.
5. Anderson BL. Psychological interventions for cancer patients to enhance the quality of life. J Consult Clin Psychol 60:552–68, 1992.
6. Tearnan BH, Ward CH, Cleeland CS. Psychological management of malignant pain. In: Tollison CD, ed. Handbook of chronic pain management. Baltimore: Williams and Wilkins, 1989:402–16.
7. Derogatis LR, Morrow GR, Fetting J, et al. The prevalence of psychiatric disorders among cancer patients. JAMA 249:751–7, 1983.
8. Ahles TA, Blanchard EB, Ruckdeschel JC. The multidimensional nature of cancer-related pain. Pain 17:277–88, 1983.
9. Sharer AU, Schreiber S, Galai T, McLoud RN. Posttraumatic stress disorder following medical events. Br J Clin Psychol 2:247–53, 1993.
10. Telch CF, Telch MJ. Group coping skills instruction and supportive group therapy for cancer patients: a comparison of strategies. J Consult Clin Psychol 54:802–8, 1986.
11. Massie MJ, Gagnon P, Holland JC. Depression and suicide in patients with cancer. J Pain Symptom Manage 9:325–40, 1994.
12. Turk DC, Meichenbaum D, Genest M. Pain and behavioral medicine. New York: Guilford Press, 1983.
13. Jacobson PB, Hann DM. Cognitive-behavioral interventions. In: Holland JC, ed. Psycho-oncology. New York: Oxford University Press, 1998:717–29.
14. Skinner BF. Science and human behavior. New York: Macmillan, 1953.
15. Pavlov IP. Conditioned reflexes. Oxford: Oxford University Press, 1927.
16. Fotopoulos SS, Graham, C, Cook MR. Psychophysiologic control of cancer pain. In: Bonica JJ, Ventrifidda V, eds.

Advances in pain research and therapy. New York: Raven Press, 1979:231–43.

17. Fotopoulos SS, Cook MR, Graham C, et al. Cancer pain: evaluation of electromyographic and electrodermal feedback. Prog Clin Biol Res 132D:33–53, 1983.

18. Barber J, Gitelson J. Cancer pain: psychological management using hypnosis. CA Cancer J Clin 30:130–6, 1980.

19. Araoz DL. Use of hypnotic techniques with oncology patients. J Psychosoc Oncol 1:47–54, 1983.

20. Barber J. Hypnotic analgesia. In: Holzman AD, Turk DC, eds. Pain management: a handbook of psychological treatment approaches. New York: Pergamon Press, 1986:151–67.

21. Hilgard ER. Hypnosis in the relief of pain. Los Altos: William Kaufman, 1975.

22. Margolis CG. Hypnotic interventions for pain management. Int J Psychosom 32:12–19, 1985.

23. Spiegel D, Bloom JR, Yalon I. Group support for patients with metastatic breast cancer. Arch Gen Psychiatry 38:527–33, 1981.

24. Spiegel D, Bloom JR. Group therapy and hypnosis reduce metastatic breast carcinoma pain. Psychosom Med 45:333–9, 1983.

25. Woolfolk RL, Lehrer PM, eds. Principles and Practice of Stress Management. New York: Guilford Press, 1984.

26. Ahles TA. Psychological techniques for the management of cancer-related pain. In: McGuire DB, Yarbro CH, eds. Cancer pain management. Orlando: Grune & Stratton, 1987:245–58.

27. Millard RW. Behavioral assessment of pain and behavioral pain management. In: Patt RB, ed. Cancer pain. Philadelphia: JB Lippincott, 1993:85–97.

28. Sloman R, Brown P, Aldana E, Chee E. The use of relaxation for the promotion of comfort and pain relief in persons with advanced cancer. Contemp Nurse 3:6–12, 1994.

29. Hyman RB, Feldman HR, Harris RB, et al. The effects of relaxation training on clinical symptoms: a meta-analysis. Nurs Res 38:216–20, 1989.

30. Wolpe I: Psychotherapy by reciprocal inhibition. Stanford, CA: Stanford University Press, 1958.

31. Jacobson E: Progressive relaxation, 2nd ed. Chicago: University of Chicago Press, 1938.

32. Bernstein DA, Carlson CR. Progressive relaxation: abbreviated methods. In: Luhrer PM, Woolfolk RL, eds. Principles and practice of stress management, 2nd ed. New York: The Guilford Press, 1993:53–88.

33. Schultz JH, Luthe W. Autogenic methods, vol 1. New York: Grune & Stratton, 1969.

34. Linden W. The autogenic training method of J.H. Schultz. In: Luhrer PM, Woolfolk RL, eds. Principles and practice of stress management, 2nd ed. New York: The Guilford Press, 1993:205–30.

35. Simonton OC, Matthews-Simonton S, Sparks TF. Psychological intervention in the treatment of cancer. Psychosomatics 21:226–33, 1980.

36. Hamilton V. Cognition and stress: an information processing model. In: Goldberger L, Breznitz S, eds. Handbook of

stress: theoretical and clinical aspects. New York: Free Press, 1982:105–20.

37. Beck AT. Cognitive approaches to stress. In: Luhrer PM, Woolfolk RL, eds. Principles and practice of stress management, 2nd ed. New York: The Guilford Press, 1993:333–72.

38. Christensen DN. Postmastectomy couple counseling: an outcome study of a structured treatment protocol. J Sex Marital Ther 9:266–74, 1983.

39. Fawzy FI, Cousins, N, Fawzy N, et al. A structured psychiatric intervention for cancer patients: 1. Changes over time in methods of coping and affective disturbance. Arch Gen Psychiatry 47:720–5, 1990.

40. Heninrich RL, Coscarelli-Schag C. Stress and activity management: group treatment for cancer patients and their spouses. J Consult Clin Psychol 53:439–46, 1985.

41. Ahles TA. Psychological approaches to the management of cancer-related pain. Semin Oncol Nur 1:141–6, 1985.

42. Meichenbaum D. Stress inoculation training. Elmsford, NY: Pergamon Press, 1985.

43. Meichenbaum D. Stress inoculation training: a 20-year update. In: Luhrer PM, Woolfolk RL, eds. Principles and practice of stress management, 2nd ed. New York: The Guilford Press, 1993:373–406.

44. Lazarus RS, Folkman S. Stress, appraisal and coping. New York: Springer-Verlag, 1984.

45. Turk DC, Rennert D. Pain and the terminally ill cancer patient: a cognitive social learning perspective. In: Sobell HJ, ed. Behavior therapy in terminal care. Cambridge, MA: Ballinger, 1981:95–123.

46. Moore K, Altmaier E. Stress inoculation training with cancer patients. Cancer Nurs 10:389–93, 1981.

47. Sobel H, Worden J. Helping cancer patients cope: a problem-solving intervention for health care professionals. New York: BMA/Guilford Press, 1981. (Audiocassette)

48. Jay SM, Elliott CH. Coping with childhood leukemia and its treatment: a parent's perspective. Urbana, IL: Carla Medical Communication, 1986. (Videotape)

49. Jay SM, Elliott CH. A stress inoculation program for parents whose children are undergoing painful medical procedures. J Consult Clin Psychol 58:799–804, 1990.

50. Fawzy FI, Fawzy NW. Psychoeducational interventions. In: Holland JC, ed. Psycho-oncology. New York: Oxford University Press, 1998: 676–93.

51. Fawzy I, Fawzy NW, Arndt LA, Pasnas RO. Critical review of psychosocial interventions in cancer care. Arch Gen Psychiatry 52:110–12, 1995.

52. Richardson JL, Shelton DR, Krailo M, Levine AM. The effect of compliance with treatment on survival among patients with hematologic malignancies. J Clin Oncol 8(2):356–64, 1990.

53. Fawzy FI, Fawzy NW, Hyun CS, et al. Malignant melanoma: effects of an early structured psychiatric intervention, coping and affective state on recurrence and survival 6 year later. Arch Gen Psychiatry 50:681–9, 1993.

54. Classen C, Sephton SE, Diamond S, Spiegel D. Studies of life-extending psychosocial interventions. In: Holland JC,

ed. Psycho-oncology. New York: Oxford University Press, 1998:730–42.

55. Sourkes BM, Massie MJ, Holland JC. Psychotherapeutic issues. In: Holland JC, ed. Psycho-oncology. New York: Oxford University Press, 1998:694–700.

56. Spiegel D, Bloom JR, Kraemer HC, Gottheil E. Effect of psychosocial treatment on survival of patients with metastatic breast cancer. Lancet 2:888–91, 1989.

57. Spiegel D. Living beyond limits. New York: Times Books, 1993.

58. Foley KM. Pain syndromes in patients with cancer. In: Bonica JJ, Ventafriddi V, Fink RB, et al., eds. Advances in pain research and therapy. New York: Raven Press, 1975:59–75.

59. Foley KM. The treatment of cancer pain. N Engl J Med 313:845, 1985.

60. Breitbart W, Holland JC. Psychiatric aspects of cancer pain. In: Foley KM, et al., eds. Advances in pain research and therapy. New York: Raven Press, 1990:73–87.

14 Rehabilitation medicine interventions

THERESA A. GILLIS
Christiana Care Health System and the Helen F. Graham Cancer Center

Introduction

Rehabilitation is a term not frequently associated with the management of cancer pain. However, the rehabilitation concept is a framework in which cancer pain management resides. Rehabilitation may be defined as the process of restoration and maximization of quality of life through enhancing function and mitigating disability. A person's function is influenced by abilities and limitations, and includes domains of physical health, emotional status, intellect/cognition, vocational and avocational activity, social activity, and role fulfillment.

The burden of pain is manifested in an individual through suffering but also through impaired function and consequent reduction in independence, as well as alterations in social roles and self-image. Successful pain management, therefore, may bring about improved mobility and function, and thus quality of life. Pain management becomes an essential step in the successful rehabilitation of the cancer patient.

Rehabilitation interventions include both pain-managing and pain-relieving techniques, as well as efforts to improve function. Functionally oriented efforts may involve the application of strengthening, coordination, balance, and other training exercises; use of therapeutic equipment; and adaptive education. This chapter focuses on those interventions directed toward pain management. Some movement-based therapies are used for pain management, although their more frequently recognized benefits are strength, coordination, endurance, and balance. The pain management and functional improvement goals are never exclusive and frequently coexist for cancer patients throughout the course of the disease.

Rehabilitation philosophy

Rehabilitation has traditionally been viewed as an intervention used after a chronologically discrete onset of disability, such as may follow a cerebrovascular accident, traumatic spinal cord injury, or amputation. This model is widely accepted in both lay and medical professional populations, and the course of functional recovery is somewhat predictable (Fig. 14.1). However, rehabilitation also plays crucial roles in chronic disease models, for which disability is more gradual, fluctuant in severity, and unpredictable in course. Pertinent examples of these include rheumatoid arthritis and other arthidities, diabetic vasculopathy and neuropathy, and Parkinson's disease, all of which may have waxing and waning courses of functional impairment requiring intensive rehabilitation or maintenance programs.

Rehabilitation services have not been universally offered to cancer patients, and rehabilitation concepts are not always incorporated in their care. There are many possible reasons for this oversight. The diagnosis of cancer still holds a mystique for many rehabilitation professionals, who equate it to a death sentence despite an

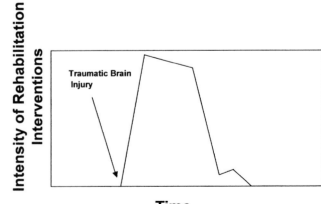

Fig. 14.1 Rehabilitation intervention following discrete pathophysiologic event, such as traumatic spinal cord injury, cerebrovascular accident, traumatic brain injury, or amputation.

overall improving survival rate. There is limited exposure to patients receiving cancer treatment during the training of many therapists and physiatrists, and therefore little experience to refute their erroneous beliefs. Anxieties provoked by these beliefs and awareness of their own knowledge deficits lead some rehabilitationists to exclude those with cancer diagnoses. Very slowly, this tide is turning and, in the United States, there is increasing interest in adding specific oncology training into therapy school curricula and physical medicine and rehabilitation physician residency education.

Both oncology professionals and rehabilitationists may be dissuaded from offering rehabilitation because of concerns that a "poor" prognosis makes rehabilitation concepts a waste of time and effort. Because "cancer" encompasses a multitude of tumor pathologies and patient-specific factors such as stage at diagnosis, tumor response to prior treatment, and morbidity from prior treatment, as well as perhaps change in tumor behavior over time, each patient is somewhat unique. It is more difficult to describe a functional ability curve as shown in Fig. 14.2 with much certainty for any given cancer

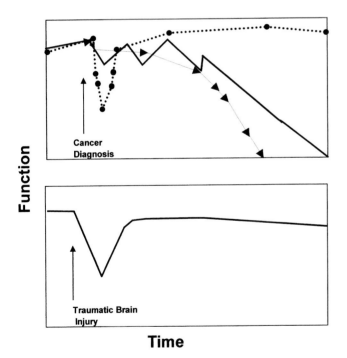

Fig. 14.2 Variability in functional abilities after cancer diagnosis compared to more predictable functional recovery after traumatic brain injury. Cancer diagnosis, histopathological factors, and individual patient characteristics create much more uncertainty in rehabilitative management. In traumatic brain injury and many other rehabilitative diagnoses, the severity of functional limitation may vary, but the recovery course and stability of function are more consistent.

patient. Understanding these factors as much as possible for a *specific* patient remains necessary to create a rehabilitation plan appropriate to his or her situation. When a patient with stage IV carcinoma of the lung with liver metastasis develops a paraplegia as a result of metastatic spinal cord compression in a high thoracic level, rehabilitation efforts should be pursued. Rehabilitation goals that included gait training, planning for work re-entry, and prescription of an electric wheelchair and van lift in order to return to work would usually be inappropriate because of the length of time required to reach those goals relative to expected survival. Appropriate rehabilitation efforts might include training in safe transfers from bed to a wheelchair to avoid injury, patient or family/caregiver education regarding protection of insensate skin, bowel and bladder management, and bathing strategies. Independent mobility within the home might include an electric wheelchair if resources permit; more often a lightweight, well-fitted wheelchair with removable arm and leg rests may be rented. It is most helpful to identify the patient's needs first, then attack as many as possible, as completely as possible, within the boundaries afforded by the patient's priorities, resources available (i.e., financial, rehabilitation, workplace, family, and community support), and disease process.

There are also biases and misconceptions regarding cancer-related disability among patients, caregivers, and the general public. Many people unnecessarily accept functional decline as a natural part of the disease process. They may also accept pain as a necessary aspect of the cancer diagnosis. Encouraging changes in public knowledge and awareness through media and Internet access has led to expectations of greater quality of life over the past several years.

Other factors may contribute to lack of use of rehabilitation services. Many oncologists and surgeons have little experience with organized rehabilitation efforts in the care of patients during their training. Some oncologists are more focused on the course of the patient's disease than the functional deficits caused by the disease and treatments. Many patients are more focused on survival during their physician visits and may not mention functional problems. Rehabilitation interventions may be inaccurately perceived as expensive care despite the fact that a therapeutic joint injection or a series of physical therapy treatments may cost less than 1 month's supply of an analgesic medication for a painful joint. These treatments are usually less expensive than "routine" diagnostic studies, many of which are obtained serially during the course of treatment. Most frequently, however, the oncology treatment team fails to recognize a problem that is amenable to rehabilitation in their patient (1).

As cancer treatments improve and patients survive longer as a result of slower disease progression, better disease management, or cure, a chronic disease model for cancer rehabilitation will become more widely understood. This model entails use of rehabilitation interventions in gradually increasing proportions as impairments increase because of cancer or cancer treatment (2). A second appropriate model incorporates repeating, and in some cases, cyclical, brief bursts of rehabilitation after acute exacerbations of disability (Fig. 14.3).

Particularly challenging to oncologists, physiatrists, and other rehabilitation professionals, and especially to patients, is the reality that overwhelming cancer pain, tremendous functional impairment, and large systemic tumor burden often go hand-in-hand. Tumor metastases to the neurological and musculoskeletal systems create direct and severe functional impairments. Other compromised systems (e.g., respiratory, gastrointestinal, integumentary) also limit function through symptoms of discomfort or inconvenience.

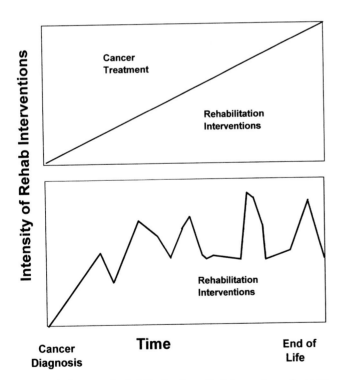

Fig. 14.3 Patterns of rehabilitation intensity between time of cancer diagnosis and end of life. Rehabilitation interventions are defined as functional restoration (mobility, activities of daily living, therapeutic exercise), education, adaptive equipment, ambulatory aids and orthoses, and pain management.

Impairments may also arise as a consequence of pain-relieving medications or procedures. Examples of these include limitations in mobility after spinal fusion, cordotomy, or use of epidural anesthetics. Patients with cancer often face disability as a direct result of their treatment. Limb salvage procedures, amputations, laryngectomies, and other surgical procedures leave readily identifiable deficits. Less frequently identified but often equally disabling consequences of treatment include joint contractures, lymphedema, leg length discrepancy, and osteoporotic fractures.

Lastly, patients do not experience cancer in a health vacuum. Co-morbidity becomes a larger and more significant concern in an aging population. Peripheral vascular disease, diabetic neuropathy, osteoarthritis, visual and auditory losses, and cognitive fragility are more frequently encountered (3). Although unrelated to the cancer diagnosis, recovery of independence may be slowed or prevented by these factors.

A rehabilitation plan may include strengthening exercises, training the patient and caregiver regarding the safe use of ambulatory aids (e.g., walkers, canes, crutches), orthoses and prostheses, adaptive equipment (e.g., bath bench, elevated commode seat), wheelchairs, and transfer assist devices (e.g., lifts, sliding boards). Medical professionals such as physiatrists, physical therapists, and occupational therapists typically provide rehabilitation interventions. Nurses, oncologists, and many other care providers also use and reinforce these and related strategies. Ultimately, patients and caregivers learn to use these strategies, with some modification, in a self-maintenance program. The ultimate goal of all rehabilitation interventions is to maximize knowledge, self-care, and health so that the patient is empowered to function as autonomously as possible.

Rehabilitation and pain management

Rehabilitation care often has much to offer in the management of cancer pain. Physiatrists and therapists may use range of motion and stretching of specific soft tissue and muscle groups to relieve contractures, improve mobility and posture, and thus reduce discomfort. Restoring muscle balance and joint or spine kinetics enhances muscular efficiency and thus reduces fatigue. Modalities can generate beneficial effects on local areas of pain and may also serve as powerful pain modulators at both the spinal and cerebral levels. Massage, transcutaneous electrical nerve stimulation (TENS), acupuncture and acupressure, and thermal modalities (ultrasound, topical heat and cold) are postulated to influence pain perception through endogenous pain modulating systems, as originally described in the gate-control theory (4). Direct effects on local tissues are also presumed to occur via alterations in blood flow and inflammatory cascades (see later).

For patients with pain caused by direct tumor invasion, physical interventions are generally adjuncts to pharmacological management. Patients with advancing cancer who prefer rehabilitation approaches over opioid analgesic medications may have anxieties about drug use that must be explored by their physicians. Some non-pharmacologic interventions, however, may ease pain perception and aid patients even with the most severe cancer pain. Music, movement, and touch are recognized by patients as helpful in coping with discomfort, and although research in these areas is not robust, it is encouraging. Because of their simplicity and ease of use, these techniques tend to be overlooked. However, taking the time to introduce these to patients and families often results in a significant contribution to their quality of life throughout their course of disease, whether cancer is cured or controlled, or death is drawing near.

When pain originates in joints, muscle, or other soft tissues that are not directly involved by tumor, physical efforts are often efficacious and may be the only intervention required to effect relief. Unfortunately, quite often physicians rely solely on pharmacological means to treat the symptom rather than physical means that may successfully address the origin.

Skeletal pain

Pain may originate from the bone and articular surfaces. Examples of non-malignant pain syndromes include fractures, rheumatoid arthritis, spondyloarthropathies (e.g., ankylosing spondylitis), spondylolisthesis, osteomyelitis, and osteoarthritis including spinal facet degeneration. These syndromes may occur in the patient with cancer. Cancer-related skeletal pain is usually related to bone metastasis. Radiotherapy and other primary treatments can be effective and rehabilitative approaches should be considered as part of the overall strategy. In the cancer population, skeletal pain also may occur as a result of osteoporotic compression fractures of the spine and insufficiency fractures of the pelvis, which may be late sequelae of hormonal ablation (both estrogen and testosterone); long-term or frequent corticosteroid treatment of cancer; the use of FK506, cyclosporine and other immunosuppressive medications (5–7); and/or local radiation treatment. Many cancer patients encounter more

than one of these risk factors, and such fractures are not uncommon. Avascular necrosis is also an etiology of treatment-related pain.

Rehabilitative options for management of these painful conditions may include use of bracing or casting to immobilize painful segments, use of cooling modalities to reduce acutely inflamed joints (although often poorly tolerated by rheumatoid patients), and use of ambulatory aids such as crutches and walkers when lower extremities are affected. Intra-articular injections of steroids can be highly effective for severely affected joints in arthritic patients.

Osteoporosis management may require treatment with calcium, vitamin D, estrogen replacement for women and testosterone for men when not contraindicated, and/or bisphosphonate therapy (e.g., alendronate sodium). Alendronate has been shown to normalize the rate of bone turnover and increase bone mass (8). *Essential* rehabilitation treatments for osteoporotic patients include postural correction exercises, strengthening of spine extension musculature, and stretching of the anterior chest, neck, and abdominal muscles. Weight training, with weights gradually increasing from as little as 1 to 2 pounds, and weight-bearing exercises (e.g., walking, Tai Chi) (9) are also helpful for maintaining strength and enhancing bone density, and lessening risk for fractures or additional fractures (10). Spinal flexion exercises and forceful forward bending or lifting of heavy weights from a flexed position must be avoided (11).

Neuropathic pain

Pain associated with direct damage of neural structures is usually characterized as burning, electrical, lancinating, or squeezing. Spinal cord, plexus, and peripheral nerves may be injured through tumor encroachment on these structures, surgical procedures, and chemotherapy agents. Postherpetic neuralgia is not uncommon among cancer patients, and phantom pains after amputation or mastectomy (12) are recognized. Dysesthesias in the distribution of the intercostobrachial nerve (along the posteromedial upper arm) after axillary dissection is sometimes a cause of anxiety among patients who have not been warned about these very common sequelae. Interventions include desensitization techniques such as massage, tapping, and patting the affected area, and electrical stimulation (TENS, "Neuroprobe") in hopes of modulating the pain at the spinal level. Compression by tight garments can ease perceptions of pain and are particularly useful for peripheral neuropathy and phantom limb sufferers.

Soft tissue pain

Non-malignant pain may originate within muscles as a result of injury, inflammation, or overuse. Frequently, this cause of pain is overlooked in cancer patients. Once bone metastasis, spinal cord compression, plexopathy, and other diagnoses detectable with imaging studies have been ruled out, physicians may be stymied as to how to proceed. Several diagnoses have been overused in a "waste-basket" manner because of this dilemma, including postthoracotomy syndrome and postmastectomy syndrome. In fact, many of these patients have rib or scapular motion limitations and not primarily neuropathic pain, and their pain may be resolved through rehabilitative treatment alone. As occurs elsewhere in the practice of medicine, the practitioner's diagnostic skills, interpretation of physical findings, philosophical framework and conceptualization of pain mechanisms, and familiarity with therapeutic options create tremendous variability in the choice of therapy and physical agents used.

Diagnosis of muscle dysfunction is difficult, relying on palpatory skills to detect tissue texture changes and sometimes subtle range of motion limitations or postural deviations. Research does support the notion that patients in pain experience changes in muscle activation. Surface electromyography (EMG) studies of patients in pain revealed failure of the dysfunctioning muscle to return to a quiet baseline electrophysiologic activity at the conclusion of movement, or a higher peak level of activity compared to paired non-painful muscles (13). However, experimentally produced muscle pain causes suppression of EMG resting activity (14).

When pain is thought to originate within a discrete muscle unit, with a trigger point and its associated referred pain pattern, injection or dry needling may be chosen. If the pain is muscular with dull, aching characteristics but without trigger point findings, and postural changes or range of motion limitations are found, stretch or massage may be chosen. Aching pains thought to originate within a spinal segment's sclerotome (vertebral body and its costal processes or neural arch) or its associated myotome may be treated through manipulation interventions.

Trigger points

Myofascial trigger points have been described as hyperirritable spots, which are generally within taut bands of skeletal muscle or the muscle's fascia (15–17). They possess fairly uniform characteristics on examination (Table 14.1) (18).

Pain refers from an active trigger point into contiguous or non-contiguous structures, often but not necessarily

Table 14.1. *Trigger point characteristics*

- Sharply circumscribed spot of exquisite tenderness
- Local twitch response with snapping palpation
- Recoil or flinching ("jump sign") with pressure
- Painful active or passive stretch of affected muscle
- Reduced range of motion or distensibility of affected muscle
- Painful contraction of affected muscle
- Reduced maximal contractile force
- Deep tenderness and dysesthesia referral
- Autonomic disturbance in reference zone (pallor, hyperemia, sudomotor, pilomotor activity with stimulation)

within the same dermatome, sclerotome, or myotome innervated by a posterior spinal root (19). It is theorized that trigger points arise in areas of increased metabolic demand, reduced circulation and local ischemia, or areas of focal nociceptor or mechanoreceptor hyperirritability. Combinations of these factors or some other antecedent pathophysiology may be postulated. They may be activated directly by acute muscular overload or overuse, direct trauma, or cold. Activation may also occur indirectly through 1) protective postural responses to nearby intra-articular inflammation, arthritides, or other active trigger points; 2) referred visceral pain, with the trigger point found in the myotome shared by the same visceral innervation; and 3) emotional distress. Trigger points are self-sustaining in that they do not resolve spontaneously, although they may become "latent" or less symptomatic with time, awaiting the next triggering event. They are often accompanied by sleep disturbance as well. Trigger points may also arise within scars, with different symptomatology; these refer burning, prickling, or lancinating pains locally and without referral patterns. There is no palpable neuroma or discrete mass at these sites.

Muscular imbalance and shortening

In the absence of trigger points, pain may also arise from shortened muscles or soft tissues, which change the muscular balance of a joint. Any given muscle has an optimal resting length and an optimal dynamic length and must work harmoniously with surrounding muscles for movement. A muscle may be overstretched because of contracted soft tissues in its accompanying nearby joint or contracted antagonist muscles. An *overstretched* muscle fibril has poor actin-myosin cross-bridging within its sarcomere and, therefore, reduced contractility, resulting ultimately in reduced strength. Muscular injury and inflammation can arise with attempts to use the overstretched muscle against resistance. *Foreshortened* muscle also fails to have optimal actin-myosin cross-bridging and thus also has reduced strength. Foreshortened muscles place their antagonist counterpart muscles at suboptimal resting and active lengths, and restrict joint range of motion; this increases the risk of tendinous, ligamentous, and articular injury. Stretching encompasses manual techniques applied by physical therapists, osteopathic physicians, chiropractors, and patients themselves. These interventions seek to move joints and muscles to restore optimal muscular length and joint mobility, and thus reduce pain and maximize strength and function.

Somatic dysfunction

Somatic dysfunction is a concept used by practitioners of manual medicine, including osteopathic physicians, chiropractors, and some physical therapists and allopathic physicians. It is defined as impaired or altered function of related components of the somatic (body framework) system; skeletal, arthrodial, and myofascial structures; and related vascular, lymphatic, and neural elements. The diagnostic criteria for somatic dysfunction include asymmetry of structure or function, impaired range of motion of a joint or region (either hypermobile or hypomobile), and tissue texture abnormality within the skin, fascia, muscle, ligament, etc. (20). Treatment of somatic dysfunction is through manipulative or manual therapy, and its goal is the restoration of maximal, pain-free movement of the musculoskeletal system in postural balance. Muscle strength testing, observation of physical symmetry during patient motion and at rest, and a thorough neurological examination are of critical importance to eliminate malignant etiologies for pain before use of manipulative therapy, owing to its high risks of severe injury.

Capsulitis, ligamentous and tendinous injuries

Intrabursal and intra-articular injections are also frequently helpful for temporary relief of pain from adhesive capsulitis of the shoulder as an adjunct to a physical therapy program (21), but should not be repeated more than once. Heating of musculature with ultrasound or more superficial methods promotes stretch of the capsule. Management of chronic bursitis may also warrant intrabursal corticosteroid injection. An acutely inflamed bursa can indicate a septic joint, and fluid analysis, including cell count, culture, and crystal detection, is warranted.

Shoulder pain in plegic or paretic upper extremities (whether spastic or flaccid) (22) is poorly understood. Anterior and inferior subluxation of the humeral head, capsular constriction, overstretch of the rotator cuff musculature, and bicipital tendonitis are likely co-existent etiologies for the pain these patients experience. Cold and heat modalities, orthosis support of the joint, gentle stretching of tight muscles, and antispasticity medications may be used.

Ligamentous and tendinous pain usually arise through acute strains or tears. Diagnosis is usually made by history; joint instability is generally not apparent because of edema and protective subconscious inhibition (splinting) by the patient. Rest, ice, and immobilization are commonly used and compression and elevation help reduce edema formation and accompanying pain.

Manual interventions

Trigger point management

Practitioners have found that needling a trigger point, either with or without injections of saline or anesthetic agents, relieves the focal pain as well as the referral. Many clinicians also follow injections with stretch of the affected muscle and related muscle groups. Some clinicians will apply forceful localized pressure during massage to these points, or use acupressure or acupuncture needle insertion into these areas. There is a correlation of 70% between classically defined acupuncture points and trigger points (23).

The diagnosis of trigger points is specific to the characteristics described previously. It is intuitive but sometimes forgotten by rehabilitationists and pain management physicians that an area of tenderness and palpable nodularity can originate from metastatic foci within soft tissues. Therefore, needling techniques must be used with caution when the possibility of soft tissue metastasis is present, and avoided when the classically defined examination findings are absent. The risk of severe hemorrhage caused by needling must also be noted if the primary cancer is hypervascular in nature, such as renal cell carcinoma.

Directed stretching of the affected muscle(s) is more successful in obtaining relief, and more useful for patients with numerous trigger points or multiple affected muscles than needling, and is non-invasive. Vapocoolant spray and ice massage may be used to both distract the patient from the discomfort of the stretch and to reduce local blood flow and inflammation, as discussed later. Scar manipulation via massage, needling with acupuncture, or injections of short-acting anesthetic agents may inactivate these points (24). Scar treatments are also routinely performed in acupuncture therapy, for both pain management and overall health maintenance, and are discussed in more detail later.

A randomized, controlled trial compared ultrasound, massage, and exercise against sham ultrasound, massage, and exercise. After a 4-week treatment period no benefit was detected for the ultrasound group, although both groups were improved over the control group. This study's findings gave mild support to the role of massage in trigger point management (25). Further study comparing modalities, massage, and specific stretching interventions are needed, as massage alone is not the primary means of trigger point treatment.

Stretch and manipulation

Osteopathic medicine was founded in the theory that disease arises from mechanical pressure on the nerves and blood vessels of the spine, and that this pressure is caused by malalignment of vertebrae or the associated musculature, and laxity or shortening (contracture) of those muscles. Chiropractic practice attends more specifically to the vertebral segments. Manipulative therapy may be defined as movement of a bone or a joint in an attempt to improve its range of motion or its alignment with other structures. Practitioners of manual medicine identify and treat somatic dysfunction (see previously). The goal of manipulation is to restore maximal, pain-free movement of the musculoskeletal system in postural balance.

Manipulation has been well accepted by the public (26). Despite a paucity of randomized controlled trials (27), these manual techniques are gaining acceptance among allopathic practitioners for the treatment of selected painful conditions.

Osteopathic and chiropractic manipulation in the cancer population is controversial. Most literature from these disciplines describe cancer as an absolute contraindication to manipulative therapy because of concerns about metastatic involvement in the spine or epidural space (28). Little mention is made in the literature of actual examples of manipulation-induced complications in cancer patients, but theoretically the risks of neurological injury or skeletal injury exist. Because of these safety considerations, manipulative therapy should be considered appropriate for neuromyotomal or myofascial pains that arise from maladaptive, compensatory postural changes in areas not directly involved by primary or metastatic disease.

In most manipulative therapy schemata, a painful joint is moved to its physiological tissue barrier and then beyond it to gain realignment and proper motion. The patient presentation and the practitioner's skills and training philosophy dictate the direction of movement, choice of direct or indirect (leveraged) technique, and the force used. Anecdotally, gentle, non-thrust, low-velocity movements are well tolerated by patients when the treated areas are not directly or indirectly compromised by tumor. Muscle energy techniques use patient movements against the resistance of the practitioner in isometric or near-isometric contractions. Because the force and duration of effort are completely controlled by the patient, muscle energy techniques can be used safely in body segments where no tumor is present and no risk of fracture is detected.

Manual and mechanical traction can also be used to achieve soft tissue and muscular stretch. Patients are generally passively stretched by these interventions. Stretch may relieve an acute episode of pain, but rehabilitation is incomplete until the opposing musculature is strengthened sufficiently to reduce recurrence of the painful process.

Massage

Evidence of massage for therapeutic purposes can be traced to ancient Chinese, Japanese, Greek, and Indian Ayurvedic health practices and was well established as a health-maintaining activity by the Romans. After the decline of the Roman Empire, little was known about its use until "Turkish massage" was reintroduced to Europe through the writings of de Chauliac in the 1300s and Pare' in the 1500s (29); Paré coined the stroke names *effleurage, pétrissage,* and *tapotement* (30). Interest in the West was heightened after French missionary work in China in the early nineteenth century. Ling in Sweden, followed by Metzger in Holland, as well as Tissot and Georgii in France, spread the use of massage through Europe. "Swedish massage" has grown in popularity; it and other forms of massage are now among the most commonly used complementary medicine interventions (26).

The most common uses of massage are promotion of relaxation and reduction in pain and anxiety or stress. Feelings of well-being are elicited, which may arise from a feeling of companionship or care from the practitioner, or a change in self-image or ability to communicate. Direct mechanical physiological changes are also thought to occur, including transiently increased local blood and lymphatic flow and venous return (31–33). Edema is mobilized and venous return is increased, allowing enhanced arterial flow into the tissue capillary beds (34). Reflexive physiological changes have been proposed by some authors, such as increased sympathetic activity with increased systolic blood pressure, heart rate, peripheral skin temperature, and decreased respiration rate (35). Others have found no consistent effects on autonomic functions (36). In one study, beta-endorphins were found to increase in subjects for 1 hour after massage, peaking at a 5-minute postmassage test (33), but Day et al. found no significant changes in endorphin levels after massage (37). Deep friction massage, although uncomfortable, can be used to release fascial limitations when these inhibit range of motion.

A recent review of randomized trials of massage therapy for non-malignant low back pain suggested that it might be a beneficial therapy but that few unflawed studies have been published (38). In three studies, massage was compared to chiropractic manipulation or electrostimulation (39), manipulation (40), and balneotherapy (spa treatments), traction, or non-treatment (41); in all cases, no significant differences were obtained between massage and the alternate therapy approaches. The case can be argued, however, that the subjects in these studies had quite heterogenous biomechanical derangements and chronicities. If study designs incorporated these more specific diagnostic descriptions and subjects were stratified accordingly, different subject diagnostic groups may have responded more favorably to specific treatments.

Although used successfully in the treatment of trigger points, myofascial pain, lymphedema, and the pain and spasm related to upper motor neuron injuries, massage has the potential to worsen inflammatory or traumatic arthritis, bursitis, phlebitis, and entrapment neuropathies. It may be associated with bleeding in patients with hemophilia or a coagulopathy (42).

Research specifically exploring the use of massage in cancer patients is also limited. Ferrel-Torry and Glick identified significant reductions in pain perception on a visual analog scale (VAS) immediately after a 30-minute massage. The intervention included effleurage, pétrissage, and trigger point massage (43). Another study found that a very brief (10-minute) massage had brief benefit in VAS pain intensity only for the male subjects. Detailed description of the massage method was not included (44).

Acupuncture

Acupuncture needles are believed to stimulate type II and type II muscle afferent nerves or A delta fibers, sending impulses to the spinal cord. In the spinal cord, acupuncture-induced release of enkephalin and dynorphin presynaptically block transmission of pain signals into the spinothalamic tract. Input to the midbrain periaqueductal gray matter and raphe nucleus can lead to the release of norepinephrine and serotonin in the spinal cord to inhibit pain presynaptically and postsynaptically in the spinothalamic tract. Pituitary stimulation releases beta-endorphin into the blood from the pituitary (45).

In Oriental medicine, acupuncture needles are placed to correct deficiencies in Qi, loosely interpreted by Westerners as one's vital energy or life force and defense against illness and disease. The location, pattern, and order of needle placement influences the balance of yin and yang within the patient, adding to or dissipating the "energy" in the organs and functions influenced by specific meridians where Qi circulates.

Electroacupuncture combines use of acupuncture needles and either high (100–200 Hz) or low (2–4 Hz) frequency electrical stimulation. High frequency stimulation has been shown to have a rapid-onset, non-cumulative, non-opioid receptor-mediated effect. Its analgesia does not outlast the treatment (46). Conversely, low frequency stimulation creates a slow onset, cumulative-benefit, naloxone-reversible effect, which persists after the treatment. Use of electrical therapy is determined by the practitioner's experience.

As mentioned previously, there is considerable overlap between trigger points and acupuncture points. Many acupuncture points are also palpably detectable hollows or anatomical tissue planes, which, in Western theory, may signify easily influenced zones of lymphaticoneurovascular bundles in the subcutaneous tissue. Peripheral endings of cranial and spinal nerves, and penetrations of neurovascular bundles through superficial fascia, have been cited as morphological findings of acupuncture points (47). Acupuncture treatment protocols are highly individualized to both patient characteristics and practitioner's style and interpretation of findings, making randomized controlled trials exceptionally difficult to achieve.

Many Oriental cultures have developed their own methods of Qi manipulation. Acupressure is the use of fingers, thumbs, and hands to stimulate acupuncture points. It has shown benefit in managing postoperative pain (48). Shiatsu, which means "finger pressure" in Japanese, is the use of heavy, perpendicular pressure applied with the fingers, palm of the hand, or heel of the foot. The treating practitioner's "energetic" characteristics are also thought to influence the degree of benefit for the patient. Mention in scientific literature is extremely limited, although mention has been made of its use in palliative care (49).

Reflex systems

Several anatomical structures have been identified in different cultures and traditions as having the ability to manifest signs of injury or disease elsewhere in the body. The hand, ear, foot, scalp, and other sites have been described as having a homuncular organization (50). In the ear, for example, organization of the anatomy on the ear follows embryological patterns. Endodermal organs are represented in the concha, mesodermal organs in the pinna, and ectodermal organs on the lobule. Sympathetic and parasympathetic nerve fibers with cell bodies in the reticular formation supply the ear, and in theory this connection allows transmission of messages from the body to the ear and vice versa. Concha innervation is primarily parasympathetic via the vagus nerve, whereas the pinna involves sympathetic fibers from the trigeminal nerve, and the lobule from the superior cervical plexus. Pain or tenderness is elicited by even superficial touch, and changes in cutaneous appearance (discoloration or pallor, flaking, hyperhidrosis or dryness, swelling, etc.) occurring in areas that correspond to the afflicted region. Changes in electrical conductance can also be detected in discrete points on the ear that correspond to areas of pain or dysfunction. "Reflexology" typically refers to treatment of the foot. Acupuncturists and other practitioners of Oriental medicine commonly use stimulation of ear points. Massage, electrical stimulation, acupuncture, and acupressure techniques are used at these areas.

Touch

Massage and stretch use touch as a means to enact the activity, whereas simple touch is an end unto itself. Laying on of hands has been understood across the centuries as a healing intervention. Companionship, compassion, and empathy are communicated by this interaction and can benefit the patient through this emotional validation. Intuitively, touch is beneficial for many patients through its influence on the suffering, emotional component of the painful experience. Its use is obviously not limited to the health care team.

Reiki is a practice ranging from the laying on of hands to healing at a distance. Its origins are also within Asia. An interesting uncontrolled pilot study of patients experiencing cancer and non-cancer pain showed significant improvements in visual analog and Likert scale ratings of pain after a single Reiki treatment (51). Obviously much more work is needed in this area before it can be identified as an effective adjuvant means of pain management.

Modalities

Humans have used modalities since the earliest of times to decrease pain and return a person to optimal physical functioning. In rehabilitation medicine, these modalities have included diathermy, spa therapy, hydrotherapy, use of cold and heat, and ultrasound. Traditionally, therapists have been taught not to use heat or ultrasound in cancer patients, as these allow for increased blood flow to and from a tumor site, possibly potentiating metastases. Unfortunately, the data supporting or refuting this claim are insufficient. Some of these modalities have gained widespread acceptance despite few well-designed supportive studies.

Superficial heat and cold

Superficial heat is recognized as a means of increasing collagen extensibility and decreasing joint fluid viscosity, as well as enhancing local metabolic activity. Superficial cold has opposite effects; its desirable effect is to reduce metabolic activity in areas of acute inflammation and pain. Modalities effect temperature change via conduction, convection, or conversion.

Hydrocollator packs are segmented canvas sacks filled with silica dioxide, which absorbs heated water (70–80° C) and then conducts heat in a therapeutic range for as long as 30 minutes. Hot packs should be wrapped in towels to absorb moisture and protect the skin. They can be quite heavy and thus difficult to tolerate on painful areas. Patients should not lie on packs because of increased temperatures generated at bony prominences and increased risk of injury focally. Commercially available gel packs can be heated in either a microwave or in hot water at the stovetop. Heating is obviously more difficult to control, with heightened risk of burns, and the duration of heat is much shorter. However, they are easy to use and well accepted by patients.

Heating lamps use tungsten or quartz heating elements to generate infrared energy. In the home, incandescent bulbs can also generate heat. Changing the distance between the bulb and the patient controls the maximum heat and rate of heating.

Heating pads may have electrical heating elements or circulating fluid. Electrical heating pads have been shown to generate peak temperatures as high as almost 52° C on merely the lowest setting, and temperature oscillations of up to 5° C were also found (52).

The dipping or immersing of distal extremities into liquified *paraffin* is another form of superficial heating.

Mineral oil and paraffin are combined in a 1:7 ratio and maintained at 52–54° C; the reservoir should be cool enough to have a rim of congealed wax at its edges to prevent burns during immersion. Home units are available but are somewhat expensive. For many patients, warm-water baths are just as comfortable and have less associated mess. Traditionally, paraffin baths have been used for contracted joints in the hands or feet resulting from rheumatoid arthritis.

Superficial heat is obviously not completely free of the risk of injury. Blood flow to the heated area increases in an attempt to dissipate heat more rapidly. Inflammatory edema and bleeding increase as a result. There is also an increased production of lymphatic fluid, which can lead to lymphedema in at-risk individuals. Heat over insensate skin can easily create severe burns. Irradiated skin dissipates heat poorly owing to changes in microcirculation and loss of sweat glands or local lymphatic glands and can easily be injured.

Cryotherapy may be used to raise pain thresholds (53), temporarily diminish muscular tone and spasticity (54,55), decrease synovial collagenase activity (56), minimize formation of edema, and diminish inflammation (57). Cooling of the skin below about 15° C (58,59) acutely causes vasoconstriction. Gradual vasodilation appears to reflexively follow vasoconstriction in an attempt to rewarm the cooled area. In the presence of sustained cold, skin temperature drops rapidly, slows in its decline, and reaches equilibrium 12–16° C below its initial point at roughly 10 minutes, whereas subcutaneous tissues fall only 3–5° C during this time (54,60). Muscle temperatures after 5 minutes of ice massage at 2 cm below the skin surface have been reduced by as much as 15° C at the biceps brachii (61). Insulation by subcutaneous fat creates individual variability in effect. When a limb is packed in ice, vasoconstriction occurs within 5 minutes and can produce decreases of blood flow as great as 30% in soft tissue and 20% in skeletal muscle by 25 minutes (58).

Ice massage involves direct stroking of tissues with ice wands or chunks, often for 5 to 10 minutes at a time. Ice packs cool more gradually through toweling and are helpful to improve tolerance in some patients. *Vapocoolant sprays* produce local analgesia and are used frequently in the treatment of trigger points (see above) (62). Spray is applied in a linear fashion and parallel to the muscle fibers. Skin temperature may drop by as much as 20° C during application (63) as a result of evaporation. *Ice and cold water* are frequently used in the home or in therapy. Gel packs are commercially available, conform to joint shapes, and are quickly refrozen. Immersion of any tissue in water cooler than 15° C is poorly tolerated. Injuries may occur quickly; responses such as Raynaud's phenomenon, cold urticaria, frostbite and frostburn, and abrupt hypotensive changes must be watched for.

Ultrasound

Most therapeutic ultrasound is between 0.8 and 3 MHz; higher frequencies attenuate more rapidly and have poor tissue penetration, whereas lower frequencies are difficult to focus. Pulsed waveform (PW) or continuous waveform (CW) may be used. CW generates heat and is limited by patient comfort and risk of injury to 2.0 to 2.5 W/cm^2. PW alternates higher intensities of ultrasound with absence of signal, which avoids the heating limitations caused by CW. PW also creates streaming and cavitation movements of molecules within tissue, which dominate at higher intensities than are tolerable in CW. The benefits of PW are not universally acknowledged, and CW has been more thoroughly investigated.

Generally, treatment is applied in overlapping sweeping or circular motions for 10 minutes, using a conducting gel or mineral oil. Non-thermal effects such as cavitation and standing waves may cause tissue damage. To avoid injury, the applicator head should be kept in constant motion and fluid-filled cavities, such as the eye and gravid uterus, should be avoided. As described previously, appropriate intensities should also be maintained. Metal prosthesis or implants of any nature may create interfaces where heat could potentially build up. The spinal cord, heart, and brain should also be avoided.

Ultrasound is often used in areas of tendon and bursa inflammation, particularly at the shoulder, elbow, and knees. Some controlled studies in this patient population have found lack of benefit or lack of superiority to oral anti-inflammatory medications regarding the desired outcome of increased joint range of motion (64,65). Study designs were hampered by murky diagnostic criteria, lack of blinding, variations in the treatment protocols, and limited numbers of subjects. Definitive conclusions could not be reached.

Ultrasound is commonly used in the treatment of joint contractures and reduced range of motion. Ultrasound has been shown capable of heating the deep structures of the hip joint, which cannot be achieved through other superficial heating modalities (66–68). The combination of heat with stretching results in superior tendon extensibility compared to either agent alone (69).

Unfortunately, the efficacy of ultrasound for the treatment of osteoarthritis and joint inflammation is not fully established. Many studies fail to adequately separate chronic joint pain patients from acute injury, and CW or PW and dosing are often not standardized.

Water-based therapy

Water is a popular means of pain management throughout the world. The buoyancy of water reduces pain associated with weight bearing and axial loading. It is an effective means of heat transfer, via either convection with agitation or conduction when static. It can also serve as a medium for exercise, providing resistance in all planes of motion. Water temperatures between 33–36° C are most commonly used and are well tolerated by most patients. Precautions against heat or cold injury, as described earlier, are just as important in water therapies. Systemic hyperthermia and hypothermia and drowning are additional risks.

Hydrotherapy is the immersion of a limb or body region in warmed, agitated water. Whirlpool baths and specialized immersion tanks such as the Hubbard tank use pumps to agitate water. Temperatures below 33° C or above 38° C are usually not used for total body immersion; the higher the percentage of body surface immersed, the lower the temperature should be within this range. Systemic hyperthermia and cardiovascular injury can occur at temperatures above 38° C. Extremities can be treated in water as warm as 45° C for short periods.

Hydrotherapy is helpful for irrigation and debridement of wounds, often with handheld sprays or directional jets for better penetration and cleansing. The warm water encourages movement in painful or stiff joints. Water movement creates a sensation of massage that may relax muscle spasm and reduce overall anxiety. Facilitated stretch can be performed on a limb within the whirlpool or tank, although heat penetration to medium and large joints may not be as effective as ultrasound.

Balneotherapy refers to the therapeutic effects of baths, most commonly mineral baths. Despite the popularity of such baths in many places around the world, and in the United States in earlier centuries, it is uncommonly used now. Its benefits are thought largely to be confined to the general sense of well-being attributable to the buoyancy and reduced effort experienced in other forms of water therapy. However, when the integrity of the skin is reduced, such as with open wounds, psoriatic lesions, or other pathology, mineral and gas solutes may achieve penetration and exert benefits not seen in intact skin. Atmospheric gases (carbon dioxide, nitrogen, and methane), calcium, magnesium, cobalt, zinc (70), and hydrogen sulfide (71) may all be present in spa waters, but little is known regarding specific benefits of these solutes. Mineral-rich hot packs were found to be associated with significant improvements in morning stiffness and grip strength when compared to depleted, mineral-poor hot packs used in arthritic patients (72).

Transcutaneous electrical nerve stimulation

TENS is infrequently mentioned as a treatment for cancer pain. Ventafridda (73) reported the use of TENS among cancer patients. Relief was noted to be significant but of short duration in 70%–80%. By the tenth day of treatment, 58% of those with initially good relief found TENS no longer effective. Pain diagnoses (e.g., visceral, neuropathic, or bone metastasis) and stimulation characteristics were not well described, however.

Application of electrical stimulation to the skin has been shown to effect analgesia for a variety of painful conditions. High frequencies (80–100 Hz) stimulate large-diameter myelinated afferent nerve fibers, producing analgesia within the stimulated region with rapid onset. This analgesia is also not reversible by the opioid antagonist naloxone (74). This sensory input appears to influence the transmission of pain messages within the spinothalamic tract, either by direct inhibition of an abnormally or inappropriately active nerve or by activation of pain modulatory systems. Low-frequency stimulation (1–4 Hz) at higher intensities (10 or more amperes) activates sensory afferents and produces a localized muscle twitch. The analgesic response in this case is slower in onset, provides more generalized relief, persists after the conclusion of stimulation, and has cumulative effects (46). This mechanism is endorphin-dependent and thus reversible with naloxone (74).

It is much more common to use TENS for the more indirect causes of cancer-related pain such as myofascial pain, muscle spasm, or chronic postsurgical neuropathic pain. Studies of TENS for these pain diagnoses are also mixed in their findings. A double-blind study of acute and chronic low back pain patients, with presumably a variety of musculoskeletal pain etiologies, was treated with either high-intensity TENS or mechanically administered massage. Pain relief was noted to be significantly greater in the TENS group in this study (75). However, TENS was not significantly superior to ice massage among a group of patients with chronic low back pain

(76). Chronic neuralgic pain often responds well to low-frequency, high-amplitude stimulation, although duration of relief is variable. Subjects with postherpetic neuralgia and peripheral nerve lesions (77) appear to achieve more sustained relief than those with plexus (78) or radicular origins (79). TENS has also been used to effectively relieve acute postoperative pain after laparotomy, thoracotomy, and laminectomy (80).

Orthoses and ambulatory aids

The function of an orthosis is to support an anatomical structure to enable function or reduce pain. Many orthoses are used in the supportive management of cancer pain, particularly pain that is exacerbated or intensified by movement. An optimal orthosis relieves pain but enables function as much as possible. Thus, although casting a limb may completely immobilize a limb and thereby avoid movement-related pain, the ability to use the limb is so compromised that it is generally a poor choice.

Skin integrity is also a consideration in cancer patients. Nutritionally depleted patients with poor subcutaneous fat stores may tolerate skin pressure poorly, necessitating careful fitting of the device. Skin may be friable and easily injured because of the effects of steroidal medications. Irradiated skin often has a reduced ability to dissipate heat buildup underneath an orthosis. Irradiated skin may have fibrotic changes that prevent normal glide over subcutaneous structures and is thus predisposed to friction injury. Once injured, these areas heal with difficulty and with a higher risk of infection.

Spinal orthoses may be prescribed when primary or metastatic lesions affect the vertebral column or adjacent soft tissues. The orthoses may support the patient before and after surgical resection and stabilization of the spine, or be offered when the patient's advanced disease or other co-morbidities prevent them from being a surgical candidate. Excellent discussions of spinal stability and surgical rationale and techniques are found in the literature (81). The thoracolumbosacral orthosis (Fig. 14.4) provides the greatest restriction in motion in lower thoracic and lumbar segments. Higher thoracic levels and cervical involvement may require use of a sternal-occipital-mandibular immobilization brace (Fig. 14.5). Halo fixation provides the most complete immobilization of most cervical levels but is infrequently used in cancer patients.

When frank spinal instability is not a concern, orthoses may be chosen for pain relief and ease of application and use. The Jewett orthosis provides three-point contact at the sternum, pubis, and lumbar region, and is useful for

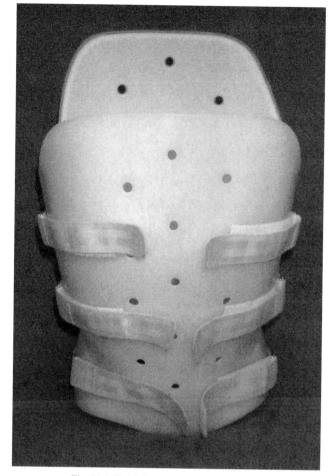

Fig. 14.4 Rigid thoracolumbosacral orthosis.

compression fractures in the thoracic and lumbar spine, when kyphosis and flexion forces on the spine need to be minimized. Rigid and soft cervical collars provide postural cues and slight reduction in range of motion, as rotation and lateral bending are not well controlled. Soft corsets provide comfort to some patients; patients however, with rib metastasis may not tolerate the pressure they exert on the thoracic cage (Fig. 14.6).

Extremity orthoses generally hold the limb in a position of function. This may be done for pain relief and improvement in safety or fatigue. An ankle-foot orthosis (AFO) creates a stable walking surface for patients with severe peripheral neuropathy and foot drop, but may also be helpful in those with weakness caused by lumbosacral plexopathy or paraparesis. The AFO reduces the energy cost of gait; without it, the patient with foot drop must hike the leg and/or excessively flex the knee during swing-through phase (steppage gait). The device also enhances proprioceptive awareness in patients with reduced sensation.

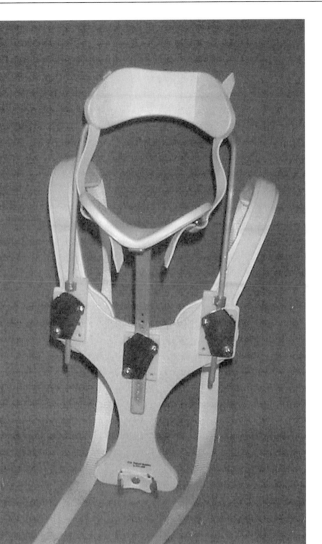

Fig. 14.5 Sternal-occipital-mandibular immobilization.

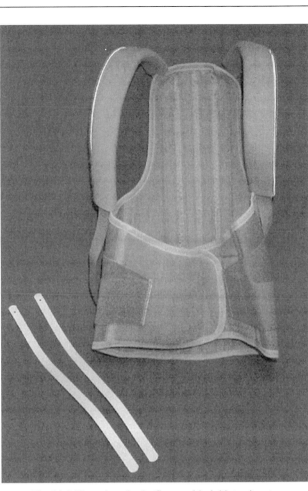

Fig. 14.6 Thoracic orthosis. Corset with rigid stay inserts.

Upper extremity devices may strive to decrease load of the limb on a painful shoulder joint and control planes of motion. The shoulder immobilizer (Fig. 14.7) or abduction pillow (Fig. 14.8) fulfills both these goals, and although the limb position is not one of optimal function, it can at least serve as a stable base of support for the contralateral limb to manipulate or hold items against. Several orthosis designs have been attempted to immobilize the scapula against the chest wall for patients with spinal accessory nerve loss or neuropraxia after cervical lymph node dissection. Without the function of the trapezius, scapular instability prevents overhead use of the ipsilateral arm.

Ambulatory aids permit transfer of the center of gravity away from painful lower extremities and decreased transmission of force through the painful limb. A wide range of devices are available (Fig. 14.9) and are prescribed by rehabilitationists based on patient-specific characteristics. Devices are fit to a patient based on height and girth, and patients require instruction by therapists for safety. Insurers and other health care payers may permit only one ambulatory aid and may not pay for revisions or changes when an improper device has been prescribed.

Compression

Compression has long been used as an intervention for acute injury, along with rest, ice, and elevation. In this use, compression retards the soft tissue swelling that accompanies the inflammatory cascade. This edema itself can be painful and may excessively slow the recovery of mobility. Compression is also often helpful in chronic conditions where pain or altered sensation exists, or edema persists. In the example of a humeral fracture brace (Fig. 14.10), the device provides mechanical stability through compression.

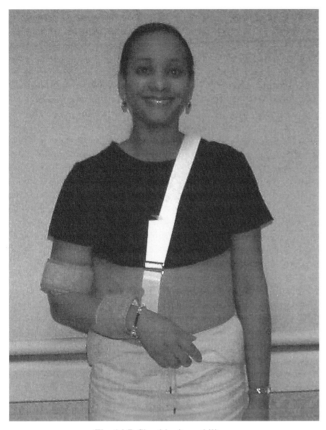

Fig. 14.7 Shoulder immobilizer.

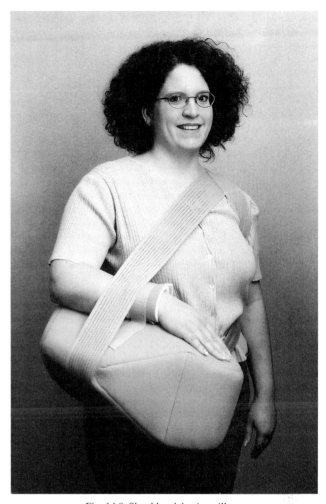

Fig. 14.8 Shoulder abduction pillow.

Use of compression garments or devices often help patients with allodynia or dysesthesias related to peripheral neuropathies, plexopathies, or radicular or other peripheral nerve injuries. Activation of endogenous pain modulatory systems may explain the diminished pain perception anecdotally experienced by these patients. However, while donning tight garments or custom-fitted sleeves or stockings, some patients experience exacerbation of pain. Although tight garments may also enhance sensory perception in the presence of peripheral neuropathies, possibly improving kinesthetic awareness, insensate skin must frequently be evaluated for the development of pressure injury, and patients and caregivers must monitor and inspect skin at least twice daily.

Compression garments, sleeves, and stockings are frequently used to attempt to control lymphatic edema. Lymphedema is not reversed but may accumulate more slowly in the presence of these garments. Optimal lymphedema treatment combines manual lymphatic drainage massage, a specific and superficially directed form of massage, with low-stretch compression bandaging and exercises for the affected limb. Treatment continues on a daily basis for several weeks until limb measurements have reached a stable degree of reduction and/or a caregiver can demonstrate independence in performing basic massage and bandaging techniques for the patient. Once limb size stabilizes, patients take on a more independent means of measuring and caring for the limb, including daytime wear of an appropriately sized or custom-fitted compression garment, and nighttime bandaging, if possible.

Pneumatic compression pumps have been used for many years in the treatment of chronic lymphedema of the extremities. Sequential, gradient pressure air chambers within the pneumatic sheath push lymphatic fluid into the axilla or groin. Concerns have been voiced about the potential for exacerbation of lymphatic injury through their use. Critics suggest that compression pumps force lymph into already overwhelmed proximal lymphatic vessels, promoting further injury and inflammation with repeated use.

The presence of tumor in axilla or groin is a general contraindication to the use of pneumatic pumps or lymphatic massage, owing to fears of tumor dissemination.

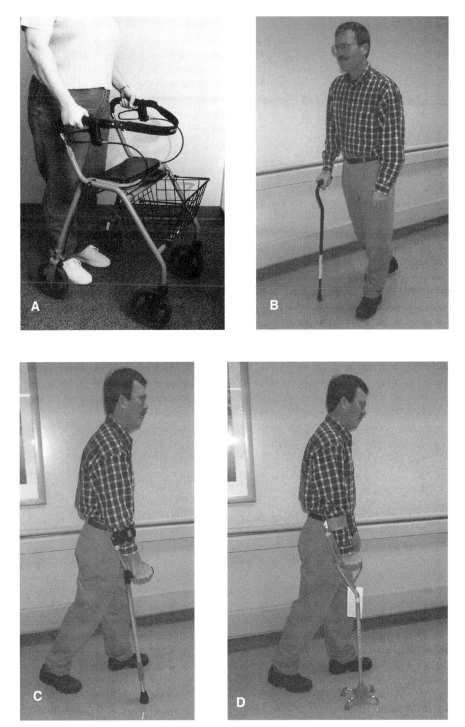

Fig. 14.9 (A) Rolling walker with brakes and seat. (B) Single-point cane. (C) Forearm crutch. (D) Quad-base care with forearm cuff.

Clinical experience has shown that pumps may exacerbate malignant pleural or pericardial effusions because of the rapidity of fluid shifting. Compressive bandaging is often used for palliation of malignant lymphedema, particularly if the edema causes pain, immobility, and/or recurrent infection. Descriptive studies of palliative treatment for malignant lymphedema are needed.

Energy conservation

The concept of "energy conservation" is frequently misunderstood, but may prove helpful to some patients experiencing cancer pain. Rather than resorting to bed rest and inactivity, the intervention encourages activity toward pleasurable or purposeful goals. Fundamental compo-

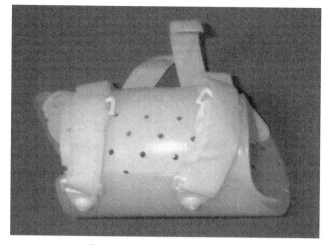

Fig. 14.10 Humeral fracture brace.

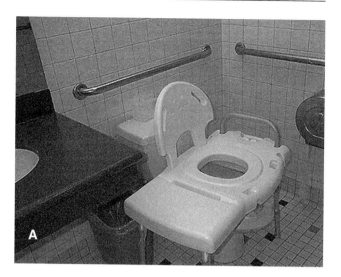

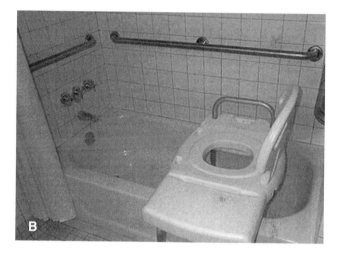

nents include planning and pacing to prevent overexertion and redundant, wasteful efforts. Prioritization of tasks can reduce distress when pain or fatigue limits a patient's endurance. Adaptive equipment items, such as those shown in Fig. 14.11 can also reduce the number and severity of "energy sinks," which occur during painful or inefficient activities. In this manner, energy conservation is compatible with exercise programs and enhanced activity; it entails "working smarter" rather than cutting back. Commonly used as a therapeutic intervention in chronic neurological diseases (multiple sclerosis, post-polio syndrome) and rheumatoid arthritis, it is gaining familiarity among oncology professionals.

Therapeutic exercise

Exercise may be prescriptive or self-initiated. Prescriptive exercise is directed toward enhancement or restoration of function, generally in strength, coordination, or speed. Specific muscle groups and joints may be targeted as well as overall performance. The mode (e.g., weight-lifting, bicycling), frequency, duration, and goals are all components of the prescription. Among those with pain related to cancer, prescriptive exercise may be warranted after surgery or other treatments when function is compromised.

A variety of self-initiated exercises may benefit patients with cancer-related pain, through enhancement or maintenance of endurance, coordination, or postural control, or promotion of a sense of well-being. Some may increase cardiopulmonary fitness or flexibility. Studies indicate that some patients use exercise to combat fatigue. Exercise is well recognized to benefit pain management for patients with primary fibromyalgia syndrome, osteoarthritis, and other painful chronic conditions. Use

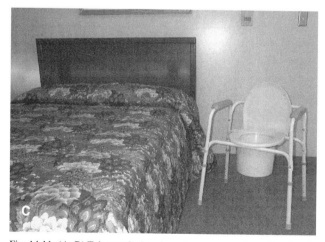

Fig. 14.11 (A, B) Tub transfer bench used over commode and in tub. (C) Bedside commode that can also be placed in a shower. (D, E) Dressing stick. (F) Long-handled shoe horn. (G) Sock aid.

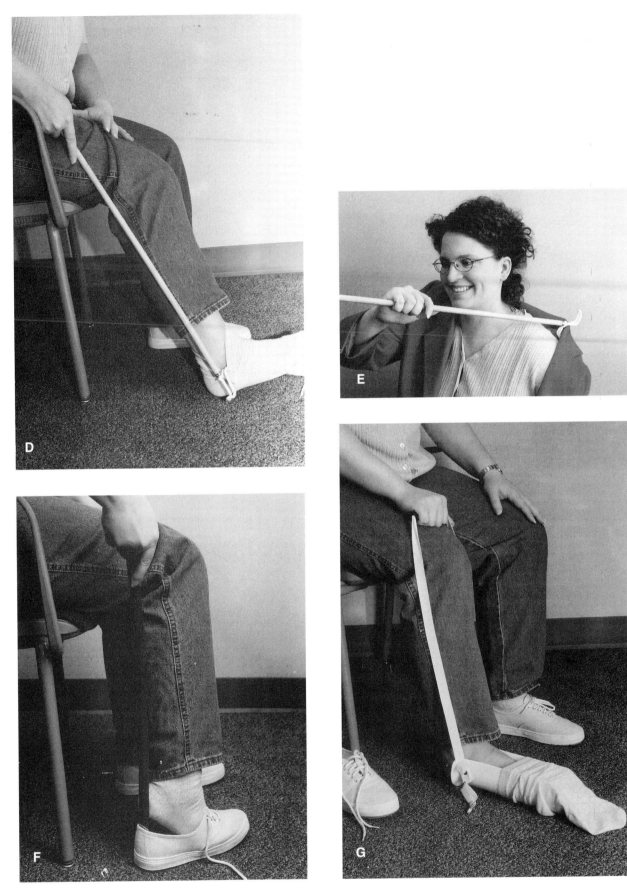

Fig. 14.11 *Continued*

of these interventions may be limited in patients with severe pain or advanced/metastatic disease that directly affects mobility, such as bone metastasis, spinal cord compression, or brain metastasis. Elderly patients are often less familiar or experienced in movement therapies, may be more sedentary or less inclined toward exercise, are generally less flexible, and are therefore at higher risk of injury. With instructors who are able to modify and adapt programs for a patient's specific needs, however, almost all but those in severe pain or very near the end of life can participate in these therapies to some extent.

Walking, swimming, stationary bicycling, and other familiar means are not specifically discussed. For patients with sedentary lifestyles before the diagnosis of cancer, traditional exercises may be intimidating or unrealistic. Other movement therapies, such as those described in this section, can provide novel, group-oriented activity, and perhaps enhanced compliance or lifestyle changes. Unless specifically noted, there is little information on the formal study of these therapies in cancer patients.

Tai Chi

Tai Chi, or Tai Chi Chuan, is a practice of movement with origins during the late Ming and early Qing dynasties more than 3000 years ago. Initially a martial art, it has gradually become popularized in China as a means of maintaining health and well-being. Its 108 movements, or forms, are used to balance yin and yang, and strengthen Qi, the life force or vital energy, which wards off illness and disease. An emphasis is placed on relaxing unnecessary tension in the body, controlled but fluid weight-shifting from one leg to another, maintaining a flexed-knee position, and heightened but relaxed kinesthetic and breathing awareness. Increased popularity in the West has also led to an impressive array of literature, including randomized controlled trials.

Tai Chi has been shown to have impressive and significant benefits over cycle ergometry in ventilatory frequency, and ratio of dead space ventilation to tidal volume. When compared to sedentary matched individuals, Tai Chi practitioners had significantly higher oxygen uptake, pulse oximetry, and work rate (82), and experienced less decline in maximal oxygen uptake and pulse oximetry than control subjects at a 2-year follow-up evaluation (83). Other comparison studies showed practitioners to have significantly greater peak oxygen uptake, greater flexibility, and lower percentage of body fat when compared to sedentary subjects (84).

None of these benefits have been specifically identified in cancer patients. Most relevant to the management of wellness despite chronic, painful disease is a study of patients with rheumatoid arthritis. In this study, those who practiced Tai Chi once or twice a week for 10 weeks had no further deterioration in their joint mobility and symptomatology compared to a control group (85).

Yoga

Yoga is a practice of specific postures and breathing techniques, accompanied by mental quietude, concentration, or focus. It is used as a means of achieving well-being for its participants, and in healthy volunteers was associated with higher life satisfaction, lower excitability, aggressiveness, emotionality, and somatic complaints (86). A study of patients with osteoarthritis of the hands (87) involved eight 1-hour sessions of yoga, and the intervention group showed statistically significant improvements in finger joint tenderness, pain with activity, and finger range of motion over the control group. A similar study design involving patients with carpal tunnel syndrome found significant improvements in grip strength and pain intensity compared with control subjects receiving splinting and stretching (88).

Pilates

Joseph Pilates (1880–1967) developed a form of therapy emphasizing kinesthetic awareness, particularly in the pelvic and truncal muscles, and the notion of a "stable core" from which movement must arise. Areas of injury are weak links in the body's kinetic chain and must work in harmony with the entire structure. Awareness and strength are developed through specific exercises, often using eccentric muscle contractions. Exercise equipment uniquely designed to facilitate this development is also incorporated. Strength and coordination are progressively increased through more challenging tasks on these devices.

Alexander

The Alexander Technique refers to a rationale of movement awareness wherein the student engages the mind in the conscious choice between beneficial and automatic, and non-beneficial postures (89). F. M. Alexander (1869–1955) thought that bad postural habits could be broken only after they were understood with both body and mind. Students develop an awareness of the dynamic relationship between the head, neck, and torso during rest and activity termed "the means-whereby" (90). Students then learn to sense and stop automatic, inhibitory muscle contractions that impede smooth movement and increase effort and risk of injury. Instructors use verbal and tactile guidance to aid learning of proper alignment during movement. Group or individual instruction may be offered. Benefits have been identified in the treatment of patients with back pain (91).

Feldenkrais

Moshe Feldenkrais (1880–1967) led students to discover alternate, pain-free means of performing functional tasks. Re-education of body movements is learned by either awareness through movement (ATM) or functional integration (FI). ATM occurs in classes where students notice patterns of their own muscle tension and habits during activity and are led to find less restrictive options for their usual movements. FI is generally individualized, with tactile cues from the instructor during repetitive movements. Feldenkrais methods place less emphasis on the cognitive contribution to movement; rather, development of the automatic but correct pattern of movement is the goal.

Mind–body techniques

Although not within the usual scope of practice for many rehabilitationists, these interventions are commonly practiced but little discussed or researched. They are included as reminders of their adjunctive but often helpful role in pain management.

Music

It has been postulated that music may diminish the awareness of pain by the distraction it provides. In another theory, pleasant and uplifting music may stimulate the brain to release endorphins that relieve pain centrally. Music can elicit the relaxation response, lessen anxiety, and reduce muscle tension. For some, it is a means to facilitate guided imagery techniques. Music can evoke memories, increase or decrease emotional states, and change moods.

Although most clinicians are intuitively aware of the effects music holds for them personally, the notion of prescriptive music is still not widely accepted. In the United States, the National Association for Music Therapy and the American Music Therapy Association are striving for increased recognition of formalized music interventions. Incorporating appropriate music into treatment areas and home environments seems a natural enhancement that is frequently overlooked. Some studies have in fact investigated the addition of soothing music to chemotherapy infusion and found reductions in the incidence of nausea and emesis (92). Music therapy has also been recommended for the control of postoperative nausea and vomiting (93). Case reports (94) and anecdotal experience suggest that pain perceptions can be altered through music therapy.

Relaxation and imagery

Imagery refers to the mental exercise of visualizing positive surroundings or circumstances. This may refer to pleasant vistas previously experienced or purely imaginary but very soothing locations. Participants may also create mental images of their cancer being battled successfully, with metaphoric representations or allegorical qualities. Relaxation techniques can include deep breathing, breathing awareness, progressive muscular relaxation moving from one section of the body to another, and active muscle contraction followed by relaxation.

Several studies have described encouraging results from this intervention in patients with cancer. Syrjala et al. (95) found that mucositis pain in bone marrow transplant recipients improved during a 5-week study in subjects treated with relaxation and imagery but not in those participating in a therapist support group or in a control group. *Hypnosis* may promote physiological and cognitive characteristics that are similar to progressive relaxation, imagery, and meditation.

Meditation and prayer

Both meditation and prayer involve focused attention and may attempt to exclude negative or random thoughts. In addition to the spiritual outlook and beliefs that may benefit from prayer or meditation, both may be associated with a relaxation response, with attendant reductions in heart rate, respiratory rate, and blood pressure (96). Whereas meditation generally involves focusing inward, prayer often looks outward to a larger purpose or higher power.

Prayer does not necessarily imply disdain for medical knowledge. Conventional medical views may consider religious beliefs in miraculous healing through prayer as incompatible with rational thought. However, those who pray may seek healing not only through cure but through hope in the next life and in a merciful God (97). In a survey of women with gynecological cancer, 49% felt they had become more religious after their diagnosis, and none felt less religious. More than 90% of these patients said their religious lives helped them sustain their hopes (98).

Shapiro (99) assessed a small group of long- and short-term meditators and found a 62.9% incidence of at least one adverse event within the group, without significant differences between them. These adverse effects included disorientation, confusion, depression, increased awareness of one's negative qualities and emotions, increased fears and anxiety, boredom, pain, and withdrawal from daily activities in order to pursue meditation. Most noted a greater sense of relaxation and lower levels of perceived stress, more positive thinking, self-confidence, compassion, and tolerance of oneself and others (100).

Therapeutic touch

Therapeutic touch (TT) has gained some attention as a means of affecting health or painful conditions. This discipline in fact does not involve touching but rather use of the practitioner's hands to detect alterations in energy and temperature in the patient's body from a distance of 4 to 5 centimeters. The theory is that the body emits freely flowing energy that is unimpeded in health but diminished or blocked in the ill. By delineating abnormal gradients in the patient's energy characteristics, a practitioner is then postulated to alter these through their own energy field. There has also been some discussion as to whether TT is, in fact, a religious practice based on its construct of the individual and the world (101), or the interpretation of it as a means of spiritual healing (102).

Applications of TT have included the treatment of acute symptoms of headache and postoperative pain as well as chronic pain associated with arthritis. TT has purportedly accelerated the rate of wound healing (103). A recent case report described the beneficial use of TT in a patient with a below-normal degree of hypnotic responsiveness, suggesting an effect not dependent on patient suggestibility (104). A study comparing TT with sham TT among acute burn unit patients found improvements in pain and anxiety VAS ratings in the TT group, but no significant difference in opioid usage (105). A small, unblinded study of terminal cancer patients suggested improvements in well-being after 20 minutes of TT when compared to subjects who rested quietly (106). Other authors found encouraging results in pain and function in a single-blinded randomized controlled trial in osteoarthritic patients (107). Many of these studies were not properly powered or well designed, however.

It remains unclear whether the benefit patients receive is through social contact, placebo response, or energy field changes. A placebo response would not necessarily indicate that TT is not a beneficial adjuvant intervention (108). Obviously much more work must be done with this intervention to establish its efficacy in a variety of diagnoses. Controversy will likely continue until more robust scientific research can elucidate its effects on the body.

Conclusion

Rehabilitation disciplines have much to offer cancer patients in pain. Unfortunately, access to rehabilitation disciplines is frequently limited by knowledge gaps among oncologists, patients, and rehabilitationists themselves. There are few rehabilitationists with familiarity and comfort in identifying and managing sequelae of cancer or cancer treatment, including pain. There are also few rehabilitationists with established relationships with cancer treatment facilities and oncologists. Many patients and cancer treatment teams are unaware how physiatrists, physical and occupational therapists, and other professionals can ameliorate functional deficits as well as pain.

Patients with a diagnosis of cancer may experience pain from a variety of etiologies. Malignant and non-malignant origins may coexist within the same patient. Attribution of any and every pain experienced by a cancer patient to the cancer itself leads to missed opportunities for partial or full pain relief through non-pharmacological means. Physiatrists and other rehabilitation disciplines are ideally positioned to assist in the management of pain of soft tissue and neuropathic and skeletal origin once they have acquired knowledge and familiarity with fundamental principles of oncology and the complications and deficits progressive disease may create.

References

1. Lehmann JF, DeLisa JA, Warren CG, et al. Cancer rehabilitation: assessment of need, development and evaluation of a model of care. Arch Phys Med Rehabil 59:410–9, 1978.
2. World Health Organization. Cancer pain relief and palliative care. Technical Report Series No. 804. Geneva: WHO, 1990:17.
3. Gillis TA. Rehabilitation of the elderly cancer patient. Cancer Bull 47:245–9, 1995.
4. Melzack R, Wall PD. Pain mechanisms: a new theory. Science 150:971–9, 1965.
5. Hodgson SF. Corticosteroid-induced osteoporosis. Endocrin Metab Clin North Am 19:95–111, 1990.
6. Buchsel PC, Leum EW, Randolph SR. Delayed complications of bone marrow transplantation: an update. Oncol Nurs Forum 23:1267–91, 1996.
7. Rodino MA, Shane E. Osteoporosis after organ transplantation. Am J Med 104:459–69, 1998.
8. Chesnut CH III, McClung MR, Ensrud KE, et al. Alendronate treatment of the postmenopausal osteoporotic woman: effect of multiple dosages on bone mass and bone remodeling. Am J Med 99:144–52, 1995.
9. Sinaki M, Fitzpatrick LA, Ritchie CK, et al. Site-specificity of bone mineral density and muscle strength in women: Job-related physical activity. Am J Phys Med Rehabil 77:470–6, 1998.

10. Sinaki M, Wahner HW, Bergstralh EJ, et al. Three-year controlled, randomized trial of the effect of dose-specified loading and strengthening exercises on bone mineral density of spine and femur in non-athletic, physically active women. Bone 19:233–44, 1996.

11. Sinaki M, Mikkelsen BA. Postmenopausal spinal osteoporosis: flexion versus extension exercises. Arch Phys Med Rehabil 65:593–6, 1984.

12. Kroner K, Knudsen UB, Lundby L, Hvid H. Long-term phantom breast syndrome after mastectomy. Clin J Pain 8:346–50, 1992.

13. Fowler RS, Kraft GH. Tension perception in patients having pain associated with chronic muscle tension. Arch Phys Med Rehabil 55:28–30, 1974.

14. Graven-Nielsen T, Svensson P, Arendt-Nielsen L. Effects of experimental muscle pain on activity and coordination during static and dynamic motor function. Electroencephalogr Clin Neurophysiol 105:156–64, 1997.

15. Sola AE, Bonica JJ. Myofascial pain syndromes. In: Bonica JJ, ed. The management of pain. Philadelphia: Lea & Febiger, 1990:352–67.

16. Cailliet R. Soft tissue pain and disability. Philadelphia: FA Davis, 1977:32–5.

17. Melzack R. Relation of myofascial trigger points to acupuncture and mechanisms of pain. Arch Phys Med Rehabil 62:114–7, 1981.

18. Travell JG, Simon DG. Myofascial pain and dysfunction: the trigger point manual. Baltimore: Williams & Wilkins, 1983:16.

19. Travell JG, Simon DG. Myofascial pain and dysfunction: the trigger point manual. Baltimore: Williams & Wilkins, 1983:14.

20. Greenman PE. Principles of manual medicine, 2nd ed. Philadelphia: Williams & Wilkins, 1996:11.

21. Rizk TE, Pinals RS, Talavier AS. Corticosteroid injections in adhesive capsulitis: investigation of the value and site. Arch Phys Med Rehabil 72:20–2, 1991.

22. Van Ouwenaller C, Laplace PM, Chantraine A. Painful shoulder in hemiplegia. Arch Phys Med Rehabil 67:23–6, 1986.

23. Melzack R, Stillwell DM, Fox EJ. Trigger points and acupuncture points for pain: correlations and implications. Pain 3:3–23, 1977.

24. Travell JG, Simon DG. Myofascial pain and dysfunction: the trigger point manual. Baltimore: Williams & Wilkins, 1983:19.

25. Gam AN, Warming S, Larsen LH, et al. Treatment of myofascial trigger-points with ultrasound combined with massage and exercise—a randomised controlled trial. Pain 77(1):73–9, 1998.

26. Eisenberg DM, Kessler RC, Foster C, et al. Unconventional medicine in the United States. Prevalence, costs, and patterns of use. N Engl J Med 328:246–52, 1993.

27. Koes BW, Assendelft WJ, van der Heijden GJ, et al. Spinal manipulation and mobilization for back and neck pain: a blinded review. BMJ 303:1298–1303, 1991.

28. Greenman PE. Principles of manual medicine, 2nd ed. Philadelphia: Williams & Wilkins, 1996:52.

29. McPartland J, Miller B. Bodywork therapy systems. Phys Med Rehabil Clin North Am 10(3):583–602, 1999.

30. Pare A. Oeuvres completes. Paris: JB Balliere, 1948.

31. Goats GC, Keir KA. Connective tissue massage. Br J Sports Med 25:131–3, 1991.

32. Wakim K, Marin F, Terrier J, et al. The effects of massage on the circulation on normal and paralyzed extremities. Arch Phys Med Rehabil 30:135–44, 1949.

33. Kaada B, Torsteinbo O. Increase of plasma beta-endorphins in connective tissue massage. Gen Pharmacol 20(4):487–9, 1989.

34. Carrier EB. Studies on physiology of capillaries: reaction of human skin capillaries to drugs and other stimuli. Am J Physiol 61:528–47, 1922.

35. Barr JS, Taslitz N. The influence of back massage on autonomic functions. Phys Ther 50:1679–91, 1970.

36. Reed BV, Held JM. Effects of sequential connective tissue massage on autonomic nervous system of middle-aged and healthy adults. Phys Ther 68:1231–4, 1988.

37. Day JA, Mason RR, Chesrown SE. Effect of massage on serum level of beta-endorphin and beta-lipotropin in healthy adults. Phys Ther 67:926–30, 1987.

38. Ernst E. Massage therapy for low back pain: a systematic review. J Pain Symptom Manage 17:65–9, 1999.

39. Godrey CM, Morgan PP, Schatzker J. A randomized trial of manipulation for low-back pain in a medical setting. Spine 9:301–4, 1984.

40. Hoehler FK, Tobis JS, Buerger AA. Spinal manipulation for low back pain. JAMA 245:1835–8, 1981.

41. Konrad K, Tatrai T, Hunka A, et al. Controlled trial of balneotherapy in treatment of low back pain. Ann Rheum Dis 51:820–2, 1992.

42. Tan, JC. Physical modalities. In: Practical manual of physical medicine and rehabilitation. St. Louis: Mosby, 1998:133–55.

43. Ferrell-Torry AT, Glick OJ. The use of therapeutic massage as a nursing intervention to modify anxiety and the perception of cancer pain. Cancer Nurs 16:93–101, 1993.

44. Weinrich SP, Weinrich MC. The effect of massage on pain in cancer patients. Appl Nurs Res 3(4):140–5, 1990.

45. Pomeranz B. The scientific basis for acupuncture. In: Stux G, Pomeranz B, eds. Acupuncture textbook and atlas. Berlin: Springer-Verlag, 1987:1–34.

46. Pomeranz B. Electroacupuncture and transcutaneous electrical nerve stimulation. In: Stux GG, Pomeranz B, eds. Basics of acupuncture, 2nd ed. Berlin: Springer-Verlag, 1991:250–60.

47. Helms JM. Acupuncture energetics: a clinical approach for physicians. Berkeley: Medical Acupuncture Publishers, 1995:26–9.

48. Felhendler D, Lisander B. Pressure on acupoints decreases postoperative pain. Clin J Pain 12:326–9, 1996.

49. Stevensen C. The role of shiatsu in palliative care. Complement Ther Nurs Midwifery 1:51–8, 1995.

50. Soliman N, Frank BL, Nakazawa H, et al. Acupuncture reflex systems of the ear, scalp and hand. Phys Med Rehabil Clin North Am 10:547–71, 1999.

51. Olson K, Hanson J. Using Reiki to manage pain: a preliminary report. Cancer Prev Control 1(2):108–13, 1997.

52. Diller KR. Analysis of burns caused by long-term exposure to a heating pad. J Burn Care Rehabil 12:214–7, 1991.

53. Curkovic B, Vitulic V, Babic-Naglic D, Durrigl T. The influence of heat and cold on the pain threshold in rheumatoid arthritis. Z Rheumatol 52:289–91, 1993.

54. Hartviksen K. Ice therapy in spasticity. Acta Neurol Scand 38:79–84, 1962.

55. Miglietta O. Action of cold on spasticity. Am J Phys Med 52:198–205, 1973.

56. Harris ED, McCroskery PA. The influence of temperature and fibril stability on degradation of cartilage collagen by rheumatoid synovial collagenase. N Engl J Med 290:1–6, 1974.

57. Schmidt KL, Ott VR, Rocher G, Schaller H. Heat, cold and inflammation (a review). Z Rheumatol 38:391–404, 1979.

58. Ho SS, Illgen RL, Meyer RW, et al. Comparison of various icing times in decreasing bone metabolism and blood flow in the knee. Am J Sports Med 23(1):74–6, 1995.

59. Taber C, Contryman K, Fahernbruch J, et al. Measurement of reactive vasodilation during cold gel pack application to non-traumatized ankles. Phys Ther 72(4):294–9, 1992.

60. Lehmann JF, de Lateur BJ. Diathermy and superficial heat and cold therapy. In: Kottke FJ, Stillwell GK, Lehmann JF, eds. Krusen's handbook of physical medicine and rehabilitation, 3rd ed. Philadelphia: WB Saunders, 1982:275–350.

61. Lowdon BJ, Moore RJ. Determinants and nature of intramuscular temperature changes during cold therapy. Am J Phys Med 54(5):223–33, 1975.

62. Travell J. Ethyl chloride spray for painful muscle spasm. Arch Phys Med Rehabil 33:291–8, 1952.

63. Oosterveld FG, Rasker JJ. Effects of local heat and cold treatment of surface and articular temperature of arthritic knees. Arthritis Rheum 37(11):1578–82, 1994.

64. Haker E, Lundeberg T. Pulsed ultrasound treatment in lateral epicondylagia. Scand J Rehabil Med 23(3):115–8, 1991.

65. Nykanen M. Pulsed ultrasound treatment of the painful shoulder. A randomized, double-blind, placebo controlled study. Scand J Rehabil Med 27(2):105–8, 1995.

66. Lehman JF, Erickson DJ, Martin GM, Krusen FH. Comparison of ultrasonic and microwave diathermy in the physical treatment of periarthritis of the shoulder. Arch Phys Med Rehabil 35:627–34, 1954.

67. Lehmann JF, Fordyce WE, Rathbun LA, et al. Clinical evaluation of a new approach in the treatment of contracture associated with hip fracture after internal fixation. Arch Phys Med Rehabil 42:95, 1961.

68. Lehmann JF, McMillan JA, Brunner GD, Blumberg JB. Comparative study of the efficiency of short-wave, microwave and ultrasonic diathermy in heating the hip joint. Arch Phys Med Rehabil 40:510–2, 1959.

69. Lehmann JF, Masock AJ, Warren CG, et al. Effect of therapeutic temperatures on tendon extensibility. Arch Phys Med Rehabil 51(8):481–7, 1970.

70. Rishler M, Brostovski Y, Yaron M. Effect of spa therapy in Tiberias on patients with ankylosing spondylitis. Clin Rheumatol 14(1):21–5, 1995.

71. Forster MM. Mineral springs and miracles. Can Fam Physician 40:729–37, 1994.

72. Sukenik S, Buskila D, Neumann L, Kleiner-Baungarten A. Mud pack therapy in rheumatoid arthritis. Clin Rheumatol 11(2):243–7, 1992.

73. Ventafridda V. Transcutaneous nerve stimulation in cancer pain. In: Bonica JJ, Ventafridda V, eds. Advances in pain research and therapy, vol. 2. New York: Raven Press, 1979:509–15.

74. Sjölund BH, Eriksson MB. The influence of naloxone on analgesia produced by peripheral conditioning stimulation. Brain Res 173(2):295–301, 1979.

75. Melzack R, Vetere P, Finch L. Transcutaneous electrical nerve stimulation for low back pain. A comparison of TENS and massage for pain and range of motion. Phys Ther 63(4):489–93, 1983.

76. Melzack R, Jeans ME, Stratford JG, Monks RC. Ice massage and transcutaneous electrical stimulation: comparison of treatment for low-back pain. Pain 9(2):209–17, 1980.

77. Ericksson MB, Sjölund BH, Nielzen S. Long-term results of peripheral conditioning stimulation as an analgesic measure in chronic pain. Pain 6(3):335–47, 1979.

78. Wynn Parry CB. Pain in avulsion lesions of the brachial plexus. Pain 9(1):41–53, 1980.

79. Sindou M, Keravel Y. Pain relief through transcutaneous electrical nerve stimulation (TENS). Results on painful neurological disorders in 180 cases. Neurochirurgie 26(2):153–7, 1980.

80. Cotter DJ. Overview of transcutaneous electrical nerve stimulation for treatment of acute postoperative pain. Med Instrum 17(4):289–92, 1983.

81. Holdsworth F. Fractures, dislocations and fracture-dislocations of the spine. J Bone Joint Surg Am 52(8):1534–51, 1970.

82. Lai JS, Wong MK, Lan C, et al. Cardiorespiratory responses of Tai Chi Chuan practitioners and sedentary subjects during cycle ergometry. J Formos Med Assoc 92(10):894–9, 1993.

83. Lai JS, Lan C, Wong MK, Teng SH. Two-year trends in cardiorespiratory function among older Tai Chi Chaun practitioners and sedentary subjects. J Am Geriatr Soc 43(11):1222–7, 1995.

84. Lan C, Lai JS, Wong MK, Yu ML. Cardiorespiratory function, flexibility, and body composition among geriatric Tai Chi Chuan practitioners. Arch Phys Med Rehabil 77(6):612–6, 1996.

85. Kirsteins AE, Dietz F, Hwang SM. Evaluating the safety and potential use of a weight-bearing exercise, Tai Chi Chuan, for rheumatoid arthritis patients. Am J Phys Med Rehabil 70(3):136–41, 1991.

86. Schell FJ, Allolio B, Schonecke OW. Physiological and psychological effects of Hatha-Yoga exercise in healthy women. Int J Psychosom 41(1–4):46–52, 1994.

87. Garfinkel MS, Schumacher HR Jr, Husain A, et al. Evaluation of a yoga based regimen for treatment of osteoarthritis of the hands. J Rheumatol 21(12):2341–3, 1994.

88. Garfinkel MS, Singhal A, Katz WA, et al. Yoga-based intervention for carpal tunnel syndrome: a randomized trial. JAMA 280(18):1601–3, 1998.

89. Cotter AC. Western movement therapies. Phys Med Rehabil Clin North Am 10(3):603–16, 1999.

90. Alexander FM. The resurrection of the body. New Hyde Park, NY: Delta/Dell, 1974.

91. Elkayam O, Ben Itzhak S, Avrahahami E, et al. Multidisciplinary approach to chronic back pain; prognostic elements of the outcome. Clin Exp Rheumatol 14(3):281–8, 1996.

92. Standley J. Clinical applications of music therapy and chemotherapy: the effects on nausea and emesis. Music Therapy Perspectives 9:91–6, 1992.

93. Thompson HJ. The management of post-operative nausea and vomiting. J Adv Nurs 29(5):1130–6, 1999.

94. Magill-Levreault L. Music therapy in pain and symptom management. J Palliat Care 9(4):42–8, 1993.

95. Syrjala KL, Donaldson GW, Davis MW, et al. Relaxation and imagery and cognitive-behavioral training reduce pain during cancer treatment: a controlled clinical trial. Pain 63(2):189–98, 1995.

96. Benson H. The relaxation response: history, physiological basis and clinical utility. Acta Med Scand 660:231–7, 1982.

97. Hufford DJ. Epistemologies in religious healing. J Med Philos 18(2):175–94, 1993.

98. Roberts JA, Brown D, Elkins T, et al. Factors influencing views of patients with gynecological cancer about end-of-life decisions. Am J Obstet Gynecol 176(1):166–72, 1997.

99. Shapiro DH Jr. Adverse effects of meditation: a preliminary investigation of long-term meditators. Int J Psychosom 39(1–4):62–7, 1992.

100. Shapiro DH Jr. Overview: clinical and physiological comparison of meditation with other self-control strategies. Am J Psychiatry 139(3):267–74, 1982.

101. Bullough VL, Bullough B. Should nurses practice therapeutic touch? Should nursing schools teach therapeutic touch? J Prof Nurs 14(4):254–7, 1998.

102. Mackereth P, Wright J. Therapeutic touch: nursing activity or form of spiritual healing? Complement Ther Nurs Midwifery 3(4):106–10, 1997.

103. Wirth DP. Complementary healing intervention and dermal wound reepithelialization: an overview. Int J Psychosom 42:493–502, 1996.

104. Leskowitz ED. Phantom limb pain treated with therapeutic touch: a case report. Arch Phys Med Rehabil 81(4):522–4, 2000.

105. Turner JG, Clark AJ, Gauthier DK, Williams M. The effect of therapeutic touch on pain and anxiety in burn patients. J Adv Nurs 28(1):10–20, 1998.

106. Giasson M, Bouchard L. Effect of therapeutic touch on the well-being of persons with terminal cancer. J Holistic Nursing 16(3):383–98, 1998.

107. Gordon A, Merenstein JH, D'Amico F, Hudgens D. The effects of therapeutic touch on patients with osteoarthritis of the knee. J Fam Pract 47(4):271–7, 1998.

108. Meehan TC. Therapeutic touch as a nursing intervention. J Adv Nurs 28(1):117–25, 1998.

15 Neurosurgical techniques in the management of cancer pain

SAMUEL J. HASSENBUSCH AND LAUREN JOHNS
The University of Texas M. D. Anderson Cancer Center

Introduction

Neurosurgical procedures for pain management in cancer patients are at a crossroad. Although the intracranial operations traditionally have been used as later options, there is a movement toward applications of these techniques in earlier stages of disease. It is estimated that 10% or more of cancer patients do not receive adequate relief with pharmacological treatment options because they are often troubled by dose-limiting side effects such as nausea or cognitive dysfunction (1). Earlier use is now suggested by improvements in accuracy as well as the cost-containment benefits and ease of discomfort that these techniques provide. One-time procedures, performed with the patient under local anesthesia, allow for short hospital stays and low morbidity rates and are now useful, if not desirable, because of their cost-containment considerations. Although many of these procedures are old, recent improvements and technological innovations have renewed interest in their use (Fig. 15.1). Some of these improvements, such as focused radiotherapy, allow almost non-invasive interventional pain techniques at the intracranial level. Despite newer developments, the role of spinal ablative procedures, with their low risks, remains stable in overall pain management.

The relative roles of ablative and augmentative procedures are still controversial in neurosurgical pain management. Many of these ablative procedures have been available for 40 to 50 years, yet, in many situations, they have been replaced by newer augmentative procedures over the past 10 years. Pain relief from ablative procedures may be of shorter duration than that resulting from stimulation and may be accompanied by deafferentation pain (2). More recently, however, older techniques for intracranial ablative procedures have been updated. With the use of improved stereotactic equipment and guidance

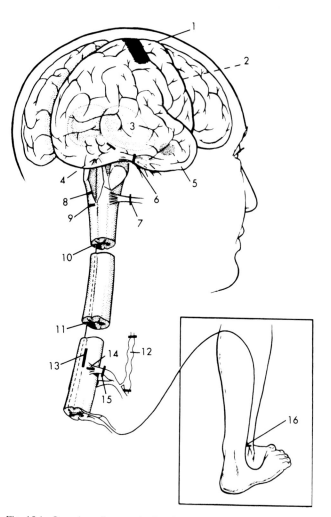

Fig. 15.1. Overview of anatomic sites for pain procedures in the central nervous system. (From Raj PP. Practical management of pain, St. Louis: Mosby, 2000:793.)

by computed tomography (CT) and magnetic resonance imaging (MRI), the accuracy of intracranial procedures has been improved and the need for ventriculography largely eliminated. The procedures can be performed with the patient under local anesthesia, perhaps with intravenous sedation, and require only a twist drill hole, rather than a burr hole or a craniotomy.

Patients generally must have severe pain that is not relieved adequately by systemic medications or simple neurolytic procedures. Though some of the procedures, such as thalamotomy and cingulotomy often have been used for pain of non-cancer causes, these operations are still quite beneficial to the cancer patient (3–7). As with long-term spinal infusions of morphine, it remains unclear whether delayed recurrence of pain represents extension of the underlying tumor to new anatomic areas or late failure of the procedure (8,9).

Although the neurosurgical procedures are used for both nociceptive and neuropathic pain, it appears that, with the exception of thalamotomy, nociceptive pain responds better to intracranial procedures, which also cover larger body areas. Neuropathic pain often responds better to spinal procedures that have more limited areas of coverage. In addition to logistical issues, choice of a specific operation also needs to take into consideration the type of pain, severity, location, and primary cause of the painful sensation.

Techniques

Though neurosurgical approaches to lesion placement are fairly standard, the requisite tools have changed as technology has progressed. Originally, ablations were placed using open surgical techniques (10). Air or contrast ventriculography for intracranial lesions was the traditional, accurate method for placing lesions at coordinates defined by the anterior commissure-posterior commissure (AC-PC) line (11,12). General anesthesia was often required to perform the procedure, which could not adjust for interpatient variability in anatomy. Now, however, closed operations using stereotaxis under ventriculogram, CT, or MRI guidance have become dominant.

CT and MRI for stereotactic guidance eliminate the need for ventriculography and also increase the surgeon's ability to correct for individual patient variation in anatomy (13,14). For example, by using MRI, the actual trajectory for the electrode placement can be planned in relation to other brain structures. Special angled slices that correspond to the trajectory for the electrode placement can be performed, allowing identification of the tar-

get site and the actual trajectory through various brain structures on these slices. CT has a high resolution and accuracy but also a more limited level of resolution, thus making direct observation of the target difficult (15). MRI is especially useful in the identification of relevant anatomy but does suffer from a somewhat lower accuracy because of magnetic field inhomogeneity (16,17). Although there are statistically significant differences between CT- and MRI-derived coordinates, the actual discrepancies are small enough that the MRI can be used alone for target localization (15). Because neither method is entirely exact, a variety of intraoperative procedures are often used to confirm lesion placement (15). Such techniques include the use of "reversible" lesions, allowing intraoperative testing of the area without causing permanent damage, low-frequency stimulation that aids determination of the function of the region surrounding the target, and single-unit microelectrode recording to ensure preservation of critical structures in the area (15).

Radiosurgery using the GammaKnife, for example, is increasingly used to create ablative lesions for treatment of chronic pain and functional disorders. This method is particularly useful for sites found deep within the brain (2). Targets in the thalamus and the anterior limb of the internal capsule have been frequently reported (18–20). The radiosurgical technique for these pain-relieving lesions uses a similar technique to that for focused radiation (radiosurgery) of a brain tumor. Although radiosurgery is non-invasive to the brain, the extent that lesions become smaller and the degree of pain relief that can be expected at various time points after the radiation exposure are unclear.

Description of specific procedures

The following procedures either are currently being practiced or, based on past reports, offer significant efficacy of relief with minimal morbidity. As seen from the descriptions that follow, some of these procedures treat specific pain areas such as the head or legs, whereas others treat more generalized areas of pain. The various approaches have been divided into ablative and augmentative techniques and listed within each group beginning with the most commonly used technique first.

Ablative techniques—intracranial
Hypophysectomy   The mechanism by which lesions of the pituitary gland bring pain relief is unclear, although it is generally agreed that neither the limbic system nor areas controlling affective responses are manipulated.

Current research supports three theories for hormonal, hypothalamic, and neurotransmitter release mechanisms. A postulated hormonal mechanism involves changes in a humoral substance in the cerebrospinal fluid or hormonal changes via a direct neural mechanism (21,22). Contrary to this proposal, it has been noted that pain relief occurs almost immediately without any regard for tumor regression. Relief can also occur in the thalamic pain regions and hormonally unresponsive tumors on a scale that could not be inferred given the degree of pituitary ablation experienced (23–27). Still, very small amounts of tumor regression cannot be discounted (28).

Modalities used to perform a hypophysectomy lend credence to the hypothalamic mechanism theory. A possible relation to the pain relief properties of the posteromedial hypothalamus can be observed, although the morphological effects of hypophysectomy, regardless of the technique used to create the lesions, center in the anterior hypothalamus, specifically in the supraoptic and paraventricular nuclei (28,29). Projections from the paraventricular nucleus to the periaqueductal gray, rostral ventral medulla, and lamina I of dorsal horn have been noted, linking the area to crucial elements in the descending antinociceptive system (31–33). Information suggesting the particularly strong impact that pituitary ablations have on the paraventricular nucleus, coupled with knowledge of anatomical connections between this area and antinociceptive regions of the brain, suggests the role of endogenous neurotransmitters. It has been observed, however, that naloxone does not reverse pain relief as it does with opioid-based relief. Although plasma concentrations of beta-endorphin were elevated in one study, no changes have been found in cerebrospinal fluid concentrations of metenkephalin or beta-endorphin.

Techniques for open surgery on the area include the transcranial hypophysectomy (34) and the open microsurgical hypophysectomy (22,26,35,36). As technology has improved stereotactic methods, percutaneous stereotactic lesions are being created using radiofrequency thermal techniques, cryotherapy, or interstitial placement of radioactive seeds. The success of focused radiation therapy (e.g., GammaKnife) on pituitary tumors has led to the use of this non-invasive modality to create similar lesions for pain relief.

Of these various techniques for hypophysectomy, stereotactic instillation of alcohol into the pituitary gland is one of the best described and most common techniques at this time. Alcohol has been shown to pass to the floor of the third ventricle, hypophyseal portal vessels, and the hypothalamus (27). The use of stereotaxy for chemical hypophysectomy enables an injection of alcohol volumes between 1 and 5 ml, a method first described in 1957 (37). Better results have been achieved using alcohol volumes extending to the upper volumes of this range that are clearly greater than the volume of the sella (28).

After placing the patient under general anesthesia and securing the stereotactic frame, the surgeon locates the superoposterior part of the sella as the initial target. An 18-gauge, 6-inch spinal needle is introduced in a transnasal trajectory that passes through the floor of the sphenoid sinus. This needle is then replaced by a 20-gauge spinal needle directed through the sellar wall, with its progression observed by means of lateral x-ray fluoroscopy. Injection of 1 to 2 ml of alcohol in aliquots of 0.1 ml follows placement of the needle tip. After withdrawing the needle halfway to the floor of the sella, another 1 to 2 ml of alcohol is injected (28). The needle is completely withdrawn after this last injection. Throughout the procedure, the eyes are monitored for compression of cranial nerves in the cavernous sinus as evidenced by changes in pupil size or movement of eyes from the midline.

Other methods used to perform a hypophysectomy, such as stereotaxic radiofrequency hypophysectomy, stereotaxic cryohypophysectomy, and interstitial irradiation use standard stereotactic methods of intracranial operations (7,25,38–40).

Hypophysectomy is generally recommended for patients with severe cancer pain such as metastatic breast or prostate carcinoma with diffuse areas of pain. It can also be effective for hormonally unresponsive tumors (21,27,41–43). In two different series of more than 100 patients each, chemical hypophysectomy appeared to provide significant pain relief. Excellent pain relief was reported in 45%–65% of all patients, and 75%–85% of patients ceased using opioids. The mean postoperative survival time was 5 months, and the mean length of pain relief was 3 months. This length of pain relief was accomplished with one additional alcohol injection in 25%–30% of patients and with two additional injections in another 3%–9% (21,28,44). Of the patients treated with alcohol injections, those suffering from breast or prostate carcinoma (50%–75% of patients) appeared to have slightly better pain relief than those with other types of tumors (28). Approximately 25% of patients had at least one significant exacerbation of pain after the procedure, and one third of these patients had more than one exacerbation (28).

Common complications included hormonal deficiency, such as diabetes insipidus, in 5%–20% of patients, cerebrospinal fluid leak in 1%–10% of patients, and ocular nerve palsy or temporal field visual loss in 2%–10% of patients (28,45). Most of these changes were temporary (28). Other problems associated with the procedure on a far less frequent basis were meningitis in 0.5%–1% of patients, hypothalamic changes, headaches, and carotid artery damage in approximately 0.5% of patients (45). Despite a reported 2%–5% mortality rate, it seems likely that these numbers have been significantly lowered with the adoption of newer percutaneous and stereotactic methods (39,45).

Thalamotomy   The thalamus is the termination site of the spinothalamic tract (lateral nucleus and central lateral nucleus of the medial thalamus), the pathway responsible for transmitting information about pain and temperature from the body to higher areas in the brain (2). The lateral thalamus seems to be principally involved with sensory discrimination aspects of pain, whereas the medial thalamic nuclei has more to do with affective responses (2). In the late 1930s and early 1940s, there were increasing reports of the use of thalamotomy in the treatment of patients with Parkinson's disease. In his attempt to create a means to preserve involuntary movements through an open pallidotomy, Meyers also based his work on these ideas. Using the effectiveness of pallidal lesions as corroborating evidence, investigators reasoned that lesions of their thalamic projections in the ventrolateral nucleus of the thalamus would also be effective (46). Advances in human stereotaxic procedures have led to a resurgence in use of the thalamotomy.

Despite its development for non-cancer pain, thalamotomy can be highly effective for and has been reported in the treatment of cancer pain (6,46). Thalamotomy is generally considered for intermittent shooting and hyperpathic or allodynic pain and not considered very effective for steady, burning, or dysesthetic components of central or deafferentation pain (46). The targets have been the basal thalamus, medial thalamus, and dorsomedian thalamus affecting extralemniscal fibers, and thalamic projections terminating in the intralaminar nucleus, centromedianum nucleus, and the frontal lobe (47). One of the most effective sites appears to be the inferior posteromedial thalamus, containing the intralaminar, centromedianum, and parafascicularis nuclei, all of which might affect the paleospinothalamic tract (48). More recent literature has proposed that the medial thalamus is related to the spinoreticular tract, the descending passageway responsible for conducting impulses to many of the motor neurons (2). Ablations of the lateral thalamus,

particularly the ventrocaudal parvocellular nucleus, attempt to destroy the pain-receiving nucleus itself. Combination lesions, such as centromedianum and parafasicularis lesions with dorsomedial nucleus or the thalamic pulvinar lesions, might provide better long-term results (48). Although lesion size is an important component of this type of operation, a standard does not truly exist because many surgeons have personal preferences. Specific cases may dictate a particular lesion size so as not to inflict damage on the surrounding areas (46).

Currently, a thalamotomy includes the use of stereotactic methods, frame imaging, referencing, target location(s) selection, and careful introduction of the probe so that sensitive motor structures remain intact (46). These operative steps are followed by physiological testing to confirm the site (46). The interactive nature of these tests requires the use of local anesthesia to ensure patient cooperation. The testing site according to Tasker (46) should be approximately in the 15-mm sagittal plane or the tactile representation of the contralateral manual digits. A 2-inch diameter head shave and prep is made for the entry point.

Two types of physiological testing can be used to determine target accuracy. Macrostimulation requires nominal instrumentation with quick progression and total identification of the brain and the spectrum of structures at variable distances from the probe. The process can be executed simultaneously with deep brain recording using the same electrode. The microelectrode recording technique is capable of identifying a limited group of structures. Located on the arc of the stereotactic frame, the microelectrode extends from its protective tubing with the aid of a hydraulic microdrive (46). Actual stimulation with the microelectrode occurs every 1.0 mm at 300 Hz, 100 mA, 0.1 ms, until responses occur below about 15 mA (46). A bipolar concentric electrode, 1.1 mm in diameter with a 0.5 mm tip separated by a 0.5 mm ring, monitors the stimulation. In the medial thalamus, neurons that fire spontaneously in a burst fashion provide clear hallmarks of the region, whereas an absence of touch-responsive neurons signals the proximity to the ventrocaudal parvocellular nucleus in the lateral thalamus (2). Both types of stimulation effects are used to minimize damage, procedural failure, and any morbidity resulting when a lesion is made in a position other than the anticipated anatomical target. A documented example of this can be seen in Nashold's work where he implanted electrodes as a testing method before performing a thalamotomy (40). The implanted electrodes permitted an accurate direction for the placement of the thalamotomy electrode tip during the actual operation (40).

Complications often depend on the problem necessitating the operation and include paresis, cognitive disorders, infection and mortality (although rare in nociceptive pain cases), seizures, speech disturbance, and other matters related to specific areas of disease. Both medial and lateral lesions of the thalamus are moderately effective (approximately 60% pain relief) in dealing with cancer pain, but lateral thalamotomy carries with it higher rates of complication, nearly 32% (2). In treatment of nociceptive pain, thalamotomy has been reported to produce transient loss of all contralateral sensory modalities after the operation and also pseudoparesis in many of the cases studied by Tasker. The patients seemed to lose the appreciation of position and vibration sense owing to the lesions in the ventrocaudal nucleus (46). Though lesions do not seem to affect cognitive ability, studies have shown that left-sided lesions affect language and the dominance of the right ear in listening exercises (right ear advantage) (2). Enthusiasm for the use of thalamotomy, however, has waned over the past few years because of concerns of pain recurrence after 6 to 12 months. Because of this decreased efficacy and the significant risks, more recent reports have suggested that thalamic stimulation should be carried out before considering the creation of a lesion (46).

Cingulotomy Dating back to 1948, the method calling for the creation of lesions in the cingulate gyrus originated when Cairns removed a portion of the anterior cingulate gyrus in an open operation (50). The use of the open cingulotomy in the 1940s and 1950s produced significant improvements in psychiatric symptoms in most patients (10). In 1962, Foltz first described the application of stereotaxy to bilateral anterior cingulate lesions for pain relief, and Ballantine began to use ventriculogram-guided stereotaxy to create smaller lesions in the anterior cingulate gyrus. Although a cingulotomy has most often has been applied to patients with affective disorders, there are numerous reports of its use for severe pain control (3,4,51–53). The procedure has been quite successful with cancer patients suffering from diffuse or multiply located pain but has not been fully adopted because of neurosurgical stereotactic techniques required to perform the operation (1,16,17).

With the availability of technology capable of guiding closed procedures, there is no present role for open surgical techniques for cingulotomy. The specific target is the cingulate gyrus, 20 to 30 mm posterior to the anterior tip of the lateral ventricles. The target is 1.5 mm lateral to midline and 15 mm superior to the roof of the lateral ventricles (55,56) (Fig. 15.2A). The radiofrequency method is used more commonly, with each lesion being created at 75° C for 60 to 90 seconds. The result is a cylindrical lesion approximately 10 to 20 mm long and 5 to 7 mm in diameter, centered in each cingulate gyrus (Fig. 15.2B).

Although its exact role in pain transmission is unclear, the anterior cingulate cortex incorporates motor, affective, memory, and nociceptive functions, accounting for the various pathways connecting this area with the basal ganglia, frontal subsystems, and lateral frontal and parietal regions (1,57). The involvement of the cingulate gyrus in emotional processes has led to the suggestion that the anterior cingulate cortex is most notable for its role in human response to pain rather than sensitivity to pain stimuli (57). Still, studies of cingulate gyrus lesions in laboratory animals have shown a reduction contralaterally in the response to pain, particularly noxious thermal stimuli (1,58). The anterior cingulate cortex, particularly the posterior side of this region, has been shown to be particularly responsive to nociceptive signals from the thalamus (58). A recent study indicates that the anterior section of this region is activated by attention-demanding tasks. Some patients studied a year after cingulotomy were determined to have executive and attentional deficits, particularly in the areas of focused and sustained attention (57).

As many as 30% of patients were treated for severe chronic pain in the many reports of patients undergoing cingulotomy. Approximately 51% of these patients who were treated with intractable cancer pain had moderate, marked, or complete pain relief 3 months after the procedure. Like many ablative procedures, cingulotomy is more effective for patients with a shorter survival time (16,17). The main complications resulting from cingulotomy using ventriculogram guidance (in the treatment of psychiatric or pain symptoms) have been controllable seizures (9% incidence), transient mania (6% incidence), decreased memory (3% incidence), hemiplegia from intracerebral hematoma (0.3% incidence), and a low, but measurable mortality rate (0.9%) (55,59). In neuropsychiatric examination, the only abnormalities noted were occasional difficulties in copying complex figures, performing two tapping tests, and successfully completing memory components of an organized serial learning test (51,60,61). Present evidence suggests that changes in attention resulting from cingulate gyrus lesions do not significantly affect daily functioning and social behavior for patients with severe cancer pain.

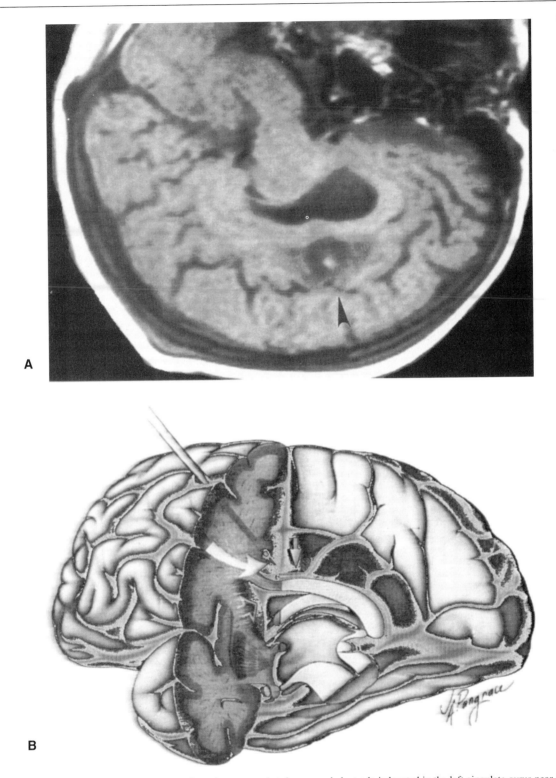

Fig. 15.2. (A) Placement of cingulotomy electrode through cortex so that the exposed electrode is located in the left cingulate gyrus near the distal portion of the anterior cerebral arteries *(closed arrow)* and lateral ventricles. (From Arbit E. Management of cancer-related pain, Mount Kisco, NY: Futura, 1993:303). (B) Postcingulotomy MRI (sagittal view) showing resultant cylindrical lesion in the cingulate gyrus *(arrow)*. (From Arbit E. Management of cancer-related pain. Mount Kisco, NY: Futura, 1993:303).

Trigeminal tractotomy   The discovery that lesions in the descending trigeminal tract affected pain and temperature without diminishing touch sensation led to the study of this area and the adjacent nucleus caudalis as a target site for the ablative treatment of trigeminal neuralgia (62). The nucleus caudalis lies on the surface of the medulla posterior to the dorsal spinocerebellar tract, lateral to the fasciculus cuneatus, and inferior to the restiform body (63). It appears to act as a relay station for pain and temperature transmission from cranial nerves II, V, IX, and X so that destruction of its oral pole decreases neuron hyperexcitability and severs the ascending multisynaptic pathways for pain (64).

Trigeminal tractotomy is used primarily for treatment of patients with head and neck cancer and with intractable pain in the distribution of the trigeminal nerve. For those patients whose pain is more diffuse in the head and neck, mesencephalotomy often is a more effective choice (65). Although trigeminal tractotomy was originally used to treat trigeminal neuralgia and postherpetic neuralgia, it is not frequently used for these conditions because of the availability of other percutaneous and open operations. Newer research indicates that, because the trigeminal, glossopharyngeal, and vagal nerves all meet at the spinobulbar juncture, ablative therapy in this region can also be used to treat vagoglossopharyngeal and geniculate neuralgias (94). Other treatment options have higher morbidity and mortality rates and more extreme complications (64).

Both percutaneous and open surgical techniques have been described for this operation. A percutaneous technique has been reported with needle penetration at the C1-foramen magnum area under stereotactic guidance (66,67). Use of CT technology in particular allows direct visualization of the target and generates measurements of the spinal cord that are patient-specific (64). An electrode with a 0.5 to 0.6 mm diameter is angled 30 degrees cephalad and placed in the spinal cord, 6 mm lateral to the midline, to a depth of 4 mm. With the patient under local anesthesia, electrical stimulation at 50 Hz should provide facial response to low voltage. Stimulation will be felt in contralateral body areas via the spinothalamic tract if placement is too ventral, and placement that is too dorsal will be felt in ipsilateral areas via the fasciulus cuneatus.

Based on the procedures described by Sjoqvist (62), the open operation uses a prone position to unilaterally remove bone from the occiput and C1. After opening the dura, a lesion is created on the nucleus caudalis, 3 to 5 mm below the surface of the cervicomedullary junction, using a transverse knife. Located 4 to 8 mm inferior to the obex, the incision extends medially from the fasciculus cuneatus to the rootlets of the spinal accessory nerve. An oblique incision that is angled from superior to inferior as it is made from posterior to anterior minimizes the chance of accidentally injuring the restiform body. Extension of the lesion to include part of both the spinothalamic tract and the fasciculus is recommended for mouth coverage. The tractotomy is often combined with other nerve and/or root sections in the same area.

Limited published reports of the results of this procedure, either with open or percutaneous techniques, suggest that about 75%–85% of patients with head and neck cancer have good pain relief. Postoperative sensory changes in the area of the pain accompanied by limited relief have been documented as well. Duration of efficacy appears to be months rather than years after the procedure (63). In some cases, pain associated with the percutaneous operation may result in termination of the procedure before completion. Temporary complications consist of changes in ipsilateral arm coordination, contralateral leg sensation, and ipsilateral arm (rarely leg) proprioception. Less frequent complications include Horner's syndrome, dysarthria, gait changes, and hiccoughs. Overall mortality has been estimated at 5%–10% in patients with advanced cancer.

Mesencephalotomy   Mesencephalic tractotomy (mesencephalotomy), the surgical production of lesions in the midbrain, has been reported to provide significant pain relief in more than 80% of cancer patients on both short- and long-term (2–4 year) follow-up evaluation (2). The longest duration of pain relief in cancer patients is in the extremities, whereas pain in the chest and abdomen does not respond adequately (68). The procedure is particularly effective in the treatment of head and neck cancer. A common target site is found by locating the spinothalamic tract (STT) and the spinoreticular tract (SRT), which are found 7 to 9 mm lateral to the midline and 4 to 7 mm lateral to the midline, respectively (carefully avoiding the medial lemniscus, which is 9 to 12 mm lateral of the midline) (2). By disrupting the junction of the STT and the SRT, the lesions on the mesencephalon disrupt two nociceptive pathways (2).

The target has been at the superior colliculus or inferior colliculus level, although it appears that the inferior colliculus target provides a lower incidence of ocular problems but perhaps with lower success (50%–70%). In the studies carried out by Bosch, the target was identified based on intraoperative ventriculography with water-soluble medium using the frontal burr-hole route (68). The usual stereotactic techniques are performed with the patient under general anesthesia to further standardize the procedure. The area of evoked pain is limited to a very small range (about 2 to 3 mm of target) and requires the use of a bipolar concentric electrode for extremely precise localized stimulation. Stimulation of the STT results in thermal or noxious sensation contralaterally, whereas stimulation of the media lemniscus results in temporary paraesthesias of the contralateral side (2).

The accuracy of the stereotactic trajectory to the rostral midbrain also reduces morbidity and other risks (69). Because of neuropathic side effects, the operation should be limited to patients with short life expectancy and lateralized nociceptive pain. With a well-defined target, the operation can produce pain relief comparable to other pain relief operations such as open anterior cordotomy, midline myelotomy, and dorsal root entry zone lesions (68). The major side effect appears to be difficulties with ocular movement and binocular vision, with mortality rates varying from 1%–7% (49,70). Postoperative dysesthesia has been reported in studies of the medial lemniscus after large mesencephalic lesions in all different types of patients (40,69). These side effects have been reduced by using a smaller electrode, neural recording, and more precise electrical stimulation (69).

The results of this operation vary because of the nature of the particular diseases. Although nociceptive pain is often sensitive to opioids, mesencephalic surgery is a successful and viable alternative.

Pulvinotomy   Pulvinotomy appears to be ideally suited to treatment of intractable cancer pain whose symptoms are similar to those indicated for cingulotomy, particularly in patients with survival times up to 18 months (71). Kudo et al. first described lesions in the pulvinar of the thalamus for pain relief in 1966, and by 1975, 30 patients had undergone this treatment. Exact mechanisms for pain relief have not yet been ascertained, but research indicates that the oral and medial parts of the pulvinar are involved in pain appreciation (72). Electrophysiologic studies in cats have demonstrated that the pulvinar is involved in an indirect route for afferent stimuli (73). From the pulvinar, afferent transmission connections have been traced to the temporal lobe and, from there, to the posterior sensory cortex (74).

Typically, lesion placement has occurred only in the medial area or in both the medial and lateral areas of pulvinar. Concentration of the lesions in the hemisphere contralateral to the site of pain appears to be less effective than lesions positioned bilaterally (38,48,71). The coordinates for pulvinar lesions have been 4 mm superior to the anteroposterior commissure line, 5 mm posterior to the posterior commissure, and lateral to the anteroposterior commissure line by either 10 to 11 mm for a medial target or 15 to 16 mm for a lateral target (71). Lesions are created using ultrasonic probes, with a setting of 75 watts and 2.5 megacycles for 30 seconds, at two to six separate sites, resulting in lesions 5 to 6 mm in diameter (71). Currently, MRI-guided stereotaxis and radiofrequency thermal tools are also used to generate lesions in the pulvinar.

Moderate to excellent pain relief has been reported in as many as 25% of patients for periods ranging from 1 to 2.5 years (71,74). When the lesions are extended backward to involve the pulvinar, the lesions, especially in the anterior pulvinar, have been found to be more effective than the centrum medianum thalamotomy (74). Extension of the lesions to a more posterior region of the pulvinar, particularly when coupled with thalamotomy lesions in the centrum medianum and parafascicularis provides an increase in pain relief (75). Preexisting pain is most affected by this operation, and there is no reported loss of somatic sensation after the procedure (48). Analysis of patients after pulvinotomy has shown no apparent changes in cognitive functions, although temporary changes in behavior, such as tendencies toward childishness, excessive excitability, and euphoria, have all been observed (76).

Hypothalamotomy   Lesions of the hypothalamus were reported initially for cancer pain control in 1971, with 28 patients reported to have received the procedure for pain control between 1971 and 1982 (77,78). Beta-endorphin concentrations in ventricular cerebrospinal fluid, believed to increase in response to nociceptive stimuli, elevate as a result of electrical stimulation of the target before actual ablation of the area and remain at a higher level for at least 2 days after the hypothalamotomy (79). A postoperative degeneration of axon fibers occurs in regions found ipsilateral to the hypothalamus, including the nucleus ventrocaudalis parvocellularis of Hassler, nucleus parafascicularis, somatosensory cortices, pallidum, and the reticular formation but not in the dorsomedial nucleus of the thalamus (80). Cancer patients suffering from diffuse pain, particularly when an emotional or visceral component is present, are good candidates for the operation (69).

Target sites had previously been localized 2 mm below the midpoint and 2 mm lateral to the lateral wall of the third ventricle, but more recent reports have suggested that a more posterior placement may provide greater pain control (80). In one series, 15 of 21 hypothalamotomy procedures were bilateral, with "good" results reported in 62% of patients (69,79). Hypothalamotomy does not seem to result in any significant complications; however, published reports are very limited.

Combined procedures As technology enables intracranial procedures to be performed with much more ease, combinations of these techniques should be increasingly used, with particular attention paid to those combinations already used to treat affective disorders. For instance, the use of cingulotomy and anterior capsulotomy, in which lesions are created in both the cingulate gyrus and the anterior limb of the internal capsule, is well reported within the realm of affective disorders. The same combination also has proved useful in the area of severe cancer-related pain, yielding better pain relief, including neuropathic pain, than cingulotomy alone (81). Targets for thalamotomy also include the pulvinar as an additional target because of the increase in pain relief that this combination brings (75). As experience and technological advances improve and become more accessible, it is hoped that interest in the research of combination therapy will result in more modalities that provide better long-term efficacy in pain control.

Ablative procedures—spinal

Cordotomy Until recently, intraspinal ablative procedures have been favored despite the variety of intracranial procedures available as the older spinal methods are "rediscovered" by using newer percutaneous techniques and CT guidance. Although the use of intraspinal ablative procedures appears to be decreasing as technological innovations focus more attention on intracranial ablative and intraspinal augmentative procedure, the most acknowledged procedure, cordotomy, is still a standard option. The aim of the operation is to disrupt the spinothalamic tract as it enters the medulla. However, the mechanism of action for this procedure has been suggested to affect more than just C-fibers because pain relief coincides with a lessened sensation of pinching skin and temperature cooling (82).

In the percutaneous method, x-ray fluoroscopy is used to position a radiofrequency electrode needle at the level of the C1-2 interspace in the lateral spinothalamic tract as determined by the area of pain (51) (Fig. 15.3). CT guidance allows for better visualization and more accurate

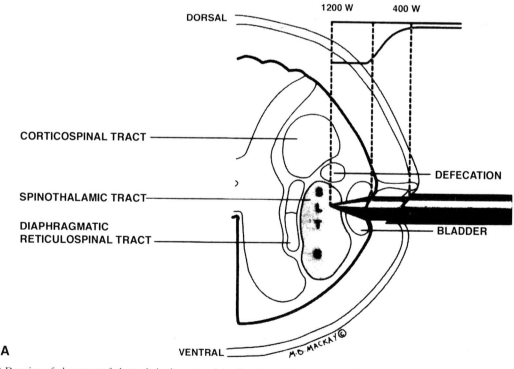

Fig. 15.3. (A) Drawing of placement of electrode in the posterolateral section of the spinothalamic tract for percutaneous cordotomy using CT guidance (From North RB, Levy RM. Neurosurgical management of pain. New York: Springer-Verlag, 1997:206.) (B) Lateral cervical spine x-ray fluoroscopy showing positioning of the cordotomy electrode anterior to the dentate ligament, which is outlined with injected contrast. (From North RB, Levy RM. Neurosurgical management of pain. New York: Springer-Verlag, 1997:203.) *(Figure continues)*

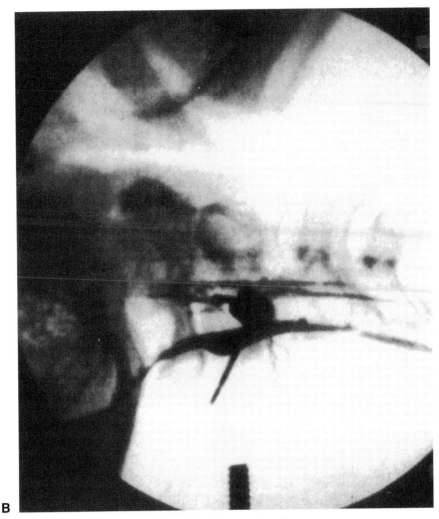

B

Fig. 15.3. *(Figure continued)*

insertion of the electrodes into the spine. A cordotomy needle puncture is made in the side of the neck contralateral to the site of pain with the aid of a questioning stimulation in which the patient is asked about sensory changes and twitching. The open surgical technique for cordotomy is similar to the percutaneous method except that it is often carried out with the patient seated in an upright position. In this procedure, the anterolateral surface of the spinal cord is viewed and an avascular area is found for the incision. The blade projects 6 mm through the cervical area and 4 to 5 mm in the thoracic area and then cuts ventrally to transect the ventral quadrant but spare the medial funiculus. The open operation is currently considered the less effective surgical option because it is associated with more risks than the percutaneous operation.

A patient's case must be exactly suited to the procedure for pain relief to be successfully achieved. Proper preoperative respiratory/pulmonary function is critical because mortality is almost always related to respiratory problems. The main complication during and after surgery is the possible loss of the sensation of temperature. Possible side effects of the percutaneous operation include contralateral limb weakness from lesioning too deep, transient Horner's syndrome, respiratory problems, and burning postcordotomy dysesthetic syndromes. Postlesional dysesthesias and new pain, either in the contralateral limb or above the level of the previous pain, have been reported. Some patients also have been reported to experience low levels of analgesia owing to the failure of the surgery or lack of adequate anatomical localization of target sites during the operation. A small group has experienced new pain formation in a similar and/or different location, whereas others did not experience relief at all. In other words, the operation is fairly successful in achieving pain relief, although many small impediments may hinder success along the way.

In the large series of Tasker, long-term success with no pain was found in 33% of patients and partial pain relief in 12%. Persistent pain was noted in 6% and a dysesthetic pain in 34%; 2.6% required a repeat cordotomy for continued pain relief. Others, however, have found that absolute pain relief has decreased through postoperative time, with only 37% having satisfactory analgesia even after 5 to 10 years (81). Complications in the Tasker series included persistent paresis (2%), bladder dysfunction (2%), temporary respiratory failure (0.5%), and death (0.5%).

Midline myelotomy   First conceived by Armour in 1927 as a way of treating a patient with tabetic abdominal pain (85), the midline myelotomy was first performed by Putnam in 1934 (86). Since its first use, the procedure has undergone many mechanical and functional adjustments for new applications. The procedure for midline myelotomy also has undergone adjustments as technologies have changed; it can now be performed with mechanical ablation, radiofrequency techniques, or carbon dioxide laser (87) to section midline fibers posterior to the central canal of the spinal cord.

The lesions are usually created at the lower thoracic spinal cord level, although Gildenberg and Hirshberg (47) and others also have reported lesions at C1. The percentage of patients reporting moderate-to-marked pain relief has been approximately 70%, with only rare complications or side effects noted. This procedure is particularly effective for visceral lower body pain in cancer patients where other procedures are inapplicable or unsuccessful. There is evidence for a tract in the anterior part of the medial borders of the posterior columns mediating both pelvic and more proximal epigastric visceral pain (88–91). Research conducted with laboratory animals has shown that lesions in the dorsal column reduce responses to noxious colorectal pain stimulation by 60%–80%, compared with the 20% reduction that results from lesioning the ventral posterolateral nucleus of the thalamus (92). Orthograde and retrograde tracers have shown the presence of a postsynaptic pathway (separate from the spinothalamic tract) that ascends in the gray matter around the central canal to the nucleus gracilis (93). From there, nociceptive stimuli are relayed to the ventral posterolateral nucleus of the thalamus using the medial lemniscus (93). A study of cancer patients with visceral pain has confirmed that punctate midline myelotomy of the midthoracic spinal cord can reduce visceral pain and use of narcotics without changes in sensation or

motor function (93). In general, analgesia from hyperpathia and background pain has been obtained without sensory loss but with preserved ability to localize and discriminate between sharp and dull stimuli (94).

A commissural myelotomy on the spinal cord aims to interrupt all decussating second-order spinothalamic fibers that are contributing to pain perception on both sides of the body through the posterior commissure of the spinal cord. Two methods are presently available for patients: open and closed. The open operation requires an incision in the spinal cord down the exact midline between the two gracilis tracts and ventrally configured down until completely divided (Fig. 15.4). This transection disconnects the two sides of the posterior half of the spinal cord so that they are now independent of each other and can no longer communicate dorsally. The closed operation involves placement of a radiofrequency electrode between the two gracilis tracts using CT guidance.

Although many different methods have been described over many decades, there continues to be a lack of knowledge about the myelotomy, particularly the mechanism of pain relief. Because the use of this procedure has been diminishing over the last 15 years, there have been only about 425 total cases reported throughout neurosurgical journals (45,84,91,93–102).

Augmentative procedures
Intraventricular infusion of opioid   The intraventricular infusion of opioids is one of the best known intracranial

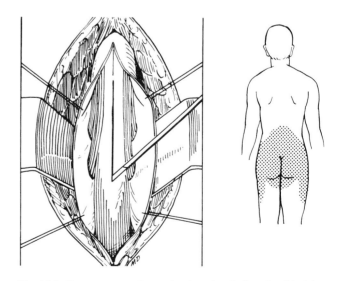

Fig. 15.4. Open exposure of posterior thoracic spinal cord and incision to create a plane between posterior columns down to the level of the central canal. Area of typical pain relief is shown. (From Bonica JJ. The management of pain. Philadelphia: Lea & Febiger, 1990:2074).

augmentative procedures. The mechanism by which it regulates pain appears to involve supraspinal pathways for analgesia. This treatment option is normally among the last resort options for a patient's treatment (106).

The opioid can be delivered by an implanted infusion pump placed subcutaneously in the anterior abdominal wall and connected by subcutaneous tubing to an implanted ventricular catheter. The length of action of the intraventricular injections appears to be significantly longer than with intraspinal delivery. Patients may be able to receive adequate relief with an implanted ventricular catheter connected to a subcutaneous Ommaya reservoir-type device with one to two injections/day (107). Morphine sulfate is the usual agent and appears to provide a marked increase in potency as compared to intrathecal or epidural infusions, with daily morphine doses for intraventricular delivery ranging from 50 to 700 μg/day (108–110)).

Recent studies using sheep indicated that certain drugs, particularly lipophilic morphine-type drugs, have problems diffusing through the cerebrospinal fluid pathways to reach distant receptors. Thus, the type of opioid must be carefully considered. Payne et al. (103) used drugs such as hydromorphine, morphine, methadone, naloxone, and then sucrose to test the spread of specific opioids in cerebrospinal fluid (CSF). Morphine, hydromorphone, and sucrose were identified at approximately 90 minutes in the lumbar CSF after an intracerebroventricular (ICV) injection (106). Hydromorphone was located after 50 minutes. Methadone was never found in the CSF because the ICV and IT dosage of lipophilic opioids creates distinctly different CSF distributions from hydrophilic drugs, such as morphine (103).

Most significantly, it has been shown that there is a rapid spread of hydrophilic compounds in CSF after lumbar intrathecal injections. The hydrophilic nature of these compounds, however, does make it more difficult for them to attach to the desired receptors. The lipophilicity of the opioid determines the extent of diffusion and concentration in the brain after ICV administration (103). Brain concentrations of the morphine persist for a few hours after injection, although the drug is unevenly dispersed in the tissue. Because morphine is hydrophilic, the movement of the drug through the ventricles of the brain is more like passive diffusion than active transport. Fentanyl, sufentanil, and etorphine, the lipophilic opioids, are cleared in the CSF after 1 hour as they bind better to lipophilic receptors (103).

This procedure appears to be best suited for head and neck cancer pain. Occasionally, it is used for patients with limited survival time (1–3 months) who develop a tolerance to intraspinal infusion of opioids despite a good initial response to the treatment. Several factors must be weighed for effective treatment with intraventricular morphine delivery via an Ommaya reservoir, such as the location of the pain, age of the patient, and the history of opioid usage. The lower limbs benefit from lumbar subarachnoid administration of morphine, whereas craniofacial or diffuse pain was more responsive to the analgesic effect of ICV delivery (111).

Seiwald et al. (112) have described in detail their experience with 20 patients (18 cases suffering from cancer) treated with ICV morphine injections between 1990 and 1993. Administration of morphine into the ventricle through a catheter-reservoir system was non-destructive and effectively relieved nociceptive pain (112). They also found that lower doses were slower to bring about pain relief. Somatogenic pain was ameliorated in 95% of the patients; however, minimal effects were seen in the management of neurogenic pain (112). The safety and side effects of the intraventricular injections or infusions are similar to intraspinal infusions with the exception of the increased risk of respiratory depression noted in the first 3 days of the intraventricular delivery (107,109).

Deep brain stimulation   Interest in stimulation swelled in the late 1960s and early 1970s as the severe morbidity rates and limited scope of some early ablative procedures came to light (113). In 1972, the first stimulation of periventricular and periaqueductal gray matter were performed in humans (113). Particularly effective in those with chronic pain that activates the paleospinothalamic tract, deep brain stimulation is currently the most useful technique for central pain caused by spinal cord lesions as well as pain that is inadequately relieved with spinal cord or peripheral nerve stimulation (113). The use of deep brain stimulation has also been reported in the relief of chronic pain of non-cancer etiology (114).

During this procedure, an electrode implant is carried out by placing the patient under local anesthesia while a burr hole is made 3 cm from the midline in the coronal structure. These burr holes are made easily with CT- and MRI-guided stereotaxis because the technology enables accurate placement of the stimulating electrodes (114). For this operation, the initial targets are either the periventricular gray/periaqueductal gray (PVG/PAG) area, the ventral posterior lateral thalamus, or the internal capsule (114). To implant an electrode in the PVG/PAG, the exploring electrode tip is placed 10 mm posterior to the midpoint of the AC-PC line at a depth of 4 to 5 mm

(113). The internal capsule can be found using the atlas of Tasker and Emmers and test stimulation performed at the junction of the thalamus and internal capsule (113).

In the PVG/PAG, stimulation sets off an endogenous opiate system, mediated primarily by beta-endorphins, that inhibits noxious pain impulses (113). Judging from failed trials with naloxone, the system in the thalamus and internal capsule does not involve opiates, although the mechanism of action is not precisely known (113). The type of pain being experienced and the severity of the situation aid in determining which target site will provide sufficient analgesia. Stimulation of the PVG/PAG is best suited to nociceptive pain, whereas stimulation of areas in and around the thalamus is thought to work better for neuropathic pain (115). The small size of thalamic targets as well as the numbness that may result from implantation have led some surgeons to prefer the internal capsule to the lateral thalamus (113). Many surgeons place electrodes temporarily in both areas and allow the patient to choose the location that best alleviates pain; others rely on intraoperative stimulation to determine placement. After 4 days, routine tests of the apparatus determine the frequencies that generate pain relief. Several days to 3 months after implantation, a radiofrequency-receiving device can be attached so that the patient can freely use the device (113).

In cancer pain, deep brain stimulation can accommodate patients with pain refractory to ablative procedures. This includes pain from diffuse bone metastases, midline or bilateral pain (especially of the lower body), brachial or lumbosacral plexopathy, and recurrent pain from head and neck cancer (116). In a series of 31 patients with cancer pain who were treated with deep brain stimulation, 87% of the patients experienced satisfactory relief, with 55% of these experiencing lasting relief until death (116). In a 15-year trial of 68 patients, 78% underwent internalization of their devices, and 79% reported long-term relief (115).

Complications are unavoidable because they are greatly influenced by the placement of the deep brain stimulator electrode. They occur less frequently when the electrode is placed in the PVG region than when it is placed in the PAG region. The most reported complication in the Kumar study resulted from hardware malfunction, although 20%–25% of patients involved in the study reported the development of migraine-type headaches. One complication specific to PVG/PAG is the development of tolerance. It has been suggested that ramp stimulation (intermittent stimulation) and administration of L-tryptophan for 2 to 3 weeks can diminish this occur-

rence (113). Although individual variations can reduce the chance for successful analgesia as a result of deep brain stimulation, the possibility of effective pain relief is both promising and realistic for most patients (115).

Conclusion

The neurosurgical options for treating intractable cancer pain are many. Advances in technology, particularly in the area of magnetic resonance guidance, have greatly improved the accuracy and ease of application of the intracranial techniques.

Over the past decade, the technology for and use of spinal procedures has remained fairly constant, and as a result information is still not complete concerning the best application of many of these procedures. Most certainly, it should be emphasized that these techniques are applied only to patients with severe pain, as many of the non-interventional options will suffice for pain that is minimal or mild in severity.

Selection of a specific technique can be based on expected survival time of the cancer patient, pain location, and/or preference toward ablative or augmentative options. Despite the praise heaped by different clinical groups on individual methods, information regarding the best modalities of treatment for specific pain syndromes is still lacking. This might be an indication that technology has outpaced our knowledge of the most effective application for each procedure. As knowledge of the efficacy of different various pain grows, it is hoped that the role of each of these neurosurgical procedures in the overall management of cancer patients experiencing severe pain will be clarified.

References

1. Wong ET, Gunes S, Guaghan E. Palliation of intractable cancer pain by MRI-guided cingulotomy. Clin J Pain 13:260–3, 1997.
2. Davis KD, Lozano AM, Tasker RR, Dostrovsky JD. Brain targets for pain control. Stereotact Funct Neurosurg 71:73–179, 1999.
3. Foltz EL, White LE. Pain "relief" by frontal cingulomotomy. J Neurosurg 19:89–100, 1962.
4. Hurt RW, Ballantine HT. Stereotactic anterior cingulate lesions for persistent pain: a report on 68 cases. Clin Neurosurg 21:334–51, 1974.
5. Mempel E, Dietrich RZ. Favorable effect of cingulotomy on gastric crisis pain. Neurol Neurochir Pol 11:611–3, 1977.
6. Sano K. Neurosurgical treatments of pain: a general survey. Acta Neurochir Suppl 38:86–96, 1987.

7. Santo JL, Arias LM, Barolat G, et al. Bilateral cingulumotomy in the treatment of reflex sympathetic dystrophy. Pain 41:55–9, 1988.

8. Coombs DW. Intraspinal analgesic infusion by implanted pump. Ann N Y Acad Sci 531:108–22, 1988.

9. Yaksh TL, Onofrio B. Retrospective consideration of the doses of morphine given intrathecally by chronic infusion in 163 patients by 19 physicians. Pain 31:211–23, 1987.

10. Lewin W. Observations on selective leucotomy. J Neurol Neurosurg Psychiatry 24:69–73, 1961.

11. Spiegel EA, Wycis H, Marks M, et al. Stereotactic apparatus for operations on the human brain. Science 106:349–50, 1947.

12. Spiegel EA. Guided brain operations. Basel, Switzerland: Karger, 1982.

13. Hadley MN, Shatter AG, Amos M. Use of the Brown-Roberts-Wells stereotactic frame for functional neurosurgery. Appl Neurophysiol 48:61–8, 1985.

14. Hassenbusch SJ, Pillay PP. Cingulotomy for intractable pain using stereotaxis guided by magnetic resonance imaging. In: Rengachary SS, Wilkins RH, eds. Neurosurgical operative atlas. Baltimore: Williams & Wilkins, 1992:449–58.

15. Holtzheimer PE III, Roberts DW, Daray TM. Magnetic resonance imaging versus computed tomography for target localization in functional stereotactic neurosurgery. Neurosurgery 45:290–8, 1999.

16. Hassenbusch SJ, Pillay PP. Cingulotomy for treatment of cancer-related pain. Mt. Kisco, NY: Futura, 1993:297–312.

17. Pillay PK, Hassenbusch SJ. Cingulotomy for cancer pain: two year experience. Stereotact Funct Neurosurg 59:33–8, 1992.

18. Leskell L. Cerebral radiosurgery: gammathalamotomy in two cases of intractable pain. Acta Chir Scand 134:585–95, 1968.

19. Steiner L, Foster D, Leksell L, et al. Gammathalamotomy in intractable pain. Acta Neurochir 52:173–178, 1980.

20. Lindquist C, Kilstrom L, Hellstrand E. Functional neurosurgery: a future for the gamma knife? Stereotact Funct Neurosurg 57:72–81, 1991.

21. Miles J. Chemical hypophysectomy. Adv Pain Res Ther 2:373–80. 1979.

22. Tindall GT, Payne NS, Nixon DW. Transsphenoidal hypophysectomy for disseminated carcinoma of the prostate gland. J Neurosurg 50:275–82, 1979.

23. Kapur TR, Dalton GA. Trans-sphenoidal hypophysectomy for metastatic carcinoma of the breast. Br J Surg 56:332–7, 1969.

24. Zervas NT. Stereotaxic radiofrequency surgery of the normal and abnormal pituitary gland. N Engl J Med 280:429–37, 1969.

25. Maddy JA, Winternitz WW, Norrell H. Cryohypophysectomy in the management of advanced prostatic cancer. Cancer 28:322–8, 1971.

26. Silverberg GD. Hypophysectomy in the treatment of disseminated prostate carcinoma. Cancer 39:1727–31, 1977.

27. Levin AB, Ramirez LF, Katz J. The use of stereotaxic chemical hypophysectomy in the treatment of thalamic pain syndrome. J Neurosurg 59:1002–6, 1983.

28. Levin AB. Hypophysectomy in the treatment of cancer pain. In: Arbit E, ed. Management of cancer related pain. Mt. Kisco, NY: Futura, 1993:281–95.

29. Daniel PM. The human hypothalamus and pituitary stalk after hypophysectomy of pituitary stalk section. Brain 95:813–24, 1972.

30. Nilaver G, Zimmerman EA, Wilkins J, et al. Magnocellular hypothalamic projections to the lower brain stem and spinal cord of the rat: immunocytochemical evidence for predominance of the oxytocin-neurophysin system compared to a vasopressin-neurophysin system. Neuroendocrinology 30:150–8, 1980.

31. Sofroniew MV. Projections from vasopressin, oxytocin, and neurophysin neurons to neural targets in the rat and human. J Histochem Cytochem 28:475–8, 1980.

32. Swanson LW, Sawchenko P. Paraventricular nucleus: a site for the integration of neuroendocrine and autonomic mechanism. Neuroendocrinology 31:410–7, 1980.

33. Silverman AJ, Zimmerman EA. Magnocellular neurosecretory system. Annu Rev Neurosci 6:357–80, 1983.

34. Kudo T, Toshii N, Shimizu S, et al. Effects of stereotactic thalamotomy to intractable pain and numbness. Keio J Med 15:191–4, 1966.

35. Gros C, Frerebeau P, Privat JM, et al. Place of hypophysectomy in the neurosurgical treatment of pain. Adv Neurosurg 3:264–72, 1975.

36. Tindall GT, Ambrose SS, Christy JH, et al. Hypophysectomy in the treatment of disseminated carcinoma of the breast and prostate gland. South Med J 69:579–83, 1976.

37. Greco T, Sparagli F, Cammilli L, et al. L'alcolizzazione della ipofisi per via transfenoidal nella terapia di particoloari tumori maligni. Settim Med 45:355–6, 1957.

38. Yoshii N, Fukuda S. Effects of unilateral and bilateral invasion of thalamic pulvinar for pain relief. Tohoku J Exp Med 127:81–4, 1979.

39. Lipton S. Percutaneous cervical cordotomy and pituitary injection of alcohol. In: Swerdlow M, ed. Relief of intractable pain. Amsterdam, The Netherlands: Elsevier, 1983:269–304.

40. Shieff C, Nashold B. Stereotactic mesencephalotomy. Neurosurg Clin North Am 1(4):825–39, 1990.

41. Perrault M, LeBeau J, Klotz B, et al. L'hypophysectomie totale dans le traitment du cancer sein: premier cas francais: avenir de la methode. Therapie 7:290–300, 1952.

42. Katz S, Levin AB. Treatment of diffuse metastatic pain by instillation of alcohol in to the sella turcia. Anesthesiology 46:115–21, 1977.

43. Williams NE, Miles JB, Lipton S, et al. Pain relief and pituitary function following injectionof alcohol into the pituitary fossa. Ann R Coll Surg Engl 62:203–7, 1980.

44. Madrid JL. Chemical hypophysectomy. Adv Pain Res Ther 2:381–91, 1979.

45. Tasker RR. Neurosurgical and neuroaugmentative intervention. In: Cancer pain. Philadelphia: Lippincott, 1993:471–500.

46. Tasker RR. Thalamotomy. Neurosurg Clin North Am 1:841–66, 1990.

47. Gildenberg PL, Hirshberg RM. Limited myelotomy for the treatment of intractable cancer pain. J Neurol Neurosurg Psychiatry 47:94–9, 1984.

48. Sweet WH. Central mechanisms of chronic pain (neuralgias and certain other neurogenic pain). Res Publ Assoc Res Nerv Ment Dis 58:287–303, 1980.

49. Shieff C, Nashold B. Stereotactic mesencephalic tractotomy for thalamic pain. Neurosurg Res 9:101–4, 1987.

50. Lewin W. Selective leucotomy: a review in surgical approaches in psychiatry. In: Laitinen LK, ed. Baltimore: University Park Press, 1972:69–73.

51. Faillace LA, Allen RP, McQueen JD, Northrup B. Cognitive deficits from bilateral cingulotomy for intractable pain in man. Dis Nerv Sys 32:171–5, 1981.

52. Ortiz A. The role of the limbic lobe in central pain mechanisms: an hypothesis relating to the gate control theory of pain. In: Laitinen LV, Livingston KE, eds. Surgical approaches in psychiatry. Baltimore: University Park Press, 1972:59–64.

53. Sharma T. Absence of cognitive deficits from bilateral cingulotomy for intractable pain in humans. Tex Med 69:79–82, 1973.

54. Sharma T. Abolition of opiate hunger in humans following bilateral anterior cingulotomy. Tex Med 70:49–52, 1974.

55. Ballantine HT. A critical assessment of psychiatric surgery: past, present, and future. In: Berger BH, ed. American handbook of psychiatry. New York: Basic Books, 1986:1029–45.

56. Ballantine HT, Bouckoms A, Thomas EK, Giriunas IE. Treatment of psychiatric illness by stereotactic cingulotomy. Biol Psychiatry 22:807–19, 1987.

57. Cohen RA, Kaplan RF, Moser DJ, et al. Impairments of attention after cingulotomy. Neurology 53:819–24, 1999.

58. Davis KD, Taub E, Duffner F, et al. Activation of the anterior cingulate cortex by thalamic stimulation in patients with chronic pain: a positron emission tomography study. J Neurosurg 92:64–9, 2000.

59. Jenike MA, Baer L, Ballantine T, et al. Cingulotomy for refractory obsessive-compulsive disorder. Arch Gen Psychiatry 48:548–55, 1991.

60. Allen RP, Faillace L. A clinical test for detecting defects of cingulate lesions in man. J Clin Psychol 28:63–5, 1972.

61. Corkin S, Twitchell TE, Sullivan EV. Safety and efficacy of cingulotomy for pain and psychiatric disorder. In: Hitchcock ER, Ballantine HT, Myerson BA, eds. Modern concepts in psychiatric surgery. New York: Elsevier North-Holland, 1979:253–72.

62. Sjoqvist O. Studies on pain conduction in trigeminal nerve: a contribution to the surgical treatment of facial pain. Acta Psychiatr Neurol Suppl 1–139, 1938.

63. White JC, Sweet W. Pain and the neurosurgeon: a forty-year experience In: C.C. Thomas ed. Springfield, IL, 1969:232–51, 314–20.

64. Kanpolat Y, Savas A, Batay F, Sinav A. CT-guided trigeminal tracheotomy–nucleotomy in the management of vagoglossopharyngeal and geniculate neuralgias. Neurosurgery 43:484–8, 1998.

65. Spiegel EA, Wycis HT. Mesencephalotomy in the treatment of "intractable" facial pain. Arch Neurol 69:1, 1953.

66. Nashold BS Jr, Crue BL. Stereotaxic mesencephalotomy and trigeminal tractotomy. In: Youmans JR, ed. Neurological surgery, 2nd ed. Philadelphia: WB Saunders, 1982:3702–16.

67. Schvarcz JR. Spinal cord stereotactic techniques re trigeminal nucleotomy and extralemniscal myelotomy. Appl Neurophysiol 41:99–112, 1978.

68. Harris B. Dorsal rhizotomy. In: Wilkins RH, ed. Neurosurgery. New York: McGraw-Hill, 1985:2430–7.

69. Amano K, Kitamura K, Sano K, et al. Relief of intractable pain from neurosurgical point of view with reference to present limits and clinical indications: a review of 100 consecutive 57 cases. Neurol Med Chir (Tokyo)16:141–53, 1976.

70. Frank F, Gais G. Stereotactic mesencephalic tractotomy in the treatment of chronic pain. Acta Neurochir (Wien) 99:38–40, 1989.

71. Yoshii N, Mizokami T, Ushikubo Y, et al. Comparative study between size of lesioned area and operative effects after pulvinotomy. Appl Neurophysiol 45:492–7, 1982.

72. Strenge H. The functional significance of the pulvinar thalami. Fortschr Neurol Psychiatry 46:491–507, 1978.

73. Kudo T, Toshi N, Shimizu S, et al. Stereotactic thalamotomy for pain relief. Tohoku J Exp Med 96:219–23, 1968.

74. Laitinen LV. Anterior pulvinotomy in the treatment of intractable pain. In: Sweet WH, Martin-Rodriguez JG, eds. Neurosurgical treatment in psychiatry pain, and epilepsy. Baltimore: University Park Press, 1977:669–72.

75. Mayanagi Y, Bourchard G. Evaluation of stereotactic thalamotomies for pain relief with reference to pulvinar intervention. Appl Neurophysiol 39:154–7, 1976.

76. Yoshii N, Fukuda S. Several clinical aspects of thalamic pulvinotomy. Appl Neurophysiol 39:162–4, 1977.

77. Sano K. Sedative neurosurgery with reference to posteromedial hypothalamotomy. Neurol Medicochir 4:112–42, 1962.

78. Fairman D. Hypothalamotomy as a new perspective for alleviation of intractable pain and regression of metastatic malignant tumors. In: Fusek K, ed. Present limits of neurosurgery. Prague: Czech Republic, Avicenum Czechoslovakian Medical Press, 1971:525–8.

79. Mayanagi Y, Sano K, Suzuki I, et al. Stimulation and coagulation of the posteromedial hypothalamus for intractable pain, with reference to beta-endorphins. Appl Neurophysiol 45:136–42, 1982.

80. Sano K, Sekino H, Hashimoto I, et al. Posteromedial hypothalamotomy in the treatment of intractable pain. Confinia Neurol 37:285–90, 1975.

81. Hassenbusch SJ, Pillay P. Ablative intracranial neurosurgery for cancer pain: three-year experience and modification of techniques. J Neurosurg 76:396A, 1992 (abstract).

82. LaHuerta J, Campbell J. Clinical and instrumental evaluation of sensory function before and after percutaneous anterolateral cordotomy at cervical level in man. Pain 42:23–30, 1990.

83. Amano K, Kitamura K, Tatsuya T, et al. Stereotactic mes-encephalotomy for pain relief. Stereotact Funct Neurosurg 59:25–32, 1992.

84. Rosomoff HL, Papo I, Loeser JD. Neurosurgical operations on the spinal cord. In: Bonica JJ, ed. The management of pain. Philadelphia: Lea & Febiger, 1990:2067–81.

85. Armour D. Surgery of the spinal cord and its membranes. Lancet 1:691, 1927.

86. Putnam TJ. Myelotomy of the commissure. Arch Neurol Psychiatry 32:1189, 1934.

87. Fink RA. Neurosurgical treatment of non-malignant intractable rectal pain: microsurgical commissural myelotomy with the carbon dioxide laser. Neurosurgery 14:64, 1984.

88. Hirshberg RM, Al-Chaer NM, Lawand NB, et al. Is there a pathway in the posterior funiculus that signals visceral pain? Pain 67:291–305, 1996.

89. Al-Chaer ED, Lawand N, Westlund KN, Willis WD. Visceral nociceptive input into the ventral posterolateral nucleus of the thalamus: a new function for the dorsal col-umn pathway. J Neurophysiol: 2661–74, 1996.

90. Al-Chaer ED, Lawand N, Westlund KN, Willis WD. Pelvic visceral input into the nucleus gracilis is largely mediated by the postsynaptic dorsal column pathway. J Neurophysiol 76:2675–90, 1996.

91. Feng Y, Cui M, Al-Chaer ED, Willis WD. Epigastric antinociception by cervical dorsal column lesion in rats. Anesthesiology 89:411–20, 1998.

92. Willis WD, Al-Chaer ED, Quast MJ, Westlund KN. A vis-ceral pathway in the dorsal column of the spinal cord. Proc Natl Acad Sci USA 96:7675–9, 1999.

93. Nauta JW, Soukup VM, Fabian RH, et al. Punctate midline myelotomy for relief of visceral cancer pain. J Neurosurg 92:125–30, 2000.

94. Schvarcz JR. Stereotactic extralemniscal myelotomy. J Neurol Neurosurg Psychiatry 39:53–7, 1976.

95. Sunder-Plassmann M, Grunert V. Commissural myelotomy for drug resistant pain. In: Koos WT, Spetzler RF, eds. Clinical neurosurgery. Stuttgart: Georg Thieme Verlag, 1976:165–70.

96. Hitchcock E. Stereotactic myelotomy. Proc R Soc Med 67:771, 1974.

97. Seiwald M, Alesch F, Kofler A. Intraventricular morphine administration as a treatment possibility for patients with intractable pain. Wien Klin Wochenschr 108:5–8, 1996.

98. Broager B. Commissural myelotomy. Surg Neurol 2:71, 1974.

99. Cook AW, Kawakami Y. Commissural myelotomy. J Neurosurg 47:1, 1977.

100. Lippert RG, Hosobuchi Y, Nielsen SL. Spinal commissuro-tomy. Surg Neurol 2:373, 1974.

101. Papo I, Luongo A. High cervical commissural myelotomy in the treatment of pain. J Neurol Neurosurg Psychiatry 39:105, 1976.

102. King RB. Anterior commissurotomy for intractable pain. J Neurosurg 47:7, 1977.

103. Payne R, Gradert TL, Inturrisi C. Cerebrospinal fluid distri-bution of opioids after intraventricular and lumbar sub-arachnoid administration in sheep. Life Sci 59:1307–21, 1996.

104. Sweet WH. Operations in the brain stem and spinal canal, with an appendix on open cordotomy. In: Wall PD, ed. Textbook of pain. Edinburgh: Churchill Livingstone, 1984:615–31.

105. Adams JE, Lippert R, Hosobuchi Y. Commissural myelo-tomy. In: Sweet WH, ed. Current techniques in operative neurosurgery. New York: Grune & Stratton, 1988:1185–9.

106. Siegfried J. Intracerebral neurosurgery in the treatment of chronic pain. Schweiz Rundsch Med Prax 87:314–7, 1998.

107. Brazenor GA. Long-term intrathecal administration of mor-phine: a comparsion of bolus injection via reservoir with continuous infusion by implanted pump. Neurosurgery 21:484–91, 1987.

108. Tseng LF, Fujimoto J. Differential actions of intrathecal naloxone on blocking the tail flick inhibition induced by intraventricular beta-endorphin and morphine in rats. J Pharmacol Exp Ther 232:74–9, 1985.

109. Dennis GC, DeWitty RL. Long-term intraventricular infu-sion of morphine for intractable pain in cancer of the head and neck. Neurosurgery 26:404–8, 1990.

110. Lazorthes Y. Intracerebroventricular administration of mor-phine for control of irreducible cancer pain. Ann NY Acad Sci 531:123–32, 1988.

111. Karavelis A, Foroglov G, Selviaridis P, Fountzilas G. Intraventricular administration of morphine for control of intractable cancer pain in 90 patients. Neurosurgery 39:57–62, 1996.

112. Seiwald M, Alesch F, Kofler A. Intraventricular morphine administation as a treatment possibility for patients with intractable pain. Wien Klin Wochenschr 108:5–8, 1996.

113. Richardson DE. Deep brain stimulation for pain relief. In: Wilkins RH, Rengachary SS, eds. Neurosurgery. New York: McGraw-Hill, 1985:2421–6.

114. Goodman RR. Surgical management of pain. Neurosurg Clin North Am 1:701–17, 1990.

115. Kumar K, Toth C, Nath RK. Deep brain stimulation for intractable pain: a 15-year experience. Neurosurgery 40:736–45, 1997.

116. Young RF. Electrical stimulation of the brain for the treat-ment of intractable cancer pain. In: Arbit E, ed. Management of cancer-related pain. Mt. Kisco, NY: Futura, 1993:257–69.

SECTION V   THE ROLE OF ANTINEOPLASTIC THERAPIES IN PAIN CONTROL

16 Palliative radiotherapy

NORA A. JANJAN, MARC DELCLOS, CHRISTOPHER CRANE,
MATTHEW BALLO, AND CHARLES CLEELAND
The University of Texas M. D. Anderson Cancer Center

Introduction

During the past decade, 11 million cases of cancer were
diagnosed and 5 million people died from cancer.
Approximately one half the patients diagnosed with cancer
develop metastatic disease, and more than 70% of all cancer patients develop symptoms from either their primary or
metastatic disease (1–4). The decrease in the total number
of cancer deaths that occurred between 1996 and 1997 was
not sustained; there were 955 more cancer-related deaths in
1998 than in the previous year (5). As the second most
common cause of death in the United States, accounting for
23% of all deaths in 1998, cancer is the leading cause of
death among women ages 40 to 79 years old. It is estimated
that 1,268,000 new cases of cancer will be diagnosed this
year, and 553,400 will die of cancer, more than 1500 people a day. Cancer of the lung, prostate, breast, and rectum
constitute more than 50% of all cancer deaths.

Palliation represents a large component of cancer treatment and includes the use of therapeutic and supportive
care measures. Unlike other aspects of cancer therapy,
tumor control and survival are not the endpoints of therapeutic success in palliative care. Quality of life is now
recognized as an endpoint which is as important as survival (6,7). The goal of palliative care is to effectively
and efficiently relieve symptoms and maintain the maximum quality of life for the duration of the patient's life
(2–4,8–13). The effectiveness of palliative therapy can be
assessed, in part, by the percentage of patients who experience persistent/recurrent symptoms and the effort
required to control these symptoms with a variety of therapeutic modalities (12,14,15). Like other aspects of cancer care, a multidisciplinary approach is generally
needed for effective palliative care (16,17).

The debility that results from cancer and its treatment is
a significant issue on a socioeconomic level. Among more
than 9700 community-based Medicare beneficiaries,
poorer health, more limitations of the activities of daily
living, and greater levels of health utilization were documented among the 1647 individuals who had cancer (18).
Limitations in activities included difficulty walking
(38%), getting out of a chair (21%), completing heavy
housework (34%), and shopping (17%). Poorer health
was observed more frequently in patients with lung,
breast, prostate, and colon cancer. Lung, bladder, and
prostate cancers predicted increased health care utilization, and lung cancer most frequently limited the activities of daily living. The mean annual Medicare reimbursement for lung cancer was more than twice that for colon,
breast, and prostate cancers. Even though the decrease in
functional capacity for cancer patient is generally not as
prolonged as with other chronic diseases such as arthritis,
stoke, and emphysema, the annual health care costs for
cancer patient were greater than the health care costs for
other chronic diseases (19). Assuming that not all of the
individuals identified with the diagnosis of cancer in this
Medicare review had active disease at the time of the
analysis, then an even greater percentage of cancer
patients with active disease are functionally impaired and
use more health care resources.

Approximately 300,000 patients in the United States
receive palliative radiation per year at a cost of $900 mil-
lion. About 100,000 patients receive curative radiation
therapy, incurring a cost of $1.1 billion per year (20). The
National Institutes of Health estimates that the overall
cost for cancer in the year 2000 was $180.2 billion. This
included $60 billion for direct medical costs, $15 billion
resulting from lost productivity because of illness, and
$105.2 billion caused by lost productivity because of
death (5). Because health care costs represent a key economic and political issue, these analyses become increas-

ingly important. The charge is to find palliative care strategies that relieve suffering, increase personal independence, and prevent complications of the disease, and its treatment in the most cost-effective way.

It is important to recognize that terminal illness imposes substantial economic and other burdens on both patients and those who care for them. Among six randomly selected cities across the United States, 988 terminally ill patients and 893 caregivers were interviewed. Needs for transportation, nursing care, personal care, and economic costs were evaluated (21). The leading causes of terminal illness were cancer (51.8%), heart disease (18%), and chronic obstructive pulmonary disease (10.9%). The mean age was 66.5 years (range 22–109 years), and 59.4% were at least 65 years old. Among all patients, 50.2% experienced substantial pain, 17.5% were bedridden for more than 50% of the day, 70.9% had shortness of breath while walking one block or less, 35.5% had urinary or fecal incontinence, and 16.8% had depressive symptoms. In the previous 6 months, only 33.5% had not been hospitalized, 22.3% required a hospital stay that involved the intensive care unit, and 36.8% had undergone a surgical procedure. Overall, 35% of patients had substantial care needs that resulted in an expenditure of more than 10% of their household income on health care; 16% of families had to take out a loan, spend their savings, or obtain an additional job to cover medical costs. Patients with substantial needs were more likely to consider euthanasia and administering care significantly affected the life of over 35% of caregivers. Of importance, patients and caregivers assisted by physicians who listened to their needs had significantly fewer burdens of care. Only 28% of families felt burdened by the illness if the physician was involved in the needs of terminal care, as compared to 42% whose physicians did not listened to the needs of the family ($p = 0.005$).

In their medical training, physicians are not prepared to deliver excellent palliative care. Education in this area is deficient. On average, medical textbooks devote only 2% of their total pages to end-of-life care (22). A review of the 50 top-selling textbooks from multiple medical specialties found that only 24% of textbooks, and specifically only 38% of oncology textbooks, had helpful information in end-of-life care. Other barriers to effective pain treatment include lack of assessment, patient reluctance to report pain and to use analgesics, and physician reluctance to prescribe opioids (1,16,17,23–25).

Skills in pain management can be taught and can have striking results. In one clinic, for example, the mean pain score, using a numeric scale on which 10 is the worst

pain imaginable, was 5.2 among 45 inpatients referred for consultation to the pain service; 56% of patients had pain scores ≥ 5 and 20% had pain scores ≥ 8 on presentation (16). All patients had used opioids previously, and 41 were receiving opioids at the time of consultation. Within 24 hours using medical management, the mean pain intensity was 2.7 ($p < 0.05$).

Findings from 108 patients referred to an outpatient multidisciplinary bone metastases clinic affirm the need for a systematic approach to pain treatment. The median age of the population was 55 years, and 69% of the patients were less than 65 years old. The time since diagnosis of the primary tumor ranged from 2 weeks to 23 years; the median time since diagnosis was 22 months, and 30% of patients had been diagnosed within the past 6 months. Pain was the presenting symptom in 74% of patients at diagnosis. On average, pain was rated as moderate to severe in 79% and severe in 23% of patients; at its worst, pain was rated as severe by 78% and intolerable by 22% of the patients. Only 45% of patients experienced good relief from the prescribed analgesics, and 23% indicated that the prescribed analgesics were ineffective (17). Despite this, 21% of patients worked full-time and 6% were employed part-time; 13% were homemakers and only 16% considered themselves disabled.

Demographics of painful metastatic disease

The four most common cancers—lung, breast, prostate, and colorectal—have high rates of mestastases spread to bone and visceral structures (5,26–35). Occasionally, musculoskeletal pain is an indicator of an undiagnosed malignancy. Among 491 patients with new or recurrent complaints of bone pain and no known underlying malignancy, 4% of the entire group and 9% of patients ≥ 50 years old had definite evidence of metastases (28). Of the group that had any abnormality noted on bone scan, 20% had evidence of metastatic disease, and all of these occurred among patients ≥ 50 years old. Pain was localized in the back in 52%; 16% had pain in the hips or pelvis, 15% in the extremities, and diffuse pain was identified in 57% of cases. Malignancies were subsequently diagnosed in the lung (32%) and prostate (16%).

Because of an aging population and improved screening, the incidence of prostate cancer has increased dramatically since 1985. Prostate cancer represents the second leading cause of death from cancer among men (5,30,31,34,35). Pain develops in 75% of prostate cancer patients during the course of their disease (29–33). Radiographically detectable bone metastases develop in

20% of patients with stage A$_2$ (T$_{1b}$) and B (T$_2$) disease, 40% of patients with stage C (T$_3$), and 62% of patients with stage D$_1$ (T$_4$) disease presentations (32–35). In the 1970s, only 50% of cancers were confined to the prostate gland, and metastases were present in 30% of cases at diagnosis. In one population-based study where routine screening was not done and only palliative intervention was performed, there was a statistically significant relationship between the disease-specific death rate, stage of disease, and tumor differentiation (33). Of 719 new cases, 45% were diagnosed incidentally, only 31% had organ-confined disease, and 35% of patients had bone metastases at diagnosis (28,32). Symptoms at diagnosis included prostatism (42%), bone pain (12%), and fatigue (9%). The median age of diagnosis was 75 years. Age at diagnosis, however, did not influence disease-specific survival rates. Prostate cancer was the cause of death in 62% of patients, and the disease-specific survival rates at 1, 5, and 10 years were 80%, 38% and 17%, respectively (Table 16.1). Even now when patients are referred to a urologist for symptoms, only 70% of cases have disease confined to the prostate gland; pathologic confirmation of disease confined to the prostate gland occurs in only 50% of patients undergoing prostatectomy. With routine screening using digital rectal examination and prostate-specific antigen, 70% are pathologically confined to the gland.

The risk for the subsequent development of distant metastases is significantly lower when the primary tumor is controlled. Survival rates after an isolated recurrence of disease in prostate cancer are influenced by the initial stage of the disease and the disease-free interval from initial treatment (33,36,37). In more than 70% of cases of locally recurrent prostate cancer, radiation can control

symptoms that include hematuria, urinary outflow obstruction, ureteral obstruction, and lower extremity edema (36). With or without local recurrence, the survival rate is most compromised by the presence of distant metastases. The survival rates at 5 years and 10 years after pelvic recurrence alone equal 50% and 22%, respectively. With distant metastases, the survival rate at 5 years is 20% and less than 5% at 10 years (35–37).

Although any site can be involved, more than one half of palliative therapy is prescribed to relieve symptoms from bone metastases (38–40). In 1993, about 800,000 patients were estimated to have metastatic disease, and bone metastases are the most frequent symptomatic site (38). Reflecting the systemic spread of disease, metastatic involvement of a solitary bony site of or only the bones is rare and occurs in less than 10% of patients. Among hospitalized patients, severe pain was experienced by more than 50% of patients with bone metastases (4). One of the most important goals in the treatment of bone metastases is to relieve suffering and return the patient to independent function (38–40). The location of the metastasis, however, can influence the degree of pain relief achieved with palliative interventions. Metastatic involvement of weight-bearing bones and bones responsible for ambulation and activities of daily living are often less likely to respond completely to palliative interventions. Pain relief is achieved with radiation therapy in 73% of spine metastases, 88% of limb lesions, 67% of pelvic metastases, and 75% of metastases to other parts of the skeleton (14).

Prognostic factors influencing palliative therapies

Prognosis is influenced by the overall metastatic burden and the number and location of the sites involved by disease. When metastases are also found in the lung, liver, and/or central nervous system, the prognosis is especially poor. Quality-of-life measurements have been shown to predict survival and add to the prognostic information derived from the Karnofsky Performance Status (KPS) and extent of disease (41–45). Physical symptoms that include pain, dry mouth, constipation, change in taste, lack of appetite and energy, feeling bloated, nausea, vomiting, weight loss, and feeling drowsy or dizzy portend a poorer prognosis (41). Among 208 patients with terminal cancer, the overall median survival was 15 weeks. Shorter survival times were independently associated with the following factors: primary site (lung cancer vs. breast and gastrointestinal cancers), liver metastases, comorbidities, weight loss of greater than 8 kg in the previous 6 months, and clinical estimation of a less than

Table 16.1. *Disease-specific survival rates at 5 and 10 years based on stage of disease and tumor differentiation among 623 patients with prostate cancer treated only with palliative intent*

Stage of disease[a]	5 years	10 years
T$_{1a}$	84%	74%
T$_{1b}$	60%	29%
T$_2$	47%	12%
T>2	20%	4%
T1-2, Nx, M0	71%	42%
T>2, Nx, and/or M1	20%	4%
Tumor grade[a]		
G1	65%	42%
G2	42%	12%
G3	21%	8%

[a] $p < 0.0001$

2-month survival by the treating physician. Laboratory assessments including serum albumin levels of less than 3.5 dg/L, lymphocyte counts of less than 1×10^9/L, and lactate dehydrogenase levels of more than 618 U/L also were associated with a poor prognosis (42). After these independent factors were accounted for in the analysis, other factors, such as the performance status, symptoms other than nausea and vomiting, tumor burden, and socioeconomic characteristics, did not have an independent impact on prognosis.

Some of the uncertainties in predicting prognosis were addressed in a project, the Study to Understand Prognoses and Preferences for Outcomes and Risks of Treatments (SUPPORT). This study first retrospectively evaluated and developed a model to predict prognosis based on the outcomes of 4301 patients. The model was then prospectively tested on 4028 patients (45). Once developed, the model to predict prognosis was applied by physicians in 1757 cases to estimate the likelihood that a patient would survive 2 to 6 months. Among the cases analyzed were 406 patients with advanced colon cancer, 764 patients with lung cancer, and 594 patients with multiple-organ system failure with malignancy. Using this model, physician estimates were within 7.5% of the model estimates, the model was always within 3% of the actual survival, and the physicians were within 9% of the actual survival. Although physicians were generally accurate in predicting prognosis, patients with metastatic cancer generally overestimated their survival in this study. However, once patients acknowledged that they had a 10% chance of dying within 6 months, they were much more likely to prefer comfort care to life extension. Despite this and efforts to educate physicians and patients about palliative care options and about end-of-life issues, many patients in this recent study continued to receive ineffective cancer treatments, and they died in the hospital.

After bone metastases are diagnosed, the median survivals are 12 months for breast cancer, 6 months with prostate cancer, and 3 months with lung cancer. In breast cancer, the median survival rate is 48 months when metastases are confined to the skeletal system, but it decreases to only 9 months if visceral metastases are also present (26,27). In prostate cancer, the distribution of bone metastases has prognostic significance (37,46,47). The rate of survival is significantly longer when the metastases are restricted to the pelvis and lumbar spine, and among patients who respond to salvage hormone therapy (37,46). Any metastatic involvement outside the pelvis and lumbar spine results in lower rates of survival

irrespective of response to salvage hormone therapy. A bone scan index (BSI) has been formulated based on the weighted proportion of tumor involvement in individual bones. The BSI was then related to known prognostic factors and survival in patients with androgen-independent prostate cancer (47). In multiple-variable proportional hazards analyses, only the BSI, age, hemoglobin level, and lactate dehydrogenase level were associated with survival. Survival rates were 18.3 months for a BSI of <1.4%, 15.5 months for a BSI of 1.4 to 5.1%, and 8.1 months for a BSI > 5.1%.

The site of the primary disease and the presence of a solitary metastatic site are predictive of a more prolonged survival (41,48–51). However, the presence of bone metastases predicts progression of disease to other sites. Bone metastases also are the most common cause of cancer-related pain (5,26,27,33,37,46). The median length of survival is critical to evaluating response to, and determining the appropriate recommendations for, palliative therapy.

The economics of palliative care

Most of health care costs for cancer patients are incurred in the last months of life. For a number of reasons, only a small percentage of patients with extensive disease receive innovative therapies as part of a clinical trial. In palliative care, cancer is treated like a chronic disease. Cancer symptoms are controlled through the direct treatment of the symptoms (e.g., opioids for pain) and by treating the cause of the symptoms. As palliative therapy, antineoplastic treatment is administered to shrink the tumor as much as possible to reduce symptoms.

Cancer treatment often does not significantly improve survival and is given to maintain comfort. Physicians must communicate what can be reasonably achieved with palliative care to patients and families and begin discussions about end-of life issues. There is a growing recognition that physicians must be trained better in end-of-life issues, including hospice care. The physician must knowledgeably and compassionately discuss these issues with the patient and family. The physician needs to reassure the family that the patient will not be abandoned and that care will continue. Keeping the goals of palliative care in mind, palliative therapy needs to target symptomatic areas or areas at risk for incurring morbidity with progressive disease. Aggressive therapeutic approaches should be limited to patients with an extended prognosis, those whose goal is to maintain functional integrity (e.g., surgical stabilization of a pathologic fracture), and those participating in a clinical trial. Ineffective therapies that incur morbidity and cost and provide little or no palliative benefit should not be administered.

The roles of systemic agents, such as chemotherapy, hormonal therapy, bisphosphonates, and radiopharmaceuticals, alone or in combination with localized palliative radiation still have not been fully defined. Nonetheless, there has been an increased interest in the role of palliative chemotherapy. Palliative chemotherapy is defined as the administration of chemotherapy, such as gemcitabine, to relieve tumor-related symptoms when no or only a modest survival advantage is expected (52,53). These interventions can be helpful, but chemotherapy related side effects should be minimized.

Although palliation constitutes a large part of radiotherapeutic practice, radiation is generally underutilized in palliative care. At M.D. Anderson Cancer Center, about 25% of all radiation treatments were administered with palliative intent. This pattern of practice has been stable for more than 40 years (40). Consistent with radiotherapeutic practice in the United States, palliative radiotherapy for bone metastases was administered to approximately 25% of all radiotherapy patients in Sweden; however, this corresponded to only 10% of all Swedish cancer patients (54). With more than one half of patients with prostate, breast, and lung cancer developing symptoms of metastases, palliative radiation therapy is greatly underutilized.

Part of the difficulty in determining the best multidisciplinary approach relates to the various types of clinical problems that require palliative care. Even among patients with bone metastases, a number of different clinical problems, such as pathologic fracture and spinal cord compression, will require different multidisciplinary considerations. Issues that specifically need to be addressed are how therapies can be combined to achieve additive or synergistic effects, and how to address treatment of visceral and bone metastases. Like the approach used in curative therapies by combining chemotherapy and radiation, studies are needed that evaluate the combination of radiation (external beam radiation and radiopharmaceuticals) with chemotherapy, hormonal therapy, and bisphosphonates for the purposes of symptom control. Furthermore, there are significant cost–benefit issues to be considered. As an example, the Trans-Canada study that evaluated localized radiation alone or in combination with strontium-89 demonstrated that combined therapy was more cost effective (55–57).

Areas for specific consideration of cost–benefit in radiation therapy are single fraction radiation, radio-

pharmaceuticals, and systemic therapies. Although more abbreviated radiation courses may result in cost savings, the response to therapy must be critically analyzed to ensure that treatment efficacy is not compromised. These analyses must be specific to the type of primary tumor, location, and extent of the metastases, and prognosis. Ineffective palliative therapy given by any means is especially costly because of the continued need for analgesics, functional limitation, and need for systemic therapies and surgery because of unrelieved pain and disability (58,59).

Much controversy surrounds the cost-effective use of bisphosphonates for bone metastases. One study showed that the cost of pamidronate exceeded the cost savings from the prevented adverse events. The projected net cost to prevent an adverse skeletal-related event was $3940 with chemotherapy and $9390 with hormonal therapy (60). The cost per unit benefit was $108,200 with chemotherapy and $305,300 with hormonal therapy per quality-adjusted year. A cost analysis study in Canada showed similar findings. Over a 12-month time frame, the total costs in the pamidronate arm were 44% higher than in the placebo arm (61). Without surgical intervention, pamidronate increased costs by $31,600 per quality adjusted life year. When the cost of surgical intervention, required by 6% of the study group, was included the use of pamidronate increased costs by $13,300 per quality-adjusted life year. Based on the number of breast cancer patients that would meet clinical indications to receive pamidronate, the added cost for bisphosphonates would exceed $10 million (Canadian) per year in Ontario. Studies are clearly needed to optimize the use of bisphosphonates in combination with other therapeutic modalities to improve the overall cost profile.

Radiotherapy is highly cost effective when compared to analgesic therapy. The costs for radiotherapy were evaluated among 66 patients who underwent palliative radiation totaling 30 Gy in 10 fractions (72%) or 20 Gy in 5 fractions. Pain scores decreased about 4 points (0 to 10 scale) after radiotherapy, from a median level of 5.58 before radiation to 1.55 after treatment (62). Likewise, incident pain (pain with movement) decreased 5 points, from 7.32 before treatment to 1.94 after treatment. The estimated cost of radiotherapy ranged from $1200 to $2500 per patient. With durable pain relief for 9 months, the estimated cost of analgesics over the same time period would have totaled $9000 to $36,000. In this study, a brief course of radiation therapy proved to significantly reduce pain and was cost effective when compared with the continued need for analgesics. This is a particularly important consideration for the treatment of hospice patients.

In other trials, bisphosphonates were used to overcome the limitations of response with systemic therapy and either delayed or decreased the number of patients referred for palliative radiation. In these studies, radiation therapy was given only in cases of symptomatic progressive disease while bisphosphonates and systemic therapy were being administered. Although statistically significant improvements were observed, fewer than one half the original cohort of breast cancer patients completed the first year of the trial and fewer than one third continued the randomized therapy for 2 years (63–71). The reason for discontinuing therapy included adverse events, poor response to therapy, or refusal to continue treatment in nearly one half of patients (65,66). Almost one half of these patients developed a skeletal event on bisphosphonates. Although statistical benefit was shown, research is needed to determine the optimal schedule of administration for bisphosphonates and how they can best be combined with other modalities in light of the issues related to cost effectiveness (70,72).

Symptom relief in locally advanced or metastatic disease

Symptoms must be controlled whether treatment is administered with curative or palliative intent, and radiation oncologists must be knowledgeable in the management of cancer-related pain. Control of pain facilitates simulation and administration of palliative therapy. Furthermore, in the United States, the Joint Commission on Accreditation of Healthcare Organizations (JCAHO) issued a new set of standards for the assessment and management of pain that went into effect January 1, 2001. These standards indicate that all patients have the right to appropriate assessment and management of pain, and that patients be taught that pain management is a part of treatment.

These new standards of care will significantly affect the practice of medicine. In all oncologic specialties, cancer-related pain continues to be inadequately treated. Even though palliation represents a significant proportion of radiotherapeutic practice, many radiation oncologists do not have an adequate base of knowledge about analgesic therapy. In a survey of Radiation Therapy Oncology Group (RTOG) physicians, 83% believed that the majority of cancer patients with pain were undermedicated. In their practice, 40% reported that pain management was of poor or fair quality. Opioid analgesics would not be used

by 23% until the patient had an estimated survival of 6 months or less. Barriers to adequate pain management included poor pain assessment (77%), patient reluctance to report pain (60%), patient reluctance to take analgesics (72%), and physician reluctance to prescribe opioids (41%). For 72% of the RTOG physicians, the prescription of opioid analgesics was prompted by the failure to respond to palliative radiotherapy (43). The results proved not to be substantially different than the responses to the same survey among Eastern Cooperative Oncology Group physicians 7 years earlier (25) before the publication of the Agency for Health Care Policy and Research Guidelines on Cancer Pain Management (2,3).

Clinical considerations in palliative radiotherapy

Curative treatment attempts to render the patient disease-free. Curative therapy can be applied to either primary or metastatic disease. The prognosis of a patient who is rendered disease-free after resection of a single liver metastasis from rectal cancer is better than a patient who has an extensive, inoperable lung cancer who does not have metastatic disease.

Unlike curative therapy, in which a high total dose of radiation is administered to eradicate tumor, a hypofractionated schedule is generally prescribed in palliative radiation. Hypofractionated radiation schedules for palliative therapy range from 2.5 Gy per fraction administered over 3 weeks for a total dose of 35 Gy, 20 Gy in 1 week, to a single 4 to 8 Gy dose of radiation. Most frequently in the United States, 30 Gy is administered in 10 fractions over 2 weeks (12,38,39,73–76). The dose fractionation schedule used depends on prognosis, volume, and site to be irradiated.

Treatment with palliative intent is intended to control the symptoms of disease when the disease cannot be eradicated. Effective antineoplastic therapy provides the most palliative benefit for locally advanced or metastatic cancer in any organ. Radiation can be used alone or in combination with other antineoplastic therapies. The symptoms most commonly relieved by radiation are pain, bleeding, and obstruction. The palliative interventions recommended depend on the patient's clinical status, burden of disease, and location of the symptomatic site. For either locally advanced or metastatic disease, these factors are indexed to the relative effectiveness, durability, and morbidity of each palliative intervention. Prognosis represents the single most important factor in deciding palliative therapy.

A number of clinical, prognostic, and therapeutic factors must be considered to determine the optimal treatment regimen for a course of palliative radiotherapy. The clinical status is accounted for in the treatment setup and in the number of treatments prescribed. The radiation dose-fractionation schedule and technique also should consider the integration of other therapies. Many radiotherapeutic options exist for tumors that cause localized symptoms. Brachytherapy and application of conformal and intensity modulated radiation therapy can better localize radiation dose and reduce side effects, especially in a previously irradiated area (12,13,15,36,39,75,77–79).

Issues regarding reirradiation are especially important in palliative therapy. Experimental data suggest that acute responding tissues recover radiation injury in a few months and can tolerate another full course of radiation therapy. However, there is considerable variability in recovery from radiation among late-reacting tissues (78). The heart, bladder, and kidney do not exhibit any recovery of any late radiation effects; but the skin, mucosa, lung, and spinal cord do recover subclinical radiation injury. This recovery depends on the organ irradiated, the size of the initial dose of radiation, and the interval between doses of radiation. Clinical correlates exist and limited toxicities have generally been reported with reirradiation (79).

The symptomatic site becomes more important to the palliative approach than whether it results from locally advanced or metastatic tumor. In general, radiation portals are used to palliate bronchial obstruction resulting from a primary lung cancer, recurrent breast cancer, or metastatic melanoma. The number of radiation fractions prescribed for treatment with palliative intent depends more on prognosis than on primary histology. Common sites palliated by radiation, either alone or in combination with other treatments, include tumor involvement of the lung, pelvis, skin and subcutaneous tissues, brain, and bone. Symptoms resulting from cancer in these sites include pain, bleeding, visceral obstruction, and lymphatic obstruction.

The limited radiation tolerance of the normal tissues, such as the spinal cord, that are adjacent to a bone metastasis makes it impossible to administer a large enough dose of radiation to eradicate a measurable volume of tumor. Palliative radiation should result in sufficient tumor regression of critical structures to relieve symptoms for the duration of the patient's life. Symptoms that recur after palliative radiation most commonly result from localized regrowth of tumor. Control of cancer-related pain with the use of analgesics is imperative to allow comfort during and while awaiting response to therapeutic interventions. Pain represents a sensitive

measure of disease activity. Close follow-up monitoring should be done after any palliative therapeutic intervention to ensure control of cancer and treatment-related pain, and to initiate diagnostic studies to identify progressive or recurrent disease.

Bone metastases

Bone metastases in prostate and breast cancers involve the axial skeleton more than 80% of the time because of the predilection of these tumors to involve the red marrow. Metastatic invasion of the bone cortex rarely happens without red marrow involvement (80–84). For this reason, the spine, pelvis, and ribs are generally involved before metastases become evident in the skull, femurs, humeri, scapulae, and sternum. The mechanisms involved in the metastatic spread of cancer to the bone are complex. The predilection of specific types of tumors, such as prostate cancer, that metastasize to bone is not well understood.

Bone is unique because it is continuously remodeled by local and systemic growth factors. The process involved in bone remodeling includes an increase in osteoclast activity followed by an increased attraction and proliferation of osteoblast precursors, which mature and lay down new bone (80–88). Tumors can release osteoclastic stimulatory factors either locally or systemically, including parathyroid hormone-related protein, transforming growth factor-alpha, transforming growth factor-beta, prostaglandins, and cytokines (88). Tumors can also indirectly stimulate bone loss through the activation of immune mechanisms that release cytokines, including tumor necrosis factor and interleukin-1. Metastases to bone result from a synergistic relationship between the cancer cell and the bone that results in increased bone resorption resulting from release of mediators from the cancer cells or leukocytes. Factors released during bone resorption promote growth of the cancer through activation of proliferation associated oncogenes.

The relationship between bone invasion and bone pain is unknown. Pain may result from the stimulation of nerve endings from the release of factors such as prostaglandins, bradykinin, histamine, or substance P in areas of bone involvement (84). Mass effect from stretching of the periosteum, pathologic fracture, or direct tumor growth into adjacent nerves and tissues may be the mechanism for pain in larger metastatic deposits.

Multidisciplinary evaluation of patients with metastatic disease to the bone allows comprehensive management of the associated symptoms, determines the risk for pathological fracture, and helps coordinate administration of a wide range of available antineoplastic therapies (9,17,53,89–91). Bone scintigrams are the most sensitive and specific method of detecting bone metastases, but magnetic resonance imaging (MRI) is the best available technique for evaluating the bone marrow, neoplastic invasion of the vertebrae, the central nervous system, and peripheral nerves (92–95). Bone or other metastases rarely fail to be detected when radiographic diagnosis is pursued. When radiographic confirmation of malignancy is equivocal, bone biopsy should be considered (80,81,96).

Bone metastases can be treated with localized and/or systemic therapies. Because radiation provides treatment only to a localized symptomatic site of disease, it is frequently used in coordination with systemic therapies such as chemotherapy, hormonal therapy, and bisphosphonates. Radiopharmaceuticals are another systemic option that treats diffuse symptomatic bone metastases (55,56,97–108). Because the radiation is deposited directly at the involved area in the bone, radiopharmaceuticals such as strontium-89 can also be used to treat bone metastases when symptoms recur in a previously irradiated site. Radiopharmaceuticals can also act as an adjuvant to localized external beam irradiation and reduce the development of other symptomatic sites of disease.

There are two major sets of experience with palliative radiation for bone metastases. The RTOG conducted a prospective trial that included a variety of treatment schedules. To account for prognosis, patients were stratified on the basis of whether they had a solitary or multiple sites of bony metastases. The initial analysis of the study concluded that low-dose, short-course treatment schedules were as effective as high-dose protracted treatment programs (109). For solitary bone metastases, there was no difference in the relief of pain when 20 Gy using 4 Gy fractions was compared to 40.5 Gy delivered as 2.7 Gy per fraction (Table 16.2). Relapse of pain occurred in 57% of patients at a median of 15 weeks after completion of therapy for each dose level. In patients with multiple bone metastases, the following dose schedules were compared: 30 Gy at 3 Gy per fraction, 15 Gy given as 3 Gy per fraction, 20 Gy using 4 Gy per fraction, and 25 Gy using 5 Gy per fraction. No difference was identified in the rates of pain relief between these treatment schedules. Partial relief of pain was achieved in 83%, and complete relief occurred in 53% of the patients studied. More than 50% of these patients developed recurrent pain, the fracture rate equaled 8%, and the median duration of pain control

Table 16.2. *Percentage of patients who responded to radiation relative to time, designated in weeks after completion of radiation therapy*

Total dose (Gy)	Dose per fraction (Gy)	Tumor dose at 2 Gy/fx	Weeks post XRT			
			< 2	2–4	4–12	12–20
Solitary mets						
40.5	2.7	42.9	7%	29%	53%	77%
20.0	4	23.3	16%	50%	66%	82%
Multiple mets						
30.0	3	32.5	19%	48%	73%	84%
15.0	3	16.2	34%	70%	84%	93%
20.0	4	23.3	28%	53%	75%	88%
25.0	5	31.25	22%	41%	72%	80%

This prospective trial, conducted by the RTOG, randomized radiation dose and number of fractions and stratified the randomization on the basis of solitary or multiple bone metastases (79,80). Also listed is the radiobiological equivalent dose if administered at 2 Gy per fraction.

was 12 weeks for all the radiation schedules used for multiple bony metastases. Prognostic factors for response included the initial pain score and site of the primary.

In a reanalysis of the data, a different definition for complete pain relief was used and excluded the continued administration of analgesics. By using this definition, the relief of pain was significantly related to the number of fractions and the total dose of radiation that was administered (110). Complete relief of pain was achieved in 55% of patients with solitary bone metastases who received 40.5 Gy at 2.7 Gy per fraction as compared to 37% of patients who received a total dose of 20 Gy given as 4 Gy per fraction (Table 16.3). A similar relationship was observed in the reanalysis of patients who had multiple bone metastases. Complete relief of pain was achieved in 46% of patients who received 30 Gy at 3 Gy per fraction versus 28% of patients treated to 25 Gy using 5 Gy fractions. In most cases, the interval to response was 4 weeks for both complete and minimal relief of symptoms.

Three important issues are identified from the RTOG experience. First, results of the reanalysis demonstrate the importance of defining what represents a response to therapy. Second, this revised definition of response showed that the total radiation dose did influence the degree that pain was relieved (109,110). The response rates and the radiobiologically equivalent doses are listed from the reanalysis in Table 16.2 for each of the treat-

Table 16.3. *Dose-response evaluation from the reanalysis of the RTOG Bone Metastases Protocol (79)*

	Dose/fx (Gy)	Total dose (Gy)	Tumor dose at 2 Gy/fx	CR	*p* value
Solitary bone mets	2.7	40.5	42.9	55%	*p* < 0.0003
	4.0	20.0	23.3	37%	
Multiple bone mets	3.0	30.0	32.5	46%	*p* < 0.0003
	3.0	15.0	16.2	36%	
	4.0	20.0	23.3	40%	
	5.0	25.0	31.25	28%	

Listed are the dose per fraction (dose/fx), total radiation dose, the radiobiological equivalent dose if administered at 2 Gy/fx, the complete response rate (CR) using the definition that excludes the use of analgesics and that accounts for retreatment.

ment schedules used. Showing that higher radiation doses result in higher rates of pain relief, these results also correspond well to the results in another study with breast, prostate, and lung cancer patients (Table 16.4). Patients treated with total doses of 40 Gy or more had a 75% rate of complete pain relief versus a 62% rate of complete pain relief for patients treated with total doses of less than 40 Gy (14). Third, the RTOG experience identified the amount of time that was needed to experience relief of pain after radiation for bone metastases (Table 16.4). It is important to note that only half the patients who were going to respond had relief of symptoms at 2 to 4 weeks after radiation (109,110). This underscores the need for continued analgesic support after completing radiation. Consistently, it took 12 to 20 weeks after radiation to accomplish the maximal level of relief. That period may reflect the time needed for reossification. Radiographic evidence of recalcification is observed early in about one fourth of cases, and in 70%, recalcification is seen within 6 months of completing radiation and other palliative therapies (84–87). Therefore, determining the time to response and defining the parameters of response are critical to an evaluation of

Table 16.4. *Rate of complete response (CR) after treatment of bone metastases with conventional fractionation (2 Gy per fraction)*

	CR	< 40 Gy	≥ 40 Gy
Breast	66%	41%	71%
Prostate	73%	62%	75%
Lung	57%	44%	63%

The overall CR rate and CR rate stratified to total radiation dose administered are presented (10).

outcome. The total dose of radiation may also be a significant factor for complete pain relief.

Similar issues were observed when pretreatment pain characteristics were used to determine the efficacy of palliative radiation. Among patients who had a life expectancy of only a few months, fewer than 25% of patients had a complete response to palliative radiation. In this case, a complete response was defined as becoming pain-free within 28 days after the start of treatment with stable analgesic consumption. A partial response was achieved in 35% of patients, and 42% had no response to palliative radiation. Pretreatment evidence of neuropathic pain was the only significant prognostic or clinical variable that predicted for failure to respond to palliative radiation; severe neuropathic symptoms were present in 33% of patients treated (48,111–113).

A variety of radiation schedules have been evaluated in palliative therapy for bone metastases. One trial compared 30 Gy in 10 fractions to 15 Gy in 3 fractions given as 2 fractions per week among 217 breast cancer patients. No difference was observed in pain scores, analgesic use, treatment side effects, or survival. At 12-month follow-up evaluation, about 70% had little to no limitation in activity (114). Consistent with other reports, survival was 45% at 3 months, 33% at 6 months, and only 20% at 1 year.

Response of the cancer to treatment may be the most important prognostic factor in the specific management of bone metastases. A prospective randomized trial compared 30 Gy given as 2 Gy fractions to 20 Gy with 4 Gy fractions among 100 patients with a median follow-up time of 12 months. The primary tumor was located in the breast (43%), lung (24%), and prostate (14%). The pelvis (31%), vertebrae (30%), and ribs (20%) were the most common sites treated. These characteristics were equally distributed between the study groups. The biologically effective dose (BED) was 28 Gy_{10} and 36 Gy_{10} for the treatment arms. No significant differences were observed in the frequency, duration of pain relief, mobility, or pathological fractures based on the radiation schedule (115). The mean interval from the completion of radiation to pain relief was approximately 10 days in both groups. The mean duration of pain relief was 245 days in each group, and it lasted up to 84% of the remaining survival time. Of importance, responders had a highly significant ($p < 0.0001$) improvement in survival. Other factors that affected overall survival were primary tumor site ($p < 0.0001$), performance status ($p < 0.0001$), age ($p < 0.03$), and BED ($p < 0.04$).

The importance of pain control on survival was unexpectedly seen in a trial comparing best medical management of pain with placement of an intrathecal catheter for pain control in locally advanced and recurrent cancer. The majority of patients in the trial had lung or ovarian cancer (116). Corresponding with improvements in pain control, a highly significant survival benefit was observed among patients who underwent intrathecal catheter placement. It is possible that survival may be linked to improved mobility afforded by pain control. It is unknown whether pain, through its effects on sleep and other functions, also affects cytokine release and other immunologic parameters that may ultimately affect survival. This is an area of active research.

It is unknown if a dose-response relationship actually exists. Published results do not control for histology, type (blastic or lytic), or location of the metastases, or the type of pain (neuropathic, mechanical, somatic). Many of the older reports do not include validated pain surveys or account for analgesic use. Definition and duration of response are variable (117,118). It is unclear how many patients statistically assigned to a high-dose arm completed therapy, and how many assigned to the low-dose arm actually received a high-dose of radiation as a result of retreatment. Three reports, Gillick and Goldberg (119), Blitzer (110), and Jeremic et al. (120), suggest a dose-response relationship for bone metastases.

The RTOG study (109,110) demonstrated that the level of pain also correlated with prognosis among patients with multiple bone metastases. This survival difference may be an important observation because unrelieved pain and the resultant sequelae of immobility may contribute to mortality as well as morbidity (18,19,37,41,49,111,116). Larger data sets that include prognostic factors in multivariate analysis are required to determine the effect of pain and response to therapy on quality of life and survival outcomes.

Further research may determine that the radiation dose schedules should be specific to the primary tumor, site of metastases, and type of pain to maximize response. No matter which radiation schedule is used, retreatment should be considered at the first sign of progressive symptoms to achieve the maximum and most durable level of palliation. Pain management should be optimized given intriguing reports of its relationship to survival. Future research should target level of pain relief and cost effectiveness. Although equal rates of response are observed between single and multiple fractions of radiation, future analyses should evaluate survival and durability of response. Criteria need to be established to determine which clinical presentation would best benefit from single or multifraction therapy (121–124). Most

important, these analyses should assess the efficacy and costs of treating symptoms that recur in an irradiated field.

Single fraction radiation

Single fraction radiation has been applied extensively in Europe and is the subject of an RTOG trial. Because of convenience, cost effectiveness, and the ability to reirradiate, it is of significant interest in palliative care; however, many in the United States remain concerned about efficacy. The benefit of lesser cost and greater convenience with a shorter course of radiation may be lost through the continued need for analgesics. For example, a cost-effectiveness comparison was conducted among 1171 patients who were randomized to receive either 8 Gy in 1 fraction or 24 Gy × 6 fractions. The two treatment arms were equivalent in terms of palliation, including analgesic use (125). However, 25% of the 8 Gy arm required retreatment as compared to 7% in the 24 Gy multifraction arm. A cost analysis showed that the 8 Gy arm cost $1734 (Euro) as compared to $2305 (Euro) for the multifraction arm, representing a 25% cost difference. However, when the costs of retreatment were included in the analysis, this cost difference was reduced to only 8%, but an economic advantage continued to exist because of the need for decreased radiotherapy capacity.

Radiobiologically, a single 8 Gy fraction would give the same side effects to late reacting tissues as if 18 Gy were given over nine treatments at 2 Gy per fraction (126). The radiobiologically equivalent dose to the tumor for a single 8 Gy fraction would be 12 Gy if 2 Gy fractions were used. The most common dose fractionation schedule used for palliative radiation in the United States is 30 Gy over 10 fractions. Radiobiologically, this is equivalent to 36 Gy at 2 Gy per fraction for late-reacting tissues and 32.5 Gy to the tumor.

When a single dose of radiation was compared to a radiation schedule in a number of studies with multiple radiation fractions, no difference was reported in either how quickly symptoms resolved or the duration of pain relief (115,125,127–130). In each case, symptom relief lasted 3 months in 70% of patients, 6 months in 37%, and 12 months in 20% of cases. As in the RTOG study, in this study about 69% of patients responded at 4 weeks, and response rates plateaued, totaling 80%, at 8 weeks (109,110,125,127,130–133). Complete response rates after a single 8 Gy fraction are 15% at 2 weeks, 23% at 4 weeks, 28% at 8 weeks, and 39% at 12 weeks postradiation.

The Bone Pain Trial Working Party (128) conducted a trial among 765 patients with skeletal metastases comparing a single 8 Gy fraction to either 20 Gy/5 fractions or 30 Gy/10 fractions. Pain severity and analgesic requirements were recorded before treatment, 2 weeks after treatment, and at 1-, 2-, 3-, 4-, 5-, 6-, 8-, 10-, and 12-month follow-up evaluation. Pain relief was the primary endpoint. In both groups, pain management with analgesics before radiotherapy was inadequate. Consistent with other data, 70% of patients presented to radiation therapy with moderate to severe pain despite the fact that 70% were prescribed opioid analgesics. No difference was identified in the time to first improvement in pain, time to complete pain relief, time to pain recurrence, risk for spinal cord compression or pathological fracture, nausea/vomiting, or in analgesic requirements between the two schedules of radiation. In both groups, 57% experienced a complete response to radiation. At 6- and 12-month in follow-up evaluation, however, about 55% of patients still required opioid analgesics. Retreatment, however, was twice as common in the 8 Gy arm (23% vs. 10%), although this did not result in overall differences in pain relief. The authors believed that physicians were more likely to administer retreatment after a single 8 Gy course of radiation than after a multiple fraction course of therapy.

Reirradiation for persistent or recurrent pain is often precluded when higher radiation doses are administered. Because the radiobiological dose is relatively low when a single fraction of radiation is administered, reirradiation is generally possible (15,126,132). Reirradiation was necessary, however, in 25% of patients who received a single 8 Gy radiation fraction, but all of these patients were reported to respond to the second dose of radiation. When a single fraction of 4 Gy was compared to a single 8 Gy fraction, the rate of response was slightly lower and fewer acute radiation reactions were noted, but a greater proportion of patients required reirradiation (133). With reirradiation, the overall rate of response was equivalent for 8 Gy and 4 Gy fractions.

Reirradiation with a single 4 Gy fraction also yields a 74% response rate, including a 31% complete response rate (132). Pain relief was also achieved in 46% of patients who did not initially respond to a single 4 or 8 Gy fraction. Patients who had a previous complete response to therapy were more likely to respond to reirradiation when compared to the group that previously experienced a partial response (85% vs. 67%).

A shorter radiation schedule, such as a single fraction, is advantageous for patients with poor prognostic factors. First, it is easier for patients with a poor performance sta-

tus to complete therapy. Second, response rates are equal for single and multifraction therapy at 3 months because median survival is less than 6 months among patients with poor prognostic factors (12,37–39,74,75,113,123,125, 127–130,133). The option of retreatment after a single fraction of radiation may also provide an advantage among patients with good prognostic factors as a means to periodically reduce tumor burden and control symptoms in noncritical anatomic sites. Higher radiation doses that provide more durable pain relief are considered warranted for patients with good prognostic factors who require treatment over the spine and other critical sites (134–140).

The projected length of survival is the critical issue to determine the optimal radiation dose and schedule for palliative radiation. In one study, only 12 of 245 patients were alive at the time of analysis, with approximately 50% alive at 6 months, 25% at 1 year, 8% at 2 years, and 3% at 3 years after palliative radiation. For patients with breast cancer, the survival rates at these time points after palliative radiation were 60%, 44%, 20%, and 7%, respectively. For prostate cancer, the survival rates were 60% at 6 months, 24% at 1 year, and no patients survived 2 years (141). In the RTOG trial, the median survival for solitary bone metastases was 36 weeks, and median survival for the group with multiple bone metastases was 24 weeks (109,110).

It may not matter that the response to radiation therapy is optimized either through a more protracted course, if a dose-response relationship exists, or through retreatment (62). Significant consideration must be given to patient accessibility, convenience, and cost effectiveness. It is clear that a durable and significant response from radiation, not the schedule of administration, is the key issue in palliative radiation.

Pathologic fracture

The most significant morbidity of bone metastases relates to pathological fracture and spinal cord compression. Pain that persists or that recurs after palliative radiation should be evaluated to exclude progression of disease, possible extension of disease outside the radiation portal that results in referred pain, and bone fracture. Reduced cortical strength can result in compression, stress, fractures, or microfractures. Plain radiographs have a 91% concordance rate in detecting posttreatment disease progression and fractures in comparison to the 57% specificity rate of bone scans performed after radiotherapy (86). Pathologic fractures occur in 8% to 30% of patients with bone metastases (90,142–146). Proximal long bones are more commonly involved than distal bones. Consequently, 50% of pathologic fractures occur in the femur, and 15% occur in the humerus (Fig. 16.1). The femoral neck and head are the most frequent locations for pathological fracture because of the propensity for metastases to involve proximal bones and the stress of weight placed on this part of the femur. More than 80% of pathologic fractures occur in breast (50%), kidney, lung, and thyroid cancers.

Approximately 10% to 30% of metastatic lesions in long bones develop a pathologic fracture that will require surgical intervention. Patients with pathologic fracture resulting from bone metastases have clinical outcomes after surgical repair that are comparable to patients sustaining a traumatic fracture (90,143,144). Prognosis is generally poor if hypercalcemia is present and if parenteral opioids are required to control pain from other

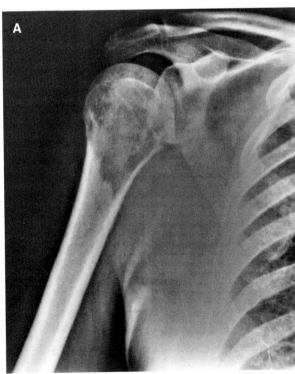

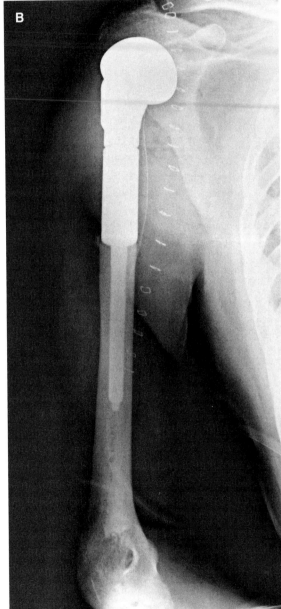

Fig. 16.1. (A) An extensive lytic lesion in the proximal humerus. (B) Prophylactic internal fixation was performed to prevent pathological fracture. This patient, who complained primarily of pain in the hip, would have been placed on crutches to reduce stress on the involved femur. A bone scan and x-ray study, obtained to exclude other sites of metastatic involvement, identified this lesion in the humerus. The humerus would have certainly fractured if all the patient's weight had been displaced to the upper extremities with the use of crutches.

sites of bone metastases; in these cases, the decision for surgical intervention should be based on of the severity of, and the symptoms associated with the fracture (143). As shown in Fig. 16.2, postoperative radiation is often given after surgical fixation of a pathologic fracture to reduce risk of progressive disease in the bone that could result in instability of the internal fixation (90).

Treatment of pathologic fracture or impending fracture depends on the bone involved and the clinical status of the patient. Indications for surgical intervention of pathologic fracture or impending fracture include these factors: 1) an expected survival of more than 6 weeks, 2) an ability to accomplish internal stability of the fracture site, 3) no co-existent medical conditions that preclude early mobilization, 4) metastases involving weight-bearing bones, 5) and lytic lesions more than 2 to 3 cm in size or metastases that destroy more than 50% of the cortex (142–146). It is unclear whether osteolytic metastases are more likely to fracture than osteoblastic lesions because

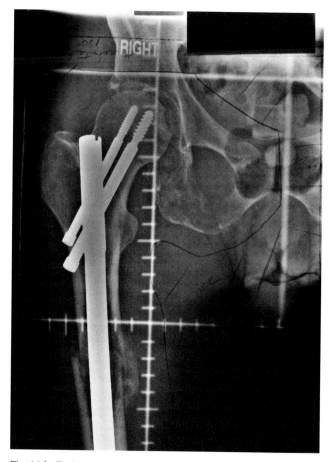

Fig. 16.2. Typical radiation portal after fixation of a pathologic fracture of the femur. Radiation is administered to treat residual disease around the internal fixation device, pubis, and acetabulum.

osteoblastic lesions, by definition, have an osteolytic component so that new bone can be formed.

Spinal cord compression

The vertebral column is involved by metastatic tumor in 40% of patients who die of cancer. Approximately 70% of vertebral metastases involve the thoracic spine, 20% the lumbosacral region, and 10% the cervical spine. The time from the original diagnosis of cancer to the development of metastatic spinal disease averages 30 months. Median survival among patients with spinal cord compression is 7 months, with a 36% probability for a 1-year survival. After epidural spinal cord compression is diagnosed, the mean survival time is 14 months for breast cancer, 12 months for prostate cancer, 6 months for malignant melanoma, and 3 months for lung cancer (5,134,142); the overall median survival time is 5 months.

Pain is the initial symptom in approximately 90% of patients with spinal cord compression. Paraparesis or paraplegia occurs in more than 60% of patients, sensory loss is noted in 70% to 80%, and bladder and/or bowel disturbances are noted in 14%–77% of patients (75,91, 147–151). The extent of the epidural mass influences prognosis because a complete spinal block results in greater residual neurologic impairment than a partial block.

Weakness can signal the rapid progression of symptoms, and 30% of patients with weakness become paraplegic within 1 week. Rapid development of weakness, defined as occurring in less than 2 months, most commonly occurs in lung cancer; breast cancer and prostate cancer can progress more slowly. Neurological deficits can develop within a few hours in up to 20% of patients with spinal cord compression (91,134,137,139,147,148,151). The severity of weakness at presentation is the most significant factor for recovery of function. Ninety percent of patients who are ambulatory at presentation will be ambulatory after treatment. Only 13% of paraplegic patients will regain function, particularly if paraplegia is present for more than 24 hours before the initiation of therapy. More than 30% of patients who develop spinal cord compression are alive 1 year later, and 50% of these patients will remain ambulatory with appropriate therapy.

Pain can be present for months to days before neurological dysfunction evolves. Unlike pain caused by degenerative joint disease, which primarily occurs in the low cervical and low lumbar regions, pain resulting from epidural spinal cord compression can occur anywhere in the spinal axis, and is aggravated by recumbency. Epidural metastases are most common in the thoracic spine, followed by the lumbar and then cervical regions. Lung and breast cancers tend to metastasize more commonly to the thoracic spine, and colon and pelvis tumors have a predilection for the lumbosacral region (91).

Any cancer patient with back pain, especially with known metastatic involvement of the vertebral bodies, should be suspected as having spinal cord compression. The risk of spinal cord compression exceeds 60% among patients with back pain and plain film evidence of vertebral collapse resulting from metastatic cancer (91,134,147, 149–153,188). Epidural spinal cord disease is documented in 17% of asymptomatic patients who have an abnormal bone scan but normal plain films; 47% of asymptomatic patients with vertebral metastases noted on both bone scan and plain film will also have associated epidural disease (134). Symptomatic patients with a normal vertebral contour and osteoblastic changes on plain film and bone scan should also be evaluated for spinal cord compression (Fig. 16.3).

Radiographic determination of the involved spinal levels is critical to radiation treatment planning. Clinical determination of the location of epidural spinal cord compression in 33% of cases is incorrect (134–136,154). Plain film radiographs will show involvement of more than one spinal level in about one third of patients. Destruction of the pedicles is the most common finding on plain radiographs that identifies spine metastases. In contrast, computed tomography (CT) shows that the initial anatomic location of metastases is in the posterior portion of the vertebral body and that destruction of the pedicles occurs only in combination with involvement of the vertebral body (Fig. 16.4) (155). Osteoblastic bony expansion, commonly seen in both prostate and breast cancers, can result in spinal cord compromise as well as osteolytic vertebral compression fractures (150).

If the results of MRI, tomographic studies, and surgical findings are included, more than 85% of patients will have multiple sites of vertebral involvement (135,136,139,156,174). Multiple sites of epidural involvement are also common; 10% to 38% of epidural metastases involve multiple non-contiguous levels (91). A review of 337 patients evaluated between 1985 and 1993 studied the benefit of complete spinal imaging. When the entire spine was radiographically evaluated, 32% of patients had multiple sites of epidural involvement; when imaging was limited to the symptomatic site, only 18% of cases detected multiple areas of epidural tumor spread (156). Although failure to image the cervical spine would have missed only 1% of epidural tumor deposits, this rate increased to 21% if either the thoracic

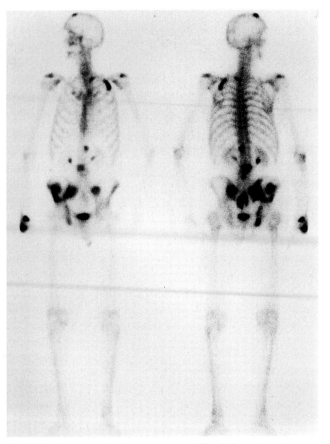

Fig. 16.3. Bone scan that demonstrates multifocal disease involvement. Metastatic involvement in weight-bearing areas such as the pelvis and lower lumbar area significantly affects mobility.

or lumbar regions were not fully imaged. The presence of multiple epidural tumor deposits was an independent prognostic factor for poorer survival. Secondary epidural tumor deposits were included 93% of the time within the radiation portals.

Treatment of spinal cord compression includes corticosteriods, radiotherapy, and/or neurosurgical intervention. Radiotherapy is the treatment of choice for most cases of spinal cord compression; depending on the circumstances, this can be a radiotherapeutic emergency (91,151) (Fig. 16.5). Functional outcome is dependent on the clinical findings at the time radiation is administered. The outcomes of 166 patients who presented to a cancer center with spinal cord compression confirmed on MRI were reviewed relative to performance and neurological status. More than 50% of patients had prostate or breast cancer; 13% had lung cancer. The thoracic spine was most commonly involved, either alone (57%) or with lesions in the lumbar region (11%). Multiple levels of epidural involvement were documented in 28% of patients.

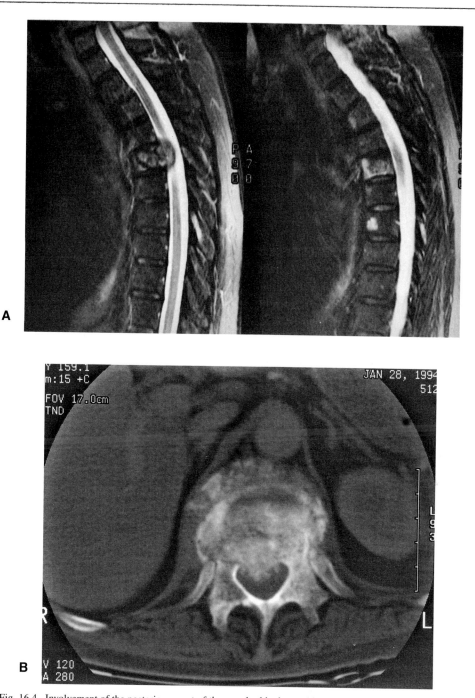

Fig. 16.4. Involvement of the posterior aspect of the vertebral body resulting in partial spinal cord compression.

Symptoms included back pain in 122 patients, limb weakness in 128 patients, sensory loss in 90 patients, and sphincter disturbance in 53 patients; more than 50% of the group had moderate to major neurological disturbances. Radiotherapy was given to 92% of patients. Median survival from confirmation of spinal cord compression was 82 days (range 1–1349 days). The performance status improved in 16%, and the neurological status improved in only 20% of cases; 55% to 60% of patients remained the same and 25% were worse after treatment (151). Death in the hospital occurred in 32% of patients. Of the remaining 68%, patients returned home in most of the cases, with only 11% sent to another hospital, 4% to a rehabilitation center, and 5% to a hospice. The pretreatment performance and neurological status were highly predictive of outcome. Because of continued disability and pain after

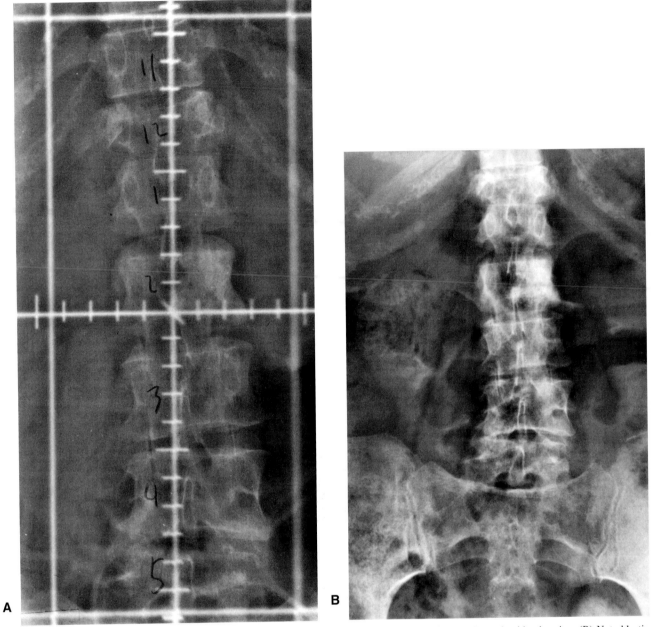

Fig. 16.5. (A) A typical radiation portal to treat multifocal areas of disease involvement in the vertebral bodies and epidural region. (B) Note blastic lesions in the pedicles especially at L₂.

treatment, continued medical intervention is especially needed to assist in home care efforts.

Spinal cord compression resulting from metastatic tumor can be prevented or effectively treated when diagnosed early (91,134–140,147,148). Most commonly, 30 Gy in 10 fractions is administered in the treatment of spinal cord compression and carcinomatous plexopathy. Pain relief can be accomplished in 73% of patients after treatment (147,148). Although more prolonged courses of radiation have been given to treat spinal cord compres-

sion, a short course of radiotherapy was evaluated in a patient group with a poor overall prognosis. Among the 53 patients treated, 11 had lung cancer, 11 prostate, 9 with gastrointestinal, 5 with renal cell, and 3 with breast cancer. Pain was present in 96%, weakness was evident in 84% (41% were unable to walk and 12% were paraplegic). Radiotherapy consisted of a single 8 Gy fraction; a second 8 Gy fraction was given 1 week to responders or stable patients (157). The median field size was 136 cm², and all patients treated to the upper abdomen were premedicated. Pain relief was accomplished in 67%, and motor function improved in 63%. Early diagnosis and therapy were important in predicting response to radiotherapy. Ability to ambulate and maintain continence was preserved in 91% and 98%, respectively. Only 38% of non-ambulatory patients and 44% of those with bladder incontinence improved. Median survival time was 5 months; 30% survived 1 year. Survival was significantly better for ambulatory patients. For patients with spinal cord compression and poor prognostic factors, short course radiotherapy appeared to provide efficient and effective palliation.

Surgical intervention should be considered for patients presenting with a high-grade epidural lesion caused by a neoplasm with poor radiosensitivity. Surgery may also be considered in cases of tumor progression in a previously irradiated area, for stabilization of the spine, in paraplegic patients with limited disease and good probability of survival, and for establishing a diagnosis (76,91,134, 135,137,139,147,148,152,155). Adjuvant radiotherapy is often given to treat microscopic residual disease after neurosurgical intervention among previously unirradiated patients. Surgical restoration of the vertebral alignment may be required because of neurologic compromise and pain caused by progressive vertebral collapse. Vertebral collapse may occur because of cancer or vertebral instability after cancer therapy (Fig. 16.6). Appropriate intervention should be pursued because the neurologic compromise and pain from vertebral instability can be as devastating as that with epidural spinal cord metastases (139,155,158).

Paravertebral masses are most commonly associated with lung cancer and are rare in prostate cancer (152,159). Approximately 20% of patients with epidural cord compression will have an associated paravertebral mass. Surgical resection combined with radiation therapy has been suggested to improve functional outcome when a paravertebral mass is associated with spinal cord compression because radiation alone is less effective with larger tumor burdens.

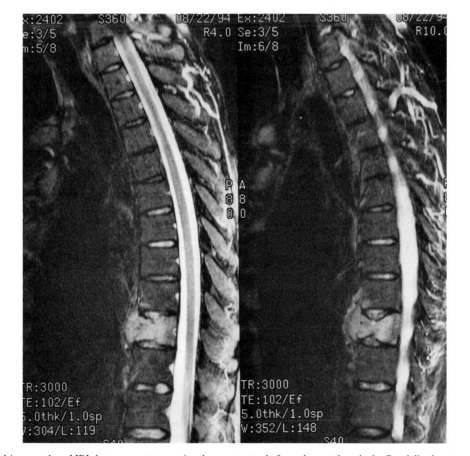

Fig. 16.6. Spinal cord is normal on MRI, but recurrent tumor involvement extends from the vertebrae body. Specialized treatment planning needs to ensure adequate radiation doses to the involved region.

Radiation tolerance of the spinal cord

The potential for the development of radiation myelitis with total radiation doses that exceed 40 Gy at 2 Gy per fraction represents the limiting factor in the treatment of large tumor burdens near or involving the spinal canal. Furthermore, the length of spinal cord that needs to be irradiated significantly affects the radiation tolerance of the spinal cord (160–162). Histopathologic changes, experimentally observed after fractionated irradiation of the spinal cord include white matter necrosis, massive hemorrhage, and segmental parenchymal atrophy that are consistently associated with abnormal neurologic signs (162). Other pathologic responses involve focal fiber loss and white matter vacuolation. Experimental data also have shown that the time course and extent of long-term recovery from radiation are dependent on the specific type and age of tissue (160,162).

Radiation tolerance is based on the dose per fraction, total dose, and the volume of tissue treated. The dose per fraction is the most important factor in the tolerance of tissues to radiation. Clinical and experimental experience has failed to demonstrate any difference in radiosensitivity in different segments of the spinal cord (160,163). The risk of radiation myelitis in the cervicothoracic spine is less than 5% when 6000 cGy is administered at 172 cGy per fraction, or 5000 cGy is given with daily fractions of 200 cGy per fraction. Especially among patients who have received chemotherapy or have had spinal injury, the total dose to the spinal cord is generally limited to 4000 cGy administered at 200 cGy per fraction to minimize any risk of irreversible radiation injury to the spinal cord. The total dose is also an extremely important factor defining the radiation tolerance of the spinal cord. A steep curve based on total radiation dose predicts the risk of developing radiation myelopathy; a small increase in total radiation dose can result in a large increased risk for radiation myelopathy (160,162). However, using the linear quadratic model, no progressive myelopathies have been identified with doses of 60 Gy in 2 Gy fractions to the spinal cord. Concerns have been raised that the conservative limit of radiation dose to the spinal cord has compromised tumor control. With conventional fractionation of 1.8 to 2 Gy fractions, the incidence of myelitis at 5 years was 0.2% after 45 Gy, and 1%–5% after 60 Gy (163). These determinations from the linear-quadratic model have correlated well with clinical data.

Retreatment of a previously irradiated segment of spinal cord results in high risk for radiation-induced myelopathy because other neurological pathways cannot compensate for an injury to a specific level of the spinal cord. Within 6 months, there is an approximate 30% repair of spinal tissue. If 50 Gy was administered initially, this represents 85% of the tolerance dose to the spinal cord (163,164). With 1 to 2 years between radiation treatments to allow repair, tolerance dose to the spinal cord is determined to be about 135% with reirradiation. Therefore, a total dose of 75 to 81 Gy given in two radiation courses with conventional fractionation spaced 1 to 2 years apart should not result in significant injury. Conformal techniques along with spinal cord recovery provide an option for reirradiation (165,166). Included are approaches with intensity modulated radiation therapy. Especially if the patient is not a surgical candidate, reirradiation may be the only viable option to maintain neurological integrity for the remainder of the patient's life. Because of the limited overall prognosis, risk for long-term radiation injury is small.

The radiation tolerance of the spinal cord can be compromised by prior injury. Vasogenic edema of the spinal cord and nerve roots can be caused by compression injury along with venous hemorrhage, loss of myelin, and ischemia. Synthesis of prostaglandin E_2 is increased with vasogenic edema and can be inhibited by steroids or nonsteroidal anti-inflammatory agents (91,160,161). Two separate mechanisms of radiation injury can occur and result from white matter damage and vasculopathies. White matter damage is associated with diffuse demyelination and swollen axons that can be focally necrotic and have associated glial reaction. Vascular damage experimentally has been shown to be age-dependent and can result in vascular necrosis.

Six major types of injury have been shown experimentally to result from radiation to the spinal column. Five of these occur in the spinal cord and one in the dorsal root ganglia. The most severe spinal lesions, all of which are due to vascular damage and result in neurological dysfunction, include white matter necrosis, hemorrhage, and segmental parenchymal atrophy. The two less severe spinal lesions included focal fiber loss and scattered white matter vacuolation resulting from damage to glial cells, axons, and/or the vasculature; these less severe sequelae are seen with lower total doses of radiation and are less likely to result in neurological dysfunction. In dorsal root ganglia, radiation damage included intracytoplasmic vacuoles and loss of neurons and satellite cells that could affect sensory function. These findings are distinct from the demyelination of the posterior columns associated with the self-limiting Lhermitte's syndrome (161). Meningeal thickening and fibrosis can also be observed after radiation, but the clinical significance of this is unknown. Ependymal and nerve root damage from radiation is rare.

Experimental studies have shown that high-dose steroids are more effective than lower dose medications in reversing edema and improving neurologic function. Consistent with this are clinical data including a well-designed randomized trial that administered radiation therapy either with high-dose corticosteroids or placebo. In their trial, the group that received corticosteroids was more likely to retain or regain ambulation (91). Pain relief is also more rapid and complete with high-dose steroids (initial bolus of 100 mg followed by 4–24 mg dexamethasone four times daily for the duration of radiation therapy) among patients suspected to have spinal cord compression.

Persistent pain after spinal radiation

Persistent or recurrent pain after radiotherapy for vertebral metastases should be investigated to exclude the possibility of progressive disease inside or outside the radiation portal, or mechanical spinal instability because of a vertebral compression fracture. Radiation-induced neural injury generally does not result in pain. Compression fractures that occur shortly after completing radiation are related to bony insufficiency with tumor cell kill rather than radiation effects (Fig. 16.7). Changes seen in the bone marrow on MRI after palliative radiotherapy usually can be distinguished from those seen with progressive disease (93–95,167,168). Trials are also underway to determine therapeutic response among lytic bone lesions with bone mineral density evaluations (169).

Based on clinical and radiographic grounds, leptomeningeal carcinomatosis must also be considered in the diagnostic evaluation of persistent or recurrent pain. Leptomeningeal carcinomatosis occurs more commonly than expected. For example, only one half the cases of breast cancer with leptomeningeal carcinomatosis will be diagnosed before patient death (134,148,152,153,175). Performing a lumbar puncture is a relative barrier to the diagnosis; at least three cerebrospinal fluid (CSF) samples are necessary to cytologically exclude the diagnosis of leptomeningeal disease because in 10% to 40% of patients, the initial CSF sample fails to document tumor cells (170). MRI can identify leptomeningeal disease among patients with normal CSF cytology and is sensitive and specific in locating regions of nodular leptomeningeal involvement. Except in the case of nodular leptomeningeal involvement where localized radiotherapy may be of benefit as an adjuvant, intrathecal chemotherapy is generally the treatment of choice (153).

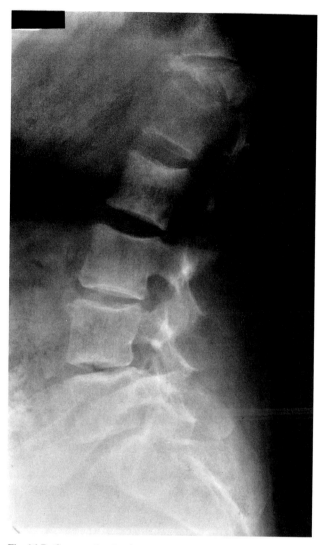

Fig. 16.7. Compression fraction of the 12th thoracic vertebral body after an initial pain-free interval after palliative radiation. Vertebral weakness with rapid tumor regression resulting in the compression fracture, which caused recurrent back pain as a result of spinal instability.

Diffuse bone metastases

Other therapeutic approaches, including wide field radiotherapy, systemic radionuclides, and bisphosphonates have been used among patients with disseminated bone metastases. Both approaches are useful in augmenting the therapeutic effect of localized radiation and in preventing asymptomatic bony lesions from progressing. Although usually not a significant consideration in localized irradiation, adequate bone marrow reserve is required for wide field radiotherapy and systemic radionuclides. Bone marrow scans can be performed to determine the volume of functioning marrow and assess the feasibility of delivering wide field radiotherapy or radionuclides (55–57,171–175).

Wide-field radiotherapy

Hemibody irradiation has been used to treat diffuse bone metastases by administering 6 to 10 Gy in one fraction to the upper, mid, or lower body. Response rates are consistently reported to be greater than 70%, and more than 20% of patients have complete relief of pain. In patients with prostate cancer, the overall response rate is 80%, and complete relief of pain is 30% (165,172,177). About one half of patients experience relief of pain within 48 hours of treatment, and the overall response rates is 80% for all types of primary tumors. More than one half the patients treated did not require further palliative irradiation for recurrent bone pain over the duration of their lives. For prostate cancer patients, the mean duration of pain relief is 15 weeks, and mean survival time is 25 weeks.

An RTOG study demonstrated that hemibody radiation reduced the time to disease progression and decreased the need for subsequent palliative radiation of bone metastases at 1 year follow-up evaluation when compared to local field irradiation alone. These results from the RTOG study are consistent with other reported experience using hemibody irradiation (171,172). Median survival time after hemibody irradiation was significantly longer among patients who present with a good performance status. Approximately 90% of patients with a complete response and 70% of patients with a partial response had a good to excellent performance status before radiotherapy. Prior systemic therapy does not influence response to wide field radiotherapy. Symptomatic bone metastases, which are also refractory to chemotherapy or hormonal therapy, had complete response rates of 70% and partial response rates of 24% with hemibody radiation (165). Symptoms were palliated in 88% of cases when a previously treated area was reirradiated. Significant toxicity was observed in less than 10% of patients, and 50% experienced stabilization of disease at 1 year. With current strategies, acute toxicities associated with hemibody irradiation are manageable. Premedication prevents nausea, and partial shielding minimizes lung dose and the risk for radiation pneumonitis. Acute hematologic depression is limited.

Because of the potential toxicity to visceral structures and the difficulty in treatment setup, hemibody radiation is not routinely used to palliate multifocal bone metastases. Concerns regarding the permanent effects on bone marrow reserve also exist relative to the subsequent need for chemotherapy. For these reasons, radiopharmaceuticals, which have no systemic toxicities other than the effect on blood counts, have gained popularity over hemibody radiation in the treatment of multifocal bone metastases. However, radiopharmaceuticals are most useful in blastic bony lesions, and hemibody radiation may be an important palliative option among patients with diffuse lytic bone metastases that are refractory to other therapies.

Radiopharmaceuticals

An alternative to hemibody irradiation for the treatment of widely disseminated bone metastases is the use of systemic radioisotopes. The most commonly used radiopharmaceuticals for the treatment of bone metastases are strontium-89 and samarium-153 (Table 16.5). Strontium-89 combines with the calcium component of hydroxyapatite in osteoblastic lesions. Many reports indicate effective palliation of pain lasting up to 6 months in 60% to 80% of patients with breast and prostate cancers (55–57,173–175). Improvements in functional status and quality of life have been observed, and about 20% of patients have complete resolution of pain. Pain control has been reported to be superior among patients with disseminated prostate cancer treated both with strontium-89 and local radiotherapy as compared to localized irradiation alone (56,57). Because the activity of strontium-89 is limited to bone, use of radiopharmaceuticals is contraindicated when epidural disease is associated with ver-

Table 16.5. *Characteristics of radiopharmaceuticals used to treat bone metastases*

Radioisotope	Radiation type	Half-life (days)	Typical response rate (%)	Typical time to response (days)	Typical duration of response (months)	Myelo-suppression
Phosphorus-32	↑ Energy beta	14	78	14	1.5–11.3	3+
Strontium-89	↓ Energy beta	50	70–80	7–20	≤ 6	1+
Samarium-153	Beta/gamma	2	65	7–21	3–4	3+
Rhenium-186	Beta/gamma	4	80	7–21	2	1+
Tin-117m	Beta/gamma	14	—	—	—	?
Iodine-131	↓ Energy beta	8	72	—	≤ 2	0 to +1

From Friedland J. Local and systemic radiation for palliation of metastatic disease. Urol Clin North Am 26:391–402, 1999.

tebral metastases. Myelotoxicity, resulting in a 25% decline of initial platelet and white blood cell counts, is usually transient and represents the only significant toxicity associated with strontium-89 (55,56,102). Experience from a number of clinical trials has demonstrated strontium-89 to be an effective therapy that is easily administered in an outpatient setting. The radiation dose absorbed by the bone marrow is 2 to 50 times less than the dose administered by strontium-89 to the osteoblastic lesion. Radiation doses to metastatic bony lesions with strontium-89 can range from 3 Gy to more than 300 Gy.

Clinical response to strontium-89 is comparable to wide field radiotherapy. Response to strontium-89 therapy has been documented both subjectively and objectively. Subjective response, manifested as symptomatic improvement, was reported in a validated survey by more than 80% of patients with prostate cancer. Objective evidence of response was documented by reductions in alkaline and acid phosphatase levels that were also associated with a decrease in the uptake in metastatic lesions on sequential bone scans (55,56,102,104). Prior therapies for prostate cancer, including local radiation therapy and systemic chemotherapy or hormone therapy, do not influence toxicity or affect clinical response to strontium-89. Administered as an adjuvant to localized external beam radiotherapy in metastatic prostate cancer, strontium-89 has been shown to improve pain relief and delay progression of disease in prospective randomized clinical trials. Almost twice as many patients treated with strontium-89 were reported to be pain-free at 3-month follow-up evaluation when compared to patients treated with localized external beam radiation. Analgesics were no longer required by 17% of patients treated with strontium-89, whereas only 2% of the patients treated with localized radiotherapy alone were able to discontinue analgesic use. Quality-of-life assessments demonstrated increased physical activity along with improved pain relief after strontium-89 was administered in conjunction with localized external beam radiation therapy. Cost–benefit analysis has also suggested an advantage to the administration of strontium-89 with reductions in costs of hospitalization for tertiary care (55,56,107).

Several other radiopharmaceuticals are available for clinical application including samarium-153, gallium nitrate, phosphorus-32, and rhenium-186 (173–175). The therapeutic mechanism of action relates to the physical and biologic half-life in the bony lesion, mean energy, and delivered dose of the radiopharmaceutical. Table 16.5 summarizes some of the physical characteristics and clinical data for various radionuclides. Phosphorus-32 and strontium-89 emit pure beta rays (little penetration in tissue), and rhenium-186 and samarium-153 emit both beta rays and relatively high-energy gamma-ray photons that penetrate tissue for some distance.

Because samarium-153 has a gamma-ray component, it is possible to directly image the distribution of the radiation dose. The scans after injection of samarium-153 are comparable to diagnostic scans obtained with technitium-99m. The mean skeletal uptake is more than 50% of the dose (106). Non-skeletal sites receive negligible radiation doses, and complete clearance of radiation not absorbed by the radiation occurs within 6 to 8 hours of administration (105). In a double-blind placebo controlled clinical trial, samarium-153 was shown to be an effective agent in palliating painful bone metastases in patients with breast cancer. Pain relief occurred within 1 week and lasted at least 16 weeks after administration (101). Approximately 65% of patients responded within the first 4 weeks, and 43% had relief of pain of at least 16 weeks' duration. No significant bone marrow toxicities were observed. Recommended doses range between 1.0 and 1.5 mCi/kg. In more than one third of patients, multiple administrations are possible (108).

Rhenium-186 concentrates selectively in bone; the mechanism of action is similar to that of technetium diphosphonate-99m, which is used in diagnostic bone scans. This characteristic allows direct imaging of the deposition of rhenium-186 in bony metastases. The metastatic lesion receives tens of Gy in dose after administration of rhenium-186, and the radiation dose to the marrow is limited to 0.75 Gy (97,175). Thrombocytopenia appears to be the dose-limiting toxicity. Similar to the reports of strontium-89 among patients with prostate cancer, decreases in prostate-specific antigen have also been observed after administration of rhenium-186 (175).

Phosphorus-32 has been used to treat bone metastases in patients with prostate cancer for more than 30 years, with 77% of patients experiencing significant pain relief (97). The response rates and duration of response with phosphorus-32 are similar to wide field radiation and strontium-89. However, the main disadvantage of phosphorus-32 is that more than 30% of patients develop severe hematologic toxicity.

Marrow suppression caused by radioisotopes is caused by either penetrating gamma radiation or a radioisotope with a long half-life. For example, transient cytopenia is observed with strontium-89 because it has a fairly long half-life of 51 days, even though it emits a beta particle of low penetrance and low energy (1.46 MeV) (Table 16.5). Hematotoxicity is more pronounced in patients with pretreatment platelet counts of $\leq 60 \times 10^3$, whereas blood counts of $\leq 2.5 \times 10^3$ or $\geq 30\%$ involvement of the red marrow bearing bone (99,102). Compromise of the red marrow bearing bone can be a consequence of tumor or prior radiation and chemotherapy.

Comparative clinical trials are necessary to determine if any difference exists in the onset and pattern of response between samarium-153, strontium-89, and other radiopharmaceuticals. Clinical data for rhenium-186 and other radiopharmaceuticals are still limited, and these agents are in various stages of clinical investigation (97,99–102,174,175). Several strategies have been proposed to further enhance the therapeutic response of radiopharmaceutical agents. These options include further dose intensity studies, adjunctive administration of bisphosphonates, and concurrent administration with chemotherapy (103). Although bone marrow toxicity is relatively limited in the doses of radiopharmaceuticals currently administered, either alone or in combination with other agents, future dose intensity studies may require temporary hematological support with colony-stimulating factors.

Sequential radiographs and bone scintigrams after hormonal and radiopharmaceutical therapy for breast and prostate cancers demonstrate an osteoblastic response that reflects remodeling of the bone in osteolytic osseous metastases (86,87). Approximately one third of patients will have evidence of increased tracer uptake on bone scans (flare) obtained 8 to 16 weeks after treatment. Of these patients with a flare response on bone scan, 72% will experience a response to treatment. By comparison, only 36% will have a response to treatment when a limited to no flare response is observed.

Radiopharmaceuticals have several advantages in their ease of administration, low rates of toxicity, and possibility for reirradiation. Future clinical studies target administration of radiopharmaceuticals earlier in the course of metastatic disease and in combination with other therapies. For example, strontium-89 has been combined with a number of chemotherapeutic agents in prostate cancer, and early reports suggest synergistic effects in both analgesia and cytotoxicity (174). Other needed areas of research involve radiopharmaceutical dose, schedule of administration, and selection of the radiopharmaceutical that will provide the optimal response based on tumor type and other factors.

Brain metastases

Radiation is used to relieve the symptoms of headache, seizure, nausea/vomiting, and neurologic dysfunction associated with brain metastases. Surgery, either alone or in combination with radiation, is often performed when a solitary brain metastasis is present, if the performance status is good, and if the cancer burden is otherwise limited. Radiation is generally given over 2 to 3 weeks, with daily fractions of 2.5 Gy to 3 Gy per day; total radiation doses range from 25 Gy after resection to 30 Gy with unresectable disease and a poor prognosis (76).

Reirradiation of brain tumors and brain metastases is common. The role of radiosurgery in 156 recurrent brain tumors and brain metastases was evaluated in a RTOG study. Between 1990 and 1994, recurrent brain tumors constituted 36% of the group, with a median prior dose of radiation totaling 60 Gy; the median prior radiation dose among the 64% of patients with recurrent brain metastases was 30 Gy. The maximum tolerated doses for tumors ≤ 2 cm, 2 to 3 cm, and 3 to 4 cm were 24 Gy, 18 Gy, and 15 Gy, respectively (166). Maximum tumor diameter was associated with a significantly increased risk for $\geq$ grade 3 neurotoxicity; tumors between 2 and 4 cm were 7 to 16 times more likely to develop $\geq$ grade 3 neurotoxicity. The incidence of radionecrosis was 5%, 8%, 9%, and 11% at 6, 12, 18, and 24 months, respectively. Patients with recurrent brain tumors and those treated on a linear accelerator instead of a gamma knife had a 2.8 times greater risk of progression in the radiosurgical target volume. This finding was not related to patient group because 61% of patients with recurrent brain tumors, as compared to 30% of patients with brain metastases, were treated on the gamma knife (79).

External beam therapy has been used to re-treat patients with persistent symptoms resulting from brain metastases and who are not candidates to receive radiosurgery. In general, if symptoms recur within 3 to 4 months of radiation, reirradiation is unlikely to be effective. Additional therapy may benefit patients, however, who develop recurrent neurological symptoms 6 to 9 months later and who have a KPS of > 50. With steroid administration and reirradiation, 60% response rates have been reported. Generally, a total dose of 25 to 30 Gy is prescribed with 2 to 2.5 Gy fractions (79). Risk for late toxicity depends on the total cumulative dose, volume reirradiated, and interval between the first and second course of radiation (78). A 14% risk for necrosis exists with ≥ 86 Gy using 2 Gy fractions.

Reirradiation with external beam therapy for recurrent gliomas was investigated among 24 patients who had previously received a median dose of 60 Gy. With reirradiation, the total cumulative dose was limited to 92 Gy; reirradiation was given with 1.5 Gy fractions and oral

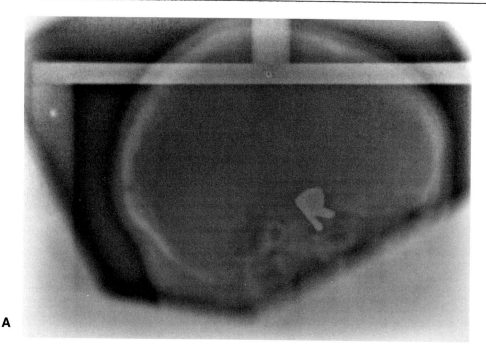

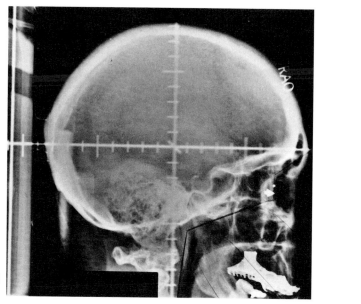

Fig. 16.8. (A) A typical radiation portal used to treat brain metastases. (B) A simulation film that comprehensively encompasses the base of the skull.

CCNU (130 mg/m^2 every 6 weeks). Response equaled 57%, and two patients survived more than 5 years. Median time to progression and overall survival were 8 and 14 months, respectively. Using this approach, no significant neurological toxicity was reported (79).

Brachytherapy has also been used for recurrent brain tumors. This technique has been applied in highly selected patients with good neurological function and well-defined tumors located within 5 cm of midline (176). The primary complication has been necrosis that

necessitated reoperation in 49% of patients. Median survival time was 54 weeks with glioblastoma multiforme.

Prognosis also can be determined from the mini-mental status examination (MMSE) before and after palliative radiation for brain metastases. In a RTOG study, 445 patients with brain metastases received 1.6 Gy bid to a total dose of 54.4 Gy, or a radiotherapy regimen totaling 30 Gy in 10 fractions to the entire brain. Having a range of scores between 11 and 30, the average MMSE before radiation was 26.5; 16% of patients had scores < 23, indicating significant cognitive impairment before radiation therapy (176). Median survival was 4.2 months and 37% were alive at 6 months. On multivariate analysis, the pretreatment MMSE and KPS were predictive of outcome; survival of 81% at 6 months and 66% at 1 year was observed among patients whose MMSE scores before and after radiation were > 23. Death from brain metastases was associated with a declining MMSE and primary site (breast vs. lung cancer). Overall, 30 Gy administered over 2 weeks proved to be an effective regimen for brain metastases, and no significant advantage was observed with a more prolonged course of therapy.

Lung

Locally advanced primary or metastatic involvement of the lung often requires palliative intervention. A variety of symptoms, some of them emergent, can manifest because of tumor involvement of the lung and mediastinum (177). Pain can result from tumor invasion of the ribs and nerve roots of the chest wall (Fig. 16.9). Vertebral involvement can be associated with spinal cord compression. Obstructive pneumonitis and hemoptysis can result from bronchial obstruction. Mediastinal infil-

tration can cause superior vena cava syndrome. All of these clinical presentations can be palliated with external beam radiation that encompasses the disease that is evident on diagnostic images and that treats pain referred along involved nerve roots. Radiation schedules that administer 30 Gy in 10 fractions over 2 to 3 weeks are typically prescribed to previously unirradiated sites. Using this type of palliative radiation schedule among 65 patients with non–small-cell lung cancer, hemoptysis decreased in 79%, arm/shoulder pain decreased in 56%, chest wall pain decreased in 53%, cough decreased in 49%, dyspnea decreased in 39%; minimal improvement was observed in fatigue (22%) and loss of appetite (11%). Decreases in dyspnea were highly correlated with radiographic evidence of response (178). Although palliative radiation is effective, most patients will have residual symptoms that require medical management.

If the area has been previously irradiated, techniques that exclude critical anatomic structures, like the spinal cord, are applied. Among a review of more than 1500 cases of lung cancer from 1982 to 1997, 23 patients underwent reirradiation for relief of symptoms. Median follow-up time was 3.2 months, and the range was 0 to 17.5 months. Consistent with other published reports,

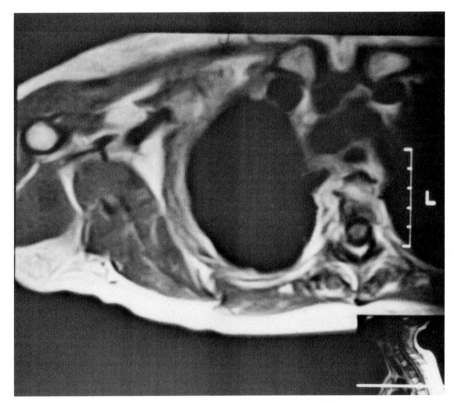

Fig. 16.9. Tumor masses invading the chest wall.

hemoptysis decreased or resolved in all of 6 symptomatic patients, 4 of 5 patients had reduced pain, 9 of 15 had a reduction in cough, and 11 of 15 had decreased dyspnea (179). The risk for radiation pneumonitis can be decreased by creating narrower margins around the radiation portal.

Other approaches, such as brachytherapy, can be used when the symptomatic site is well localized and accessible. In these cases, large doses of radiation can be delivered over a few minutes by a high-dose rate brachytherapy unit (77,165). Brachytherapy can be used as a boost to external beam therapy, or to re-treat a previously irradiated area. Precise details of techniques and radiation doses vary, but most are in the range of 6 to 10 Gy every 1 to 2 weeks for up to 3 fractions of a single fraction of 10 to 20 Gy. Overall symptom response ranges between 70% and 90%, and palliation is durable in 60% of patients (165). Relief of specific symptoms included 54% for hemoptysis, 94% for cough, 86% for dyspnea, and 51% for pulmonary collapse (77). Those with recurrent symptoms can be treated with brachytherapy again or by other methods. The incidence of radiation bronchitis and stenosis was 17%; fatal hemoptysis occurred in 5.5%. Tumor of the right mainstem bronchus and the right upper-lobe bronchus appear to be more susceptible to develop fatal hemorrhage than do left-sided lesions.

Dyspnea should be palliated with medical management while awaiting a response to radiotherapy. Oxygen therapy, maintaining adequate hemoglobin levels, and the use of opioids are effective measures; opioids will not produce respiratory depression if appropriately dosed. Although frequently used, benzodiazepine agents were found to be ineffective in four of five randomized trials (180).

Brachytherapy has also been used in treatment of esophageal cancer. Relief of dysphagia ranges between 70% and 85% in a number of published reports. A combination of a short course of external beam radiation (30 Gy in 10 fractions) plus brachytherapy as a boost relieves dysphagia for 3 to 6 months. Relative contraindications include a tumor length of 10 cm or more, extension to the gastroesophageal junction or cardia, skip lesions, extensive extraesophageal spread, macroscopic regional adenopathy, tracheoesophageal fistula, cervical esophageal involvement, or stenosis that cannot be bypassed (77).

Head and neck cancers

Palliation of locally advanced head and neck malignancies often requires more protracted radiation schedules because of the sensitive structures, such as the arytenoids and cervical spinal cord, in the radiation field. Quality of life parameters were evaluated before, during, and at 3-month intervals after chemoradiation for locally advanced head and neck cancer. Because of severe treatment-related toxicities, all quality of life and functional domains declined (181). By 12 months, marked improvement was observed although up to one third of patients continued to experience difficulty swallowing, hoarseness, and mouth/throat pain that were comparable to pretreatment symptom levels. Significant increases in dry mouth (58% vs. 17%), impaired taste (32% vs. 8%), and need for a soft food diet (82% vs. 42%) were documented after chemoradiation. Quality of life was best predicted by the pretreatment quality of life level and was irrespective of residual side effects or functional impairment.

Aggressive management of treatment-related side effects can improve tolerance to head and neck radiation (182). Using a specific pain management regimen that included opioid analgesics, symptoms caused by head and neck radiation were effectively controlled. With the regimen, pain noted more than 12 hours per day decreased by 35%, and mean weight loss of more than 5 kg decreased by 41%. Moderate to severe pain during the first week of radiation was noted in 15%. Significant improvements were observed with opioid analgesics when compared to traditional means of controlling symptoms with codeine elixirs. By the 3rd week of radiation, pain was reduced by 11%; it decreased by 24% during the 5th week and by 26% during the 7th week of radiation. At the end of radiation, pain intensity at its worst was mild in 43%, moderate in 23%, and severe in 6%; frequency of the pain was occasionally in 46%, most of day in 17%, and always in 6%. Aggressive pain management effectively relieved the severe symptoms associated with head and neck radiation.

Late radiation effects are of particular concern with reirradiation of recurrent head and neck cancers. The total biological effect after retreatment of recurrent nasopharyngeal cancers has been evaluated. The severity of damage during the initial course of radiation was the major determinant of complications associated with retreatment. Repair of normal tissues, especially when there was an interval of 2 or more years between courses of radiation, was evident because the tolerated doses were higher than expected with a single course of radiation (164). The complication-free survival rate at 5 years was actually lower in the retreatment group (81%), when compared to a group treated with a single course of radiation (48%). A 20% risk of complications at 5 years would occur with a total biologically equivalent dose of 143 Gy_3 with retreatment, or 111 Gy_3 among patients treated with a single course.

Pelvis

Hemorrhage, visceral or lymphatic obstruction, and nerve root injury present most commonly with locally advanced or metastatic disease in the pelvis. Treatment may require emergent radiotherapeutic and/or surgical interventions. Hemorrhage is commonly associated with tumors involving the rectum and genitourinary tracts. As with tumors in the lung, radiation is an effective means of stopping active bleeding. Colorectal cancers are often diagnosed among patients with unexplained bleeding.

Colorectal tumor involvement may also result in obstruction requiring stent placement to maintain the integrity of the visceral lumen while administering radiation (177,183). Occasionally a diverting colostomy will be required to bypass intestinal obstruction or fistula formation. If these procedures are not performed, intestinal colic can be palliated quickly with opioids and anticholinergics (e.g., scopolamine and atropine), which decrease peristalsis in the smooth muscle of the intestinal tract (183,184). Intestinal obstruction can also result in nausea and vomiting, which can be palliated with nasogastric decompression and pharmacological agents. Octreotide, an analog of somatostatin, reduces gastrointestinal secretions, motility, and splanchnic blood flow; has a proabsorptive effect on water and ions; and may inhibit the secretion of vasoactive intestinal peptide. These actions help to disrupt the distention-intestinal secretion-peristalsis cycle and bleeding (184,185).

Because these tumors are generally locally advanced, preoperative radiation is given with conventional fractionation if limited or no metastatic disease is evident; this is intended to stop bleeding, render the patient operable, and provide a chance for cure.

With extensive metastatic disease, 30 to 35 Gy can be given over 2 to 3 weeks to palliate symptoms of bleeding and obstruction. Fractionation has included 35 Gy/14 fractions, 30 Gy/10 fractions, and 30 Gy/6 fractions given twice weekly for 3 weeks (186). On one study, diverting colostomy was required by 16% of patients before radiation. No significant treatment-related toxicities were observed. Whether radiation is administered as conventional or hypofractionated with infusional 5-fluorouracil, symptoms from the primary tumor resolved in 94% of cases, and the endoscopic complete response rate was 36%. The colostomy-free survival rate was 87% among patients who underwent palliative chemoradiation

and 51% among patients who received preoperative chemoradiation. When surgery was performed, the 2-year survival was 46% as compared to 11% with palliative chemoradiation. Symptomatic pelvic control was not significantly different and was 81% for palliative chemoradiation and 91% for preoperative chemoradiation (187). Predictors for control of pelvic disease included pelvic pain at presentation, a biologically equivalent dose < 35 Gy at 2 Gy per fraction, and poor pathological differentiation. Poor pathologic differentiation and selection for palliative chemoradiation predicted for a worse overall survival.

Tumors involving the cervix can hemorrhage and require emergent radiotherapeutic intervention. Superficial radiographs are applied directly to the bleeding cervix through a cone that treats the bleeding site and does not compromise later radiation of other pelvic structures. Radiation doses between 5 and 10 Gy are usually administered in one to three applications of cone therapy. Brachytherapy can also be used to treat gynecologic tumors, especially in the vagina, cervix, and endometrium.

Bladder cancers or tumors that secondarily invade the bladder can also result in significant bleeding that can be palliated by external beam radiation. Urinary obstruction commonly occurs with locally advanced pelvic cancers, especially with prostate and cervical cancers. Occasionally placement of a urinary stent or urostomy/nephrostomy will be required until sufficient tumor regression can be accomplished by radiation to reestablish integrity of the urinary tract (177). As with the bowel and gynecologic tracts, a vesical fistula, resulting from either the tumor itself or from tumor regression, remains a concern.

Palliative radiation administered as 35 Gy/10 fractions or 21 Gy/3 fractions was evaluated among 272 patients with bladder cancer. With a minimum of 3-month follow-up time, 68% achieved symptomatic improvement; this included 71% for 35 Gy and 64% for 21 Gy (188). No difference was noted in efficacy, toxicity, or survival between the two radiation schedules. Overall survival was approximately 77% at 3 months, 35% at 12 months, and 19% at 24 months.

The pelvic lymph nodes and major blood vessels may become obstructed by tumor. Obstruction is seen most often when tumor arises in pelvic structures but can also occur with pelvic metastases from breast and other cancers. Lymphatic obstruction results in painful edema that is refractory to diuretic and other therapies; when severe, fluid and electrolyte imbalances can occur. Pelvic radiation can relieve lymphatic obstruction through tumor regression.

Pelvic tumors can also invade the sacral plexus and result in intractable pain. Tumor can track along nerve roots and can be associated with bony invasion of the sacrum. Pain resulting from visceral and/or lymphatic obstruction often responds more rapidly to palliative radiation than the neuropathic pain seen with sacral plexus involvement. Other radiotherapeutic approaches, such as brachytherapy, are extremely limited when the cancer persists or recurs after external beam radiation. Interventional pain management techniques are frequently required to control pain associated with sacral plexus involvement.

Reirradiation of the pelvis for symptomatic recurrence has generally been well tolerated, although data are limited. Care must be taken to exclude the intestines from the radiation portals given a 3.9 increased risk for late small bowel toxicity. Data are limited with regard to treatment volume, but the cumulative radiation dose, reirradiation dose, and the time interval between courses was not related to late toxicity (79).

Skin and subcutaneous tissues

Tumors can cause ulceration of the skin and subcutaneous tissues, which may be painful, distressing because of constant drainage, and which may become a source for the development of sepsis in immunocompromised patients. Localized radiation can be applied to destroy tumor and allow reepithelialization of the skin. Radiation that treats only the skin and subcutaneous tissues (electron beam therapy) is generally used to avoid radiation side effects to underlying uninvolved normal structures. Although usually 10 radiation treatments are given, the course of radiation can be abbreviated further, ranging from 1 to 5 days. Occasionally these lesions are treated with brachytherapy. The radioactive sources can be placed in a mold that sits on top of the tumor and delivers treatment over a few minutes (high-dose rate) or a few days (low-dose rate).

Conclusion

Radiation remains an important modality in palliative care. A number of clinical, prognostic, and therapeutic factors must be considered to determine the most optimal treatment regimen in palliative radiotherapy. Adequate management of cancer-related pain is important both during and after completing palliative irradiation. Efficient and effective palliative treatment is imperative for locally advanced and metastatic cancer to relieve symptoms, improve function, and minimize disease-related morbidity.

Radiation therapy is an important means of treating localized symptoms related to tumor involvement by providing a wide range of therapeutic options. Radiobiological principles, the radiation tolerance of adjacent normal tissues, and the clinic77al condition influence the selection of radiation technique, dose, and fraction size. The optimal dose and treatment schedule, however, is not fully defined for palliative radiation. Further study is necessary to integrate validated pain scores, analgesic use, prognostic factors, and radiobiological principles to better define the most efficient and efficacious treatment schedule according to the clinical presentation.

References

1. Cleeland CS, Gonin R, Hatfield AK, et al. Pain and its treatment in outpatients with metastatic cancer. N Engl J Med 330:592–6, 1994.
2. Jacox AK, Carr DB, Payne R, eds. Management of cancer pain. Clinical practice guideline no. 9. Rockville, MD: Agency for Health Care Policy and Research, 1994 (AHCPR publication no. 94-0592).
3. Jacox A, Carr DB, Payne R. New clinical practice guidelines for the management of pain in patients with cancer. N Engl J Med 330:651–5, 1994.
4. Brescia FJ, Portenoy RK, Ryan M, et al. Pain, opioid use, and survival in hospitalized patients with advanced cancer. J Clin Oncol 10:149–55, 1992.
5. Greenlee RT, Hill-Harmon MB, Murray T, Thun M. Cancer statistics, 2001. CA Cancer J Clin 51:15–36, 2001.
6. Anonymous. Outcomes of cancer treatment for technology assessment and cancer treatment guidelines. J Clin Oncol 14:671–9, 1996.
7. Cassel EJ. The nature of suffering and the goals of medicine. N Engl J Med 306:639–45, 1982.
8. Porzsolt F. Goals of palliative cancer therapy: scope of the problem. Cancer Treat Rev 19(Suppl A):3–14, 1993.
9. Rubens RD. Approaches to palliation and its evaluation. Cancer Treat Rev 19(Suppl A):67–71, 1993.
10. Porzsolt F, Tannock I. Goals of palliative cancer therapy. J Clin Oncol 11(2):378–81, 1993.
11. Cella DF, Tulsky DS. Quality of life in cancer: definition, purpose, and method of measurement. Cancer Invest 11:327–36, 1993.
12. Janjan NA. Radiation for bone metastases-conventional techniques and the role of systemic radiopharmaceuticals. Cancer 80:1628–45, 1997.
13. Liu L, Meers K, Capurso A, et al. The impact of radiation therapy on quality of life in patients with cancer. Cancer Practice 6:237–42, 1998.
14. Arcangeli G, Micheli A, Arcangeli F, et al. The responsiveness of bone metastases to radiotherapy: the effect of site, histology and radiation dose on pain relief. Radiother Oncol 14:95–101, 1989.
15. Mithal NP, Needham PR, Hoskin PJ. Retreatment with radiotherapy for painful bone metastases. Int J Radiat Oncol Biol Phys 29:1011–14, 1994.

16. Manfredi PL, Chandler S, Pigazzi A, Payne R. Outcomes of cancer pain consultations. Cancer 89:920–4, 2000.

17. Janjan NA, Payne R, Gillis T, et al. Presenting symptoms in patients referred to a multidisciplinary clinic for bone metastases. J Pain Symptom Manage 16:171–8, 1998.

18. Stafford RS, Cyr PL. The impact of cancer on the physical function of the elderly and their utilization of health care. Cancer 80:1973–80, 1997.

19. Cohen HJ. Cancer and the functional status of the elderly. Cancer 80:1883–6, 1997.

20. Hanks GE. The crisis in health care costs in the United States: some implications for radiation oncology. Int J Radiat Oncol Biol Phys 23:203–6, 1992.

21. Emanuel EJ, Fairclough DL, Slutsman J, Emanuel LL. Understanding economic and other burdens of terminal illness: the experience of patients and their caregivers. Ann Intern Med 132:451–9, 2000.

22. Rabow MW, Hardie GE, Fair JM, McPhee SJ. End of life care content in 50 textbooks from multiple specialties. JAMA 283:771–8, 2000.

23. Morita T, Tsunoda J, Inoue S, Chihara S. Contributing factors to physical symptoms in terminally-ill cancer patients. J Pain Symptom Manage 18:338–46, 1999.

24. Pargeon KL, Hailey BJ. Barriers to effective cancer pain management: a review of the literature. J Pain Symptom Manage 18:358–68, 1999.

25. Von Roenn JH, Cleeland CS, Gonin R, et al. Physicians attitudes and practice in cancer pain management: a survey from the Eastern Cooperative Oncology Group. Ann Intern Med 119:121–6, 1993.

26. Sherry MM, Greco FA, Johnson DH, Hainsworth JD. Breast cancer with skeletal metastases at initial diagnosis-distinctive clinical characteristics and favorable prognosis. Cancer 58:178–2, 1986.

27. Sherry MM, Greco FA, Johnson DH, Hainsworth JD. Metastatic breast cancer confined to the skeletal system. Am J Med 81:381–6, 1986.

28. Jacobson AF. Musculoskeletal pain as an indicator of occult malignancy. Arch Intern Med 157:105–9, 1997.

29. Vuorinen E. Pain as an early symptom in cancer. Clin J Pain 9:272–8, 1993.

30. Pienta KJ, Esper PS. Risk factors for prostate cancer. Ann Intern Med 118:793–803, 1993.

31. Abbas F, Scardino PT. The natural history of clinical prostate carcinoma. Cancer 80:827–33, 1997.

32. Chisholm GD, Rana A, Howard GCW. Management options for painful carcinoma of the prostate. Semin Oncol 20(Suppl 2):34–7, 1993.

33. Borre M, Nerstrom B, Overgaard J. The natural history of prostate carcinoma based on a Danish population treated with no intent to cure. Cancer 80:917–28, 1997.

34. Soloway MS, Hardeman SW, Hickey D, et al. Stratification of patients with metastatic prostate cancer based on extent of disease on initial bone scan. Cancer 61:195–202, 1988.

35. Yamashita K, Denno K, Ueda T, et al. Prognostic significance of bone metastases in patients with metastatic prostate cancer. Cancer 71:1297–1302, 1993.

36. Perez CA, Cosmatos D, Garcia DM, et al. Irradiation in relapsing carcinoma of the prostate. Cancer 71:1110–22, 1993.

37. Lai PP, Perez CA, Lockett MA. Prognostic significance of pelvic recurrence and distant metastases in prostate carcinoma following definitive radiotherapy. Int J Radiat Oncol Biol Phys 24:423–30, 1992.

38. Rose CM, Kagan AR. The final report of the expert panel for the Radiation Oncology Bone Metastasis Work Group of the American College of Radiology. Int J Radiat Oncol Biol Phys 40:1117–24, 1998.

39. Powers WE, Ratanatharathorn V. Palliation of bone metastases. In: Perez CA, Brady LW, eds. Principles and practice of radiation oncology, 3rd ed. Philadelphia: Lippincott Raven, 1998:2199–219.

40. Janjan NA. An emerging respect for palliative care in radiation oncology. J Palliat Med 1:83–8, 1998.

41. Chang VT, Thaler HT, Polyak TA, et al. Quality of life and survival-the role of multidimensional symptom assessment. Cancer 83:173–9, 1998.

42. Vigano A, Bruera E, Jhangri GS, et al. Clinical survival predictors in patients with advanced cancer. Arch Intern Med 160:861–8, 2000.

43. Cleeland CS, Janjan NA, Scott CB, et al. Cancer pain management by radiotherapists: a survey of Radiation Oncology Group physicians. Int J Radiat Oncol Biol Phys 47:203–8, 2000.

44. Lamont EB, Christakis NA. Some elements of prognosis in terminal cancer. Oncology 13:1165–70, 1999.

45. Zhong Z, Lynn J. Review of the Lamont/Christakis article. Oncology 13:1172–3, 1999.

46. Knudson G, Grinis G, Lopez-Majano V, et al. Bone scan as a stratification variable in advanced prostate cancer. Cancer 68:316–20, 1991.

47. Sabbatini P, Larson SM, Kremer A, et al. Prognostic significance of extent of disease in bone in patients with androgen-independent prostate cancer. J Clin Oncol 17:948–57, 1999.

48. Grabowski CM, Unger JA, Potish RA. Factors predictive of completion of treatment and survival after palliative radiation therapy. Radiology 184:329–32, 1992.

49. Reuben DB, Mor V, Hiris J. Clinical symptoms and length of survival in patients with terminal cancer. Arch Intern Med 148:1586–91, 1988.

50. Fielding LP, Henson DE. Multiple prognostic factors and outcome analysis in patients with cancer-communication from the American Joint Committee on Cancer. Cancer 71:2426–9, 1993.

51. Portenoy RK, Miransky J, Thaler HT, et al. Pain in ambulatory patients with lung or colon cancer. Cancer 70:1616–24, 1992.

52. Archer VR, Billingham LJ, Cullen MH. Palliative chemotherapy: no longer a contradiction in terms. The Oncologist 4:470–7, 1999.

53. Oh WK, Kantoff PW. Treatment of locally advanced prostate cancer: is chemotherapy the next step? J Clin Oncol 17:3664–75, 1999.

54. SBU-The Swedish Council on Technology Assessment in Health Care. Acta Oncol 35[(Suppl 6); Vol 1]:89–97, 1997.

55. Porter AT, Ben-Josef E. Strontium-89 in the treatment of bony metastases. In: DeVita VT, Hellman S, Rosenberg SA, eds. Important advances in oncology 1995. Philadelphia: Lippincott, 1995:87–94.

56. Porter AT, McEwan AJB, Powe JE, et al. Results of a randomized Phase III trial to evaluate the efficacy of strontium-89 adjuvant to local field external beam irradiation in the management of endocrine resistant metastatic prostate cancer. Int J Radiat Oncol Biol Phys 25:805–13, 1993.

57. Porter AT, McEwan AJB. Strontium-89 as an adjuvant to external beam radiation improves pain relief and delays in disease progression in advanced prostate cancer: results of a randomized controlled trial. Semin Oncol 20:38–43, 1993.

58. Dale RG, Jones B. Radiobiologically based assessments of the net costs of fractionated radiotherapy. Int J Radiat Oncol Biol Phys 36:739–46, 1996.

59. Janjan NA. Radiotherapeutic approaches to cancer pain management. Highlights Oncol Practice 14:103–13, 1997.

60. Hillner BE, Weeks JC, Desch CE, Smith TJ. Pamidronate in prevention of bone complications in metastatic breast cancer: a cost-effectiveness analysis. J Clin Oncol 18:72–9, 2000.

61. Dranitsaris G, Hsu T. Cost utility analysis of prophylactic pamidronate for the prevention of skeletal related events in patients with advanced breast cancer. Support Care Cancer 7:271–9, 1999.

62. Macklis RM, Cornelli H, Lasher J. Brief courses of palliative radiotherapy for metastatic bone pain. Am J Clin Oncol 21:617–22, 1998.

63. Hortobagyi GN, Theriault RL, Porter L, et al. Efficacy of pamidronate in reducing skeletal complications with breast cancer and lytic bone metastases. N Engl J Med 335:1785–91, 1996.

64. Hortobagyi GN, Theriault RL, Lipton A, et al. Long-term prevention of skeletal complications of metastatic breast cancer with pamidronate. J Clin Oncol 16:2038–44, 1998.

65. Theriault RL, Lipton A, Hortobagyi GN, et al. Pamidronate reduces skeletal morbidity in women with advanced breast cancer and lytic bone lesions: a randomized, placebo-controlled trial—Protocol 18 Aredia Breast Cancer Study Group. J Clin Oncol 17:846–54, 1999.

66. Lipton A, Theriault RL, Hortobagyi GN, et al. Pamidronate prevents skeletal complications and is effective palliative treatment in women with breast carcinoma and osteolytic bone metastases. Cancer 88:1082–90, 2000.

67. Body JJ, Bartl R, Burckhardt P, et al. Current use of bisphosphonates in oncology. J Clin Oncol 16:3890–9, 1998.

68. Bloomfield DJ. Should bisphosphonates be part of the standard therapy of patients with multiple myeloma or bone metastases from other cancers? An evidence-based review. J Clin Oncol 16:1218–25, 1998.

69. Lipton A. Bisphosphonates and breast cancer. Cancer 80:1668–73, 1997.

70. Hillner BE. The role of bisphosphonates in metastatic breast cancer. Semin Radiat Oncol 10:250–3, 2000.

71. Diel IJ, Solomayer EF, Costa SD, et al. Reduction in new metastases in breast cancer with adjuvant clodronate treatment. N Engl J Med 339:357–63, 1998.

72. Thames HD, Buchholz TA, Smith CD. Frequency of first metastatic events in breast cancer: implications for sequencing of systemic and local-regional treatment. J Clin Oncol 17:2649–58, 1999.

73. Ratanatharathorn V, Powers WE, Moss WT, Perez CA. Bone metastases: review and critical analysis of random allocation trials of local field treatment. Int J Radiat Oncol Biol Phys 44:1–18, 1999.

74. Bates T, Yarnold JR, Blitzer P, et al. Bone metastases consensus statement. Int J Radiat Oncol Biol Phys 23:215–6, 1992.

75. Bates T. A review of local radiotherapy in the treatment of bone metastases and cord compression. Int J Radiat Oncol Biol Phys 23:217–21, 1992.

76. Kagan AR. Palliation of brain and spinal cord metastases. In: Perez CA, Brady LW, eds. Principles and practice of radiation oncology, 3rd ed. Philadelphia: Lippincott Raven, 1998:2187–98.

77. Shasha D, Harrison LB. The role of brachytherapy for palliation. Semin Radiat Oncol 10:221–39, 2000.

78. Nieder C, Milas L, Ang KK. Tissue tolerance to reirradiation. Semin Radiat Oncol 10:200–9, 2000.

79. Morris DE. Clinical experience with retreatment for palliation. Semin Radiat Oncol 10:210–21, 2000.

80. Nielsen OS, Munro AJ, Tannock IF. Bone metastases: pathophysiology and management policy. J Clin Oncol 9:509–24, 1991.

81. Hendrix RW, Rogers LF, Davis, TM Jr. Cortical bone metastases. Radiology 181:409–13, 1991.

82. Garrett IR. Bone destruction in cancer. Semin Oncol 20(Suppl 2):4–9, 1993.

83. Orr FW, Kostenuik P, Sanchez-Sweatman OH, Singh G. Mechanisms involved in the metastasis of cancer to bone. Br Cancer Res Treat 25:151–63, 1993.

84. Mercadante S. Malignant bone pain: pathophysiology and treatment. Pain 69:1–18, 1997.

85. Ford HT, Yarnold JR. Radiation therapy–pain relief and recalcification. In: Stoll BA, Parbhoo S, eds. Bone metastases: monitoring and treatment. New York: Raven, 1983:343–54.

86. Hortobagyi GN, Libshitz HI, Seabold JE. Osseous metastases of breast cancer-clinical, biochemical, radiographic, and scintigraphic evaluation of response to therapy. Cancer 53:577–82, 1984.

87. Vogel CL, Schoenfelder J, Shemano I, et al. Worsening bone scan in the evaluation of antitumor response during hormonal therapy of breast cancer. J Clin Oncol 13:1123–8, 1995.

88. van der Pluijm G, Lowik C, Papapoulos S. Tumour progression and angiogenesis in bone metastasis from breast cancer: new approaches to an old problem. Cancer Treat Rev 26:11–27, 2000.

89. Conte PF, Latreille J, Mauriac L, et al. Delay in progression of bone metastases in breast cancer patients treated with intraveneous pamidronate: results from a multinational randomized controlled trial. J Clin Oncol 14:2552–9, 1996.

90. Townsend PW, Smalley SR, Cozad SC, et al. Role of post-operative radiation therapy after stabilization of fractures caused by metastatic disease. Int J Radiat Oncol Biol Phys 31:43–9, 1995.

91. Quinn JA, De Angelis LM. Neurologic emergencies in the cancer patient. Semin Oncol 27:311–21, 2000.

92. Bilsky MH, Lis E, Raizer J, Lee H, Boland P. The diagnosis and treatment of metastatic spinal tumor. The Oncologist 4:459–69, 1999.

93. Steiner RM, Mitchell DG, Rao VM, Schweitzer ME. Magnetic resonance imaging of diffuse bone marrow disease. Radiol Clin North Am 31:383–409, 1993.

94. Algra PR, Bloem JL, Tissing H, et al. Detection of vertebral metastases: comparison between MR imaging and bone scintigraphy. Radiographics 11:219–32, 1991.

95. Le Bihan DJ. Differentiation of benign versus pathologic compression fractures with diffusion-weighted MR imaging: a closer step toward the "holy grail" of tissue characterization? Radiology 207:305–7, 1998.

96. Albright JA, Gillespie, TE, Butaud TR. Treatment of bone metastases. Semin Oncol 7:418–33, 1980.

97. Holmes RA. Radiopharmaceuticals in clinical trials. Semin Oncol 20:22–6, 1993.

98. Robinson RG, Preston DF, Baxter KG, et al. Clinical experience with strontium 89 in prostatic and breast cancer patients. Semin Oncol 20:44–8, 1993.

99. Robinson RG, Preston DF, Schiefelbein M, Baxter KG. Strontium 89 therapy for the palliation of pain due to osseous metastases. JAMA 274:420–4, 1995.

100. Krishnamurthy GT, Swailem FM, Srivastava SC, et al. Tin-117m[4+]DTPA: pharmacokinetics and imaging characteristics in patients with metastatic bone pain. J Nucl Med 38:230–7, 1997.

101. Serafini AN, Houston SJ, Resche I, et al. Palliation of pain associated with metastatic bone cancer using samarium-153 lexidronam: a double-blind placebo-controlled clinical trial. J Clin Oncol 16:1574–81, 1998.

102. Rogers CL, Speiser BL, Ram PC, et al. Efficacy and toxicity of intravenous strontium-89 for symptomatic osseous metastases. J Brachytherapy International 14:133–42, 1998.

103. Sciuto R, Maini CL, Tofani A, et al. Radiosensitization with low-dose carboplatin enhances pain palliation in radioisotope therapy with strontium-89. Nucl Med Commun 17:799–804, 1996.

104. Bolger JJ, Dearnaley DP, Kirk D, et al. Strontium-89 (metastron) versus external beam radiotherapy in patient with painful bone metastases secondary to prostatic cancer: preliminary report of a multicenter trial. Semin in Oncol 20(Suppl 2):32–3, 1993.

105. Eary JF, Collins C, Stabin M, et al. Samarium 153-EDTMP biodistribution and dosimetry estimation. J Nucl Med 34:1031–6, 1993.

106. Bayouth JE, Macey DJ, Kasi LP, Fossella FV. Dosimetry and toxicity of samarium-153-EDTMP administered for bone pain due to skeletal metastases. J Nucl Med 35:63–9, 1994.

107. McEwan AJB, Amyotte GA, McGowan DG, et al. A retrospective analysis of the cost-effectiveness of treatment with metastron in patients with prostate cancer metastatic to bone. Eur Urol 26(Suppl 1):26–31, 1994.

108. Alberts AS, Smit BJ, Louw WKA, et al. Dose response relationship and multiple dose efficacy and toxicity of samarium-153-EDTMP in metastatic cancer to bone. Radiother Oncol 43:175–9, 1997.

109. Tong D, Gillick L, Hendrickson FR. The palliation of symptomatic osseous metastases-final results of the study by the Radiation Therapy Oncology Group. Cancer 50:893–9, 1982.

110. Blitzer PH. Reanalysis of the RTOG study of the palliation of symptomatic osseous metastasis. Cancer 55:1468–72, 1985.

111. Rutten EHJM, Crul BJP, van der Toorn PPG, et al. Pain characteristics help to predict the analgesic efficacy of radiotherapy for the treatment of cancer pain. Pain 69:131–5, 1997.

112. Kelly JB, Payne R. Pain syndromes in the cancer patient. Neurol Clin 9:937–53, 1991.

113. Portenoy RK. Cancer pain management. Semin Oncol 20:19–35, 1993.

114. Gaze MN, Kelly CG, Kerr GR, et al. Pain relief and quality of life following radiotherapy for bone metastases: a randomised trial of two fractionation schedules. Radiother Oncol 45:109–16, 1997.

115. Rasmusson B, Vejborg I, Jensen AB, et al. Irradiation of bone metastases in breast cancer patients: a randomized study with 1 year follow-up. Radiother Oncol 34:179–84, 1995.

116. Pool GE, Smith TJ, Staats P, Deer T, Stearns L, Coyne PJ, Rauch R, Boortz-Marx RL, Buchser E. Impact of pain therapy with an implantable drug delivery system on systemic opioid dose and toxicity in cancer patients. Proceedings of ASCO; abstract 1461. J Clin Oncol 21:366a; 2002.

117. Dawson R, Currow D, Stevens G, et al. Radiotherapy for bone metastases: a critical appraisal of outcome measures. J Pain Symptom Manage 17:208–18, 1999.

118. Chandler SS, Sarin R. Single fraction radiotherapy for bone metastases: are all questions answered? Radiother Oncol 52:191–3, 1999.

119. Gillick LS, Goldberg S. Technical Report No 185R. Final analysis of RTOG protocol No. 74-02. Boston: Department of Biostatistics, Sidney Farber Cancer Institute, 1981.

120. Jeremic B, Shibamoto Y, Adimovic L, et al. A randomized trial of three single-dose radiation therapy regimens in the treatment of metastatic bone pain. Int J Radiat Oncol Biol Phys 42:161–7, 1998.

121. Nielsen OS. Palliative radiotherapy of bone metastases: there is now evidence for the use of single fractions. Radiother Oncol 52:95–6, 1999.

122. Niewald M, Tkocz HJ, Abel U, et al. Rapid course radiation therapy vs. more standard treatment: a randomized trial for bone metastases. Int J Radiat Oncol Biol Phys 36:1085–9, 1996.

123. Awan AM, Weichselbaum RR. Palliative radiotherapy. Hematol Oncol Clin North Am 4:1169–81, 1990.

124. Ben-Josef E, Shamsa F, Williams AO, Porter AT. Radiotherapeutic management of osseous metastases: a survey of current patterns of care. Int J Radiat Oncol Biol Phys 40:915–21, 1998.

125. Steenland E, Leer J, van Houselingen H, et al. The effect of a single fraction compared to multiple fractions on painful bone metastases: a global analysis of the Dutch Bone Metastasis Study. Radiother Oncol 52:101–9, 1999.

126. Barton M. Tables of equivalent dose in 2 Gy fractions: a simple application of the linear quadratic formula. Int J Radiat Oncol Biol Phys 31:371–8, 1995.

127. Nielsen OS, Bentzen SM, Sandberg E, et al. Randomized trial of single dose versus fractionated palliative radiotherapy of bone metastases. Radiother Oncol 47:233–40, 1998.

128. Bone Pain Trial Working Party. 8 Gy single fraction radiotherapy for the treatment of metastatic skeletal pain: randomised comparison with a multifraction schedule over 12 months of patient follow-up. Radiother Oncol 52:111–21, 1999.

129. Cole DJ. A randomized trial of a single treatment versus conventional fractionation in the palliative radiotherapy of painful bone metastases. Clin Oncol 1:59–62, 1989.

130. Price P, Hoskin PJ, Easton D, et al. Prospective randomised trial of single and multifraction radiotherapy schedules in the treatment of painful bone metastases. Radiother Oncol 6:247–55, 1986.

131. Barak F, Werner A, Walach N, Horn Y. The palliative efficacy of a single high dose of radiation in treatment of symptomatic osseous metastases. Int J Radiat Oncol Biol Phys 13:1233–5, 1987.

132. Jeremic B, Shibamoto Y, Igrutinovic I. Single 4 Gy re-irradiation for painful bone metastasis following single fraction radiotherapy. Radiother Oncol 52:123–7, 1999.

133. Hoskin PJ, Price P, Easton D, et al. A prospective randomised trial of 4 Gy or 8 Gy single doses in the treatment of metastatic bone pain. Radiother Oncol 23:74–8, 1992.

134. Boogerd W, van der Sande JJ. Diagnosis and treatment of spinal cord compression in malignant disease. Cancer Treat Rev 19:129–50, 1993.

135. Byrne TN. Spinal cord compression from epidural metastases. N Engl J Med 327:614–9, 1992.

136. Grant R, Papadopoulos SM, Greenberg HS. Metastatic epidural spinal cord compression. Neurol Clin 9:825–41, 1991.

137. Maranzano E, Latini P, Checcaglini F, et al. Radiation therapy in metastatic spinal cord compression–a prospective analysis of 105 consecutive patients. Cancer 67:1311–7, 1991.

138. Janjan NA. Radiotherapeutic management of spinal metastases. J Pain Symptom Manage 1:47–56, 1996.

139. Loblaw DA, Laperriere NJ. Emergency treatment of malignant extradural spinal cord compression: an evidence-based guideline. J Clin Oncol 16:1613–24, 1998.

140. Boogerd W. Central nervous system metastasis in breast cancer. Radiother Oncol 40:5–22, 1996.

141. Madsen EL. Painful bone metastasis: efficacy of radiotherapy assessed by the patients: a randomized trial comparing 4 Gy x 6 versus 10 Gy x 2. Int J Radiat Oncol Biol Phys 9:1775–1779; 1983.

142. Paterson AHG. Bone metastases in breast cancer, prostate cancer and myeloma. Bone 8(Supp 1):17–22, 1987.

143. Bunting RW, Boublik M, Blevins FT, et al. Functional outcome of pathologic fracture secondary to malignant disease in a rehabilitation hospital. Cancer 69:98–102, 1992.

144. Heisterberg L, Johansen TS. Treatment of pathologic fractures. Acta Orthop Scand 50:787–90, 1979.

145. Fidler M. Incidence of fracture through metastases in long bones. Acta Orthop Scand 52:623–7, 1981.

146. Oda MAS, Schurman DJ. Monitoring of pathological fracture. In: Stoll BA, Parbhoo S, eds. Bone metastases: monitoring and treatment. New York: Raven, 1983:271–88.

147. Turner S, Marosszeky B, Timms I, Boyages J. Malignant spinal cord compression: a prospective evaluation. Int J Radiat Oncol Biol Phys 26:141–6, 1993.

148. Boogerd W, van der Sande JJ, Kroger R. Early diagnosis and treatment of spinal metastases in breast cancer: a prospective study. J Neurol Neurosurg Psychiatry 55:1188–93, 1992.

149. Peteet J, Tay V, Cohen G, MacIntyre J. Pain characteristics and treatment in an outpatient cancer population. Cancer 57:1259–65, 1985.

150. Wada E, Yamamoto T, Furuno M, et al. Spinal cord compression secondary to osteoblastic metastasis. Spine 18:1380–1, 1993.

151. Cowap J, Hardy JR, A'Hearn R. Outcome of malignant spinal cord compression at a cancer center: implications for palliative care services. J Pain Symptom Manage 19:257–64, 2000.

152. Bach F, Agerlin N, Sorensen JB, et al. Metastatic spinal cord compression secondary to lung cancer. J Clin Oncol 10:1781–7, 1992.

153. Russi EG, Pergolizzi S, Gaeta M, et al. Palliative radiotherapy in lumbosacral carcinomatous neuropathy. Radiother Oncol 26:172–3, 1993.

154. Algra PR, Heimans JJ, Valk J, et al. Do metastases in vertebrae begin in the body or the pedicles? Imaging study in 45 patients. Am J Roentgenol 158:1275–9, 1992.

155. Landmann C, Hunig R, Gratzi O. The role of laminectomy in the combined treatment of metastatic spinal cord compression. Int J Radiat Oncol Biol Phys 24:627–31, 1992.

156. Schiff D, O'Neill BP, Wang CH, O'Fallion JR. Neuroimaging and treatment implications of patients with multiple epidural spinal metastases. Cancer 83:1593–601, 1998.

157. Maranzano E, Latini P, Perrucci E, et al. Short-course radiotherapy (8 Gy × 2) in metastatic spinal cord compression: an effective and feasible treatment. Int J Radiat Oncol Biol Phys 38:1037–44, 1997.

158. Saip P, Tenekeci N, Aydiner A, et al. Response evaluation of bone metastases in breast cancer: value of magnetic resonance imaging. Cancer Invest 17:575–80, 1999.

159. Kim RY, Smith JW, Spencer SA, et al. Malignant epidural spinal cord compression associated with a paravertebral

mass: its radiotherapeutic outcome on radiosensitivity. In J Radiat Oncol Biol Phys 27:1079–83, 1993.

160. Jeremic B, Djuric L, Mijatovic L. Incidence of radiation myelitis of the cervical spinal cord at doses of 5500 cGy or greater. Cancer 68:2138–41, 1991.

161. Wen PY, Blanchard KL, Block CC, et al. Development of Lhermitte's sign after bone marrow transplantation. Cancer 69:2262–6, 1992.

162. Powers BE, Thames HD, Gillette SM, et al. Volume effects in the irradiated canine spinal cord: do they exist when the probability of injury is low? Radiother Oncol 46:297–306, 1998.

163. Fowler JF, Bentzen SM, Bond SJ, et al. Clinical radiation doses for spinal cord: the 1998 international questionnaire. Radiother Oncol 55:295–300, 2000.

164. Lee AWM, Foo W, Law SCK, et al. Total biological effect on late reactive tissues following reirradiation for recurrent nasopharyngeal carcinoma. Int J Radiat Oncol Biol Phys 46:865–72, 2000.

165. Barton R, Kirkbride P. Special techniques in palliative radiaion oncology. J Palliat Med 3:75–83, 2000.

166. Shaw E, Scott C, Souhami L, et al. Single dose radiosurgical treatment of recurrent previously irradiated primary brain tumors and brain metastases: final report of RTOG Protocol 90–05. Int J Radiat Oncol Biol Phys 47:291–8, 2000.

167. Sugimura H, Kisanuki A, Tamura S, et al. Magnetic resonance imaging of bone marrow changes after irradiation. Invest Radiol 29:35–41, 1994.

168. Yankelevitz DF, Henschke C, Knapp PH, et al. Effect of radiation therapy on thoracic and lumbar bone marrow: evaluation with MR imaging. Am J Roentgenol 157:87–92, 1991.

169. Shapiro CL, Keating J, Angell JE, et al. Monitoring therapeutic response in skeletal metastases using dual-energy x-ray absorptiometry: a prospective feasibility study in breast cancer patients. Cancer Invest 17:566–74, 1999.

170. Bach F, Bjerregaard B, Soletormos G, et al. Diagnostic value of cerebrospinal fluid cytology in comparison with tumor marker activity in central nervous system metastases secondary to breast cancer. Cancer 72:2376–82, 1993.

171. Salazar OM, Rubin P, Hendrickson FR, et al. Single dose half-body irradiation for palliation of multiple bone metastases from solid tumors–final Radiation Therapy Oncology Group Report. Cancer 58:29–36, 1986.

172. Poulter CA, Cosmatos D, Rubin P, et al. A report of RTOG 8206: a phase III study of whether the addition of single dose hemibody irradiation to standard fractionated local field irradiation is more effective than local field irradiation alone in the treatment of symptomatic osseous metastases. Int J Radiat Oncol Biol Phys 23:207–14, 1992.

173. Friedland J. Local and systemic radiation for palliation of metastatic disease. Urol Clin North Am 26:391–402, 1999.

174. Silberstein EB. Systemic radiopharmaceutical therapy of painful osteoblastic metastases. Semin Radiat Oncol 10:240–9, 2000.

175. De Klerk JMH, Zonnenberg BA, van het Schip AD, et al. Dose escalation study of rhenium-186 hydroxyethylidene disphosphonate in patients with metastatic prostate cancer. Eur J Nucl Med 21:1114–20, 1994.

176. Murray KJ, Scott C, Zachariah B, et al. Importance of the mini-mental status examination in the treatment of patients with brain metastases: a report from the Radiation Therapy Oncology Group Protocol 91–04. Int J Radiat Oncol Biol Phys 48:59–64, 2000.

177. Kagan AR. Palliation of visceral recurrences and metastases. In: Perez CA, Brady LW, eds. Principles and practice of radiation oncology, 3rd ed. Philadelphia: Lippincott Raven, 1998:2219–26.

178. Langenduk JA, ten Velde GPM, Aaronson NK, et al. Quality of life after palliative radiotherapy in non-small cell lung cancer: a prospective study. Int J Radiat Oncol Biol Phys 47:149–55, 2000.

179. Gressen EL, Werner-Waski M, Cohn J, et al. Thoracic reirradiation for symptomatic relief after prior radiotherapeutic management for lung cancer. Am J Clin Oncol 23:160–3, 2000.

180. Ripamonti C. Management of dyspnea in advanced cancer patients. Support Care Cancer 7:233–43, 1999.

181. List MA, Siston A, Haraf D, et al. Quality of life and performance in advanced head and neck cancer patients on concomitant chemoradiotherapy: a prospective examination. J Clin Oncol 17:1020-8, 1999.

182. Janjan NA, Weissman DE, Pahule A. Improved pain management during radiation therapy for head and neck carcinoma. Int J Radiat Oncol Biol Phys 23:647–52, 1992.

183. Mancini I, Bruera E. Constipation in advanced cancer patients. Support Care Cancer 6:356–64, 1998.

184. Rousseau P. Management of malignant bowel obstruction in advanced cancer: a brief review. J Palliat Med 1:65–72, 1998.

185. Gagnon B, Mancini I, Pereira J, et al. Palliative management of bleeding events in advanced cancer patients. J Palliat Care 14:50–4; 1998.

186. Janjan NA, Breslin T, Lenzi R, et al. Avoidance of Colostomy Placement in Advanced Colorectal Cancer with Twice Weekly Hypofractionated Radiation Plus Continuous Infusion 5-Fluorouracil. J Pain Symptom Manage 20:266–72, 2000.

187. Crane CH, Janjan NA, Abbruzzese JL, et al. Effective pelvic symptom control using initial chemoradiation without colostomy in metastatic rectal cancer. Int J Radiat Oncol Biol Phys 49:107–16, 2001.

188. Duchesne GM, Bolger JJ, Griffiths GO, et al. A randomized trial of hypofractionated schedules of palliative radiotherapy in the management of bladder carcinoma: results of medical research council trial BA09. Int J Radiat Oncol Biol Phys 47:379–88, 2000.

17 Palliative systemic antineoplastic therapy

MICHAEL J. FISCH

The University of Texas M. D. Anderson Cancer Center

Introduction

Palliative care for patients with advanced cancer involves a focus on alleviating suffering and promoting quality of life. Understandably, the emphasis of palliative care is on mitigating the impact of the malignancy on the individual rather than persisting in the direct battle against the cancer. In this shift toward palliation, patients and providers sometimes lose sight of the potential value that anticancer therapy can provide in terms of relieving symptoms and preserving function. Clearly, systemic anticancer therapy such as chemotherapy, hormonal therapy, or other modalities (monoclonal antibody infusion, gene therapy, etc.) may introduce significant risks to the patient with advanced cancer. There are not only the risks related to toxicity, but also the risk of added expense and the loss of valuable time and energy, which are precious and could be used in other ways. The uncertainty regarding outcomes and the complexity involved in making treatment decisions have made the issue of palliative systemic therapy controversial and sometimes a source of conflict between providers and/or family members.

This chapter outlines the therapeutic rationale for considering palliative systemic therapy, including how to select patients who are most likely to benefit from therapy, how to ascertain patient preferences, and how to choose the appropriate time to initiate therapy as well as discontinue it. Basic information related to chemotherapy, hormonal therapy, and monoclonal antibody therapy is also reviewed.

Determining whether palliation is the appropriate goal

The first step in selecting patients for palliative systemic therapy is to ensure that the patient is not being prematurely offered palliative therapy when a realistic chance of cure is still available. Although this is generally not a problem for medical oncologists, it can be difficult for other specialists involved in palliative care to recall which dis-

seminated malignancies are currently considered curable under some circumstances. Table 17.1 summarizes the response categories for first-line systemic therapy for

Table 17.1. *Response categories for first-line systemic therapy for metastatic cancer*

Potentially Curable
Acute myeloid leukemia
Acute lymphocytic leukemia (childhood)
Chronic myelogenous leukemia
Myelodysplastic syndrome
Hodgkin's disease
Non-Hodgkin's lymphoma (some subsets)
Hairy cell leukemia
Germ cell tumors

Highly Responsive (Response Rates ≥ 50%)
Breast carcinoma
Ovarian carcinoma
Androgen-dependent prostate cancer (hormonal therapy)
Small cell lung carcinoma
Lymphoma (some subsets)
Multiple myeloma

Moderately Responsive (Response Rates ≥ 30%)
Non–small-cell lung cancer
Colorectal cancer
Transitional cell carcinoma of the urothelial tract
Sarcoma (some subsets)
Endometrial carcinoma (hormonal therapy)

Poorly Responsive (Response Rates ≤ 30%)
Gastric carcinoma
Esophageal carcinoma
Head and neck carcinoma
Pancreatic carcinoma
Androgen-independent prostate cancer
Osteogenic sarcoma

First-Line Therapy Frequently Omitted (Notoriously Resistant)
Hepatocellular carcinoma
Renal cell carcinoma
Malignant melanoma
Mesothelioma
Anaplastic thyroid cancer
Islet cell and carcinoid tumors

metastatic cancer. With the exception of hairy cell leukemia and germ cell cancer, which are usually cured with conventional dose chemotherapy, each of those diseases has been shown to be amenable to dose-intense chemotherapy (1). There are other malignancies for which cure with systemic therapy is more than an anecdotal event, but it happens in less than 10% of patients. These diseases (such as renal cell carcinoma, malignant melanoma, and bladder cancer) can create significant confusion. Patients may receive inconsistent messages about the intent of therapy, sometimes hearing the word "cure," and on other occasions the intent of therapy may be framed in palliative terms only. Generally speaking, these diseases are sometimes curable for patients in good general health with mostly low bulk disease in favorable sites. Finally, there are some diseases for which complete resection of isolated metastatic sites can produce long-term survival. Examples of this situation include metastatic colorectal cancer with resectable liver metastases, metastatic sarcoma, melanoma, or renal cell carcinoma with resectable lung metastases, and relapsed, refractory germ cell cancer with resectable pulmonary or retroperitoneal metastases. In each instance, the goal is to render the patient disease-free by surgery. When this is feasible, as many as 20% of patients obtain long-term survival.

Performance status is a powerful predictor of prognosis and treatment outcome

Performance status refers to a judgment about the level of activity that a patient exhibits. It is also referred to as *functional status*. In clinical trials of chemotherapy the first and most widely used measure was the Karnofsky Performance Status (KPS) measure described in 1948 as part of an outcome evaluation of nitrogen mustard use in the treatment of unresectable bronchogenic carcinoma (2). Another activity scale was developed in 1960 by Zubrod et al. (3) and later adapted by the Eastern Cooperative Oncology Group (ECOG) for use in various chemotherapy trials (4). These performance status measures are summarized in Table 17.2. For the purpose of most clinical trials, "good" performance status is considered ECOG level 0 or 1 (KPS ≥ 70%), ECOG level 2 is considered borderline, and ECOG levels 3 and 4 are considered "poor" performance status. Measurement of performance status is limited by the fact that it involves only a crude, unidimensional quantification of activity levels, and that it is observer-rated rather than self-reported. Physicians tend to underestimate symptoms and overestimate function relative to patients (5). However, it has the advantage of being easy to administer, and its interpretation is straightforward.

Table 17.2. *Performance status by ECOG and Karnofsky Criteria*

Grade	Description
0	Fully active, able to carry on all predisease performance without restriction (Karnofsky 90–100)
1	Restricted in physically strenuous activity, but ambulatory and able to carry out work of a light or sedentary nature such as light housework or office work (Karnofsky 70–80)
2	Ambulatory and capable of all self-care, but unable to carry out any work activities. Up and about more than 50% of waking hours (Karnofsky 50–60)
3	Capable of only limited self-care, confined to bed or chair more than 50% of waking hours (Karnofsky 30–40)
4	Completely disabled. Cannot carry on any self-care. Totally confined to a bed or chair (Karnofsky 10–20)

Performance status has been shown to be a powerful prognostic factor for outcome in a variety of diseases (6–14) as well as a predictive factor for response to therapy (15). For these reasons, performance status is commonly used as a stratification factor in clinical trials or as an eligibility criterion. For example, one might limit the generalizability of a trial of combination chemotherapy because the trial only included (or only benefited) patients with good performance status. There are also numerous examples where performance status is used as an outcome measure, including in Karnofsky's original article.

Patients with better performance status tend to have fewer symptoms, live longer, and are also more likely to respond to therapy. Patients most likely to benefit from palliative chemotherapy for lung cancer are those with ECOG performance status of 0 or 1 (16). This rule of thumb is potentially applicable for other patients with advanced solid tumors that exhibit only modest response rates (30%–50%) with chemotherapy. Patients with ECOG performance status level 2 are generally less likely to benefit, and those with poor performance status tend to have an unfavorable risk-benefit ratio when offered conventional chemotherapy for advanced cancer compared to supportive care alone. The exceptions to this rule are patients with diseases that have rapid doubling times and are also known to be very sensitive to chemotherapy (response rates ≥ 50%). Patients with leukemia, high- or intermediate-grade lymphoma, gastrointestinal stromal tumors, or untreated small cell lung cancer or breast cancer are often offered chemotherapy despite poor performance status. Such patients will occasionally respond and improve dramatically. These responders are usually debilitated because of the cancer itself, rather than because of severe infection or underlying co-morbid medical problems.

Not all metastatic sites are equal—some respond better than others

For patients with advanced solid tumors, the volume of metastatic disease and the multiplicity of anatomical sites are usually related to both prognosis and likelihood of response to therapy. It is quite easy to understand why a patient with only one small metastatic lesion would have a better prognosis than a patient with bulky disease in multiple sites. However, it is less obvious but equally evident that patients with metastatic disease to visceral sites such as the bone, liver, or brain have a worse prognosis and are less likely to respond to systemic therapy than to patients who have involvement of other sites such as pulmonary parenchyma, lymph nodes, or skin. This observation has been noted for more than 20 years. Early in the cisplatin era, the series of trials using cisplatin-based chemotherapy for germ cell cancer involved the Indiana Staging System (17). This staging system was originally based on the clinical observation that not only was the number of metastatic sites and size of the lesions important to outcome, but also that visceral sites carry a worse prognosis. As such, patients with bone, liver, or brain metastases were considered to have advanced extent disease, regardless of other prognostic factors. Two decades later, this observation was confirmed in a more rigorous, evidence-based update of the staging system for germ cell cancer (18). This same observation has been made in less responsive solid tumors as well (6, 8, 19). Another important observation is that systemic therapy is not as effective for local control of primary sites as it is for treatment of metastatic sites. This fact was also established more than 20 years ago. Using data from the Eastern Clinical Drug Evaluation Program from 1961–1965, Slack and Bross (20) reviewed response and location data from six primary tumor sites and six metastatic sites. With the exception of breast cancer, metastases were found to respond better than the advanced primary tumors from which they were derived (20). New advances in molecular oncology may eventually yield clues to the biological basis of this observation.

The impact of prior therapy—the first shot is the best shot

Medical oncologists never save their bullets—the first attempt at systemic therapy is the best opportunity for achieving a response and accomplishing the treatment goal of prolongation of survival and/or palliation of symptoms. Table 17.1 lists the current expectations for response for first-line systemic therapy for adults with metastatic cancer. Of course, medical oncology is a discipline in rapid evolution. Detection of new molecular targets leads to drug development and discovery. Realistic expectations for response to treatment can shift in any given disease. At this point, the first-line systemic therapy is combination chemotherapy for most malignant disorders. In hormonally responsive tumors such as prostate cancer, breast cancer, endometrial cancer, and papillary thyroid cancer, hormonal manipulations are often appropriate as the initial treatment. Renal cell carcinoma and malignant melanoma are somewhat unusual in that they share a profound resistance to combination chemotherapy and a better response rate to biological therapy using agents such as alpha-interferon or interleukin-2 (alone or in combination). For these tumors, the response rates remain poor despite biological therapy, but there are a small percentage of patients (5%–10%) who achieve a response that can be amazingly durable (measured in years rather than months).

Patients who progress after first-line therapy generally have a poor prognosis, and the expected response rates for further therapy are quite low. Only a handful of metastatic cancers remain at least moderately responsive to second-line systemic therapy (Table 17.3). In this setting, not only are bulk of disease, multiplicity of sites, and type of metastatic sites important for predicting prognosis and response to therapy, but so is the type of response to first-line therapy and the duration of that response. For example, a patient with advanced breast cancer who achieves a complete remission lasting 14 months with adriamycin-based chemotherapy is more likely to respond to second-line therapy than is a patient who failed to respond to initial therapy or whose initial response lasted only 3 months. There are dramatically fewer clinical trials that address the use of systemic therapy in the setting of progression after first-line treatment

Table 17.3. *Metastatic cancers moderately responsive to second-line systemic therapy*

Breast carcinoma
Ovarian carcinoma
Acute and chronic leukemias (most subsets)
Lymphoma (some subsets)
Germ cell carcinoma
Multiple myeloma

compared to studies of previously untreated patients. As such, it can be difficult to formulate realistic expectations when faced with the choice of salvage therapy. As a general rule-of-thumb, most solid tumors show response rates to second-line therapy that are one-third to one-half the response rate in the first line setting. For example, a patient with advanced transitional cell carcinoma of the bladder with lung metastases might have an expected initial response rate with combination chemotherapy of 40%, and with second-line therapy using an active single agent to which the patient has not been exposed, the expected response rate is less than 25% and the expected duration of response is similarly reduced. It is not clear whether this rule-of-thumb applies equally well to patients treated with regimens containing one or more novel agents that are distinct from traditional cytolytic chemotherapy.

Age and its impact on treatment outcome

Most systemic therapy for advanced cancer carries a significant risk of toxicity. The impact of a patient's age on the expected outcome of treatment is an area of controversy in medicine. One can argue against age discrimination in medical oncology based on data available from older prospective studies in cancer patients that show the effect of age is diminished or absent when multiple regression analysis is applied (21,22). More recent prospective studies in cancer patients (23) and in seriously ill hospitalized adults (24) suggest that there is indeed a modest, independent effect of age on treatment outcome. The underlying explanation for this age effect is not only that treatment risk often increases with age, but also that advancing age brings with it other, competing health risks (25). For example, a treatment that can effectively reduce the 5-year mortality rate from a given cancer from 50% to 25% would have less impact on the average, vigorously health 80-year-old man compared to a similarly healthy 70-year-old man.

The effect of competing risks is important to consider when making a decision about whether to pursue systemic anticancer therapy, but once a decision is made to proceed with therapy, older adults with cancer benefit from full-dose treatment. Attempts to modify the dose and schedule of palliative chemotherapy below standard thresholds have had inferior outcomes for older adults. This is evident in a variety of diseases including small-cell lung cancer, non-Hodgkin's lymphoma, and breast cancer.

It is difficult to palliate the asymptomatic patient: the importance of symptom assessment

Combination chemotherapy or other aggressive treatment of cancer may bring palliation by virtue of reducing the burden of tumor. Often, the goal of aggressive therapy is cure or prolongation of survival or local control of vital areas, and palliation is a secondary benefit. Indeed, the toxicity of aggressive therapy may worsen the overall health of the patient on a temporary or permanent basis. Strictly speaking, palliative chemotherapy is treatment that is directed primarily at relief of one or more bothersome symptoms, with the goal of improving the overall quality of life for the patient. Improved survival, objective response, and/or effective local control are possible outcomes of palliative chemotherapy for some individuals, but it is not the primary intent; that is, one might consider the treatment successful with or without any of those outcomes. Within this conceptualization of palliation, palliative chemotherapy would rarely apply to the asymptomatic patient. Likewise, a patient with symptoms that are easily manageable with supportive care is also not ideal for palliative chemotherapy. For example, consider a patient with a head/neck tumor that produced pain that was easily relieved with acetaminophen plus codeine given on an occasional basis. Contrast this with a patient whose tumor appears less alarming, but who requires high doses of opioids to obtain partial relief from the nociception caused by the tumor. The latter patient might benefit from palliative chemotherapy with the intent of providing better analgesia and possibly reducing the dose of opioids and side effects of the opioids. The patient with good pain control on low doses of opioids is much less likely to benefit from chemotherapy with palliative intent. Some oncologists contend that chemotherapy may be appropriate for the patient with manageable symptoms to prevent the worsening of symptoms in the future. This approach is valid for diseases that are potentially curable or highly sensitive to systemic therapy. In addition, for metastatic non–small-cell lung cancer and colorectal cancer, diseases which are in the category of moderately responsive to systemic therapy, there are data to support use of chemotherapy (for patients with good performance status) combined with "best" supportive care (26–28). For most other cancers that are either moderately or poorly responsive to systemic therapy, the use of chemotherapy to prevent or delay the onset of symptoms may be appropriate under some circumstances (depending on the patient's preference style), but the evidence to support a palliative benefit for the average patient is lacking. Likewise, even for specific clinical settings for which use of systemic anticancer therapy is supported based on the available evidence, the program may not be appropriate in an individual patient. This is particularly true when there are important co-morbid conditions, mitigating social circumstances, or strongly held patient and/or family beliefs that such therapy will not be beneficial on this occasion.

Elegant use of palliative chemotherapy requires the oncologist to identify the bothersome symptoms and to assess the symptoms in a disciplined fashion. Without such an assessment, the endpoint of therapy is unclear and the decisions about the duration of therapy become difficult. Pain is the most significant single symptom in patients with advanced cancer, as more than two thirds of outpatients with metastatic cancer report pain or recent analgesia use (29). Guidelines for management of cancer pain stress comprehensive pain assessment at regular intervals, including quantification of pain intensity on a 10-centimeter visual analog scale or a 0 to 10 numerical rating scale (30). A commonly used instrument for pain assessment is the Brief Pain Inventory (31). This instrument was developed in 1983 and has now been validated in at least seven different languages. The rationale for using chemotherapy to improve pain relief is not simply to reduce tumor burden and to alleviate the mechanical effects of the cancer on normal structures, but also to diminish tumor function and production of nociceptive chemicals. For instance, chemotherapy may be indicated to treat hypercalcemia associated with parathyroid hormone-like protein associated with solid tumors such as squamous and renal cell carcinomas.

For most patients with advanced cancer, pain is just one of several co-occurring symptoms (32–38). Prevalent symptoms other than pain include fatigue, anorexia, constipation, and dyspnea. The number of symptoms tends to increase as performance status declines. For example, in a series of hospice inpatients with advanced cancer, the median number of symptoms was 3.6 with KPS over 60, 5.7 for KPS of 30–50, and 7.4 for KPS of 10–20 (33). Because of the complexity involved in trying to assess palliation in patients with multiple symptoms, it is often helpful to use a multidimensional assessment tool rather than an instrument tailored to assess one symptom. Several reliable and valid instruments are feasible for clinical use and for research. Many of these instruments are described as "quality of life" measures, although the appropriateness of that description is sometimes argued (39). Seven of the most widely used multidimensional assessment tools for cancer patients are listed in Table 17.4. Many of these

Table 17.4. *Multidimensional scales for cancer patients*

Edmonton Symptom Assessment Scale—ESAS (102)
Functional Assessment of Cancer Therapy—FACT (103)
European Organization for Research and Treatment of Cancer Quality of Life Questionnaire—EROTC QLQ-C30 (104)
Rotterdam Symptom Check List—RSCL (105)
Cancer Rehabilitation Evaluation Systems—CARES (106)
Functional Living Index Cancer—FLIC (107)
Medical Outcomes Study Short Form—MOS SF (108)
Memorial Symptom Assessment Scale—MSAS (109, 110)

instruments have also been validated in other languages. The Edmonton Symptom Assessment Scale is particularly easy to use in the outpatient setting, as it consists of nine visual analog scales (which are easily understood by most patients), and it involves only one page. Overall, a disciplined and thorough approach to assessment of patients with advanced cancer allows for rational decision making regarding initiation of palliative chemotherapy or the adjustment of the dosage, frequency, or total duration of therapy. Just as performance status is a valuable predictor of prognosis and response to therapy, so is quality of life as measured by a multidimensional assessment (23, 40).

Ascertainment of patient preferences

An important aspect of making treatment decisions regarding palliative chemotherapy is the ascertainment of patient preferences. The patient's preferences with respect to information style, participation in decision making, and care toward the end of life need to be explored in a straightforward manner. Some physicians use a previsit questionnaire to elucidate some of these preferences; others simply ask about these issues in the first one or two visits. In the United States, more than 80% of patients are avid for full disclosure of information about their illness (41, 42), and the courts have upheld that physicians have a duty to tell the truth (although a patient can waive the right to information) (43). Regarding autonomy in decision making, there is a trend for older and sicker patients to desire less autonomy (42, 44), but most patients in the United States prefer some form of shared decision making. Regarding use of chemotherapy, at least in tertiary care settings, older adults are as likely as their younger counterparts to accept chemotherapy, although they are less likely to trade off current quality of life for potential survival benefit (45).

It is often surprising to nurses and physicians how much risk patients are willing to accept for what appears to be a slim chance of benefit. It is often assumed that patients have been misled or misinformed by their oncologists. However, there are data to support the conclusion that cancer patients tend to have a more risk-taking style compared to their oncologists, nurses, radiotherapists, and the general public. Slevin and colleagues (46) explored this issue in a prospective study of 100 cancer patients with newly diagnosed solid tumors who were surveyed about their preferences about a set of hypothetical chemotherapy treatments. Patients' responses were compared to 100 control subjects matched for age, sex, ethnic origin, and occupation. Also surveyed were 60 oncologists, 88 radiotherapists, and 790 general practitioners. Patients were clearly most willing to accept chemotherapy for a small chance of benefit. The median benefit required of cancer patients in order to accept mild chemotherapy was a 1% chance of cure, 1% chance of symptom relief, and a 3-month prolongation of survival. The next most aggressive group were oncologists, who required a median of a 10% chance of cure, 25% chance of symptom relief, and 6 months of survival benefit in order to accept mild chemotherapy. Cancer nurses, general practitioners, radiotherapists, and control subjects were all substantially more conservative than patients or oncologists. In a similar study performed in 1995, Bremnes and colleagues (47) found that patients under age 40 years were willing to accept toxic treatment for median benefits of 7% chance of cure, 8% chance of symptom relief, and 3 months of survival benefit.

One of the most difficult aspects of dealing with patient preferences involves the role of family members in the decision-making process. Most physicians, at one time or another, have faced tensions with families. Common sources of conflict include disagreement between family members and/or between different physicians, misunderstanding of medical facts or misinformation from outside sources, denial of bad news, guilt from family members, issues of secondary gain, and differing religious, ethnic, or cultural traditions (48,49). The most effective physicians are able to develop an ethic of negotiation and accommodation that involves active listening and careful, complete discussion of the diagnosis, prognosis, and treatment options (49).

Finally, any consideration of systemic anticancer therapy for palliation necessarily involves two very difficult tasks: prognostication and bad news breaking. Oncologists or palliative care specialists are often the local experts on prognostication and bad news breaking for advanced cancer patients and may be consulted to deliver that information skillfully. Prognostication refers

to outlining the possible outcomes for the disease and the frequency with which they occur, as well as using characteristics of a particular patient to more accurately predict that patient's eventual outcome (50). Clinicians sometimes use actuarial methods for prediction based on the medical literature. Prognostic information in the cancer literature is most valid when there is a representative and well-defined sample of patients studied at a similar point in the disease, follow-up that is sufficiently long and complete, use of objective and unbiased outcome criteria, and adjustment for important prognostic factors (50). Prognostic data should be reproducible, which means the system is still accurate when it is applied to different patients from the same underlying population. Ideally, these data are also transportable, which refers to a data system that is still accurate when the sample is drawn from a different but related population or when the data are collected by slightly different methods (51).

When there are no applicable or readily available actuarial data, clinicians often use clinical prediction—a method that arises from intuition and personal experience alone. For clinical prediction performed by patients, there tends to be an optimistic bias. In data derived from the Study to Understand Prognoses and Preferences for Outcomes and Risks of Treatments (SUPPORT), the subset of 917 cancer patients were examined and the ROC curve area developed from the patient estimates of survival was only 0.66, with the inaccuracies clearly biased toward more favorable outcomes (52). In this study, patients who expected their survival to exceed 6 months were more likely to seek life-extending therapy (odds ratio 2.6, CI 1.8–3.7), but the actual 6-month survival rate was not improved for those who favored life-extending therapy (52). Physicians' clinical prediction of survival produced an ROC curve area of 0.78, which was significantly superior to patients' predictions (52). Physicians did not demonstrate an optimistic bias; they were as likely to underestimate survival as to overestimate it (53). The mean of the physician estimates was always within 7.5% of the SUPPORT model estimates and always within 9% of actual survival (53). Overall, the ability of physicians or patients to accurately predict survival outcomes is limited. Nevertheless, physicians are in a position to evaluate and use published actuarial data and are generally able to produce superior clinical estimates of survival. Disclosure of prognostic information can be useful for patients and families for making treatment decisions in the setting of advanced malignancy.

How should physicians communicate difficult information about prognosis or limited treatment efficacy without

Table 17.5. *Techniques for breaking bad news*

Control of Session
- Convenient time with no interruptions
- Presence of significant others to comfort the patient
- Quiet, comfortable environment
- Sit forward and use eye contact

Style of Delivery
- Convey warmth, empathy, respect
- Avoid jargon; use simple language
- Provide the news at the patient's pace

Content of the Message
- Ascertain what the patient already knows
- Give a warning shot
- Provide realistic information and time frame
- Acknowledge uncertainty
- Provide realistic hope
- Allow for the patient's emotional reactions
- Ask patients what they want to accomplish
- Recommend taking care of personal and business affairs
- Provide realistic assurance of your continuity
- Allow for questions

eradicating hope in a way that is antipalliative? There have been numerous recent reviews of techniques to break bad news effectively (54–58). General tips for breaking bad news are summarized in Table 17.5. Bad news breaking is a clinical skill that can be developed through practice, and there are a growing number of workshops available to help physicians improve on this aspect of care.

Basic principles of palliative systemic therapy for cancer

The field of medical oncology has grown tremendously since 1970 when there were roughly 13 commonly used drugs that could be divided according to four main mechanisms of action (59). In 1971 medical oncology was recognized as a distinct discipline of the American Board of Internal Medicine, and over the past 30 years there has been significant growth in the number of therapeutic agents available. Table 17.6 outlines the general categories of the most widely used anticancer therapeutics, including biotherapy and hormonal therapy. In the past few years, new therapeutic agents have been introduced, many of which involve "targeted therapy," which takes advantage of newly discovered aspects of basic cellular and cancer biology. Any published list of the anticancer armamentarium is destined to be incomplete in this environment of rapid change in medical oncology. Some of the newer agents are available as oral agents, but most systemic therapy requires parenteral administration. Administration of parenteral systemic therapy requires not only specific cognitive and technical skills acquired by training, but also an appropriate infrastructure. The American Society of Clinical Oncology guidelines for high quality chemotherapy administration includes the following: necessary infrastructure including physical space and equipment, medical and nursing staff with

Table 17.6. *Categories of common anticancer therapeutics*

Classic alkylating agents	*Alkylating agents (other)*	*Vinca alkaloids*	*Miscellaneous*	Flutamide
Cyclophosphamide	Procarbazine	Vincristine	Suramin	Bicalutamide
Ifosfamide	Estramustine	Vinblastine	Asparaginase	Nilutamide
Carmustine	Dacarbazine	Vinorelbine		Liarozole
Lomustine	Temozolomide		*Monoclonal AB*	Aminoglutethimide
Semustine	Mitotane	*Antibiotics*	Rituximab	Ketoconazole
Melphalan	Streptozotocin	Bleomycin	Herceptin	
Chlorambucil		Dactinomycin	Tositumomab	*Androgens*
Busulfan	*Platinum compounds*	Mitomycin-C		Testosterone
Mechlorethamine	Carboplatin		*Biotherapy*	Danazol
Thio-TEPA	Cisplatin	*Newer agents or classes*	Interferon	
	Oxaliplatin	Retinoids	Interleukin-2	*Antiestrogens*
Antimetabolites		Cancer vaccines	Denileukin diftitox	Tamoxifen
5-Fluorouracil	*Taxanes*	Gene therapy		Raloxifene
Methotrexate	Docetaxel	Radiation-response	*Steroids*	Droloxifene
Capecitabine	Paclitaxel	modifiers	Prednisone	Toremifene
Gemcitabine		Antisense oligonu-	Dexamethasone	
Cladribine	*Anthracyclines*	cleotides	Methylprednisolone	*Estrogens*
Cytosine arabinoside	Doxorubicin	Antiangiogenesis targets		Diethylstilbetrol
Fludarabine	Mitoxantrone	Tyrosine kinase	*LHRH analogs*	Ethinyl estradiol
6-Mercaptopurine	Daunorubicin	Inhibitors	Leuprolide	
Deoxycoformycin		Farnesyl transferase	Goserelin	*Progestins*
Hydroxyurea	*Camptothecins*	inhibitors		Megesterol acetate
	Irinotecan	Metalloprotease	*Antiandrogens*	
	Topotecan	inhibitors	Cyproterone acetate	*Aromatase inhibitors*
			Fluoxymesterone	Anastrozole
			Finasteride	Letrozole

training and equipment for managing anaphylaxis and cardiopulmonary resuscitation, 24-hour availability of a treating physician, office support for documentation of records, and administrative support for supplies and compliance with quality assurance standards (60).

Traditional combination chemotherapy regimens are designed by combining active single agents with different mechanisms of action and non-overlapping toxicity in order to produce additive or synergistic antitumor effects without producing excessive toxicity. The appropriate doses and schedule are determined in phase I testing, and the feasibility and activity of the regimen are determined by phase II testing. There is a clear relationship for a dose-response effect for cytotoxic drugs when applied to various experimental tumor systems (61,62). In solid tumors it has been demonstrated that less than optimal dose intensity is suboptimal (63), but high-dose chemotherapy has not been found to improve outcomes (1). Outside of an investigational protocol, most oncologists will use single agents or combination chemotherapy in a dose and schedule that has been previously published. The traditional method of individualizing the dose of chemotherapy is to estimate the body surface area of the patient based on height and weight using the DuBois formula (63). The most active regimens tend to require parenteral administration of therapy. There are nearly a dozen agents available for oral use, and several additional oral agents are currently being investigated. A list of currently available oral chemotherapy agents is shown in Table 17.7. A prospective study of patients with incurable cancer demonstrated that 92 of 103 assessable patients (89%) preferred oral chemotherapy rather than parenteral therapy, but regardless of their initial preference, 70% were not willing to accept a lower response rate and 74% were not willing to accept a shorter duration of response in exchange for the convenience of oral chemotherapy (64).

Evaluation of the patient before and after initiation of systemic therapy

Once a decision has been made to initiate palliative systemic therapy, the next step is to complete a staging evaluation. The purpose of staging the patient is to evaluate the sites of disease so that a determination about response can be made after the therapy is initiated. For the purspose of evaluating solid tumors, lesions that can be measured in two dimensions by physical examination and/or by imaging are considered *measurable*. Lesions that can be detected but not measured (such as areas of uptake on a

Table 17.7. *Chemotherapy agents available orally*

Cyclophosphamide	Mercaptopurine
Chlorambucil	Methotrexate
Melphalan	Etoposide
Busulfan	Capecitabine
Hydroxyurea	Procarbazine
Temozolomide	Imatinib mesylate

bone scan) are considered *evaluable*. A complete staging evaluation involves documenting the areas of measurable and evaluable disease. As mentioned previously, a complete symptom assessment is also important so that the extent of palliation can also be assessed. The next step is to proceed with a therapeutic trial, usually 6 to 8 weeks of systemic therapy, followed by a restaging examination. A *complete response* is defined as the disappearance of all sites of measurable and evaluable disease. A *partial response* refers to a ≥ 50% decrease in the sum of the bidimensionally measurable lesions. When the lesions have decreased or increased by ≤ 25%, the patient is described as having *stable disease.* Finally, patients who develop new sites of disease and/or an increase in measurable disease of ≥ 25% are said to have *progressive disease.* Because many of the newer, targeted therapeutic agents result in disease stabilization rather than tumor shrinkage, new concepts of response are being developed. Some protocols include both traditional responders and those patients with stabilization of their disease for several months as "responders." For hematologic malignancies, response criteria are generally developed for the individual disease. For example, the criteria for response in multiple myeloma are distinct from the criteria for chronic lymphocytic leukemia. Overall, tumor response criteria may vary on the basis of the underlying disease or the nature of the therapeutic agent.

In addition to assessing the response of the tumor, the oncologist is also obliged to assess the pattern and extent of therapy-related toxicities. A common nomenclature for defining toxicities is provided by the National Cancer Institute in the United States, which publishes common toxicity criteria (http://ctep.info.nih.gov/CTC3/default. htm). The toxicities are graded on a scale of 0 (no toxicity) to 4 (severe toxicity). Selected areas of toxicity resulting from specific anticancer agents are shown in Table 17.8. Skillful supportive care during chemotherapy involves the prevention and management of treatment-related side effects. The treating physician must obtain appropriate intravenous access when necessary and should be able to recognize which agents are vesicants in

Table 17.8. *Selected areas of toxicity resulting from anticancer therapy*[a]

Encephalopathy	*Myalgias/arthralgias*	*Renal dysfunction*
Methotrexate	Paclitaxel	Cisplatin
Ifosfamide	Interferon	Carboplatin
Fludarabine	Interleukin-2	Methotrexate
Deoxycoformycin		Carmustine
Interferon alpha	*Fever/chills*	Streptozotocin
Interleukin-2	Interferon alpha	
	Interleukin-2	*Hepatotoxicity*
Cerebellar toxicity	Bleomycin	Methotrexate
Cytarabine	Etoposide	Cytarabine
5-Fluorouracil	Cladribine	Dacarbazine
		L-asparaginase
Ototoxicity		Carmustine
Cisplatin	*Nausea/vomiting*	
	Cisplatin	*Myelosuppression*
Peripheral neuropathy	Carboplatin	Paclitaxel
Cisplatin	Cyclophosphamide	Carboplatin
Paclitaxel	Doxorubicin	Doxorubicin
Docetaxel	Mechlorethamine	Daunorubicin
Vincristine	Streptozotocin	Cyclophosphamide
Vinorelbine	Dacarbazine	Ifosfamide
Vinblastine	Carmustine	Cytarabine
Interleukin-2	Dactinomycin	Mechlorethamine
		Methotrexate
Pulmonary toxicity		Dacarabazine
Bleomycin	*Stomatitis*	5-Fluorouracil
Mitomycin-C	Methotrexate	Fludarabine
Carmustine	Doxorubicin	Chlorambucil
Busulfan	Cytarabine	Melphalan
Cyclophosphamide	5-Fluorouracil	Busulfan
Chlorambucil	Hydroxyurea	Carmustine
Methotrexate		Lomustine
Cytarabine	*Diarrhea*	
Fludarabine	Irinotecan	*Depression*
	5-Fluorouracil	Prednisone
Heart failure	Cyclophosphamide	Dexamethasone
Doxorubicin	Cytarabine	Interferon alpha
Daunorubicin	Methotrexate	Leuprolide
Mitxantrone	Flutamide	Goserelin
5-Fluorouracil	Interleukin-2	Tamoxifen
Interleukin-2	Interferon alpha	
Interferon alpha		

[a] This list is not comprehensive but represents commonly used therapies that cause common toxicities.

the event of an extravasation of the chemotherapy into the skin (Table 17.9). In addition, prevention and treatment of chemotherapy-associated nausea and vomiting are extremely important. Advent of the 5-hydroxytryptamine (5-HT$_3$) blockers has greatly improved the tolerability of combination chemotherapy. In addition, the use of colony-stimulating factors to mitigate the morbidity and mortality resulting from neutropenic infections for selected patients is also a significant advance that has enabled more patients to tolerate palliative chemotherapy. There are readily available consensus statements that provide guidance for appropriate management of chemotherapy-induced emesis as well as neutropenia (65,66). It should be noted that in addition to the objective toxicities experienced by patients on chemotherapy, disruption to the patient and family related to the sheer inconvenience of frequent medical visits (expense, park-

Table 17.9. *Agents that damage skin when they extravasate (vesicants)*

Doxorubicin
Daunorubicin
Vincristine
Vinblastine
Mitomycin-C
Estramustine
Mechlorethamine

ing, need for baby-sitting, missed work, etc.) is often equally burdensome. In a study of 99 chemotherapy patients with a variety of solid tumors, the non-physical "toxicities" constituted 54% of the 15 most severe symptoms as reported by patients (67).

Landmark trials with palliative primary endpoints

The response definitions described provide the basis for generalizing data from clinical trials, and the response labels refer to the activity of the regimen against the tumor itself. Criteria for a palliative response have not been formalized and depend on the pretherapy assessment used. Two famous clinical trials have paved the way for use of palliative primary endpoints in major clinical trials. First, in 1996 Tannock and colleagues (68) reported the results of a randomized trial comparing mitoxantrone plus prednisone to prednisone alone for patients with symptomatic, hormone-resistant prostate cancer. Patients in the trial all had pain and there was an initial adjustment and stabilization of analgesic medication before beginning treatment. The primary endpoint was a palliative response defined as a 2-point decrease in pain as assessed by a 6-point pain scale (without an increase in analgesic medication) maintained for at least 3 weeks. In this trial of 161 patients, the palliative response rate in the mitoxantrone plus prednisone arm was 29% compared to 12% in the prednisone alone arm. This trial provided the basis for the Food and Drug Administration (FDA) to approve mitoxantrone for use in metastatic, hormone-resistant prostate cancer. The FDA also approved another cytolytic agent, gemcitabine, based on a trial with a palliative primary endpoint. In 1997 Burris and colleagues (69) reported the results of a randomized comparison of gemcitabine versus 5-fluorouracil for first-line therapy of advanced pancreatic cancer. Like the Tannock trial, this study included an initial lead-in period for pain stabilization. However, in this trial the measure of palliation was not as straightforward in its interpretation. These investigators defined a specific, new efficacy measure called *clinical benefit response,* which was a composite of measurements of pain (analgesic consumption and pain intensity), plus performance status and weight. To be considered a responder, a patient had to demonstrate an improvement in at least one of the three parameters (sustained for ≥ 4 weeks) without worsening any of the others. The trial included 126 patients and the gemcitabine arm showed a clinical benefit response for 23.8% compared with 4.8% of patients treated with 5-fluorouracil. Overall, these studies demonstrate a growing appreciation for the role of palliative endpoints (particularly pain) in the assessment of patients receiving systemic therapy for advanced, incurable malignancy.

Duration of therapy for the responding patient

For patients who demonstrate a complete or partial response and acceptable toxicity after a 6- to 8-week therapeutic trial of systemic therapy, the oncologist is faced with a decision about the duration of therapy. Although there is sometimes a role for maintenance chemotherapy in hematologic malignancies such as acute or chronic leukemia, most solid tumors are treated with limited chemotherapy. The rule-of-thumb is to treat with two additional cycles of therapy (usually 8 to 12 weeks) after the maximal response has been obtained. This translates into a total of four to eight cycles of therapy for most patients over the course of 4 to 8 months. There have been numerous attempts to use more prolonged courses of chemotherapy for a variety of advanced solid tumors, and that strategy has been decidedly unsuccessful (70–74). In metastatic breast cancer there are two well-known trials that evaluate the value of continuous chemotherapy. A trial involving 308 patients from Australia or New Zealand tested the hypothesis that continuous treatment with chemotherapy may be superior to limited duration therapy. In this trial, the limited duration arm involved only three cycles of chemotherapy. The study arms were not significantly different with respect to overall survival, but the continuous chemotherapy arm produced longer time-to-progression and improved quality of life despite the added therapy-related toxicities (75). Similarly, in 1991, Muss and colleagues (76) studied a cohort of 250 women with previously untreated metastatic breast cancer. The patients were initially treated with six cycles of cyclophosphamide, adriamycin, and 5-fluorouracil, and those with stable or responding disease were then randomized to maintenance chemotherapy with cyclophosphamide, methotrexate, and 5-fluorouracil, or observation until disease progression. In this study the patients receiving maintenance therapy did not improve in overall survival, but they did have increased nausea, vomiting, and mucositis as well as a roughly 6-month prolongation in time-to-progression. Interpretation of these data is limited because both trials may have featured suboptimal initial chemotherapy treatment. The Australian-New Zealand Breast Cancer Trials Group study used only three cycles of initial therapy, whereas most oncologists favor four to eight initial treatment cycles. In the latter study by Muss et al., the dosing algorithm involved up-front dose reductions for patients over 60 years old and those with three or more bone lesions. Again, the trend toward suboptimal initial dosing may have artificially inflated the apparent value of continuous (maintenance) chemotherapy. Nevertheless, maintenance chemotherapy is sometimes pursued for patients with metastatic breast cancer. In contrast to the situation with chemotherapy, it is important to realize that the current standard of care for patients who are responding to hormonal therapy for prostate cancer or breast cancer is to continue that therapy until the time of progression (77,78).

Treatment decisions for stable or progressive disease

The proper duration of therapy can be difficult to ascertain for patients who obtain only stable disease with aggressive therapy, and for those who have discordance between their objective and subjective response. In the case of stable disease, oncologists will often weigh the toxicities and inconvenience of therapy against the change in subjective well-being before recommending whether to continue treatment. For "close-call" situations, the patient's preference is often the determining factor. Sometimes, a patient will experience some degree of disease progression and yet report an improvement in certain symptoms and/or improved overall well-being. It may be argued that the treatment is slowing the rapid pace of progression and that further treatment is worthwhile. Generally speaking, this type of reasoning is worth avoiding. Patients and their physicians share a "good news" bias with respect to the value of therapy. There is often some psychological comfort gained for both the patient and physician for delaying a confrontation with bad news, or for simply finding some possible value in chemotherapy despite frankly progressive disease. The challenge for physicians using palliative chemotherapy is to be prepared to skillfully deliver bad news about disease progression (see Table 17.5), and to direct patients toward other sources of hope rather than continuation of ineffective therapy.

Hormonal therapy: an important treatment for advanced breast and prostate cancer

Hormonal therapy has been part of the anticancer arsenal since 1896 when Beetson first described the effects of oophorectomy on metastatic breast cancer (79). In the 1940s and 1950s, other forms of surgical ablation were developed, including bilateral adrenalectomy and hypophysectomy for breast cancer (80), and bilateral orchiectomy for prostate cancer (81). Currently, hormonal therapy for metastatic breast cancer and prostate cancer is usually accomplished with medical therapies found to be as effective as surgical forms of hormone ablation in randomized trials conducted mostly in the 1970s and 1980s. Although the exact mechanism of action of the various hormonal agents is not completely understood, these agents are known to influence steroid hormones or the steroid receptors found on breast and prostate cancer cells (and sometimes in other tumors) to either arrest cell growth or trigger cell death. There are other diseases for which hormonal therapies are sometimes used (such as endometrial cancer and thyroid cancer), but the following discussion focuses on strategies used to treat breast and prostate cancer.

Hormonal therapy for advanced breast cancer

The most widely used hormonal agent in advanced breast cancer is tamoxifen, a synthetic antiandrogen that has been used since the early 1970s (82). Tamoxifen acts by both estrogen-receptor binding and other non-receptor interactions. The response rate in unselected patients with metastatic breast cancer is in the 30%–40% range, but the response rate varies depending on whether the individual patient has a tumor that expresses estrogen-receptors (ER+) and/or progesterone receptors (PR+). The expected response rate with first-line use of tamoxifen is shown in Table 17.10 (82).

For patients with receptor-positive tumors, second-line therapy is also available. Premenopausal women who fail tamoxifen may be offered ovarian ablation (chemical, surgical, or postirradiation) or an aromatase inhibitor (83). Postmenopausal women are often treated with an aromatase inhibitor. In a phase III trial comparing two doses of the aromatase inhibitor anastrozole to megestrol acetate in women with advanced breast cancer who progressed after prior tamoxifen, the response rate for low-

Table 17.10. *Response to first-line hormonal therapy for advanced breast cancer*

Hormone receptor status	Expected response rate (%)
ER+, PR+	60–70
ER−, PR+	40–45
ER+, PR−	25–30
ER−, PR−	10

or high-dose anastrozole was 34% with the duration of response slightly more than 4 months (84). There are women with receptor-positive tumors who respond for 1 or more years and may benefit from three or four hormonal manipulations (83). Progestins are used for third-line maneuvers, and androgens or estrogens are used for fourth-line therapy in selected patients. Generally speaking, patients who have a major response that is very durable with first- or second-line therapy are the most likely to benefit from subsequent hormonal maneuvers ("winners win and losers lose"). More recently, new understanding about important categories of breast cancer have emerged since HER-2/neu receptor testing has become widely available. In addition, new hormonal agents are being developed. The proper role of hormonal agents in breast cancer continues to evolve rapidly.

Hormonal therapy for metastatic prostate cancer

Like breast cancer, most prostate cancer cells express a steroid receptor. In prostate cancer, the vast majority of prostate cancer cells in untreated patients are "androgen-sensitive," which means that those cells' growth and progression are dependent on continued androgen stimulation. The mainstay of treating metastatic prostate cancer is to proceed with testicular androgen suppression (85). Androgen ablation can be achieved medically by use of gonadotropin-releasing hormone (GnRH) analogs such as goserelin or leuprolide, or surgically by bilateral orchiectomy. Either method will achieve castrate levels of testosterone (< 20 ng/ml), but this effect is rapid with bilateral orchiectomy (i.e., within minutes) and may take several weeks with the GnRH analog. In 5%–10% of patients treated with GnRH analogs, there is a temporary increase in testosterone, which may be associated with a flare of pain or disease progression (including spinal cord compression or ureteral obstruction in vulnerable patients). This flare can be blocked by short-term (roughly 14 day), concomitant use of an antiandrogen. The prostate cancer outcomes are the same overall, regardless of whether a GnRH analog or bilateral orchiectomy is chosen—80%–90% of men achieve disease stabilization, the duration of response is 12 to 18 months, and the median survival is 24 to 36 months (86). In the early 1980s, several trials evaluated the efficacy of treating patients with both a GnRH analog and an antiandrogen (such as flutamide or bicalutamide) to suppress adrenal androgens (87). This strategy of "combined androgen blockade" became the standard of care until a confirmatory phase III trial evaluating bilateral orchiec-

tomy with or without flutamide showed no clinically important survival benefit (86) and inferior quality of life for the patients who received the combination therapy (88). The standard of care for patients who respond to androgen ablation but who later progress is to continue the suppression of the testicular androgens. This is based on retrospective data that show a modest survival advantage for this strategy (89). One possible explanation for these retrospective data is the existence of a persistent subpopulation of androgen-sensitive cells even for patients with disease progression resulting from androgen-insensitive disease.

When patients who have undergone androgen ablation develop disease progression (biochemical, radiographic, or symptomatic), the patient's disease is considered androgen-independent or "hormone-refractory." Management of asymptomatic patients without evident metastatic disease but with rising prostate-specific antigen (PSA) levels is controversial. In this setting, the use of androgen ablation is considered acceptable, but observation alone until progression to symptomatic (or at least radiographically evident) metastatic disease is also considered appropriate management (85).

Patients with symptomatic progression of hormone-refractory prostate cancer (HRPC) may be candidates for additional hormonal maneuvers. The rationale for this strategy is based on the hypothesis that certain clones of the prostate cancer cells may be stimulated to grow by small concentrations of adrenal androgens that could be medically suppressed. For patients who have not already been exposed to antiandrogens as part of a combined androgen blockade strategy, use of an antiandrogen such as flutamide or bicalutamide can produce a biochemical response and sometimes a symptomatic response. However, these second-line hormonal responses are generally short lived, with the median response duration approximately 4 months (90–92). For HRPC patients who progress while they are still receiving an antiandrogen, the first step should be an antiandrogen withdrawal maneuver. Discontinuing the antiandrogen treatment is associated with response in approximately 20% of patients with a median duration of response of 3 to 5 months (93). The mechanism of this withdrawal response is not clear but may be due to mutation of the androgen receptor. Interestingly, the phenomenon of hormone withdrawal responses (as well as flare reactions with initiation of hormonal therapy) are also sometimes seen in patients with breast cancer.

What about prostate cancer patients who progress after androgen ablation and then progress after antiandrogen withdrawal? Other third- and fourth-line hormonal maneuvers have been studied, including use of megestrol acetate, ketoconazole plus hydrocortisone, or hydrocortisone or prednisone alone. In this setting, objective responses are uncommon, and biochemical responses (i.e., a lower PSA) are infrequent and short lived (93).

Toxicity of hormonal therapy

Hormonal manipulations are appealing because the interventions are generally less cumbersome and less toxic than chemotherapy. Nevertheless, there are some disadvantages to using hormonal therapy. First, except for the surgical ablations, these maneuvers often require 1 or 2 months to achieve a satisfactory response. Hormonal therapy is not always well suited for rapidly progressive disease. Second, hormonal agents are associated with potential toxicities that can be burdensome to the patient with advanced cancer. A summary of some common toxicities of hormonal therapy is provided in Table 17.11.

Monoclonal antibody therapy

After many years of being restricted to using either chemotherapy or hormonal therapy as the only classes of systemic agents for advanced cancer, monoclonal antibodies have now emerged as a new class of exciting agents. Although numerous antibodies have been discovered and tested for therapeutic use, the two most widely used agents at this time are trastuzumab and rituximab. These drugs are administered by intravenous infusion on an outpatient basis. The targets, indications, and toxicities of these agents are outlined in Table 17.12.

Rituximab was the first monoclonal antibody to be approved for therapeutic use for any malignancy. The drug was approved by the FDA in November 1997 for management of patients with low-grade B-cell non-Hodgkin's lymphoma who have not responded to standard therapy (94). It is a chimeric, genetically engineered version of a mouse antibody that contains human IgG1 and kappa constant regions with murine variable regions. The pivotal trial involved 166 patients with relapsed low-grade or follicular lymphoma, and use of four weekly intravenous doses of this drug was associated with a 48% response rate, and the median duration of response was 13 months (95). There are now efforts to combine rituximab with chemotherapy (96) and to expand its use to other hematologic neoplasms (97).

Trastuzumab came into the international spotlight in May 1998 after abstract presentations at the annual meeting of the American Society of Clinical Oncology suggested that there was some activity (15% response rate) in a cohort of women with chemotherapy-refractory breast cancer and overexpression of the HER2 growth factor receptor on their tumor (98,99). This drug was approved by the FDA in September 1998. With single-agent activity demonstrated, there are now efforts to combine this agent with chemotherapy in earlier stages of breast cancer (100,101). One concerning observation has been that patients receiving trastuzumab combined with paclitaxel or adriamycin/cyclophosphamide chemotherapy have an increased risk of cardiotoxicity (98,100,101).

Table 17.11. *Toxicities associated with hormonal therapy*

Drug class	Toxicities
Corticosteroids	Hyperglycemia, hypertension, osteoporosis, peptic ulcer, cataracts, proximal muscle weakness, depression, lymphopenia
Estrogens	Nausea/vomiting, sodium retention, breast tenderness, venous thromboembolism, uterine bleeding (women), gynecomastia and loss of libido/impotence (men)
Androgens	Nausea/vomiting, fluid retention, cholestatic jaundice, masculinization (women)
Progestins	Weight gain, fluid retention, withdrawal bleeding (women)
LHRH	Hot flashes, nausea/vomiting, depression, osteoporosis, loss of libido/impotence, and gynecomastia and decreased muscle bulk (men)
Antiandrogens	Nausea/vomiting, hepatotoxicity, diarrhea (flutamide), slow visual adaptation to lighting changes (nilutamide), interstitial pneumonitis (nilutamide), facial flushing (bicalutamide)
Antiestrogens	Hot flashes, vaginal discharge and menstrual irregularities, and uterine cancer
Aromotase inhibitors	Nausea/vomiting, skin rash, lethargy, myalgias

Table 17.12. *Toxicities associated with monoclonal antibody therapy*

Drug (target)	Current indication	Toxicities
Trastuzumab (anti-HER2)	Breast cancer	Infusion-associated symptoms (flu-like), anemia/leukopenia, diarrhea, congestive heart failure (with anthracyclines)
Rituximab (anti-CD20)	Non-Hodgkin's lymphoma	Infusion-associated symptoms (flu-like), urticaria, nausea

Hope for the future

There has been an explosion in knowledge related to cancer biology as the tools of molecular biology have been applied to human cancer. Discoveries related to the basic mechanisms of disease have led to new targets and novel therapeutics. Clinicians and patients alike look forward to still more classes of cancer therapies such as gene therapy and signal transduction blockers. The opportunity to participate in phase I and phase II clinical trials provides not only some element of hope for patients with advanced cancer patients, but also the chance to contribute to scientific advancement for the benefit of future patients.

References

1. Savarese DM, Hsieh C, Stewart FM. Clinical impact of chemotherapy dose escalation in patients with hematologic malignancies and solid tumors. J Clin Oncol 15:2981–95, 1997.
2. Karnofsky DA, Abelmann WH, Craver LF, Burchenal JH. The use of nitrogen mustards in the palliative treatment of carcinoma. Cancer 1:634–56, 1948.
3. Zubrod CG, Schneiderman M, Frei E, et al. Appraisal of methods for study of chemotherapy of cancer in man. Comparative therapeutic trial of nitrogen mustard and triethylene thiophosphoramide. J Chron Dis 11:7–33, 1960.
4. Oken MM, Creech RH, Tormey DC, et al. Toxicity and response criteria of the Eastern Cooperative Oncology Group. Am J Clin Oncol 5:649–55, 1982.
5. Stephens RJ, Hopwood P, Girling DJ, Machin D. Randomized trials with quality of life endpoints: are doctors' ratings of patients' physical symptoms interchangeable with patients' self-ratings? Qual Life Res 6(3):225–36, 1997.
6. Van Glabbeke M, di Paola ED, Mouridsen H, et al. Response to anthracycline based chemotherapy and overall survival in patients with lung metastases from soft tissue sarcoma: a retrospective study of the EROTC soft tisse and bone sarcoma group (STBSG) [abstract]. Proc Am Soc Clin Oncol 18:542a, 1999.
7. Saxman SB, Propert KJ, Einhorn LH, et al. Long-term follow-up of a phase III intergroup study of cisplatin alone or in combination with methotrexate, vinblastine, and doxorubicin in patients with metastatic urothelial carcinoma: a cooperative group study. J Clin Oncol 15:2564–69, 1997.
8. Motzer RJ, Mazumdar M, Bacik J, et al. Survival and prognostic stratification of 670 patients with advanced renal cell carcinoma. J Clin Oncol 17:2530–40, 1999.
9. Coia LR, Minsky BD, Berkey BA, et al. Outcome of patients receiving radiation for cancer of the esophagus: results of the 1992–1994 patterns of care study. J Clin Oncol 18:455–62, 2000.
10. Finkelstein DM, Ettinger DS, Ruckdeshcel JC. Long-term survivors in metastatic non-small cell lung cancer: an Eastern Cooperative Group Study. J Clin Oncol 4:702–9, 1986.
11. Bauman G, Lote K, Larson D, et al. Pretreatment factors predict overall survival for patients with low-grade glioma: a recursive partitioning analysis. Int J Radiat Oncol Biol Phys 45(4):923–9, 1999.
12. Turesson I, Abildgaard N, Ahlgren T, et al. Prognostic evaluation in multiple myeloma: an analysis of the impact of new prognostic factors. Br J Haematol 106(4):1005–12, 1999.
13. Lee CK, Pires de Miranda M, Ledermann JA, et al. Outcome of epithelial ovarian cancer in women under 40 years of age treated with platinum-based chemotherapy. Eur J Cancer 35(5):727–32, 1999.
14. Nicolaides C, Fountzilas G, Zoumbos N, et al. Diffuse large cell lymphomas: identification of prognostic factors and validation of the International Non-Hodgkin's Lymphoma Prognostic Index. A Hellenic Cooperative Oncology Group Study. Oncology 55(5):405–15, 1998.
15. O'Connell JP, Kris MG, Gralla RJ, et al. Frequency and prognostic importance of pretreatment clinical characteristics in patients with advanced non-small cell lung cancer treated with combination chemotherapy. J Clin Oncol 4:1604–14, 1986.
16. Anonymous. Clinical practice guidelines for treatment of unresectable non-small cell lung cancer. J Clin Oncol 15:2996–3018, 1997.
17. Einhorn LH. Treatment of testicular cancer: a new and improved model. J Clin Oncol 8:1777–81, 1990.
18. Mead GM. International consensus prognostic classification for metastatic germ cell tumors treated with platinum based chemotherapy: final report of the International Germ Cell Collaborative Group [abstract]. Proc Am Soc Clin Oncol 14:235, 1995.
19. Bajorin DF, Dodd PM, Mazumdar M, et al. Long-term survival in metastatic transitional cell carcinoma and prognostic factors predicting outcome of therapy. J Clin Oncol 17:3173–81, 1999.
20. Slack NH, Bross ID. The influence of site of metastasis on tumour growth and response to chemotherapy. Br J Cancer 32(1):78–86, 1975.
21. Begg CB, Carbone PP. Clinical trials and drug toxicity in the elderly. The experience of the Eastern Cooperative Oncology Group. Cancer 52(11):1986–92, 1983.
22. Maltoni M, Pirovano M, Scarpi E, et al. Prediction of survival of patients terminally ill with cancer. Results of an Italian prospective multicentric study. Cancer 75(10):2613–22, 1995.
23. Coates A, Porzsolt F, Osoba D. Quality of life in oncology practice: prognostic value of EORTC QLQ-C30 scores in patients with advanced malignancy. Eur J Cancer 33(7):1025–30, 1997.
24. Hamel MB, Davis RB, Teno JM, et al. Older age, aggressiveness of care, and survival for seriously ill, hospitalized older adults. Ann Intern Med 131:721–8, 1999.
25. Welch HG, Albertson P, Nease RF, et al. Estimating treatment benefits for the elderly: the effect of competing risks. Ann Intern Med 124:577–84, 1996.

26. Cunningham D, Pyrhonen S, James RD, et al. Randomized trial of irintoecan plus supportive care versus supportive care alone after fluorouracil failure for patients with metastatic colorectal cancer. Lancet 352:1413–18, 1998.

27. Souquet PJ, Chauvin F, Boissel JP, Bernard JP. Meta-analysis of randomised trials of systemic chemotherapy versus supportive treatment in non-resectable non-small cell lung cancer. Lung Cancer 12(Suppl 1):S147–54, 1995.

28. Scheithauer W, Rosen H, Kornek GV, et al. Randomised comparison of combination chemotherapy plus supportive care with supportive care alone in patients with metastatic colorectal cancer. Br Med J 306(6880):752–5, 1993.

29. Cleeland CS, Gonin R, Hatfield AK, et al. Pain and its treatment in outpatients with metastatic cancer. N Engl J Med 330:592–6, 1994.

30. Grossman SA, Benedetti C, Payne R, Syrjala K. NCCN practice guidelines for cancer pain. Oncology 13:33–44, 1999.

31. Daut R, Cleeland C, Flanery R. Development of the Wisconsin Brief Pain Inventory to assess pain in cancer and other diseases. Pain 17:197–210, 1983.

32. Schuit KW, Sleijfer DT, Meijler WJ, et al. Symptoms and functional status of patients with disseminated cancer visiting outpatient departments. J Pain Symptom Manage 16:290–7, 1998.

33. Morita T, Tsunoda J, Inoue S, Chihara S. Contributing factors to physical symptoms in terminally ill cancer patients. J Pain Symptom Manage 18:338–46, 1999.

34. Coyle N, Adelhart J, Foley KM, Portenoy RK. Character of terminal illness in the advanced cancer patient: pain and other symptoms during the last four weeks of life. J Pain Symptom Manage 5:83–93, 1990.

35. Curtis EB, Krech R, Walsh TD. Common symptoms in patients with advanced cancer. J Palliat Care 7:25–9, 1991.

36. Donnelly S, Walsh D. The symptoms of advanced cancer. Semin Oncol 22(2): (Suppl 3):67–72, 1995.

37. Vainio A, Auvinen A. Prevalence of symptoms among patients with advanced cancer: an international collaborative study. J Pain Symptom Manage 12:3–10, 1996.

38. Ventafridda V, DeConno F, Ripamonti C, et al. Quality of life assessment during a palliative care programme. Ann Oncol 1:415–20, 1990.

39. Leplege A, Hunt S. The problem of quality of life in medicine. JAMA 278(1):47–50, 1997.

40. Cella D, Fairclough DL, Bonomi PB, et al. Quality of life in advanced non-small cell lung cancer: results from Eastern Cooperative Group Study E5592 [abstract #4]. Proc Am Soc Clin Oncol 16, 1997.

41. Degner L, Kristjanson L, Bowman D, et al. Informational needs and decisional preferences in women with breast cancer. JAMA 277:1485–92, 1997.

42. Cassileth B, Zupkis R, Sutton-Smith K, March V. Information and participation preferences among cancer patients. Ann Intern Med 92:832–6, 1980.

43. Annas G. Informed consent, cancer, and truth in prognosis. N Engl J Med 330:223–5, 1994.

44. Ende J, Kazis L, Ash A, Moskowitz M. Measuring patients' desire for autonomy: decision-making and information-seeking preferences among medical patients. J Gen Intern Med 4:23–30, 1989.

45. Yellen SB, Cella DF, Leslie WT. Age and clinical decision making in oncology. J Natl Cancer Inst 86:1766–70, 1994.

46. Slevin ML, Stubbs L, Plant HJ, et al. Attitudes to chemotherapy: comparing views of patients with cancer with those of doctors, nurses, and general public. BMJ 300:1458–60, 1990.

47. Bremnes RM, Andersen K, Wist EA. Cancer patients, doctors and nurses vary in their willingness to undertake cancer chemotherapy. Eur J Cancer 31A(12):1955–9, 1995.

48. Door Goold S, Williams B, Arnold RM. Conflicts regarding decisions to limit treatment: a differential diagnosis. JAMA 283:909–14, 2000.

49. Levine C, Zuckerman C. The trouble with families: towards an ethic of accommodation. Ann Intern Med 130:148–52, 1999.

50. Laupacis A, Wells G, Richardson WS, Tugwell P. Users' guide to the medical literature: how to use an article about prognosis. JAMA 272:234–7, 1994.

51. Justice AC, Covinsky KE, Berlin JA. Assessing the generalizability of prognostic information. Ann Intern Med 130:515–24, 1999.

52. Weeks JC, Cook EF, O'Day SJ, et al. Relationship between cancer patients' predictions of prognosis and their treatment preferences. JAMA 279:1709–14, 1998.

53. Zhong Z, Lynn J. The Lamont/Christakis article reviewed. Oncology 13:1172–73, 1999.

54. Buckman R, Kason Y. How to break bad news: a guide for health care professionals. Baltimore: Johns Hopkins University Press, 1992.

55. Baile WF, Glober GA, Lenzi R, et al. Discussing disease progression and end-of-life decisions. Oncology 13:1021–31, 1999.

56. Ptacek JT, Eberhardt TL. Breaking bad news: a review of the literature. JAMA 276:496–502, 1996.

57. Lo B, Quill T, Tulsky J. Discussing palliative care with patients. Ann Intern Med 130:744–9, 1999.

58. Loprinzi CL, Johnson ME, Steer G. Doc, how much time do I have? J Clin Oncol 18:699–701, 2000.

59. Moore C. Synopsis of clinical cancer. St. Louis: The C.V. Mosby Company, 1970.

60. Anonymous. Criteria for facilities and personnel for the administration of parenteral systemic antineoplastic therapy. J Clin Oncol 15:3416–17, 1997.

61. Frei E, Canellos GP. Dose: a critical factor in cancer chemotherapy. Am J Med 69:585–94, 1980.

62. Schabel FM, Griswold DP, Corbett TH. Increasing the therapeutic response rate to anticancer drugs by applying the basic principles of pharmacology. Cancer 50:1160–7, 1984.

63. Gurney H. Dose calculation of anticancer drugs: a review of the current practice and introduction of an alternative. J Clin Oncol 14:2590–611, 1996.

64. Liu G, Franssen E, Fitch MI, Warner E. Patient preferences for oral versus intravenous palliative chemotherapy. J Clin Oncol 15(1):110–5, 1997.

65. Anonymous. Update of recommendations for the use of hematopoietic colony stimulating factors: evidence-based practice guidelines. J Clin Oncol 14:1957–60, 1996.

66. Gralla RJ, Osoba D, Kris MG, et al. Recommendations for the use of antiemetics: evidence-based, clinical practice guidelines. J Clin Oncol 17:2971–94, 1999.

67. Coates A, Abraham S, Kaye SB, et al. On the receiving end–patient perception of the side effects of cancer chemotherapy. Eur J Cancer Clin Oncol 19:203–8, 1983.

68. Tannock IF, Osoba D, Stockler MR, et al. Chemotherapy with mitoxantrone plus prednisone or prednisone alone for symptomatic hormone-resistant prostate cancer: a Canadian randomized trial with palliative end points (see comments). J Clin Oncol 14(6):1756–64, 1996.

69. Burris HA, Moore MJ, Anderson J, et al. Improvements in survival and clinical benefit with gemcitabine as first line therapy for patients with advanced pancreas cancer: a randomized trial. J Clin Oncol 15:2403–13, 1997.

70. Eltabbakh GH, Piver MS, Hempling RE, et al. Prolonged disease-free survival by maintenance chemotherapy among patients with recurrent platinum-sensitive ovarian cancer. Gynecol Oncol 71(2):190–5, 1998.

71. Sculier JP, Joss RA, Schefer H, et al. Should maintenance chemotherapy be used to treat small cell lung cancer? Eur J Cancer 34(8):1148–55, 1998.

72. Sculier JP, Bureau G, Giner V, et al. Maintenance chemotherapy in patients with small cell lung cancer: results of a randomized trial conducted by the European Lung Cancer Working Party (Meeting abstract). Proc Annu Meet Am Assoc Cancer Res 36:A1220, 1995.

73. Shiromizu K, Matsuzawa M, Takahashi M, Ishihara O. Is postoperative radiotherapy or maintenance chemotherapy necessary for carcinoma of the uterine cervix? Br J Obstet Gynaecol 95(5):503–6, 1988.

74. Levi JA, Thomson D, Sandeman T, et al. A prospective study of cisplatin-based combination chemotherapy in advanced germ cell malignancy: role of maintenance and long-term follow-up. J Clin Oncol 6(7):1154–60, 1988.

75. Coates A, Gebski V, Bishop JF, et al. Improving the quality of life during chemotherapy for advanced breast cancer: a comparison of intermittent and continuous treatment strategies. N Engl J Med 317:1490–95, 1987.

76. Muss HB, Case LD, Richards F, et al. Interrupted versus continuous chemotherapy in patients with metastatic breast cancer. N Engl J Med 325:1342–8, 1991.

77. Kloke O, Klaassen U, Oberhoff C, et al. Maintenance treatment with medroxyprogesterone acetate in patients with advanced breast cancer responding to chemotherapy: results of a randomized trial. Essen Breast Cancer Study Group. Breast Cancer Res Treat 55(1):51–9, 1999.

78. Taylor CD, Elson P, Trump DL. Importance of continued testicular suppression in hormone-refractory prostate cancer. J Clin Oncol 11:2167–72, 1993.

79. Beatson GT. On the treatment of inoperable cases of carcinoma of the mamma: suggestions for a new method of treatment, with illustrative cases. Lancet 2:104–7, 1896.

80. Kimmick G. Current status of endocrine therapy for metastatic breast cancer. Oncology 9:877–90, 1995.

81. Huggins C, Hodges CV. Studies on prostatic cancer; the effect of castration, of estrogen and of androgen injection on serum phosphatase in metastatic carcinoma of the prostate. Cancer Res 1:293, 1941.

82. Honig SF. Hormonal therapy and chemotherapy. In: Harris JR, Lippman ME, Morrow M, Hellman S, eds. Diseases of the breast. Philadelphia: Lippincott-Raven, 1996:674–5.

83. Hortobagyi GN. Treatment of breast cancer. N Engl J Med 339:974–84, 1998.

84. Jonat W, Howell A, Blomqvist C, et al. A randomized trial comparing two doses of the new selective aromatase inhibitor anastrozole (arimidex) with megestrol acetate in postmenopausal patients with advanced breast cancer. Eur J Cancer 32A:404–12, 1996.

85. Logothetis CJ, Millikan R. Update. NCCN practice guidelines for the treatment of prostate cancer. Oncology 13:118–37, 1999.

86. Eisenberger MA, Blumenstein BA, Crawford ED, et al. Bilateral orchiectomy with or without flutamide for metastatic prostate cancer. N Engl J Med 339:1036–42, 1998.

87. Denis L, Murphy GP. Overview of phase III trials on combined androgen blockade in patients with metastatic prostate cancer. Cancer 72:3888–95, 1993.

88. Moinpour CM, Savage MJ, Troxel A, et al. Quality of life in advanced prostate cancer: results of a randomized therapeutic trial. J Natl Cancer Inst 90:1537–44, 1998.

89. Taylor CD, Elson P, Trump DL. Importance of continued testicular suppression in hormone-refractory prostate cancer. J Clin Oncol 11(11):2167–72, 1993.

90. Joyce R, Fenton MA, Rode P, et al. High dose bicalutamide for androgen independent prostate cancer: effect of prior hormonal therapy. J Urol 159:149–53, 1997.

91. Scher HI, Liebertz C, Kelly WK, et al. Bicalutamide for advanced prostate cancer: the natural versus treated history of disease. J Clin Oncol 15:2928–38, 1997.

92. Fowler JE, Pandey P, Seaver LE, Feliz TP. Prostate specific antigen after gonadal androgen withdrawal and deferred flutamide treatment. J Urol 154:448–53, 1995.

93. Small EJ. Second-line hormonal therapy for advanced prostate cancer: a shifting paradigm. J Clin Oncol 15:382–8, 1997.

94. McLaughlin P, Hagemeister FB, Grillo-Lopez AJ. Rituximab in indolent lymphoma: the single-agent pivotal trial. Semin Oncol 26(5 Suppl 14):79–87, 1999.

95. McLaughlin P, Grillo-Lopez AJ, Link BK, et al. Rituximab chimeric anti-CD20 monoclonal antibody therapy for relapsed indolent lymphoma: half of patients respond to a four-dose treatment program. J Clin Oncol 16(8):2825–33, 1998.

96. Czuczman MS. CHOP plus rituximab chemoimmunotherapy of indolent B-cell lymphoma. Semin Oncol 26(5 Suppl 14):88–96, 1999.

97. Hagberg H. Chimeric monoclonal anti-CD20 antibody (rituximab)–an effective treatment for a patient with relapsing hairy cell leukaemia. Med Oncol 16(3):221–2, 1999.

98. Slamon D, Leyland-Jones B, Shak S, et al. Addition of herceptin (humanized anti-HER2 antibody) to first line chemotherapy for HER2 overexpressing metastatic breast cancer markedly increases anticancer activity: a randomized, multinational controlled phase III trial [abstract]. Proc Am Soc Clin Oncol 17:98a, 1998.

99. Cobleigh MA, Vogel CL, Tripathy D, et al. Efficacy and safety of herceptin (humanized anti-HER2 antibody) as a single agent in 222 women with HER2 overexpression who relapsed following chemotherapy for metastatic breast cancer [abstract]. Proc Am Soc Clin Oncol 17:97a, 1998.

100. Trastuzumab and capecitabine for metastatic breast cancer. Med Lett Drugs Ther 40(1039):106–8, 1998.

101. Jerian S, Keegan P. Cardiotoxicity associated with paclitaxel/trastuzumab combination therapy (letter). J Clin Oncol 17(5):1647–8, 1999.

102. Bruera E, Kuehn N, Miller MJ, et al. The Edmonton Symptom Assessment System (ESAS): a simple method for the assessment of palliative care patients. J Palliat Care 7(2):6–9, 1991.

103. Cella DF, Tulsky DS, Gray G, et al. The Functional Assessment of Cancer Therapy scale: development and validation of the general measure. J Clin Oncol 11(3):570–9, 1993.

104. Aaronson NK, Ahmedzai S, Bergman B, et al. The European Organization for Research and Treatment of Cancer QLQ-C30. A quality of life instrument for use in international clinical trials in oncology. J Natl Cancer Inst 85:365–76, 1993.

105. Watson M, Law M, Maguire GP, et al. Further development of a quality of life measure for cancer patients. The Rotterdam Symptom Checklist (revised). Psycho-oncology 1:35–44, 1992.

106. Ganz P, Schag C, Lee J, Sim M. The CARES: a generic measure of health-related quality of life for patients with cancer. Qual Life Res 1:19–29, 1992.

107. Schipper H, Clinch J, McMurray A, Levitt M. Measuring the quality of life of cancer patients: The Functional Living Index-Cancer: development and validation. J Clin Oncol 2:472–83, 1984.

108. Ware JE, Sherbourne CD. The MOS 36-Item Short Form Health Status Survey (SF-36): 1. Conceptual framework and item selection. Med Care 30:473–83, 1992.

109. Chang VT, Hwang SS, Corpion C, Feuerman M. Validation of the Memorial Symptom Assessment Scale short form (MSAS-SF) (Meeting abstract). Proc Am Soc Clin Oncol 16:A165, 1997.

110. Portenoy RK, Thaler HT, Kornblith AB, et al. The Memorial Symptom Assessment Scale: an instrument for the evaluation of symptom prevalence, characteristics and distress. Eur J Cancer 30A(9):1326–36, 1994.

SECTION VI   PAIN IN SPECIAL POPULATIONS

18 Cancer pain management in the chemically dependent patient

STEVEN D. PASSIK, KENNETH L. KIRSH, AND VINCENT MULLEN
University of Kentucky

The challenge

Substance abuse and addiction are difficult problems both theoretically and clinically in pain management and palliative care. Cancer patients with histories of substance abuse are often seen by palliative care specialists, especially in community-based settings. Whereas concurrent drug abuse is problematic, there is the additional problem regarding the diagnosis and understanding of the less obvious aberrant drug-taking behaviors sometimes in evidence in the treatment of patients without formal psychiatric histories of substance use disorders. Such aberrant drug-taking behavior can be manifest, for example, when a patient with advanced disease and pain is unilaterally escalating drug doses, is using medications to treat other symptoms, or when prescriptions are being mishandled. The clinician is challenged to understand such circumstances and plan interventions accordingly. Once these aberrant behaviors are identified the clinician must decide on a course of action that is fair and in the best interests of the patient as well as his or her own career. Thus, the problem of chemical dependence and drug abuse spans a continuum from formal psychiatric disorders to problematic behaviors in the absence of these disorders.

With the pressure of regulatory scrutiny and our duty to treat pain but contain abuse or diversion, clinicians often think that they must avoid being duped by those abusing prescription pain medications at all costs. Thus, although the differential diagnosis of aberrant drug-related behavior is complex, clinicians tend to simplify the assessment of this issue to either addiction or not addiction. It is important to note, however, that the clinician attempting to diagnose the meaning of aberrant drug-related behaviors during pain management may not be correct in the final assessment. The fear of regulatory oversight makes practitioners feel as if they must be right—that if the aberrant behavior presents even the possibility of drug diversion or abuse, they have to "see through" the patient or family's denials to guard against the possibility of being duped. Undertreatment and avoidance of prescribing are often the results. Yet that is not what the existing laws or guidelines on prescribing opioids mandate. The clinician has an obligation to be thorough, thoughtful, logically consistent, and careful (not to mention humane and caring), but not necessarily right. Indeed there are multiple possibilities in the differential diagnosis of aberrant drug-taking behaviors, with criminal intent and diversion being only one of the more remote possibilities. Clinical management can be tailored for the multiple possibilities that might be giving rise to the behaviors noted in the assessment, and asserting control over prescriptions can be accomplished without necessarily terminating entirely the prescribing of controlled substances. In the treatment of cancer pain, clinicians do not have the same latitude not to prescribe simply because of abuse concerns. The clinical, ethical, and even moral imperatives to treat pain in patients can create difficult clinical dilemmas if patients (or someone around them) are abusing medications. These situations defy simple solutions. We attempt to address these issues in the clinical section of this chapter.

Prevalence

Nearly one third of the U.S. population has used illicit drugs, and an estimated 6%–15% have a substance use disorder of some type (1–3). As a result of this high prevalence, and the association between drug abuse and life-threatening diseases such as acquired immunodeficiency syndrome (AIDS), cirrhosis, and some types of cancer (4), problems related to abuse and addiction are commonly encountered in palliative care settings. In diverse patient populations with progressive life-threatening diseases, a remote or current history of drug abuse presents a constellation of physical and psychosocial issues that carry a stigma that can both complicate the management of the underlying disease and undermine palliative therapies. Clearly, the interface between the therapeutic use of potentially abusable drugs and the abuse of these drugs is complex and must be understood to optimize palliative care.

Substance abuse appears to be uncommon among cancer patients. In 1990, only 3% of inpatient and outpatient consultations performed by the Psychiatry Service at Memorial Sloan-Kettering Cancer Center were requested for management of issues related to drug abuse. This prevalence is much lower than the prevalence of substance use disorders in society at large, in general medical populations, and in emergency medical departments (1–3,5,6). This relatively low prevalence was also reported in the Psychiatric Collaborative Oncology Group study, which assessed psychiatric diagnoses in ambulatory cancer patients from several tertiary care hospitals (6). After structured clinical interviews, less than 5% of 215 cancer patients met the Diagnostic and Statistical Manual for Mental Disorders (DSM) 3rd Edition criteria for a substance use disorder (7).

The relatively low prevalence of substance abuse among cancer patients treated in tertiary care hospitals may reflect institutional biases or a tendency for patient underreporting in these settings. Many drug abusers are poor, feel alienated from the health care system, may not seek care in tertiary centers, and may be disinclined to acknowledge the stigmatizing history of drug abuse. For all these reasons, the low prevalence of drug abuse in cancer centers may not be representative of the true prevalence in the cancer population overall. In support of this conclusion, a recent survey of patients admitted to a palliative care unit observed findings indicative of alcohol abuse in more than 25% of respondents. Additional studies are needed to clarify the epidemiology of substance abuse and addiction in cancer patients and others with progressive medical diseases. These patients can be adequately and successfully treated only when their addiction problems are noted by staff and their special needs can be addressed (8).

Current definitions of abuse and addiction

What is meant by the terms *abuse* and *addiction,* and how does that apply to oncology patients? Both epidemiologic studies and clinical management depend on an accepted, valid nomenclature for substance abuse and addiction. Unfortunately, this terminology is highly problematic. The pharmacologic phenomena of tolerance and physical dependence are commonly confused with abuse and addiction. All the definitions applied to medical patients have been developed from addict populations without medical illness, as well as sociocultural considerations, which may lead to mixed messages in the clinical setting. The clarification of this terminology is an essential step in improving the diagnosis and management of substance abuse in the palliative care setting.

Tolerance, a pharmacologic property defined by the need for increasing doses to maintain effects (9,10), has been a particular concern during opioid therapy. Clinicians and patients both commonly express concerns that tolerance to analgesic effects may compromise the benefits of therapy and lead to the requirement for progressively higher, and ultimately unsustainable, doses. Additionally, the development of tolerance to the reinforcing effects of opioids, and the consequent need to increase doses to regain these effects, has been speculated to be an important element in the pathogenesis of addiction (11).

Notwithstanding these concerns, an extensive clinical experience with opioid drugs in the medical context has not confirmed that tolerance causes substantial problems (12,13). Although tolerance to a variety of opioid effects can be reliably observed in animal models (14), and tolerance to non-analgesic effects, such as respiratory depression and cognitive impairment (15), occurs routinely in the clinical setting, analgesic tolerance does not appear to routinely interfere with the clinical efficacy of opioid drugs. Numerous surveys have demonstrated that most patients can attain stable doses associated with a favorable balance between analgesia and side effects for prolonged periods. Dose escalation, when it is required, usually heralds the appearance of a progressive painful lesion (16–22). Unlike tolerance to the side effects of the opioids, clinically meaningful analgesic tolerance appears to be a rare phenomenon and is rarely the cause for dose escalation.

Clinical observation also fails to support the conclusion that analgesic tolerance is a substantial contributor to the development of addiction. It is widely accepted that addicts without a medical disorder may or may not have any of the manifestations of analgesic tolerance. The occasional opioid-treated patient who presents findings consistent with analgesic tolerance typically does so without evidence of abuse or addiction.

Physical dependence is defined solely by the occurrence of a withdrawal syndrome after abrupt dose reduction or administration of an antagonist (9,10,23). Neither the dose nor duration of administration required to produce clinically significant physical dependence in humans is known. Most practitioners assume that the potential for withdrawal exists after opioids have been administered repeatedly for only a few days.

There is great confusion among clinicians about the differences between physical dependence and addiction. Physical dependence, like tolerance, has been suggested to be a component of addiction (24,25), and the avoidance of withdrawal has been postulated to create behavioral contingencies that reinforce drug-seeking behavior (11). These speculations, however, are not supported by experience acquired during opioid therapy for chronic pain. Physical dependence does not preclude the uncomplicated discontinuation of opioids during multidisciplinary pain management of non-malignant pain (26), and opioid therapy is routinely stopped without difficulty in the cancer patients whose pain disappears after effective antineoplastic therapy. Indirect evidence for a fundamental distinction between physical dependence and addiction is even provided by animal models of opioid self-administration, which have demonstrated that persistent drug-taking behavior can be maintained in the absence of physical dependence (27).

Concerns over current definitions

These definitions of tolerance and physical dependence highlight deficiencies in the current nomenclature applied to substance abuse. The terms *addiction* and *addict* are particularly troublesome. In common parlance, these labels are often inappropriately applied to describe both aberrant drug use (reminiscent of the behaviors that characterize active abusers of illicit drugs) and phenomena related to tolerance or physical dependence. Clinicians and patients may use the word *addicted* to describe compulsive drug taking in one patient and nothing more than the possibility for withdrawal in another. It is not surprising, therefore, that patients, families, and staff become very concerned about the outcome of opioid treatment when this term is applied.

The labels *addict* and *addiction* should never be used to describe patients who are only perceived to have the capacity for an abstinence syndrome. These patients must be labeled *physically dependent*. Use of the word *dependent* alone also should be discouraged. Its use fosters confusion between physical dependence and psychological dependence, which is a component of addiction. For the same reason, the term *habituation* should not be used.

Sociocultural influences

By definition, the use of an illicit drug, or the use of a prescription drug without a medical indication, is abuse. If either type of drug is used in a compulsive manner that continues despite harm to the user or others, a diagnosis of addiction may be appropriate. These definitions are consonant with the social and cultural norms of drug taking.

The ability to categorize questionable behaviors (e.g., consuming a few extra doses of a prescribed opioid, particularly if this behavior was not specifically proscribed by the clinician, or using an opioid drug prescribed for pain as a nighttime hypnotic) as outside the social or cultural norm also presupposes that there is certainty about the parameters of normative behavior. In the area of prescription drug use, there are no empirical data that define these parameters. If a large proportion of patients were discovered to engage in a specific behavior, it may be normative, and judgments about deviance would be influenced accordingly. This issue was recently highlighted in a pilot survey performed at Memorial Sloan-Kettering Cancer Center, which revealed that inpatients with cancer harbor attitudes supporting misuse of drugs in the face of symptom management problems and that women with human immunodeficiency virus (at Sloan-Kettering for palliative care) commonly engage in such behaviors (28). The prevalence of such behaviors and attitudes among the medically ill raises concern about its predictive validity as a marker of any diagnosis related to substance abuse. Clearly, there is a need for empirical data that illuminate the prevalence of drug-taking attitudes and behaviors in different populations of medically ill patients.

The importance of social and cultural norms, in turn, raises the inevitable possibility of bias in determinations of aberrancy. Bias against a social group, even if subtle, could influence the willingness of clinicians to label a questionable drug-related behavior as aberrant when performed by a member of that group. Clinical observation suggests that this type of bias is common in the assessment of drug-related behaviors of patients with substance abuse histories. Questionable behaviors by such patients may be promptly labeled as abuse or addiction, even if the drug abuse history was in the remote past. In a similar way, the possibility of bias in the assessment of drug-related behaviors exists for patients who are members of racial or ethnic groups different from that of the clinician.

Disease-related variables

The core concepts used to define addiction may also be problematic as a result of changes induced by a progressive disease. Deterioration in physical or psychosocial functioning caused by the disease and its treatment may be difficult to separate from the morbidity associated with drug abuse. This may particularly complicate efforts to evaluate the concept of "use despite harm," which is critical to the diagnosis of addiction. For example, the nature of questionable drug-related behaviors can be difficult to discern in the patient who develops social withdrawal or cognitive changes after brain irradiation for metastases. Even if impaired cognition is clearly related to the drugs used to treat symptoms, this outcome might only reflect a narrow therapeutic window, rather than a desire on the patient's part for these psychic effects.

The accurate assessment of drug-related behaviors in patients with advanced medical disease usually requires detailed information about the role of the drug in the patient's life. The existence of mild mental clouding or the time spent out of bed may be less meaningful than other outcomes, such as noncompliance with primary therapy related to drug use, or behaviors that jeopardize relationships with physicians, other health care providers, or family members.

An alternative approach for defining abuse and addiction in the medically ill

Previous definitions that include phenomena related to physical dependence or tolerance cannot be the model terminology for medically ill populations who receive drugs with the potential for abuse for legitimate medical purposes. A more appropriate model definition of addiction notes that it is a chronic disorder characterized by "the compulsive use of a substance resulting in physical, psychological or social harm to the user and continued use despite that harm" (29). Although this definition was developed from experience in addict populations without medical illness, it appropriately emphasizes that addiction is fundamentally a psychological and behavioral syndrome. Any appropriate definition of addiction must include the concepts of loss of control over drug use, compulsive drug use, and continued use despite harm.

The spectrum of aberrant drug-taking behavior

Even appropriate definitions of addiction will have limited utility, however, unless operationalized for a clinical setting. The concept of "aberrant drug-related behavior" is a useful first step in operationalizing the definitions of abuse and addiction, and recognizes the broad range of behaviors that may be considered problematic by pre-

scribers. Although the assessment and interpretation of these behaviors can be challenging, as discussed previously, the occurrence of aberrant behaviors signals the need to re-evaluate and manage drug taking, even in the context of an appropriate medical indication for a drug.

If drug-taking behavior in a medical patient can be characterized as aberrant, a differential diagnosis for this behavior can be explored. A true addiction (substance dependence) is only one of several possible explanations. Of the behaviors likely to represent true addiction, some recent research suggests that multiple unsanctioned dose escalations and obtaining opioids from multiple prescribers may have some specific relevance. The challenging diagnosis of pseudo-addiction must be considered if the patient is reporting distress associated with unrelieved symptoms (30). Behaviors such as aggressively complaining about the need for higher doses, or occasional unilateral drug escalations, may be signs that the patient's pain is undermedicated.

Impulsive drug use may also indicate the existence of another psychiatric disorder, which may have therapeutic implications. Patients with borderline personality disorder can express fear and rage through aberrant drug taking and behave impulsively and self-destructively during pain therapy. Passik and Hay (31) reported a case in which one of the more worrisome aberrant drug-related behaviors, forging of a prescription for a controlled substance, was an impulsive expression of fears of abandonment having little to do with true substance abuse in a borderline patient. Such patients are challenging and most often require firm limit setting and careful monitoring to avoid impulsive drug taking. Similarly, patients who self-medicate anxiety, panic, depression, or even periodic dysphoria and loneliness can present as aberrant drug takers. In such instances careful diagnosis and treatment of these additional problems can at times obviate the need for such self-medication. Occasionally, aberrant drug-related behavior appears to be causally related to a mild encephalopathy, with confusion about the appropriate therapeutic regimen, and may be a concern in the treatment of the elderly patient. Low doses of neuroleptic medications, simplified drug regimens, and help with organizing medications can address such problems. Rarely, problematic behaviors indicate criminal intent. Such is the case when patients report pain but intend to sell or divert medications. These diagnoses are not mutually exclusive. A thorough psychiatric assessment is critically important both in the population without a prior history of substance abuse and in the population of known abusers, who have a high prevalence of psychiatric co-morbidity (32).

In assessing the differential diagnosis for drug-related behavior, it is useful to consider the degree of aberrancy. The less aberrant behaviors (such as aggressively complaining about the need for medications) are more likely to reflect untreated distress of some type, rather than addiction-related concerns. Conversely, the more aberrant behaviors (such as injection of an oral formulation) are more likely to reflect true addiction. Although empirical studies are needed to validate this conceptualization, it may be a useful model when evaluating aberrant behaviors.

Empirical validation of the aberrant drug-taking concept

The spectrum of aberrant drug-taking has been used as a heuristic to guide the assessment of problematic drug taking in several recent studies. The studies performed to date all involve small samples, although they have shown the utility of the spectrum concept as an assessment tool yielding important implications for clinicians.

The first study examined the relationship between aberrant drug-taking behaviors and compliance-related outcomes in patients with a history of substance abuse receiving chronic opioid therapy for nonmalignant pain. Dunbar and Katz (33) examined outcomes and drug taking in a sample of 20 patients with diverse histories of drug abuse who underwent a year of chronic opioid therapy. During the year of therapy, 11 patients were compliant with the drug regimen and 9 were not. The authors examined patient characteristics and aberrant drug-taking behaviors that differentiated the two groups. The patients who did not abuse the therapy were current abusers of alcohol only (or had remote histories of polysubstance abuse), were in a solid drug-free recovery as evidenced by participation in 12-step programs, and had good social support. The patients who abused the therapy were polysubstance abusers, were not participating in 12-step programs, and had poor social support. The specific behaviors that were recorded more frequently by those who abused the therapy were unscheduled visits and multiple phone calls to the clinic, unsanctioned dose escalations, and obtaining opioids from more than one source.

A second study examined the relationship between aberrant drug taking and the presence or absence of a psychiatric diagnosis of substance use disorder in pain patients. Compton and colleagues (34) studied 56 patients seeking pain treatment in a multidisciplinary pain program whom were referred for "problematic drug taking." The patients all underwent structured psychiatric interviews, and the sample was divided between those qualifying and not qualifying for psychiatric diagnoses of substance use disorders. The authors then examined the subjects' reports of aberrant drug-taking behaviors on a structured interview assessment. Patients who qualified for a substance use disorder diagnosis were more likely to have engaged in unsanctioned dose escalations, received opioids from multiple sources, and have the subjective impression of loss of control of their prescribed medications.

Passik and colleagues (28) examined the self-reports of aberrant drug-taking attitudes and behaviors in samples of patients with cancer ($n = 52$) and AIDS ($n = 111$) on a questionnaire designed for the purposes of the study. Reports of past drug use and abuse were more frequent than present reports in both groups. Current aberrant drug-related behaviors were seldom reported. Attitude items, however, revealed that patients would consider engaging in aberrant behaviors, or would possibly excuse them in others, if pain or symptom management were inadequate. It was found that aberrant behaviors and attitudes were endorsed more frequently by the women with AIDS than by the cancer patients. Overall, patients greatly overestimated the risk of addiction in pain treatment. Experience with this questionnaire suggests that both cancer and AIDS patients respond in a forthcoming fashion to drug-taking behavior questions and describe attitudes and behaviors, which may be highly relevant to the diagnosis and management of substance use disorders.

Such studies will help us to better understand the particular diagnostic meanings of the various behaviors so that clinicians may recognize which are the true "red flags" in a given population. Far too often anecdotal accounts shape the way clinicians view these behaviors. Some behaviors are regarded almost universally as aberrant despite limited systematic data to suggest that this is the case. Consider for example the patient who requests a specific pain medication, or a specific route or dose. Such behavior often reflects a patient who is knowledgeable about what works for him or her but is almost always greeted with suspicion on the part of practitioners. Other behaviors may be found to be common in nonaddicts, and although they seem aberrant based on their face value, they may have little predictive value for true addiction. That many non-addicted cancer patients might use anxiolytic medications prescribed for a friend or other, this more than likely reflects the undertreatment and underreporting of anxiety in oncology patients rather than true addiction.

Addiction in patients with drug abuse history versus those without

It is interesting to explore the differences inherent in populations of patients with and without histories of drug abuse or addiction. The following discussion highlights the known differences while also highlighting the fact that we have a long way to go regarding true understanding of the effects of prior abuse and addiction on current treatments for oncology patients.

Abuse and addiction in patients without prior drug abuse

An extensive worldwide experience in the long-term management of cancer pain with opioid drugs has demonstrated that opioid administration in cancer patients with no prior history of substance abuse is only rarely associated with the development of significant abuse or addiction (35–48). Indeed, concerns about addiction in this population are now characterized by an interesting paradox: Although the lay public and inexperienced clinicians still fear the development of addiction when opioids are used to treat cancer pain, specialists in cancer pain and palliative care widely believe that the major problem related to addiction is not the phenomenon itself, but rather the persistent undertreatment of pain driven by inappropriate fear that it will occur (49).

The very sanguine experience in the cancer population has contributed to a desire for a reappraisal of the risks and benefits associated with the long-term opioid treatment of chronic non-malignant pain (22,50). The traditional view of this therapy is negative; and early surveys of addicts, which noted that a relatively large proportion began their addiction as medical patients administered opioid drugs for pain (51–53), provided some indirect support for this perspective. The most influential of these surveys recorded a history of medical opioid use for pain in 27% of white male addicts and 1.2% of black male addicts (53).

Surveys of addict populations, however, do not provide a valid measure of the addiction liability associated with chronic opioid therapy in populations without known abuse. Prospective patient surveys are needed to define this risk accurately. The Boston Collaborative Drug Surveillance Project evaluated 11,882 inpatients who had no prior history of addiction and were administered an opioid while hospitalized; only four cases of addiction could be identified subsequently (54). A national survey of burn centers could find no cases of addiction in a sample of more than 10,000 patients without prior drug abuse history who were administered opioids for pain (55), and a survey of a large headache clinic identified opioid abuse in only three of 2369 patients admitted for treatment, most of whom had access to opioids (56).

Other data suggest that the typical patient with chronic pain is sufficiently different from the addict without painful disease that the risk of addiction during therapy for pain is likely to be low. For example, surveys of cancer patients and postoperative patients indicate that euphoria, a phenomenon believed to be common during the abuse of opioids, is extremely uncommon after administration of an opioid for pain; dysphoria is observed more typically, especially in those who receive meperidine (57). Although the psychiatric co-morbidity identified in addict populations could be an effect, rather than a cause, of the aberrant drug taking, the association suggests the existence of psychological risk factors for addiction. The likelihood of genetically determined risk factors for addiction also has been suggested by a twin study that demonstrated a significant concordance rate for aberrant drug-related behaviors (58).

Favorable surveys of pain patients are not definitive, of course, and there are conflicting data collected by multi-disciplinary pain management programs that suggest a high prevalence of abuse behaviors among the patients referred to this setting (59–67). The latter surveys, however, are subject to an important selection bias, and this bias, combined with other methodological concerns (68), limit the generalizability of these data to the large and heterogeneous populations with chronic non-malignant pain.

Overall, the evidence generally supports the view that opioid therapy in patients with chronic pain and no history of abuse or addiction can be undertaken with a very low risk of these adverse outcomes. This is particularly so in the older patient, who has had ample time to reveal a propensity for abuse. There is no substantive support for the view that large numbers of individuals with no personal or family history of abuse or addiction, no affiliation with a substance-abusing subculture, and no significant premorbid psychopathology, will develop abuse or addiction de novo when administered potentially abusable drugs for appropriate medical indications.

The inaccurate perception that opioid therapy inherently yields a relatively high likelihood of addiction has encouraged assumptions that are not supportable in populations without a prior history of substance abuse. For example, agonist–antagonist opioid analgesics are less likely to be abused by addicts than pure mu agonist opioids, and, consequently, some clinicians view the agonist–antagonist drugs as safer in terms of addiction liability. There is no evidence for this conclusion in populations without drug abuse histories, and the extensive experience with long-term opioid therapy for cancer pain and chronic non-malignant pain (19–22,69–71) has relied on the pure mu agonists. Similarly, there is a common perception that short-acting oral opioids and opioids delivered by the parenteral route carry a relatively greater risk of addiction because of the rapid delivery of the drug. Again, these perceptions derive from observations in the healthy addict population and are not relevant to the treatment of pain in medical patients with no prior history of substance abuse.

Risk of abuse and addiction in populations with current or remote drug abuse

There is little information about the risk of abuse or addiction during, or after, the therapeutic administration of a potentially abusable drug to patients with a current or remote history of abuse or addiction. Anecdotal reports have suggested that successful long-term opioid therapy in patients with cancer pain or chronic non-malignant pain is possible, particularly if the history of abuse or addiction is remote (33,72,73). Indeed, a recent study showed that patients with AIDS-related pain were able to be successfully treated with morphine whether they were substance users or non-users. In fact, the major difference found was that substance users required considerably more morphine to reach stable pain control (74). However, a modicum of caution should be used. For example, although there is no empirical evidence that the use of short-acting drugs or the parenteral route is more likely to lead to problematic drug-related behaviors than other therapeutic approaches, it may be prudent to avoid such therapies in patients with histories of substance abuse.

Clinical management

Out-of-control aberrant drug taking among palliative care patients (with or without a prior history of substance abuse) represents a serious and complex clinical occurrence. Perhaps the more difficult situations involve the patient who is actively abusing illicit or prescription drugs or alcohol concomitantly with medical therapies. The following guidelines can be useful whether the patient is an active drug abuser, has a history of substance abuse, or is not complying with the therapeutic regimen. The principles outlined help the clinician establish structure, control, and monitoring so that they can prescribe freely and without prejudice.

Multidisciplinary approach

A multidisciplinary team approach is recommended for the management of substance abuse in the palliative care setting. Mental health professionals with specialization in the addictions can be instrumental helping palliative care team members develop strategies for management and patient treatment compliance, although often such professionals are not readily available. Providing care to these patients can lead to feelings of anger and frustration among staff. Such feelings can unintentionally compromise the level of patient care surrounding the patient's pain management and contribute to feelings of isolation and alienation by the patient. A structured multidisciplinary approach can be effective in helping the staff better understand the patient's needs and develop effective strategies for controlling pain and aberrant drug use simultaneously. Staff meetings can be helpful in establishing treatment goals, facilitating compliance, and coordinating the multidisciplinary team.

Assessment

The first member of the medical team (frequently a nurse) to suspect problematic drug taking or a history of drug abuse should alert the patient's palliative care team, thus beginning the multidisciplinary assessment and management process (75). A physician should assess the potential of withdrawal or other pressing concerns and begin involving other staff (i.e., social work and/or psychiatry) to begin planning management strategies. Obtaining as detailed as possible a history of duration, frequency, and desired effect of drug use is crucial. Frequently, clinicians avoid asking patients about substance abuse out of fear that they will anger the patient or that they are incorrect in their suspicion of abuse. However, such approaches will likely contribute to continued problems with treatment compliance and frustration among staff. Empathic and truthful communication is always the best approach. The use of a careful, graduated interview approach can be instrumental in slowly introducing the assessment of drug use. This approach entails starting the assessment interview with broad questions about the role of drugs (e.g., nicotine, caffeine) in the patient's life and gradually becoming more specific in focus to include illicit drugs. Such an approach is helpful in reducing the denial and resistance that the patient may express. This interviewing style also assists in the detection of co-existing psychiatric disorders that may be present. Co-morbid psychiatric disorders can significantly contribute to aberrant drug-taking behavior. Studies suggest that 37%–62% of alcoholics have one or more co-existing psychiatric disorders. Anxiety, personality disorders, and mood disorders are the most commonly encountered (76,77). The assessment and treatment of co-morbid psychiatric disorders can greatly enhance management strategies and reduce the risk of relapse. The patient's desired effects from illicit drugs can often be a clue to co-morbid psychiatric disorders (i.e., drinking to quell panic symptoms).

Development of a multidisciplinary treatment plan

Drug abuse is often a chronic, progressive disorder. Therefore, development of clear treatment goals is essential for the management of drug abuse. Team members should not expect a complete remission of the patient's substance use problems. The distress of coping with a life-threatening illness and the availability of prescription drugs for symptom control can make complete abstinence an unrealistic goal (78). Rather, a harm reduction approach should be used that aims to enhance social support, maximize treatment compliance, and contain harm done through episodic relapse. The following guidelines are recommended for the management of patients with a substance disorder. The clinician should first establish a relationship based on empathic listening and accept the patient's report of distress. Second, it is important to use non-opioid and behavioral interventions when possible, but not as substitutes for appropriate pain management. Third, the team should consider tolerance, route of administration, and duration of action when prescribing medications for pain and symptom management. Preexisting tolerance should be taken into account for patients who are actively abusing drugs or are being maintained on methadone maintenance programs. Failure to realize any existing tolerance can result in undermedication and contribute to the patient's attempts to self-medicate. Fourth, the team should consider using longer acting drugs (e.g., fentanyl patch and sustained-release opioids). The longer duration and slow onset may help to reduce aberrant drug-taking behaviors when compared to the rapid onset and increased frequency of dosage associated with short-acting drugs. Finally, the team should make plans to frequently reassess the adequacy of pain and symptom control.

Outpatient management plan

There are a number of strategies for promoting treatment compliance in an outpatient setting. A written contract between the team and patient helps to provide structure to the treatment plan, establishes clear expectations of the roles played by both parties, and outlines the consequences of aberrant drug taking. The inclusion of spot urine toxicology screens in the contract can be useful in maximizing treatment compliance. Expectations regarding attendance of clinic visits and the management of one's supply of medications should also be stated. For example, the clinician may wish to limit the amount of drug dispensed per prescription and make refills contingent on clinic attendance. When prescribing pain medications and other drugs used in symptom control, the patient should receive clear instructions about the parameters of responsible drug taking. This practice can help to reduce hesitation by the clinician to prescribe drugs for pain and symptom management if the patient manages their medication responsibly. The clinician should consider requiring the patient to attend 12-step programs, and have the patient document attendance as a condition for ongoing prescribing. With the patient's consent, the clinician may wish to contact the patient's sponsor and make him or her aware that the patient is being treated for chronic illness that requires medications (e.g., opioids). This action will reduce the potential for stigmatization of the patient as being non-compliant with the ideals of the 12-step program. Finally, the team should involve family members and friends in the treatment to help bolster social support and functioning. Becoming familiar with the family may help the team identify family members who are themselves drug abusers and who may potentially divert the patient's medications and contribute to the patient's noncompliance. Mental health professionals can help family members with referrals to drug treatment and co-dependency groups as a way to help the patient receive optimal medical care.

Inpatient management plan

Management of a patient with substance abuse problems, who has been admitted to the hospital for treatment of a life-threatening illness, expands on the guidelines discussed above for the outpatient settings. These guidelines aim to promote the safety of patient and staff, contain manipulative behaviors by patients, enhance the use of medication appropriately used for pain and symptom management, and communicate an understanding of pain and substance abuse management. The first point of order is to discuss the patient's drug use in an open manner. In addition, it is necessary to reassure the patient that steps will be taken to avoid adverse events such as drug withdrawal. For certain specific situations, such as for preoperative patients, patients should be admitted several days in advance when possible for stabilization of the drug regimen. Also, it is important to provide the patient with a private room near the nurses' station to aid in monitoring the patient and to discourage attempts to leave the hospital for the purchase of illicit drugs. Further, the team should require visitors to check in with nursing staff before visitation. In some cases, it may be necessary to search the packages of visitors to stem the patient's access to drugs. As a final point, the team should collect daily urine specimens for random toxicology analysis and frequently reassess pain and symptom management.

As with pain regimens, management approaches should be tailored to reflect the clinician's assessment of the severity of drug abuse. Open and honest communication between the clinician and patient reassures the patient that these guidelines were established in the patient's best interest. In some cases, these guidelines may fail to curtail aberrant drug use despite repeated interventions by staff. At that point, the patient should be considered for discharge, but our experience suggests that this is only necessary in the most recalcitrant of cases. The clinician should involve members of the staff and administration for discussion about the ethical and legal implications of such a decision.

Urine toxicology screening

Clinicians must control and monitor drug use in all patients, a daunting task in some active abusers. In some cases, a major issue is compliance with treatments for the underlying disease, which may be so poor that the substance abuse actually shortens life expectancy by preventing the effective administration of primary therapy. Prognosis may also be altered by the use of drugs in a manner that negatively interacts with therapy or predisposes to other serious morbidity. The goals of care can be difficult to define when poor compliance and risky behavior appear to contradict a reported desire for disease-modifying therapies.

Urine toxicology screening has the potential to be a useful tool to the practicing clinician both for diagnosing potential abuse problems and for monitoring patients with an established history of abuse. However, recent

work suggests that urine toxicology screens are used infrequently in tertiary care centers (79). In addition, when they are ordered, documentation tends to be inconsistent regarding the reasons for ordering as well as any follow-up recommendations based on the results. Indeed, the survey found that nearly 40% of the charts surveyed listed no reason for obtaining the urine toxicology screen, and the ordering physician could not be identified nearly 30% of the time. Staff education efforts can help to address this finding and may ultimately make urine toxicology screens a vital part of treating pain in oncology patients.

Methadone

Oral methadone is a potent opioid that can be successfully used to replace oral morphine in cancer patients (80), although continuous assessment is necessary for proper use to avoid toxic effects (81). Practitioners should consider using methadone with cancer patients because of several of its outstanding properties. First, it is well absorbed enterally and, therefore, retains much of its analgesic efficacy. Second, it readily crosses the blood-brain barrier and has a relatively long half-life of approximately 25 hours, with analgesia effects of approximately 6 to 8 hours. Third, tolerance develops rather slowly, leading to more persistent effects. Finally, it is associated with less irritability compared to shorter-acting, euphoria-producing opioids (82). Equianalgesic doses are usually found in ratios from 1:1 to 4:1 for oral morphine to methadone (83).

It must be stressed that patients who have addiction concerns with opioids such as heroin cannot be given methadone as both an analgesic and as part of a maintenance recovery program. Practitioners sometimes assume that patients receiving methadone from a maintenance program do not need further pain medication, but this is simply not true (84). Methadone-maintained patients in a recovery program are fully tolerant of the maintenance dose and experience no analgesic effect from the methadone (85). Therefore, other routes of pain control must be explored (see next section).

Patients in recovery

Pain management with patients in recovery presents a unique challenge. Depending on the structure of the recovery program (e.g., Alcoholics Anonymous, methadone maintenance programs), a patient may fear ostracism from the program's members or may have an increased fear regarding susceptibility to readdiction. The first choice should be to explore non-opioid therapies with these patients, which may require referral to a pain center (84). Alternate therapies may include the use of non-steroidal anti-inflammatory drugs, anticonvulsants (for neuropathic components), biofeedback, electrical stimulation, neuroblative techniques, acupuncture, or behavioral management. If the pain condition is so severe that opioids are required, care must be taken to structure their use with opioid management contracts, random urine toxicology screens, and occasional pill counts. If possible, attempts should be made to include the patient's recovery program sponsor to garner cooperation and aid in successful monitoring of the condition.

The patient with advanced disease

Managing addiction problems in patients with advanced cancer is labor intensive and can be extremely time consuming. This begs the question as to why a clinician should even bother to address such a complex health concern in the patient with advanced disease. In fact, many clinicians might opt to overlook a patient's use of illicit substances or alcohol entirely, viewing these behaviors as a last source of pleasure for the patient. However, addiction has a deleterious impact on palliative care efforts. Proper addiction management plays an important part in the success of palliative efforts to reduce suffering. Addiction behaviors may result in increased stress for family members, family concern over the misuse of medication, a potential for masking symptoms important for the patient's care, poor compliance with the treatment regimen, and diminished quality of life. Complete abstinence may not be a realistic outcome, but reduction in use can certainly have positive effects for the patient (86).

Conclusion

Although the most prudent actions on the part of clinicians cannot obviate the risk of all aberrant drug-related behavior, clinicians must recognize that virtually any drug that acts on the central nervous system and any route of drug administration can be abused. The problem does not lie in the drugs themselves. Effective management of patients with pain who engage in aberrant drug-related behavior necessitates a comprehensive approach that recognizes the biological, chemical, social, and psychiatric aspects of substance abuse and addiction, and provides practical means to manage risk, treat pain effectively, and ensure patient safety.

An accepted nomenclature for abuse and addiction, and an operational approach to the assessment of patients with medical illness, are prerequisite to an accurate definition of risk in populations with and without histories of substance abuse. Unfortunately, there are limited data relevant to risk assessment in the medically ill. Most data relate to the risk of serious abuse or addiction during long-term opioid treatment of chronic pain in patients with no history of substance abuse. There is almost no information about the risk of less serious aberrant drug-related behaviors, the risk of these outcomes in populations that do have a history of abuse, or the risk associated with the use of drugs with the potential for abuse other than opioids.

References

1. Colliver JD, Kopstein AN. Trends in cocaine abuse reflected in emergency room episodes reported to DAWN. Publ Health Rep 106:59–68, 1991.
2. Groerer J, Brodsky M. The incidence of illicit drug use in the United States, 1962–1989. Br J Addiction 87:1345, 1992.
3. Regier DA, Meyers JK, Dramer M, et al. The NIMH epidemiologic catchment area program. Arch Gen Psychiatry 41:934, 1984.
4. Wells KB, Golding JM, Burnam MA. Chronic medical conditions in a sample of the general population with anxiety, affective, and substance use disorders. Am J Psychiatry 146:1440, 1989.
5. Burton RW, Lyons JS, Devens M, Larson DB. Psychiatric consults for psychoactive substance disorders in the general hospital. Gen Hosp Psychiatry 13:83, 1991.
6. Derogatis LR, Morrow GR, Fetting J, et al. The prevalence of psychiatric disorders among cancer patients. JAMA 249:751, 1983.
7. American Psychiatric Association. Diagnostic and Statistical Manual for Mental Disorders—III. Washington, DC: American Psychiatric Association, 1983.
8. Bruera E, Moyano J, Seifert L, et al. The frequency of alcoholism among patients with pain due to terminal cancer. J Pain Symptom Manage 10(8):599, 1995.
9. Dole VP. Narcotic addiction, physical dependence and relapse. N Engl J Med 286:988, 1972.
10. Martin WR, Jasinski DR. Physiological parameters of morphine dependence in man–tolerance, early abstinence, protracted abstinence. J Psychiatr Res 7:9, 1969.
11. Wikler A. Opioid dependence: mechanisms and treatment. New York: Plenum Press, 1980.
12. Portenoy RK. Opioid tolerance and efficacy: basic research and clinical observations. In: Gebhardt G, Hammond D, Jensen T, eds. Proceedings of the VII World Congress on Pain. Progress in pain research and management, vol. 2. Seattle: IASP Press, 1994:595.

13. Foley KM. Clinical tolerance to opioids. In: Basbaum AI, Besson J-M, eds. Towards a new pharmacotherapy of pain. Chichester: John Wiley & Sons, 1991:181.

14. Ling GSF, Paul D, Simantov R, Pasternak GW. Differential development of acute tolerance to analgesia, respiratory depression, gastrointestinal transit and hormone release in a morphine infusion model. Life Sci 45:1627, 1989.

15. Bruera E, Macmillan K, Hanson JA, MacDonald RN. The cognitive effects of the administration of narcotic analgesics in patients with cancer pain. Pain 39:13, 1989.

16. Twycross RG. Clinical experience with diamorphine in advanced malignant disease. Int J Clin Pharmacol Ther Toxicol 9:184, 1974.

17. Kanner RM, Foley KM. Patterns of narcotic drug use in a cancer pain clinic. Ann NY Acad Sci 362:161, 1981.

18. Chapman CR, Hill HF. Prolonged morphine self-administration and addiction liability: evaluation of two theories in a bone marrow transplant unit. Cancer 63:1636, 1989.

19. France RD, Urban BJ, Keefe FJ. Long-term use of narcotic analgesics in chronic pain. Soc Sci Med 19:1379, 1984.

20. Portenoy RK, Foley KM. Chronic use of opioid analgesics in non-malignant pain: report of 38 cases. Pain 25:171, 1986.

21. Urban BJ, France RD, Steinberger DL, et al. Long-term use of narcotic-antidepressant medication in the management of phantom limb pain. Pain 24:191, 1986.

22. Zenz M, Strumpf M, Tryba M. Long-term opioid therapy in patients with chronic nonmalignant pain. J Pain Symptom Manage 7:69, 1992.

23. Redmond DE, Krystal JH. Multiple mechanisms of withdrawal from opioid drugs. Ann Rev Neurosci 7:443–78, 1984.

24. World Health Organization. Technical report no. 516, youth and drugs. Geneva: World Health Organization, 1973.

25. American Psychiatric Association. Diagnostic and Statistical Manual for Mental Disorders—IV. Washington, DC: American Psychiatric Association, 1994.

26. Halpern LM, Robinson J. Prescribing practices for pain in drug dependence: a lesson in ignorance. Adv Alcohol Substance Abuse 5:184, 1985.

27. Dai S, Corrigal WA, Coen KM, Kalant H. Heroin self-administration by rats: influence of dose and physical dependence. Pharmacol Biochem Behav 32:1009, 1989.

28. Passik S, Kirsh, KL, McDonald M, et al. A pilot survey of aberrant drug-taking attitudes and behaviors in samples of cancer and AIDS patients. J Pain Symp Manage 19:274–86, 2000.

29. Rinaldi RC, Steindler EM, Wilford BB, Goodwin D. Clarification and standardization of substance abuse terminology. JAMA 259:555, 1988.

30. Weissman DE, Haddox JD. Opioid pseudoaddiction–an iatrogenic syndrome. Pain 36:363, 1989.

31. Passik S, Hay J. Symptom control in patients with severe character pathology. In: Portenoy RK, Bruera E, eds. Topics in palliative care, vol. 3. New York: Oxford University Press, 1998:213–27.

32. Khantzian EJ, Treece C. DSM-III psychiatric diagnosis of narcotic addicts. Arch Gen Psychiatry 42:1067, 1985.

33. Dunbar SA, Katz NP. Chronic opioid therapy for nonmalignant pain in patients with a history of substance abuse: report of 20 cases. J Pain Symptom Manage 11:163, 1996.

34. Compton P, Darakjian J, Miotto K. Screening for addiction in patients with chronic pain with "problematic" substance use: evaluation of a pilot assessment tool. J Pain Symptom Manage 16:355–63, 1998.

35. Jorgensen L, Mortensen M-J, Jensen N-H, Eriksen J. Treatment of cancer pain patients in a multidisciplinary pain clinic, The Pain Clinic 3:83, 1990.

36. Cleeland C, Gonin R, Hatfield A, et al. Pain and its treatment in outpatients with metastatic cancer. N Engl J Med 330:592, 1994.

37. Moulin DE, Foley KM. Review of a hospital-based pain service. In: Foley KM, Bonica JJ, Ventafridda V, eds. Advances in pain research and therapy, vol. 16, Second International Congress on Cancer Pain. New York: Raven Press, 1990:413.

38. Schug SA, Zech D, Dorr U. Cancer pain management according to WHO analgesic guidelines. J Pain Symptom Manage 5:27, 1990.

39. Schug SA, Zech D, Grond S, et al. A long-term survey of morphine in cancer pain patients. J Pain Symptom Manage 7:259, 1992.

40. Ventafridda V, Tamburini M, DeConno F. Comprehensive treatment in cancer pain. In: Fields HL, Dubner R, Cervero F, eds. Advances in pain research and therapy, vol. 9, Proceedings of the Fouth World Congress on Pain. New York: Raven Press, 1985:617.

41. Ventafridda V, Tamburini M, Caraceni A, et al. A validation study of the WHO method for cancer pain relief. Cancer 59:850, 1990.

42. Walker VA, Hoskin PJ, Hanks GW, White ID. Evaluation of WHO analgesic guidelines for cancer pain in a hospital-based palliative care unit. J Pain Symptom Manage 3:145, 1988.

43. World Health Organization. Cancer pain relief and palliative care. Geneva: World Health Organization, 1990.

44. Health and Public Policy Committee, American College of Physicians. Drug therapy for severe chronic pain in terminal illness. Ann Intern Med 99:870, 1983.

45. Agency for Health Care Policy and Research, U.S. Dept. of Health and Human Services: Clinical Practice Guideline Number 9: Management of Cancer Pain. Washington, DC: U.S. Dept. of Health and Human Services, 1994.

46. Ad Hoc Committee on Cancer Pain, American Society of Clinical Oncology. Cancer pain assessment and treatment curriculum guidelines. J Clin Oncol 10:1976, 1992.

47. American Pain Society. Principles of analgesic use in the treatment of acute pain and cancer pain. Skokie, IL: American Pain Society, 1992.

48. Zech DFJ, Grond S, Lynch J, et al. Validation of the World Health Organization guidelines for cancer pain relief: a 10 year prospective study. Pain 63:65, 1995.

49. Breitbart W, Rosenfeld BD, Passik SD, et al. The undertreatment of pain in ambulatory AIDS patients. Pain 65:239, 1996.

50. Portenoy RK. Opioid therapy for chronic nonmalignant pain: current status. In: Fields HL, Liebeskind JC, eds. Progress in pain research and management, vol. 1. Pharmacological approaches to the treatment of chronic pain: new concepts and critical issues. Seattle: IASP Publications, 1994:247.

51. Kolb L. Types and characteristics of drug addicts. Ment Hygiene 9:300, 1925.

52. Pescor MJ. The Kolb classification of drug addicts. Washington, DC: Public Health Rep Suppl 155, 1939.

53. Rayport M. Experience in the management of patients medically addicted to narcotics. JAMA 156:684, 1954.

54. Porter J, Jick H. Addiction rare in patients treated with narcotics. N Engl J Med 302:123, 1980.

55. Perry S, Heidrich G. Management of pain during debridement: a survey of U.S. burn units. Pain 13:267, 1982.

56. Medina JL, Diamond S. Drug dependency in patients with chronic headache. Headache 17:12, 1977.

57. Kaiko RF, Foley KM, Grabinski PY, et al. Central nervous system excitatory effects of meperidine in cancer patients. Ann Neurol 13:180, 1983.

58. Grove WM, Eckert ED, Heston L, et al. Heritability of substance abuse and antisocial behavior: a study of monozygotic twins reared apart. Biol Psychiatry 27:1293, 1990.

59. Buckley FP, Sizemore WA, Charlton JE. Medication management in patients with chronic non-malignant pain. A review of the use of a drug withdrawal protocol. Pain 26:153, 1986.

60. Finlayson RD, Maruta T, Morse BR. Substance dependence and chronic pain: profile of 50 patients treated in an alcohol and drug dependence unit. Pain 26:167, 1986.

61. Finlayson RD, Maruta T, Morse BR, Martin MA. Substance dependence and chronic pain: experience with treatment and follow-up results. Pain 26:178, 1986.

62. Maruta T. Prescription drug-induced organic brain syndrome. Am J Psychiatry 135:376, 1978.

63. Maruta T, Swanson DW, Finlayson RE. Drug abuse and dependency in patients with chronic pain. Mayo Clin Proc 54:241, 1979.

64. Maruta T, Swanson DW. Problems with the use of oxycodone compound in patients with chronic pain. Pain 11:389, 1981.

65. McNairy SL, Maruta T, Ivnik RJ, et al. Prescription medication dependence and neuropsychologic function, Pain 18:169, 1984.

66. Ready LB, Sarkis E, Turner JA. Self-reported vs. actual use of medications in chronic pain patients. Pain 12:285, 1982.

67. Turner JA, Calsyn DA, Fordyce WE, Ready LB. Drug utilization pattern in chronic pain patients. Pain 12:357, 1982.

68. Fishbain DA, Rosomoff HL, Rosomoff RS. Drug abuse, dependence, and addiction in chronic pain patients. Clin J Pain 8:77, 1992.

69. Gardner-Nix JS. Oral methadone for managing chronic non-malignant pain. J Pain Symptom Manage 11:321, 1996.

70. Tennant FS, Uelman GF. Narcotic maintenance for chronic pain: medical and legal guidelines. Postgrad Med 73:50–73, 1983.

71. Taub A. Opioid analgesics in the treatment of chronic intractable pain of non-neoplastic origin. In: Kitahata LM, Collins D, eds. Narcotic analgesics in anesthesiology. Baltimore: Williams & Wilkins, 1982:199.

72. Macaluso C, Weinberg D, Foley KM. Opioid abuse and misuse in a cancer pain population [abstract]. J Pain Symptom Manage 3:S24, 1988.

73. Gonzales GR, Coyle N. Treatment of cancer pain in a former opioid abuser: fears of the patient and staff and their influence on care. J Pain Sypmtom Manage 7:246, 1992.

74. Kaplan R, Slywka J, Slagle S, et al. A titrated analgesic regimen comparing substance users and non-users with AIDS-related pain. J Pain Symptom Manage 19:265–71, 2000.

75. Lundberg JC, Passik SD. Alcohol and cancer: a review for psycho-oncologists. Psychooncology 6:253–66, 1997.

76. Regier DA, Farmer ME, Rae DS, et al. Comorbidity of mental disorders with alcohol and other drug abuse. JAMA 264:2511–18, 1978.

77. Penick E, Powell B, Nickel E, et al. Comorbidity of lifetime psychiatric disorders among male alcoholics. Alcoholism. Clin Exp Res 18:1289–93, 1994.

78. Passik SD, Portenoy RK. Substance abuse issues in palliative care. In: Berger A et al., eds. Principles and practice of supportive oncology. Philadephia: Lippincott Raven Publishers, 1998.

79. Passik S, Schreiber J, Kirsh KL et al. A chart review of the ordering and documentation of urine toxicology screens in a cancer center: do they influence patient management? J Pain Symptom Manage 19:40–4, 2000.

80. Ripamonti C, Groff L, Brunelli D, et al. Switching from morphine to oral methadone in treating cancer pain: what is the equianalgesic dose ratio? J Clin Oncol 16:3216–21, 1998.

81. Mercadante S, Sapio R, Serretta M, et al. Patient-controlled analgesia with oral methadone in cancer pain: preliminary report. Ann Oncol 7:613–7, 1996.

82. Carrol E, Fine E, Ruff R, et al. A four-drug pain regimen for head and neck cancers. Laryngoscope 104:694–700, 1994.

83. Lawlor P, Turner K, Hanson J, et al. Dose ratio between morphine and methadone in patients with cancer pain: a retrospective study. Cancer 82:1167–73, 1998.

84. Parrino M. State methadone treatment guidelines. TIPS 1 DHHS Publication No. (SMA). NIAMH Press, Washington, DC: 93–1991.

85. Zweben JE, Payte JT. Methadone maintenance in the treatment of opioid dependence: a current perspective. West J Med 152:588–99, 1990.

86. Passik S, Theobald D. Managing addiction in advanced cancer patients: why bother? J Pain Symptom Manage 19:229–34, 2000.

19 Cancer pain in children

JOHN J. COLLINS
The Children's Hospital at Westmead

CHARLES B. BERDE
Harvard University Medical School

Introduction

In their experience of illness related to cancer or its treatment, children and their families report that pain is one of the most feared symptoms. Fortunately, the majority of children can achieve adequate analgesia if current pain management techniques are used. It is the rare pediatric patient who develops intractable pain. The World Health Organization (WHO) has established the principles of pain management and palliative care as a universal standard of care for all children with cancer. *Cancer Pain Relief and Palliative Care in Children* (1) is a guideline that contains information on the assessment of pain in children, analgesics and adjuvant analgesics, and the principles of non-pharmacological methods of pain control in children undergoing painful procedures (1). Recent data suggest there is room for improvement in pain management for children with cancer (2).

Epidemiology of cancer pain in children

Pain is a common symptom experienced by children with cancer. A cohort of 149 British and Australian children with cancer 7 to 12 years old were surveyed about their experience of symptoms during the preceding 48 hours (3). Approximately one third had experienced pain in the previous 48 hours. Over half of this group had pain in the medium to severe range, and one third were highly distressed by their experience (3).

As part of the validation study of Memorial Symptom Assessment Scale 10–18 (4) (MSAS 10–18), information was acquired about symptom characteristics from a heterogeneous population of children with cancer ages 10 to 18 years at Memorial Sloan-Kettering Cancer Center, New York. Children were asked about their symptoms during the preceding week. Pain was the most prevalent symptom in the inpatient group (84.4%) and was rated as moderate to severe by 86.8% and highly distressing ("quite a bit to very much") by 52.8% of these children. Pain was experienced by 35.1% of the outpatient group, of whom 75% rated it as being moderate to severe and 26.3% rated distress as "quite a bit to very much."

Pain is one of many symptoms experienced by children with cancer. Tables 19.1 (3) and 19.2 (4) demonstrate symptom prevalence, severity, frequency, and distress in children with cancer ages 7 to 12 years and 10 to 18 years, respectively. These tables give an insight into the complexity of symptoms experienced by children with cancer. Although pain is a highly prevalent symptom in children with cancer, its assessment must be considered in the light of highly symptomatic children with complex disease processes.

Table 19.1. *Prevalence and characteristics of symptoms determined by The Memorial Symptom Assessment Scale (7–12) in children with cancer aged 7–12 (N = 149) (3)*

		Degree when symptom was present		
Symptom	Overall prevalence (%)	Intensity medium amount– a lot (%)	Frequency medium amount– almost all the time (%)	Distress medium amount– very much (%)
Fatigue	53 (35.6)	51	64	5
Pain	48 (32.4)	56	54	37
Insomnia	46 (31.1)	—	—	39
Itchiness	37 (25.0)	56	54	38
Lack of appetite	33 (22.3)	—	52	12
Worry	30 (20.1)	43	43	30
Nausea	20 (13.4)	—	45	65
Sadness	15 (10.1)	60	53	50

Table 19.2. *Prevalence and characteristics of symptoms determined by The Memorial Symptom Assessment Scale in 159 children with cancer (3)*

Symptom	Overall prevalence (%)	Degree when symptom was present		
		Intensity Mod-VSev (%)[a]	Frequency A lot-AA (%)[b]	Distress QB-VM (%)[c]
Lack of energy	49.7	61.6	40.9	21.4
Pain	49.1	80.8	35.9	39.1
Feeling drowsy	48.4	64.0	34.6	18.6
Nausea	44.7	65.9	23.0	36.6
Cough	40.9	47.7	23.0	16.3
Lack of appetite	39.6	66.3	39.7	35.8
Feeling sad	35.8	59.6	17.5	39.5
Feeling nervous	35.8	56.1	28.1	23.7
Worrying	35.4	66.1	28.6	27.2
Feeling irritable	34.6	63.6	30.9	34.7
Itching	32.7	63.4	26.9	30.0
Insomnia	30.8	66.7	38.8	58.7
Dry mouth	30.8	50.2	28.6	23.5
Hair loss	28.3	66.6	NE	48.0
Vomiting	27.7	67.5	32.3	45.2
Weight loss	26.6	51.2	NE	25.0
Dizziness	24.5	55.2	15.4	21.9
Numbness/ tingling in hands/feet	22.0	36.0	28.6	22.7
Sweating	20.3	54.7	25.0	10.8
Lack of concentration	20.1	54.5	21.9	30.3
Diarrhea	20.1	61.6	28.1	33.4
Skin changes	20.1	68.8	NE	46.1
Dyspnea	16.5	69.1	22.9	29.1
Change in the way food tastes	16.5	77.0	NE	30.4
"I don't look like myself"	15.8	76.0	NE	49.5
Mouth sores	13.9	59.2	NE	56.9
Difficulty swallowing	12.6	83.8	56.3	76.1
Constipation	13.8	81.8	NE	25.9
Swelling of arms/legs	12.0	52.8	NE	8.0
Problems with urination	6.3	90.0	70	45.0

Abbreviation: NE, not evaluated.
[a] Percentage moderate to very severe.
[b] Percentage a lot to almost always.
[c] Percentage quite a bit to very much.

A study of children with cancer at the National Cancer Institute (5) found that 62% presented to their practitioners with some sort of pain complaint before their diagnosis of cancer. Pain had been present in these children for a median of 74 days before definitive anticancer treatment was begun. The duration of pain experienced was not related to the extent of disease. After initiation of therapy directed at their cancer, the majority of children had resolution of their pain, with the rare patient requiring long-term opioid therapy. Children with hematological malignancy had a shorter duration of pain than children with solid tumors (5).

Children with brain tumors often present with either symptoms of raised intracranial pressure or abnormal neurological signs (6). Most children with spinal cord tumors present with a complaint of pain (7). Spinal cord compression resulting from metastatic disease is more likely to occur late in a child's illness (8). Back pain is more common than abnormal neurological signs as a sign of spinal cord compression in children (8).

Tumor-related pain may recur at the time of relapse or when the tumor becomes resistant to treatment. As cancer treatment protocols evolve for each patient, treatment-related, rather than tumor-related, causes of pain predominate (9,10). Causes of treatment-related pain include postoperative pain, mucositis, phantom limb pain, infection, antineoplastic therapy-related pain, and procedure-related pain (e.g., bone marrow aspiration, needle puncture, lumbar puncture, removal of central venous line).

At relapse, or at a time when tumors become resistant to treatment, tumor-related pain frequently recurs. Palliative chemotherapy and radiation may be instituted as modalities of pain control in terminal pediatric malignancy, depending on tumor type and sensitivity. Severe pain in terminal pediatric malignancy occurs more commonly in patients with solid tumors metastatic to the central or peripheral nervous system (11).

A variety of non-malignant chronic pain conditions have been encountered in young adult survivors of childhood cancer (12). The etiology of these conditions include causalgia of the lower extremity, phantom limb pain, avascular necrosis, and mechanical pain resulting from failure of bony union after tumor resection, and rarely postherpetic neuralgia. Some patients require opioids for the management of non-malignant pain.

Non-pharmacological methods of pain control in children with cancer

Non-pharmacological methods of pain control include techniques categorized as physical (e.g., heat, cold stimulation, electrical nerve stimulation, acupuncture, massage), behavioral (e.g., relaxation, biofeedback, modeling, desensitization, art and play therapy), or cognitive (e.g., distraction, imagery, thought stopping, hypnosis, music therapy), according to whether the intervention is focused on modifying an individual's sensory perception, behaviors, thoughts, and coping abilities (13).

A quiet, calm environment conducive to reducing stress and anxiety, in a location separate from the child's room, is recommended. Providing a description of the steps of a given procedure and of the sensations experienced are common interventions for the preparation of a child about to undergo a painful procedure. Unexpected stress is more anxiety provoking than anticipated or predictable stress (14,15).

The decision to use a psychologic or pharmacologic approach or both depends on the knowledge of the procedure, skill of the practitioner, understanding of the child, and expectations of pain and anxiety for the particular child undergoing that procedure (14). The choice of which non-pharmacological method to use is based on the child's age, behavioral factors, coping ability, fear and anxiety, and the type of pain experienced (13). Cognitive-behavioral techniques are commonly used to decrease distress and enhance a child's ability to cope.

Distraction techniques have been shown to be effective methods of stress reduction in children undergoing painful procedures. One study enlisted the support of parents and showed not only reduction in the children's behavioral distress but also lowering of the parent's anxiety (16). Several investigators have examined and shown the effectiveness of cognitive-behavioral interventions. These have included preparatory information, relaxation, imagery, positive coping statements, modeling, and/or behavioral rehearsal (16–18). The effectiveness of hypnosis in the reduction of pain and anxiety during lumbar puncture and bone marrow aspiration in children with cancer has been confirmed by several reports (19–22).

Pharmacological management of cancer pain in children

Analgesic studies in children with cancer

Recent data indicate that pain is often not adequately assessed and treated effectively in the pediatric cancer population (2,23). Improvement in pediatric pain management will be dependent, in part, on advances in analgesic therapeutics. Unfortunately, few analgesic studies have been performed in children with cancer (24).

One difficulty in performing analgesic studies in children with cancer relates to the heterogeneous nature of pain in this population. In comparison to the adult population, it is less likely that children will have chronic cancer pain as a result of their tumor because solid tumors are less common in children than in the adult population. In addition, children often receive therapies directed at the control of their tumors until very late in the course of their illness. Consequently, these epidemiological and treatment variables make it less likely that a subpopulation of children with cancer exists that has a chronic, stable pattern of pain amenable to evaluation in an analgesic drug trial.

Most analgesic studies performed in children with cancer have been performed with small numbers of subjects (24). In addition, few were controlled studies, and only recently has self-report been used as an outcome measure for analgesic effectiveness. There have been no controlled clinical trials of adjuvant analgesics in pediatrics. Although the pharmacokinetic and the major pharmacodynamic properties of most opioids have been studied in pediatrics, little information is available about oral bioavailability and potency ratios.

Analgesics

The prescription of analgesics for children with cancer pain is based on the WHO analgesic ladder (1). This emphasizes pain intensity as the guide to the choice of analgesic. In other words, the prescription of analgesics should be according to pain severity, ranging from acetaminophen and non-steroidal anti-inflammatory drugs (NSAIDs) for mild pain to opioids (Tables 19.3 and 19.4) for moderate to severe pain. The choice of analgesic is individualized to achieve an optimum balance between analgesia and side effects (1).

Non-opioid analgesics

Acetaminophen inhibits prostaglandin synthesis primarily in the central nervous system (CNS). It is one of the most commonly used non-opioid analgesics in children and does not have the side effects of gastritis and inhibition of platelet function found with aspirin and NSAIDs. Although acetaminophen has a potential for hepatic and renal injury (25), this is uncommon in therapeutic doses. Acetaminophen does not have an association with Reye syndrome.

The antipyretic action of acetaminophen may be contraindicated in neutropenic patients in whom it is important to monitor fever. Pediatric dosing of acetaminophen is based on the dose response for antipyretic. Oral dosing of 15 mg/kg every 4 hours is recommended, with a maxi-

Table 19.3. *Opioid agonist drugs*

Drug	IM[a]	PO[a]	Half-life (hours)	Duration Action (hours)
Codeine	130	200	2–3	2–4
Dihydrocodeine		200	2–3	2–4
Oxycodone	15	30	2–3	2–4
Morphine	10	30 (repeated dose) 60 (single dose)	2–3	3–4
Hydromorphone	1.5	7.5	2–3	2–4
Methadone	10	20	15–190	4–8
Meperidine	75	300	2–3	2–4
Oxymorphone	1	10 (PR)	2–3	3–4
Levorphanol	2	4	12–15	4–8
Fentanyl (parenteral)	0.1	—	1–2	1–3
Fentanyl transdermal system[b]				48–72

Abbreviations: IM, intramuscularly; PO, by mouth; PR, per rectum.
[a] Dose (mg) Equianalgesic to 10 mg IM morphine
[b] Transdermal fentanyl 100 μm/hr = ~ 4 mg/hr
From Cherney NI, Foley KM. Nonopioid and opioid analgesics pharmacotherapy. Hematol Clin North Am 10:79–102, 1996.

mum daily dose of 90 mg/kg/day in children and 60 mg/kg/day in younger children. There are no data on the safety of chronic administration of acetaminophen in children.

In selected children with adequate platelet number and function, NSAIDs may be helpful analgesics, both alone and in combination with opioids. However, aspirin and NSAIDs are often contraindicated in pediatric oncology patients who are at risk of bleeding if they are thrombo-

cytopenic. Choline magnesium trisalicylate (Trilisate) has been recommended because of adult reports of minimal effects on platelet function in vitro and experimental studies showing minimal gastric irritation in rats, in contrast to aspirin (26). Such data should be viewed with caution, as they do not include medically frail patients with thrombocytopenia or other morbidities. There are no data on the safety, efficacy, and tolerability of COX-2 inhibitors in children with cancer.

Opioid analgesics

Codeine is a phenanthrene alkaloid derived from morphine. It is usually prescribed for moderate pain. Codeine is commonly administered via the oral route in children and is often administered in combination with acetaminophen. In equipotent doses, codeine has a similar analgesic and side effect profile to morphine. Codeine is often administered in pediatrics in oral doses of 0.5 to 1 mg/kg every 4 hours for children over 6 months old.

Oxycodone is a semisynthetic opioid and is used for moderate to severe pain in children with cancer. Oxycodone is available as a long-acting preparation and as an oral preparation in combination with acetaminophen in some countries. Oxycodone has a higher clearance value and a shorter elimination half-life ($t_{1/2}$) in children aged 2 to 20 years than in adults (27,28).

Morphine is perhaps the most widely used opioid for moderate to severe cancer pain in children. The major hepatic metabolite of morphine, morphine-6-glucuronide, produces analgesia and side effects comparable to morphine with chronic dosing. Morphine-6-glucuronide may accumulate and result in opioid side effects in patients with renal insufficiency.

Table 19.4. *Starting drug doses of commonly used opioids in pediatrics*

Drug	Usual IV starting dose (< 50 kg)	Usual IV starting dose (> 50 kg)	Usual PO starting dose (< 50 kg)	Usual PO starting dose (> 50 kg)
Morphine	0.1 mg/kg q3–4h	5–10 mg q3–4h	0.3 mg/kg q3–4h	30 mg q3–4h
Hydromorphone	0.015 mg/kg q3–4h	1–1.5 mg q3–4h	0.06 mg/kg q3–4h	6 mg q3–4h
Oxycodone	N/A	N/A	0.3 mg/kg q3–4h[a]	10 mg q3–4h
Meperidine[b]	0.75 mg/kg q2–3h	75–100 mg q3h	N/R	N/R
Fentanyl	0.5–1.5 μg/kg q1–2h	25–75 μg/kg q1–2h	N/A	N/A

Abbreviations: N/A, not available; N/R, not recommended.
[a] Smallest tablet size is 5 mg.
[b] Meperidine is not recommended for chronic use because of the accumulation of the toxic metabolite normeperidine.
From Collins JJ, Berde CB. Management of cancer pain in children. In: Pizzo PA, Poplack DG, eds. Principles and practice of pediatric oncology, 3rd ed., Philadelphia: Lippincott-Raven, 1997.

Morphine clearance is delayed in the first 1 to 3 months of life. The half-life of morphine ($t_{1/2}$) changes from 10 to 20 hours in preterm infants to 1 to 2 hours in young children (29,30). Starting doses in very young infants should be reduced by approximately 25%–30% on a per kilogram basis relative to the dosing recommended for older children. During the neonatal period for term infants, the volume of distribution is linearly related to age and body surface area (31–33). A recent study (34) suggests that when given an equivalent dose for weight, younger children are likely to have significantly lower plasma morphine and metabolite concentrations. A starting dose for oral morphine of 1.5 to 2 mg/kg/day is recommended for children with pain unrelieved by mild or moderate strength analgesics (35).

Oral morphine has a significant first pass metabolism in the liver. An oral to parenteral potency ratio of approximately 3:1 is commonly used during chronic administration (36). Typical starting intravenous morphine infusion rates are 0.02 to 0.03 mg/kg/hr beyond the first 3 months of life, and 0.015 mg/kg/hr in younger infants. Sustained release oral preparations of morphine are available for children and are usually administered at twice daily intervals. Dosing at 8-hour intervals may be appropriate in children (34). Crushing sustained-released tablets produces immediate release of morphine. This limits their use in children who must chew tablets.

Hydromorphone is an alternative opioid when the dose escalation of morphine is limited by side effects. Hydromorphone is available for oral, intravenous, subcutaneous, epidural, and intrathecal administration. A double-blinded randomized crossover comparison of morphine to hydromorphone using patient-controlled analgesia (PCA) in children and adolescents with mucositis after bone marrow transplantation showed that hydromorphone was well tolerated and had a potency ratio of approximately 6:1 relative to morphine in this setting (37). Adult studies indicate that intravenous hydromorphone is five to eight times more potent than morphine. Hydromorphone is convenient for subcutaneous infusion because of its high potency and aqueous solubility. Little is known about the pharmacokinetics of hydromorphone in infants.

Fentanyl is a synthetic opioid approximately 50 to 100 times more potent than morphine during acute intravenous administration. Fentanyl has a rapid onset after intravenous administration, because of its high lipid solubility. Fentanyl is eliminated almost entirely by hepatic metabolism. The half-life of fentanyl is prolonged in preterm infants undergoing cardiac surgery (38), but comparable values with those of adults are reached within the first

months of life (38–41). The clearance of fentanyl is higher in infants and young children than in adults (40,41).

The duration of action of fentanyl after single intravenous bolus administration is much shorter than that for morphine. These features make fentanyl useful for procedures where rapid onset and short duration are important. Fentanyl may also be used for continuous infusion for selected patients with dose-limiting side effects from morphine. Rapid administration of high doses of intravenous fentanyl may result in chest wall rigidity and severe ventilatory difficulty.

Schechter and colleagues (42) described the use of oral transmucosal fentanyl for sedation/analgesia during bone marrow biopsy/aspiration and lumbar puncture in children with cancer. This formulation was safe and effective, although the frequency of vomiting may be a limiting factor in its tolerability. In a small study using a clinical protocol, the utility, feasibility, and tolerability of transdermal fentanyl were demonstrated in children with cancer pain (43). The mean clearance and volume of distribution of transdermal fentanyl were the same for both adults and children, but the variability was higher for adults (43). A larger study is required to confirm these findings.

Meperidine is a short half-life synthetic opioid and has been used for procedural and postoperative pain in children. Neonates have a slower elimination of meperidine than children and young infants (44–48). Normeperidine, a major metabolite of meperidine, can cause CNS excitatory effects, including tremors and convulsions (49). This can occur particularly in patients with renal impairment. Meperidine is not generally recommended for children with chronic pain but may be an acceptable alternative opioid for short painful procedures. Meperidine in low doses (0.25–0.5 mg/kg IV) may be used for the prophylaxis and treatment of rigors after the infusion of amphotericin.

Methadone is a synthetic opioid that has a long and variable half-life. The oral–parenteral potency ratio is approximately 2:1. In children receiving postoperative analgesia, methadone produced equivalent but more prolonged analgesia than morphine (50,51). Because of its prolonged half-life, methadone has a risk of delayed sedation and overdosage occurring several days after the initiation of treatment.

Frequent patient assessment is the key to safe and effective use of methadone. If a patient becomes oversedated, it is recommended to stop dosing, not just reduce the dose, and to observe the patient until alertness is improved. Although "as-needed" dosing is discouraged for most patients with cancer pain, some clinicians find this approach a useful way to establish a dosing schedule for methadone

(50,51). Methadone remains a long-acting agent when administered either as an elixir or as crushed tablets.

Routes and methods of analgesic administration

Analgesics should be administered to children by the simplest, safest, most effective, and least painful route. The oral route of administration of analgesics is therefore the first choice for the majority of patients. Oral dosing is generally predictable, inexpensive, and does not require invasive procedures or technologies. The intramuscular administration of an opioid is painful and may lead to the underreporting of pain. This route of administration does not permit easy dose titration or infusion and should be avoided. Rectal administration is also discouraged in children with cancer because of concern regarding infection and the great variability of rectal absorption of drugs (52).

The eutectic mixture of local anesthetics (EMLA) is a topical preparation that provides local anesthesia to the skin, dermis, and subcutaneous tissues. It must be applied under an occlusive dressing for at least 1 hour, but depth of penetration is greater with a longer application time (90–120 minutes). EMLA has been shown to be useful for providing topical local anesthesia for procedural pain, including lumbar puncture (52) and central venous port access (53) in children with cancer. Preliminary studies of topical amethocaine for percutaneous analgesia before venous cannulation in children have demonstrated promising safety and efficacy data (54).

Intravenous administration of opioids has the advantage of rapid onset of analgesia, easier opioid dose titration, bioavailability, and continuous effect when infusions are used. The subcutaneous route is an alternative route of administration for children with poor intravenous access (55). Subcutaneous infusion rates generally do not exceed 1 to 3 ml/hr (56). A small catheter or butterfly needle (27-gauge) may be placed under the skin of the thorax, abdomen, or thigh. Subcutaneous infusion sites are changed approximately every 3 days. There are limited data on the safety, efficacy, and tolerability of transdermal fentanyl in children with cancer.

PCA has been used successfully for the management of prolonged oropharyngeal mucositis pain after bone marrow transplantation in children and adolescents (37,57,58). PCA is a method of opioid administration that permits the patient to self-administer a small bolus dose of opioid within set time limits. In postoperative use, PCA is widely used successfully by children ages 6 to 7 years and older.

PCA caters to an individual's variation in pharmacokinetics, pharmacodynamics, and pain intensity. It allows appropriate children to have control over their analgesia and allows them to choose a balance between the benefits of analgesia versus the side effects of opioids. In patients with severe mucositis, for example, opioid dosing can be timed with routine mouth care and other causes of incidental mouth pain. A controlled comparison of staff-controlled continuous infusion of morphine and PCA in adolescents with severe oropharyngeal mucositis found that the PCA group had equivalent analgesia but less sedation and less difficulty concentrating (57).

Opioid dose schedules

Unless painful episodes are truly incidental and unpredictable, analgesics should generally be administered at regular times to provide continuous pain relief. If breakthrough pain occurs, "rescues" are supplemental "as needed" doses of opioid incorporated into the analgesic regimen to allow a patient to have additional analgesia if breakthrough pain occurs. Rescue doses of opioid may be calculated, as approximately 5%–10% of the total daily opioid requirement, and may be administered every hour (59).

Opioid dose escalation may be required after opioid administration begins and periodically thereafter. The size of an opioid dose increment may be calculated as follows:

1. If greater than approximately six "rescue" doses of opioid are given in a 24-hour period, then the total daily opioid dose should be increased by the total of opioid given as "rescue" medication. For example, the hourly average of the total daily rescue opioid should be added to the baseline opioid infusion. An alternative to this method would be to increase the baseline infusion by 50% (59).
2. "Rescue" doses are kept as a proportion of the baseline opioid dose. This dose can be 5%–10% of the total daily dose (59). An alternative guideline for opioid infusions is between 50% and 200% of the hourly basal infusion rate (59).

Opioid switching

The usual indication for an opioid switch to an alternative opioid is opioid dose-limiting toxicity. In other words, the dose of opioid required to achieve adequate analgesia is limited by opioid side effects. A favorable change in opioid analgesia to side effect profile will be experienced if there is less cross-tolerance at the opioid receptors mediating analgesia than at those mediating adverse effects (60).

After long-term opioid dosing, equivalent analgesia may be attained with a dose of a second opioid that is smaller than that calculated from an equianalgesic table (Table 19.3) (60), approximately 50% for short half-life opioids. In contrast to short half-life opioids, the doses of methadone required for equivalent analgesia after switching may be on the order of 10%–20% of the equianalgesic dose of the previously used short half-life opioid. A protocol for methadone dose conversion and titration has been reported (61).

Opioid side effects

Children do not necessarily report opioid side effects voluntarily (e.g., constipation, pruritus, dreams) and should be asked specifically about these problems. An assessment of opioid side effects is included in an assessment of analgesic effectiveness. All opioids can potentially cause the same constellation of side effects (Table 19.5). If opioid side effects limit opioid dose escalation, then consideration should be given to an opioid switch. Tolerance to some opioid side effects (e.g., sedation, nausea and vomiting, pruritus) often develops within the first week of starting opioids. Children do not develop tolerance to constipation and concurrent treatment with laxatives should be considered.

Table 19.5. *Management of opioid side effects*

Side effect	Treatment
Constipation	1. Regular use of stimulant and stool softener laxatives (fiber, fruit juices are often insufficient) 2. Ensure adequate water intake
Sedation	1. If analgesia is adequate, try dose reduction 2. Unless contraindicated, add non-sedating analgesics, such as acetaminophen or NSAIDs, and reduce opioid dosing as tolerated 3. If sedation persists, try methylphenidate or dextroamphetamine 0.05–0.2 mg/kg po b.i.d. in early morning and midday 4. Consider an opioid switch
Nausea	1. Exclude disease processes (e.g., bowel obstruction, increased intracranial pressure) 2. Antiemetics (phenothiazines, ondansetron, hydroxyzine) 3. Consider an opioid switch
Urinary retention	1. Exclude disease processes (e.g., bladder neck obstruction by tumor, impending cord compression, hypovolemia, renal failure) 2. Avoid other drugs with anticholinergic effects (e.g., tricyclics, antihistamines) 3. Consider short-term use of bethanechol or Crede maneuver 4. Consider short-term catheterization 5. Consider opioid dose reduction if analgesia adequate or an opioid switch if analgesia inadequate
Pruritus	1. Exclude other causes (e.g., drug allergy, cholestasis) 2. Antihistamines (e.g., diphenhydramine hydroxyzine) 3. Consider an opioid dose reduction if analgesia adequate, or an opioid switch. Fentanyl causes less histamine release
Respiratory depression: mild–moderate	1. Awaken, encourage to breathe 2. Apply oxygen 3. Withhold opioid dosing until breathing improves, reduce subsequent dosing by at least 25%
Severe	1. Awaken if possible, apply oxygen, assist respiration by bag and mask as needed 2. Titrate small doses of naloxone (0.02 mg/kg increments as needed) stop when respiratory rate increases to 8–10/min in older children or 12–16/min in infants; do not try to awaken fully with naloxone. *Do not give a bolus dose of naloxone, as severe pain and symptoms of opioid withdrawal may ensue.* 3. Consider a low-dose naloxone infusion or repeated incremental dosing 4. Consider short-term intubation in occasional cases where risk of aspiration is high
Dysphoria/ confusion/ hallucinations	1. Exclude other pathology as a cause for these symptoms before attributing them to opioids 2. When other causes excluded, change to another opioid 3. Consider adding a neuroleptic such as haloperidol (0.01–0.1 mg/kg po/IV every 8 hours to a maximum dose of 30 mg/day)
Myoclonus	1. Usually seen in the setting of high-dose opioids, or alternatively, rapid dose escalation 2. No treatment may be warranted, if this is infrequent and not distressing to the child 3. Consider an opioid switch or treat with clonezepam (0.01 mg/kg po every 12 hours to a maximum dose of 0.5 mg/dose) or a parenteral benzodiazepine (e.g., diazepam) if the oral route is not tolerated

From Collins JJ, Berde CB. Management of cancer pain in children. In: Pizzo PA, Poplack DG. Principles and practice of pediatric oncology, 3rd ed. Philadelphia: Lippincott-Raven, 1997.
Abbreviation: NSAID, non-steroidal anti-inflammatory drug.

Adjuvant analgesics in children with cancer

Adjuvant analgesics are a heterogeneous group of medications that are analgesic in some painful conditions but have a primary indication other than pain (62). These drugs are commonly prescribed with primary analgesics. Common classes of these adjuvant agents include antidepressants, anticonvulsants, neuroleptics, psychostimulants, antihistamines, corticosteroids, and centrally acting skeletal muscle relaxants.

Antidepressants

Data from adult studies have guided the use of antidepressants as adjuvant analgesics in pediatrics. Tricyclic antidepressants have been used for a variety of pain conditions in adults including cancer pain (63). Baseline hematology and biochemistry tests and an electrocardiogram (ECG) to exclude Wolff-Parkinson-White syndrome or other cardiac conduction defects have been recommended before starting treatment with tricyclic antidepressants (64). An ECG is recommended periodically during long-term use, or if standard milligram per kilogram dosages are exceeded (65).

Psychostimulants

The use of dextroamphetamine and methylphenidate was reported in a survey of 11 children receiving opioids for a variety of indications, including cancer pain (66). Somnolence was reduced in these patients without significant adverse side effects. Dextroamphetamine potentiates opioid analgesia in postoperative adult patients (67) and methylphenidate counteracts opioid-induced sedation (68) and cognitive dysfunction (69) in advanced cancer patients. The potential side effects of methylphenidate include anorexia, insomnia, and dysphoria.

Corticosteroids

Corticosteroids may have a role in bone pain as a result of metastatic bone disease (70), cerebral edema owing to either primary or metastatic tumor (71), and epidural spinal cord compression (72). Dexamethasone tends to be the most frequently used corticosteroid because of its high potency, duration of action, and minimal mineralocorticoid effect. Corticosteroids may produce analgesia by a variety of mechanisms, including anti-inflammatory effects, reduction of tumor edema, and, potentially by a reduction of spontaneous discharge in injured nerves (73).

Anticonvulsants

The mechanism of action of anticonvulsants in controlling lancinating pain is not understood but is probably related to reducing paroxysmal discharges of neurons. Standard anticonvulsants may be problematic in children with cancer because of their potential adverse effects on the hematological profile. Gabapentin is well tolerated, appears to have a benign efficacy to toxicity ratio in children (74), and may be useful for the treatment of neuropathic pain (75).

Radionuclides

Radionuclide therapy for painful osseous metastases has been reported in the adult literature (76). One case report indicates the potential role of [131I]iodine-meta-iodobenzylguanidine ([131I]MIBG) for painful metastatic bone disease as a result of neuroblastoma in children (77). The side effects of [131I]MIBG were thrombocytopenia and cystitis.

Neuroleptics

Methotrimeprazine, a phenothiazine, is analgesic in the setting of adult cancer pain (78). It should not be used as a substitute for opioid analgesia. The mechanism by which methotrimeprazine produces analgesia and its role as an adjuvant analgesic agent in children with cancer pain is unclear. Methotrimeprazine may be useful as an adjuvant in patients with disseminated cancer who experience pain associated with anxiety, restlessness, or nausea (62).

Tolerance, physical dependence, addiction

Analgesic *tolerance* refers to the progressive decline in potency of an opioid with continued use, so that increasingly higher doses are required to achieve the same analgesic effect. Parents are often reluctant to increase dosing in their child because of a fear that tolerance will make opioids ineffective at a later date. Reassurance should be given that tolerance, in the majority of cases, can be managed by simple dose escalation, use of adjuvant medications, or perhaps by an opioid switch in the setting of dose-limiting side effects. Physical *dependence* is a physiological state characterized by withdrawal (abstinence syndrome) after dose reduction or discontinuation of the opioid, or administration of an opioid antagonist. Initial manifestations of withdrawal include yawning, diaphoresis, lacrimation, coryza, and tachycardia. *Addiction* is a psychological and behavioral syndrome characterized by drug craving and aberrant drug use.

Some parents fear that an exposure to an opioid will result in their child subsequently becoming a drug addict. The incidence of opioid addiction was examined prospectively in 12,000 hospitalized adult patients who received at least one dose of a strong opioid (79). There were only four documented cases of subsequent addiction in patients without a prior history of drug abuse. These data suggest that iatrogenic opioid addiction is an uncommon problem (79), an observation consistent with a large worldwide experience with opioid treatment of cancer pain.

References

1. World Health Organization. Cancer pain relief and palliative Care in Children. Geneva: World Health Organization, 1998.
2. Wolfe J, Grier HE, Klar N, et al. Symptoms and suffering at the end of life in children with cancer. N Engl J Med 342(5):326–33, 2000.
3. Collins JJ, Devine TB, Dick G, et al. The measurement of symptoms in young children with cancer: the validation of the Memorial Symptom Assessment Scale in children aged 7–12. J Pain Symptom Manage 23(1):10–16, 2002.
4. Collins JJ, Byrnes ME, Dunkel I, et al. The Memorial Symptom Assessment Scale (MSAS): validation study in children aged 10–18. J Pain Symptom Manage 19(5):363–77, 2000.
5. Miser AW, McCalla J, Dothage P, et al. Pain as a presenting symptom in children and young adults with newly diagnosed malignancy. Pain 29:363–77, 1987.
6. Strother DR, Pollack IF, Fisher PG, et al. Tumors of the central nervous system. In: Pizzo PA, Poplack DG, eds. Principles and practice of pediatric oncology, 4th ed. Philadelphia: Lippincott Williams & Wilkins, 2002:751–824.
7. Hahn YS, McClone DG. Pain in children with spinal cord tumors. Child Brain 11:36–46, 1984.
8. Lewis D, Packer R, Raney B. Incidence, presentation, and outcome of spinal cord disease in children with systemic cancer. Pediatrics 78:438–43, 1986.
9. Elliott SC, Miser AW, Dose AM. Epidemiologic features of pain in pediatric cancer patients: a co-operative community-based study. Clin J Pain 7:263–8, 1991.
10. Miser AW, Dothage P, Wesley RA, et al. The prevalence of pain in a pediatric and young adult population. Pain 29:265–6, 1987.
11. Collins JJ, Grier HE, Kinney HC, Berde CB. Control of severe pain in terminal pediatric malignancy. J Pediatr 126(4):653–7, 1995.
12. Berde CB, Billett AL, Collins JJ. Symptom management in supportive care. In: Pizzo PA, Poplack DG, eds. Principles and practice of pediatric oncology, 4th ed. Baltimore: Lippincott Williams & Wilkins, 2002:1301–32.
13. McGrath PA, Bush JP, Harkins SW, eds. Children in pain. New York: Springer-Verlag, 1991:83–115.
14. Zeltzer L, Jay S, Fisher D. The management of pain associated with pediatric procedures. In: Schechter NL, ed. The Pediatric Clinics of North America. Philadelphia: W.B. Saunders Company, 1989:914.
15. Siegal LJ. Preparation of children for hospitalization: a selected review of the research literature. J Pediatr Psychol 1(26):36, 1976.
16. Manne SL, Redd WH, Jacobsen P, et al. Behavioral intervention to reduce child and parent distress during venipuncture. J Consult Clin Psychol 58:565–72, 1990.
17. McGrath PA, DeVeber LL. The management of acute pain evoked by medical procedures in children with cancer. J Pain Symptom Manage 1:145–50, 1986.
18. Jay SM, Elliott C, Ozolins M, et al. Behavioral management of children's distress during painful medical procedures. Behav Res Ther 5:513–20, 1985.
19. Katz E, Kellerman J, Ellenberg L. Hypnosis in the reduction of acute pain and distress in children with cancer. J Pediatr Psychol 12:379–94, 1987.
20. Hilgard J, LeBaron S. Relief of anxiety and pain in children and adolescents with cancer: quantitative measures and clinical observations. Int J Clin Exp Hypn 30:417–42, 1982.
21. Kellerman J, Zeltzer L, Ellenberg L, Dash J. Adolescents with cancer: hypnosis for the reduction of the acute pain and anxiety associated with medical procedures. J Adolesc Health Care 4:85–90, 1983.
22. Zeltzer L, LeBaron S. Hypnosis and nonhypnotic techniques for reduction of pain and anxiety during painful procedures in children and adolescents with cancer. J Pediatr 101:1032–5, 1982.
23. Ljungman G, Kreugar A, et al. Treatment of pain in pediatric oncology: a Swedicsh nationwide survey. Pain 68:385–94, 1996.
24. Collins JJ, Portenoy RK, Bruera E, eds. Topics in palliative care. 1. Pharmacologic management of pediatric cancer pain New York: Oxford University Press, 1998:7–78.
25. Sandler DP, Smit JC, et al. Analgesic use and chronic renal disease. N Engl J Med 320:1238–43, 1989.
26. Stuart JJ, Pisko EJ. Choline magnesium trisalicylate does not impair platelet aggregation. Pharmatherapeutica 2:547, 1981.
27. Poyhia R, Seppala T. Lipid solubility and protein binding of oxycodone in vitro. Pharmacol Toxicol 74:23–7, 1994.
28. Pelkonen O, Kaltiala EH, Larmi TKL. Comparison of activities of drug metabolizing enzymes in human fetal and adult liver. Clin Pharmacol Ther 14:840–6, 1973.
29. Stanski DR, Greenblatt DJ, Lowenstein E. Kinetics of intravenous and intramuscular morphine. Clin Pharmacol Ther 24:52–9, 1978.
30. Olkkola KT, Maunuksela EL, Korpela R, Rosenberg PH. Kinetics and dynamics of postoperative intravenous morphine in children. Clin Pharmacol Ther 44(2):128–36, 1988.
31. McRorie TI, Lynn A, Nespeca MK. The maturation of morphine clearance and metabolism. Am J Dis Child 146:972–6, 1992.
32. Bhat R, Chari G, Gulati A, et al. Pharmacokinetics of a single dose of morphine in pre-term infants during the first week of life. J Pediatr 117:477–81, 1990.
33. Pokela ML, Olkkala KT, Seppala T. Age-related morphine kinetics in infants. Dev Pharm Ther 20:26–34, 1993.
34. Hunt AM, Joel S, Dick G, Goldman A. Population pharmacokinetics of oral morphine and its glucuronides in children receiving morphine as immediate-release liquid or sustained-release tablets. J Pediar 135(1):47–55, 1999.

35. Hunt AM. A survey of signs, symptoms and symptom control in 30 terminally ill children. Dev Med Child Neurol 32:347–55, 1990.

36. Cherney NJ, Foley KM, Cherney NJ, Foley KM, eds. Nonopioid and opioid analgesic pharmacotherapy of cancer pain. Philadelphia: WB Saunders, 1996:79. Hematology/Oncology Clinics of North America.

37. Collins JJ, Geake J, Grier HE, et al. Patient-controlled analgesia for mucositis pain in children: a three-period crossover study comparing morphine and hydromorphone. J Pediatr 129(5):722–8, 1996.

38. Collins C, Koren G, Crean P, et al. Fentanyl pharmacokinetics and hemodynamic effects in preterm infants during ligation of patent ductus arteriosus. Anesth Analg 64:1078–80, 1985.

39. Koren G, Goresky G, Crean P, et al. Unexpected alterations in fentanyl pharmacokinetics in children undergoing cardiac surgery: age related or disease related? Dev Pharm Ther 9:183–91, 1986.

40. Johnson K, Erickson J, Holley F, Scott J. Fentanyl pharmacokinetics in the pediatric population. Anesthesiology 61(3A):A441, 1984.

41. Gauntlett IS, Fisher DM, Hertzka RE, et al. Pharmacokinetics of fentanyl in neonatal humans and lambs: effects of age. Anesthesiology 69:683–7, 1988.

42. Schechter NL, Weisman SJ, Rosenblum M, et al. The use of oral transmucosal fentanyl citrate for painful procedures in children. Pediatrics 95:335–9, 1995.

43. Collins JJ, Dunkel I, Gupta SK, et al. Transdermal fentanyl in children with cancer: feasibility, tolerability, and pharmacokinetic correlates. J Pediatr 134:319–23, 1999.

44. Tamsen A, Hartvig P, Fagerlund C, et al. Patient-controlled analgesic therapy, part 1: pharmacokinetics of pethidine in the pre- and postoperative periods. Clin Pharmacokinet 7:149–63, 1982.

45. Hamunen K, Maunuksela EL, Seppala T, et al. Pharmacokinetics of iv and rectal pethidine in children undergoing ophthalmic surgery. Br J Anaesth 71:823–6, 1993.

46. Koska AJ, Kramer WG, Romagnoli A, et al. Pharmacokinetics of high dose meperidine in surgical patients. Anesth Analg 60:8–11, 1981.

47. Pokela ML, Olkkala KT, Kovisto M, et al. Pharmacokinetics and pharmacodynamics of intravenous meperidine in neonates and infants. Clin Pharmacol Ther 52:342–9, 1992.

48. Mather LE, Tucker GT, Pflug AE, et al. Meperidine kinetics in man: intravenous injection in surgical patients and volunteers. Clin Pharmacol Ther 17:21–30, 1975.

49. Kaiko RF, Foley KM, Grabinsky PY, et al. Central nervous system excitatory effects of meperidine in cancer patients. Ann Neurol 13:180–5, 1983.

50. Berde CB, Beyer JE, Bournaki MC, et al. Comparison of morphine and methadone for prevention of postoperative pain in 3- to 7-year-old children. J Pediatr 136–41, 1991.

51. Berde CB, Sethna NF, Holzman RS, et al. Pharmacokinetics of methadone in children and adolescents in the perioperative period. Anesthesiology 67:A519, 1987.

52. Kapelushik J, Koren G, Solh H, et al. Evaluating the efficacy of EMLA in alleviating pain associated with lumbar puncture: comparison of open and double-blinded protocols in children. Pain 42:31–4, 1990.

53. Miser AW, Goh TS, Dose AM, et al. Trial of a topically administered local anesthetic (EMLA cream) for pain relief during central venous port accesses in children with cancer. J Pain Symptom Manage 9(4):259–64, 1994.

54. Van Kan HJM, Egberts ACG, Rijnvos WPM, et al. Tetracaine versus lidocaine-prilocaine for preventing venipuncture-induced pain in children. Am J Obstet Gynecol 54:388–92, 1997.

55. Miser AW, Davis DM, Hughes CS, et al. Continuous subcutaneous infusion of morphine in children with cancer. Am J Dis Child 137(4):383–5, 1983.

56. Bruera E, Brenneis C, Michaud M, et al. Use of the subcutaneous route for the administration of narcotics in patients with cancer pain. Cancer 62:407–11, 1988.

57. Mackie AM, Coda BC, Hill HF. Adolescents use patient controlled analgesia effectively for relief for relief from prolonged oropharyngeal mucositis pain. Pain 46:265–9, 1991.

58. Dunbar PJ, Buckley P, Gavrin JR, et al. Use of patient-controlled analgesia for pain control for children receiving bone marrow transplants. J Pain Symptom Manage 10:604–11, 1995.

59. Cherny NI, Foley KM, eds. Nonopioid and opioid analgesic pharmacotherapy of cancer pain. Hematol Oncol Clin North Am 1996:79.

60. Portenoy RK, Gebhart GF, Hammond DI, Jensen TS, eds. Progress in pain research and management. Seattle: IASP Press, 1994:615–9. Opioid tolerance and responsiveness: research findings and clinical observations.

61. Inturrisi CE, Portenoy RK, Max M, et al. Pharmacokinetic-pharmacodynamic relationships of methadone infusions in patients with cancer pain. Clin Pharmacol Ther 47:565–77, 1990.

62. Portenoy RK. In Doyle D, Hanks GWC, MacDonald N (eds.). Oxford textbook of palliative medicine, 2nd ed. Oxford: Oxford University Press, 1993:181–203. Adjuvant analgesics in pain management.

63. Magni G. The use of antidepressants in the treatment of chronic pain. Drugs 42(5):730–48, 1991.

64. Heiligenstein E, Gerrity S. In Schechter NL et al. (eds.). Pain in infants, children, and adolescents. Baltimore: Williams and Wilkins, 1993:173–7. 13, Psychotropics as adjuvant analgesics. Baltimore: Williams & Wilkins, 1993:173–7.

65. Biederman J, Baldessarini RJ, Wright V, et al. A double-blind placebo controlled study of desipramine in the treatment of ADD:II. Serum drug levels and cardiovascular findings. J Am Acad Child Adolesc Psychiatry 28:903–11, 1989.

66. Yee JD, Berde CB. Dextroamphetamine or methylphenidate as adjuvants to opioid analgesia for adolescents with cancer. J Pain Symptom Manage 9:122–5, 1994.

67. Forrest WH, Brown BW, Brown CR, et al. Dextroamphetamine with morphine for the treatment of postoperative pain. N Engl J Med 296(13):712–5, 1977.

68. Bruera E, Miller MJ, Macmillan K, Kuehn N. Neuropsychological effects of methylphenidate in patients receiving a continuous infusion of narcotics for cancer pain. Pain 48:163–6, 1992.

69. Bruera E, Faisinger R, MacEachern T, Hanson J. The use of methylphenidate in patients with incident pain receiving regular opiates: a preliminary report. Pain 50:75–7, 1992.

70. Tannock I, Gospodarowicz M, Meakin W, et al. Treatment of metastatic prostatic cancer with low-dose prednisone: evaluation of pain and quality of life as pragmatic indices of response. J Clin Oncol 7(5):590–7, 1989.

71. Weinstein JD, Toy FJ, Jaffe ME, Goldberg HI. The effect of dexamethasone on brain edema in patients with metastatic brain tumors. Neurology 23:121–9, 1973.

72. Greenberg HS, Kim J, Posner JB. Epidural spinal cord compression from metastatic tumor: results with a new treatment protocol. Ann Neurology 8:361–6, 1980.

73. Watanabe S, Bruera E. Corticosteroids as adjuvant analgesics. J Pain Symptom Manage 9:442–5, 1994.

74. Khurana DS, Riviello J, Helmers S, et al. Efficacy of gabapentin therapy in children with refractory partial seizures. J Pediatr 128:829–33, 1996.

75. Mellick GA, Mellick LB. Letter. J Pain Symptom Manage 10(4):265–6, 1995.

76. Silberstein EB, Williams C. Strontium-89 therapy for painful osseous metastases. J Nucl Med 26:345–8, 1985.

77. Westlin JE, Letocha H, Jakobson S, et al. Rapid, reproducible pain relief with [131]iodine-meta-iodobenzylguanidine in a boy with disseminated neuroblastoma. Pain 60:111–4, 1995.

78. Beaver WT, Wallemstein S, Houde RW. A comparison of the analgesic effects of methotrimeprazine and morphine in patients with cancer. Clin Pharmacol Ther 7:436–46, 1966.

79. Porter J, Lick J. Addiction is rare in patients treated with narcotics (letter). N Engl J Med 302:123, 1980.

20 Cancer pain in the elderly

DAVID I. WOLLNER
Veterans Administration New York Harbor Healthcare System

Introduction

Albert Murray, an 82-year-old English teacher writes in an Op-Ed, *The Sharpest Pain,* "I'm doing more than ever, but it's harder now. I'm in constant pain. But nothing hurts more like the loss of old friends. Because I look and act so energetic in spite of the pain, people think I'm about 20 years younger than I am. That includes my doctors ... I tell them 'If I felt half as good as you say I look, I'd be in excellent shape'" (1).

These concise phrases capture the critical aspects of chronic pain in the elderly. Their lives can be busy in the face of daily pain. The loss of friends and independence amplify suffering. And physicians all too commonly fail to recognize, assess and treat pain correctly (2).

Successful aging is the primary goal for the elderly and the geriatricians who care for them: an independent, good quality of life without disability. The principles and practice of palliative medicine, geriatrics, and successful pain management are quite similar. The older person and family are at the center of an interdisciplinary team structure. The clinical goals of care and autonomy are the foundation for decision making. Psychosocial and spiritual care receive respect and a good quality of life outweighs duration of survival.

The principles and guidelines for cancer pain management cited in this text hold true for the elderly who have aged successfully. It is the frail elderly who deserve a more focused pain assessment and a more individually tailored treatment. Cognitive impairment, multiple co-morbid illnesses and their treatment, and psychosocial stressors present daunting hurdles to successful pain relief. This chapter provides information to assist clinicians in gracefully clearing these barriers.

The demographics of aging

Extraordinary changes have occurred over the past century, and none is more dramatic than the demographics of aging. Men and women are living longer. The oldest-old segment, persons aged 85 years and older, is 189 times larger than its 1900 counterpart (3). Most contemporary newborns will reach age 65 years, the very population that shoulder the majority of all cancers.

Besides the oldest old, the elderly, Americans 65 years and older, are growing in number with an increasing rate of expansion. The elderly in the United States comprise a diverse mixture of traits: sex, race, ethnicity, economic status, social characteristics, and geographic distribution. As the proportion of the working young whose tax dollars contribute to Medicare is decreasing, the population of elders in need is increasing. In light of this imbalance, the implications for governmental health care policy development are daunting.

A focus on the oldest old reveals striking information. There is exponential growth observed and predicted from 1900–2050 (Fig. 20.1). The percentage of 65-year-olds expected to survive to age 90 will have reached sevenfold by 2050. Twenty percent of Americans will be 65 or older by 2030. The oldest old demonstrates the highest degree of disability. Between one third to one half need assistance with activities of daily living (ADL), which include feeding, dressing, toileting, grooming, and assistance with ambulation.

Similar changes are seen throughout the industrialized world. The challenge to health care delivery is gigantic. Medicare legislation in the United States is now 35 years old and was originally instituted to protect seniors from catastrophic financial loss resulting from acute illness. Medicare is at the threshold of radical restructuring to successfully meet the health needs of the elderly over the years to come.

Cancer and aging

Cancer and aging are closely linked. Cancer incidence and mortality rates increase exponentially for men and

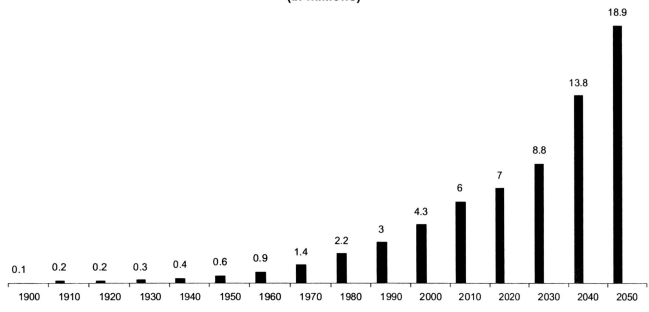

Fig. 20.1. U.S. Bureau of the Census (1993). Decennial censuses for specified years and population projections of the United States by age, sex, race, and Hispanic origin: 1993 to 2050. *Current Population Reports*, P25-1104. Washington DC: U.S. Government and Printing Office. Data from 1990 from *1990 Census of Population and Housing*, CPH-L-74, *Modified and Actual age, sex, race, and Hispanic origin data.*

women over 50 years old. Sixty percent of all cancers occur in Americans 65 years and older, and 69% of all cancer deaths are seen in the same age group. Similar patterns are seen in Italy, Japan, the United Kingdom, and throughout the industrialized world.

The Surveillance Epidemiology and End Results (SEER) Program of the National Cancer Institute (NCI) provides important epidemiologic data (4). Cancer mortality is decreasing in persons 60 years old and younger and rising in the 65 and older group. The oldest-old population has the highest number of co-morbid illnesses, incidence of dementia, and risk of adverse drug events. Therefore, a rapidly expanding population with advanced neoplastic disease and a high incidence of cognitive impairment and pain can be anticipated.

The American Cancer Society (ACS) publishes annual epidemiological data for the United States (5). The number of estimated new cancer cases during 1999 was 1221 × 10³ (623 × 10³ men, 596 × 10³ women). Eighty percent of all cancer deaths during 1995 were in men and women 60 years and older. The most common cancers causing death in older men are lung, prostate, colorectal, and pancreatic, whereas in women, lung, breast, colorectal, and pancreatic cancers predominate. Each of these more common neoplasms has strong associations with pain in early and advanced stages. Bone metastases are the most

common cause of pain when distant metastases are present. Visceral and neuropathic pain syndromes are less common and are more difficult to treat successfully.

Although the relationship between cancer incidence and aging has been established, cancer is not a normal consequence of aging. Three lines of insight provide evidence that aging is an independent variable for cancer risk. Breast cancer in women and lung cancer in both sexes decline in incidence after age 80 years (6). Autopsy information from Italy shows a decline in cancer incidence and a lesser extent of metastatic disease when cancer is found in nonagenarians and centenarians (7). Laboratory studies show that cancer is less virulent in certain older human and animal models (8).

There are two theories linking aging and cancer. Replicative senescence is observed when somatic cells in tissue culture fail to divide when stimulated after a finite period (9). Evidence reveals that replicative senescence is controlled by tumor suppressor genes (10). Senescent cells resist apoptosis (11) and therefore pose a potential threat in mitotic tissues. Soluble products may therefore stimulate initiated cells to undergo uninhibited division (12). Replicative senescence is a "double-edged sword," protecting an individual during the younger reproductive years while posing a threat in later years as a result of carcinogenesis.

Another theory relates to telomere shortening. Telomeres are terminal chromosomal structures that fortify DNA structure. Aging is associated with falling telomerase activity, and there is a relationship with telomerase decline and carcinogenesis (13). Strategies exist to counteract telomerase deficiency, thereby reducing cancer risk. Research in the laboratory and clinic will prove the worth of this theory.

Another aspect of cancer treatment specific to the aging population is the fact that treatment modalities and research protocols often fail to include the elderly. Optimal cancer treatment depends on an accurate assessment of the stage and burden of the disease. There is firm evidence that the elderly are staged and treated less often than their younger counterparts. Turner et al. (14) performed a retrospective Medline review and found that co-morbidities were difficult to co-factor and frailty had no universal definition. Earlier chemotherapy studies excluded the elderly based on age and not on functional capacity and organ function (15). Older women with advanced ovarian cancer are less likely to have debulking surgery (16). Radiotherapy is commonly used palliatively, but curative treatment is less likely to be used (17).

In the United Kingdom, an elder with cancer is less likely to see an oncologist, in part because of ageism (18). Myths about cancer in old age held by patients and their caregivers are a common barrier (19). Screening for cancer of the breast and cervix in women and colorectal cancer in both sexes can be effective in septagenarians (20).

de Rijke et al. (21) reported valuable information about age-specific differences in cancer care for the elderly based on a retrospective study of data from the Regional Cancer Registry in Limburg, the Netherlands. Cancer stage was unknown and histological confirmation of cancer was lacking most commonly in those 70 years and older. The same cohort was also less likely to receive antineoplastic therapy, and when treated with chemotherapy, less effective regimens were used.

Future needs of the elderly with cancer are tremendous. In the presence of advancing incurable disease, palliative medicine is obligated to develop research protocols to pose theses and develop a body of valid data. The issues of prevention, detection, and treatment must be explored. The union of oncology, geriatrics, and palliative care is primed to find solutions for the rapidly expanding elderly population.

Geriatric assessment tools

The application of assessment tools is the prerequisite needed to construct clinical plans of care for the elderly.

The philosophy and structure of geriatrics and palliative care assessments, therefore, are very similar.

Comprehensive Geriatric Assessment (CGA) is a fundamental screening tool in caring for the elderly. Older persons face formidable obstacles to obtaining high-caliber medical care because of fragmentation of medical, nursing, and social services (22). The CGA is an interdisciplinary process that assesses an elder's medical, psychosocial, and functional assets, as well as deficits. The CGA can be used in many settings: physician's office, hospital, long-term care (LTC) facility, and specialized geriatric clinics. The CGA may also measure ADLs, independent ADLs, and an elder's social and spiritual infrastructures.

The CGA measures four distinct sectors: functional abilities, physical health, psychological well-being, and social factors. Tools are available for each sector to further define the precise needs of an elder and how and where services are to be provided. The primary aim of the CGA is to maximize comfort and independence. A meta-analysis of controlled trials of CGA has demonstrated its value. Queries about pain can be pursued, assessments to identify its cause(s) can be made, and a treatment plan can be constructed to manage pain optimally as a result of using the CGA.

Palliative care is both a standard of care for all patients and a growing medical specialty that focuses on symptom assessment and management. The patient and family/caregivers are the central unit of care. An interdisciplinary care team assesses physical, psychosocial, spiritual, and practical needs. Clinical care is provided along the complete trajectory of any progressive and incurable disease, including care at the end of life. A good quality of life and death is the principal goal of palliative care.

Cancer pain in the elderly is best managed using a palliative care model. A medical assessment can discover the causes of pain, and a psychosocial screening can identify personal distress. A chaplain can address spiritual needs, and a caregiver may confide a relevant parcel of information that allows an interdisciplinary team to establish a plan of care for pain. The World Health Organization's (WHO) Cancer Pain and Palliative Care initiative (23) successes bear witness to a model of cancer pain control.

Extermann and Aapro (24) posited a framework for assessment of the older cancer patient. Histologic proof of cancer and disease staging are necessary first steps in any treatment plan. Surgical, radiotherapeutic, and chemotherapy fitness assessments are essential, whether the goal of care is cure or palliation. Assessment of renal, hepatic, bone marrow, and neurological function allows precise tailoring of therapies. Derivatives identical to the CGA follow: assessment of performance status, Karnofsky Performance Status, cognitive skills, and nutrition status. All prescribed, over-the-counter, and complementary and alternative medications are identified. The Moffit SAOP (Senior Adult Oncology Program) and Multidisciplinary Assessment of Cancer in the Elderly are useful but yet-to-be-validated cancer assessment tools (25).

The importance of detailed geriatric, palliative care, and oncological assessments is evident. Cancer and its treatment success pivot on successful assessments and reassessments. Pain in its many dimensions can be erased. Overarching these valuable tools is respect for an elder patient and caregiver(s) wishes. Basic ethical principles must be exercised and respected. When dilemmas arise, mechanisms for resolution exist. Post and Dubler have made an initial proposal providing a bioethical definition, principles, and guidelines of palliative care.

Long-term care

LTC facilities, commonly referred to as nursing homes, are settings where persons, primarily the elderly, receive medical, nursing, and psychosocial interventions (26). Nursing homes were originally planned as residences for the affluent and well elderly. Nursing homes are now similar to hospitals, with residents having complex medical and psychosocial needs (27). Care administered by skilled nursing facilities and certified home health agencies are the most common locations for long-term care for the elderly.

A majority of all U.S. citizens 85 years and older will spend some time in a nursing home. A cross-section of this population reveals that most have a dementing illness, a high degree of disability, and a variety of co-morbidities. The elderly make up a vast majority in LTC, and the proportion of those with dementia rises rapidly for the oldest old.

Pain is a common symptom in LTC, with a prevalence as high as 80% (28,29). Musculoskeletal disorders are the most common causes of pain, but cancer is associated with severe symptomatology (30,31). Unrelieved pain is a catalyst for a cascade of suffering manifested by depression, decline in function, social withdrawal, and increased health care costs.

Pain assessment is difficult in a nursing home resident (32,33). Clinical staff does not inquire, and residents may not report about pain. A battery of assessment tools reveals that at least one provides information about pain in the cognitively impaired (31). Depression and anxiety are common symptoms in unrelieved chronic pain. A careful physical examination is mandatory, and staff and caregivers are a valuable source of information. A brief admission to an acute care facility for procedures to diagnose and treat more complex pain is a requirement in some cases (34).

McDonald (35) published some valuable advice for evaluating the cognitively impaired elderly with cancer. Pain syndromes may present in a subtle or cryptic manner. Behavioral changes from baseline may be the only clue to pain. One interesting study showed that an around-the-clock regimen of acetaminophen and not neuroleptics yielded a 63% reduction of behavioral symptoms (36). Confusion is usually multifactorial: delirium, dementia, depression, and drug side effects can be investigated and addressed. Analgesics properly chosen, the judicious use of an antidepressant, and the discontinuation of unnecessary psychoactive medications can make a world of difference.

Complex and longer pain assessment tools are rarely useful in the cognitively impaired nursing home resident (37,38). Additionally, de Wit et al. (39) showed that a variety of pain assessment tools used in a prospective study yielded surprising results. Patients with chronic pain because of cancer were inadequately treated in a range of 16%–91%. Therefore, the measurement tool and not pain treatment per se determined the clinical outcome. The development of teaching nursing homes has shown that education, research, and good clinical care can co-exist and flourish. A recent publication reported a prospective study to determine utility of standard pain assessment tools (40). A verbal rating scale, a visual analog scale, the Wong–Baker Faces Scale, and the McGill Word Scale were administered monthly for 1 year to 37 residents. Three standard pain locator tools were administered simultaneously. Less than half of the study population could use any of the pain severity tools. Eighty-six percent, however, could locate pain on their bodies.

In a sample of 2151 nursing home residents, 64.8% could not participate in pain assessment (31). There are some strategies to facilitate assessment. A careful review of a patient's neoplastic disease history is essential, as is a complete physical examination. Simple imaging studies may be required to analyze pain etiology. Family members and friends usually provide valuable observations.

A landmark study by the Systematic Assessment of Geriatric Drug Use via Epidemiology Study Group has provided much surprising information (41). A large group (13,625) of nursing home residents with cancer 65 years and older in 1492 facilities in the United States were evaluated between 1992 and 1995. The Minimum Data Set of the Resident Assessment Instrument, an electronic database, was used. Daily pain was seen in more than 25%, and of this group, 16% received a WHO level 1 drug, 32% a WHO level 2 drug, and 26% received morphine as a level 3 analgesic. Patients over 85 years, blacks, and those with cognitive deficits were at a greater risk of receiving no analgesics. Such findings indicate that nursing homes must develop strategies to overcome the barriers to pain management (42).

Few data exist about cancer pain in elderly nursing home residents with cognitive impairment. Wynne et al. (40) studied a small population, all of whom were enrolled in an active rehabilitation program, and most of whom had pain resulting from arthritis. Nevertheless, this study showed that basic palliative care research can be successfully fulfilled in this elderly and cognitively impaired population. Larger cooperative multicenter studies can provide valuable data about cancer pain.

Caregivers provide assistance in a variety of needs of the elderly. These include direct nursing care, personal care, homemaking needs, and transportation, among others. Emanuel, et al. (43) reported on assistance given to terminal patients by caregivers. A majority of patients were older than 65 years and had advanced cancer. A large proportion required assistance and received care at home. Caregivers were family members most often and, very rarely, unrelated volunteers. Caregivers provide a lifesaving role to the elderly with incurable progressive illness and should no longer be excluded from the health care team (44).

Cognitive impairment

Confusion is a common finding in the elderly and is not a normal part of aging. Visual and auditory deficits can render pain assessment difficult. Cataract removal, treatment for macular degeneration, and cochlear implants can improve functional ability (45,46). Although these physical problems pose considerable barriers to assessing pain, dementing illnesses, delirium, and depression are the dominant impediments.

Dementia is characterized by the steady, indolent, and irreversible loss of intellectual skills. Loss of recent memory, personality changes, and withering of language (aphasia) and motor skills (apraxia) are among the most common findings in dementia. Dementia is never a part of normal aging. Dementia's clinical hallmark is a normal level of consciousness (47).

Alzheimer's disease occurs in 3%–5% of individuals older than 65 years. Prevalence approaches 45% of those over 85 years. Alzheimer's disease affects a majority of the oldest old in LTC settings (48). The Folstein Mini-Mental Status Examination is a brief and useful tool in screening for dementia (49) (Table 20.1). Alzheimer's disease is an irreversible illness whose earlier stages can be extended by the use of donepezil (50) or rivastigmine (51).

There are many dementing illnesses. Multi-infarct and Lewy body dementias, in addition to Alzheimer's disease, account for 90%–95% of all dementing illnesses. Hypothyroidism and vitamin B_{12} deficiency are easily diagnosed examples of reversible dementias. Depression is the most common affective psychiatric disease that mimics dementia (pseudodementia) (52).

Delirium is an organic neurologic syndrome characterized by fluctuating consciousness, confusion, psychomotor changes, and emotional disturbances. An altered level of consciousness and fluctuation of symptoms differentiate delirium from dementia. The Confusion Assessment Method is a simple, valid, and reliable tool that can be used to screen for delirium (53) (Table 20.2).

A total of 20%–30% of the elderly admitted to acute care settings develop delirium, and delirium affects 70%–90% of patients at the end of life (54). Underlying dementia and adverse drug events are important precipitating factors of delirium (55). The poor prognosis of delirium relative to functional status and mortality is well known (56).

Cognitive impairment is a major barrier to successful pain management in LTC. Dementia, delirium, depression, and auditory and visual sensory impairment, can act in concert to impede accurate pain assessment.

Optimal pain assessment and successful treatment can be obtained in the confused elderly. One method is to determine and treat reversible dementias. A second is to search for precipitating factors causing delirium and institute therapy (e.g., a medication review with discontinuation of offending drug[s]). Pharmacologic management of delirium requires a neuroleptic drug around the clock. Haloperidol, thioridazine, and newer atypical neuroleptic drugs are available (57) and are effective when used cautiously.

The frail oldest old in LTC is a population at high risk for pain. The probability of significant cognitive impairment in this vulnerable population is very high. There are a number of strategies to assist in leading to optimal pain management. Obtaining valid medical information, performing a precise physical examination, and pursuing history from family, friends, and caregivers are all essen-

Table 20.1. *Folstein Mini Mental State Examination (49)*

FOLSTEIN MINI MENTAL STATUS EXAM

Date: _____   Examiner: _____

Score	ORIENTATION	
( )	What is the (year) (season) (month) (date) (day)	(5 pts)
( )	Where are we? (country) (province) (city) (hospital) (floor)	(5 pts)

REGISTRATION

( )	Name 3 objects: One second to say each. Then ask the patient to repeat all three after you have said them. One point for each correct. Then repeat them until he learns them. Count trials and record _____	(3 pts)

ATTENTION AND CALCULATIONS

( )	Serial 7s. One point for each correct answer. Stop after 5 answers. *Or* spell "world" backward. (No. correct = letters before first mistake)	(5 pts)

RECALL

( )	Ask for the objects above. One point for each correct.	(3 pts)
(21)		

LANGUAGE TESTS

( )	Name: pencil, watch	(2 pts)
( )	Repeat: no ifs, ands, or buts	(1 pt)
( )	Follow a three-stage command: "Take the paper in your right hand, fold it in half, and put it on the floor."	(3 pts)
( )	Read and obey the following:	
( )	Close your eyes.	(1 pt)
	Write a sentence spontaneously below.	(1 pt)
( )	Copy design below.	(1 pt)
(9)		
_____ ( )	Total (30 pts)	

Table 20.2. *The Confusion Assessment Method (CAM) Diagnostic Algorithm[a] (53)*

Feature 1.	Acute Onset and Fluctuating Course
	This feature is usually obtained from a family member or nurse and is shown by positive responses to the following questions. Is there evidence of acute change in mental status from the patient's baseline? Did the (abnormal) behavior fluctuate during the day, that is, tend to come and go, or increase and decrease in severity?
Feature 2.	Inattention
	This feature is shown by a positive response to the following question: Did the patient have difficulty focusing attention, for example, being easily distractible, or having difficulty keeping track of what was being said?
Feature 3.	Disorganized Thinking
	This feature is shown by a positive response to the following question: Was the patient's thinking disorganized or incoherent, such as rambling or irrelevant conversation, unclear or illogical flow of ideas, or unpredictable switching from subject to subject?
Feature 4.	Altered Level of Consciousness
	This feature is shown by any answer other than "alert" to the following question: Overall, how would you rate this patient's level of consciousness? (alert [normal], vigilant [hyperalert], lethargic [drowsy, easily aroused], stupor [difficult to arouse], or coma [unarousable]).

[a] The diagnosis of delirium by CAM requires the presence of features 1 and 2 and either 3 or 4.

tial. Ferrell (58) identified additional strategies to optimize care (Table 20.3).

Depression is commonly overlooked in the elderly, and its incidence rises in the setting of progressive cancer (59). Somatic symptoms of advanced cancer are identical to those with depression. Psychologic symptoms, such as helplessness and anhedonia, are difficult to elicit in the elderly with cognitive impairment. Uncontrolled pain amplifies symptoms of depression (60). The Geriatric Depression Scale is a useful tool to assess the extent of depression in the elderly (61) (Table 20.4).

The elderly with symptomatic cancer are at high risk for depression, pseudodementia, and suicidal thoughts. Suicidality has many risk factors, including depression, unrelieved symptoms, and encephalopathy from disease and centrally active medications (62).

Depression can be treated successfully. Cognitive approaches, empathic dialog, and the bolstering of social and spiritual supports are productive initial steps. Many antidepressants are available. Tricyclics have a sedating effect that is beneficial when insomnia is present (63). The selective serotonin reuptake inhibitors have a less-sedating effect. Psychostimulants act rapidly and may be most useful in the final phase of life (64). Insomnia, tachycardia, and psychosis are potential side effects.

Apart from dementia and depression, substance abuse is a commonly overlooked cause of cognitive impairment in the elderly. Alcoholism is seen in 3%–14% of elderly in the community (65), whereas 44% of older psychiatric inpatients are alcoholics (66). Symptoms of substance abuse can mimic those of progressive cancer. Multiple symptoms from other chronic diseases make assessment more complicated.

Table 20.3. *Assessment strategies in the cognitively impaired*

Identify a comfortable and calm site
Be complete but concise with questions
Allow adequate time
    to pose questions
    to record a response
Correct for
    auditory deficit with hearing device
    visual deficit
        adequate light
        large print
Reassess frequently

Adapted from Ferrell BA. Special considerations in the management of pain in the older person. A paper presented as part of the symposium, The Management of Pain and End-Of-Life Issues in Older People: Annual Scientific Meeting of the American Geriatrics Society, May 21, 1999, Philadelphia.

Table 20.4. *Scoring: Geriatric Depression Scale (short form) with scoring*

Choose the best answer for how you have felt over the past week:
  1. Are you basically satisfied with your life? YES / **NO**
  2. Have you dropped many of your activities and interests? **YES** / NO
  3. Do you feel that your life is empty? **YES** / NO
  4. Do you often get bored? **YES** / NO
  5. Are you in good spirits most of the time? YES / **NO**
  6. Are you afraid that something bad is going to happen to you? **YES** / NO
  7. Do you feel happy most of the time? YES / **NO**
  8. Do you often feel helpless? **YES** / NO
  9. Do you prefer to stay at home, rather than going out and doing new things? **YES** / NO
 10. Do you feel you have more problems with memory than most? **YES** / NO
 11. Do you think it is wonderful to be alive now? YES / **NO**
 12. Do you feel pretty worthless the way you are now? **YES** / NO
 13. Do you feel full of energy? YES / **NO**
 14. Do you feel that your situation is hopeless? **YES** / NO
 15. Do you think that most people are better off than you are? **YES** / NO
Answers in **bold** indicate depression. Although differing sensitivities and specificities have been obtained across studies, for clinical purposes a score > 5 points is suggestive of depression and should warrent a follow-up interview. Scores > 10 are almost always depression.

Elderly alcoholics most often have a lifelong history of the disease, but for some it is a recent acquisition. An acutely intoxicated individual may be confused, have slurred speech, and may fall. A subdural hematoma may evolve with its acute and chronic neurologic sequelae. Chronic alcohol ingestion can cause many findings identical to progressive metastatic disease (67) (Table 20.5). Abstinence is the primary aim of treatment, but recognition and discussion of alcohol abuse are the necessary starting points.

In addition to alcohol, the elderly use hypnotics, opioids, cocaine, and psychostimulants. The incidence of the use of the latter is not known. As many as 1% of patients on methadone maintenance treatment programs are elderly with prior opioid addiction (68). The use of benzodiazepines, especially those with long half-lives, is problematic. In addition to the risk of addiction, physical dependence becomes evident on withdrawal of the agent (69). Delirium caused by benzodiazepine withdrawal and use looks no different from delirium seen in advanced cancer.

Loss of friends, family, and independence is a common component of aging. Depression, anxiety, and other psychological symptoms are common in the elderly. Alcohol,

Table 20.5. *Effects of chronic alcohol ingestion*

Physiological effects	Potential consequences
Decreased hydroxylation of vitamin D	Osteomalacia
Increased estrogen ratio	Fractures
	Testicular atrophy
	Spider angiomata
	Gynecomastia
	Palmar erythema
Decreased testosterone	Impotence
Thiamine deficiency	Wernicke-Korsakoff syndrome (dementia)
Altered cardiovascular function	Arrhythmias
	Congestive heart failure
B$_{12}$ malabsorption	Megaloblastic anemia
Gastritis	Atrophic gastritis
	Iron deficiency anemia
	Altered pharmacokinetics
Fatty and/or fibrotic liver	Hepatitis
	Cirrhosis
	Altered pharmacokinetics

Reprinted with permission from Gambert SR. The elderly. In: Lowinson JH, Ruiz P, Millman RB, Langrod R, eds. Substance abuse: a comprehensive textbook. Baltimore: Williams and Wilkins, 1997:692–9.

opioids, benzodiazepines, and other substances temporarily blunt these symptoms. The chronic sequelae, suffering, and, at times, death emphasize the need to diagnose and treat substance abuse in this fragile population.

Pharmacologic principles in the elderly

Pharmacological therapies play a vital role in geriatric care. The vast array of antihypertensive agents, a growing number of lipid-lowering drugs, and new, broad-spectrum antibiotics have been instrumental in extending survival and fostering successful aging. A clear understanding of the anticipated physiologic changes and status of concurrent illnesses is mandatory to ensure safe and effective drug therapies in the elderly.

In the United States, two thirds of all elders take an average of 4.5 prescription and 2.1 non-prescription drugs (70). In the LTC setting, where cognitive impairment is most likely present, an average of seven drugs is prescribed. Federal and state oversight of nursing homes has developed clear medication guidelines. A review by Beers et al. (71) showed that 40% of nursing home residents were prescribed at least one inappropriate drug, and women received a greater number than men.

Aging alters both pharmacokinetics and pharmacodynamics. Drug distribution is altered because decreased total body water and lean body mass paired with increased body fat. With chronic medical illness(es), hypoalbuminemia has an impact on the responses to drugs with high protein binding.

Liver and kidney function changes alter responses. Hepatic mass and blood flow decline, seriously affecting first-pass metabolism biotransformation of drugs. Morphine, meperidine, and some antidepressants should be used at doses 30%–40% of standard dosing. Renal mass and blood flow decline with age, reflected in decreased creatinine clearance. Tubular function declines and drugs with primary renal elimination, especially those given chronically, must be assessed frequently.

Polypharmacy refers to the use of multiple prescribed and unprescribed medications. Adverse drug events occur commonly and are easily misinterpreted as disease progression. A delirium precipitated by an anticholinergic drug in a patient with Alzheimer's disease is an example of drug-disease interaction. A drug-drug interaction can be observed when renal insufficiency results from a nonsteroidal anti-inflammatory drug (NSAID) being used with a diuretic.

Opioid and non-opioid analgesics can be used safely and effectively in the elderly. The American Geriatrics Society (AGS) has published guidelines for effective prescribing (72). Techniques are available to foster drug protocol compliance (73). General dose adjustment guidelines give some direction.

Initial dosing in an older person with cancer should be one-third to one-half that of the usual dose with drugs having a narrow therapeutic index. The BMI (body mass index) is an important factor in dosing. Dose adjustments require careful assessment. The use of an opioid and other analgesics may be a necessity. The risk of not providing adequate pain relief is far greater than any risk of side effects (74).

Cleeland et al. (75) showed astonishing underassessment and undertreatment of pain in ambulatory cancer patients. A majority of 1308 adults with metastatic cancer had had pain. Patients older than 70 had 2.4 times the risk of not receiving adequate pain control. Other studies similarly suggest undertreatment and problems with access to pain care. Symptoms of unrelated non-neoplastic illness are not addressed (76). A large number of enrollees in Medicare have no drug benefits. Health maintenance organizations increase capitations on the number of medications allowed (77). Inner-city New York City residents find serious difficulty obtaining opioids in neighborhood pharmacies (78).

These barriers must be overcome, and expertise in the pharmacological treatment of cancer pain in the elderly must be encouraged. Careful assessment, appropriate dosing, frequent monitoring, and management of side effects will improve outcomes. Until more studies are introduced and results disseminated, two adages in geriatric care are useful: "start low and go slow" (79) and prescribe "neither too much nor too little" (80).

Pain treatment

Comprehensive pain assessment is a prerequisite for successful pain management (81). Treatment planning is predicted on an accurate medical history and a precise physical examination.

Avenues of antineoplastic therapy, both curative and palliative, must be explored. Surgical resection with curative intent of a carcinoma of the sigmoid colon causing visceral pain can be effectively analgesic. Radiotherapy for locoregionally advanced head and neck neoplasms can be accomplished using external beam and/or interstitial ionizing radiation (82,83). Hormonal therapies play a vital role in the palliation of advanced breast and prostate cancer, providing objective responses in a large proportion of older patients (84,85). Proper multidimensional assessment allows systemic chemotherapy to be administered effectively in some lymphoproliferative diseases (86,87). Gemcitabine and mitoxantrone (in combination with hydrocortisone) provide palliation of pain in surgically unresectable pancreatic cancer (88) and hormone refractory metastatic prostate cancer (89), respectively.

Bone metastases are the most common cause of somatic pain syndromes in advanced cancer. An individualized plan of care can be developed (90). In addition to non-opioid and opioid analgesics, external beam radiotherapy is the most common modality used to palliate bone pain. Short-course, large-fraction courses are effective as longer 2- or 3-week protocols (91). Radiopharmaceuticals are beneficial in multifocal pain syndromes. Isotopes of phosphorus (92), strontium (93), and samarium (94) are available, and those of rhenium (95) and tin (96) are under investigation. Adjuvant co-analgesic medications are very important, especially corticosteroids and a bisphosphonate. The growing number of potent bisphosphonates can provide both analgesia and prevention of adverse skeletal events. Orthopedic procedures in lytic disease in the long bones and in spinal instability can provide excellent palliation in selected cases.

Opioids are the primary analgesics used in cancer pain. Guidelines published by the Agency for Healthcare Policy and Research (81), now the Agency for Healthcare Research and Quality, is one of a growing number of resources for cancer pain treatment. There are many opioids available for use. Morphine is the most commonly used opioid, but many are effective and well tolerated.

Cleary (97) published a practical three-phase approach in devising a therapeutic opioid regimen. Initial treatment and titration require immediate-release drugs in the opioid-naïve population. Extended-release opioids can be initiated in patients currently using immediate-release preparations. Consolidating treatments as pain is relieved usually involves an extended-release opioid with an immediate-release form for breakthrough pain. Oral transmucosal fentanyl citrate is a recent and effective addition for the management of breakthrough pain (98). Prophylaxis of opioid toxicities, especially constipation, should occur when opioid treatment becomes scheduled. The final phase of an opioid regimen is maintenance, during which doses and/or dosing intervals are adjusted to obtain optimal pain relief. Monitoring of side effects, constipation, nausea and vomiting, sedation, and confusion continues on a frequent basis.

Opioids can be administered through many routes. The oral route is the most common and the most preferred. Dysphagia resulting from mechanical obstruction or neuromuscular disease requires the use of other routes of administration. One extended-release morphine product is composed of granules that can be sprinkled on food or administered through a gastrostomy tube (99).

Although a small number of the elderly participated in initial clinical trials, transdermal fentanyl patches are safe and effective (100). Patch removal and replacement require dexterity and good vision that may be deficient in the frail elderly. Transdermal fentanyl is useful when an oral route is not possible with the administration of an immediate-release opioid rectally for breakthrough pain.

The rectal route has been used effectively (101) and is commonly underused. Suppository preparations of morphine, hydromorphone, and oxymorphone are available, and each can be used in a safe and effective manner (102). Active inflammatory disease, fecal incontinence, and neutropenia are relative contraindications to this route. There is no strong evidence that sustained-release opioids can be used effectively by rectal administration.

The subcutaneous route of opioid administration given by continuous infusion reduces peaks and valleys in serum opioid concentrations. When used in conjunction with a patient-controlled analgesia device, certain opioid side effects can be avoided, and breakthrough pain can be managed (103). Most opioids can be given via this route, and both fentanyl and sufentanil are advantageous because of their enhanced potency and lipid solubility relative to morphine (104). Residents in LTC facilities rarely have access to the subcutaneous continuous infusion route. The frail elderly at home with moderate cognitive deficits would require astute supervision if this route were used.

Intranasal (105), inhaled (106), and topical opioids (107) have been used and studied in small clinical trials. There is no clear and convincing evidence that any of these routes is superior to enteral and parenteral opioid administration.

Interventional pain therapies and intraspinal opioid infusions are rarely required. Residents in LTC facilities and those in certified home health agency programs have limited access to high-quality pain services. In highly selected elders, when standard opioid regimens are ineffective and/or side effects are overwhelming, these techniques may be both effective, safe, and at times economical (108). Clonidine can be used intraspinally as a co-analgesic with an opioid (109). Orthostatic hypotension is a side effect of significance when autonomic dysfunction is present. Addition of bupivacaine to intraspinal opioids may provide analgesia when high doses of parenteral opioids are not efficient (110).

Non-opioid analgesics and adjuvant analgesics play a critical role in achieving adequate pain relief, especially when opioid side effects become intolerable. NSAIDs include a large number of agents. Most are given orally and both gastrointestinal and renal toxicities are important and potentially life threatening when left unmonitored. The more recent cyclo-oxygenase-2 selective inhibitors have lesser, but still present gastrointestinal toxicities (111); there is no evidence of reduced toxicity to kidneys.

Adjuvant analgesics form a large number of diverse drug classes (112). They can be used in neuropathic and bone pain syndromes. There are few randomized, controlled studies proving their worth, and sequential trials may be required in selecting an optimal adjuvant drug. Cognitive impairment may result from the use of most of these agents and, therefore, require careful monitoring during their administration.

Other strategies are available and can be used concomitantly with analgesics. Physiatric techniques include cutaneous stimulation, gentle or deep massage, as well as the use of heat or cold (113). A program of maintenance physical therapy may postpone deconditioning and lessen fatigue. Psychological avenues are helpful in the cognitively intact elderly (114). Family-caregiver interventions are necessary in patients with dementing illnesses with or without superimposed delirium. The spiri-

tual needs of patients and their families can be assessed easily. Near the end of life, spiritual assessment and care are essential for all dimensions of cancer pain.

Complementary and alternative therapies are popular among patients with cancer (115). They are used in conjunction with standard therapies most often, although a small number of patients use them exclusively. Understanding which complementary treatments are used and what their meaning is to patients should be a standard part of comprehensive pain assessment.

Opioid side effects

Opioid side effects can be a serious problem in the elderly. The literature in this area is growing but still is quite sparse. Analgesic studies exclude the more frail cancer patient. The variety of side effects seen during opioid administration is common to those of other medical conditions and treatments for the elderly (116).

Constipation is common in the elderly. This is due to a suppressed gastrointestinal reflex and poor dietary fiber intake (117). Many medical conditions will exacerbate constipation, including immobility, depression, and hypothyroidism. All anticholinergics, calcium channel blockers, and sedatives are important additive factors. Autonomic neuropathy and cauda equina metastases are further etiologies. A daily regimen of a stool softener and laxative, proper review of medications when opioid therapy starts, and frequent reassessments will help avoid this distressing and, at times, threatening symptom.

Opioid administration does not cause dementia, but confusion is a common finding in the elderly patient with advanced cancer (118). Delirium resulting from medical illness and medication toxicities is almost universal in older hospitalized patients. An acute confusional state may be the sole indication of pain. A number of maneuvers may be used if an opioid is a possible cause of confusion (119). They include reduction of opioid dose, addition of an adjuvant analgesic, and switching to another opioid. If the symptom is refractory to all attempts, assessment for neuraxial opioids may be needed.

Lethargy and fatigue are common findings that may be opioid induced. Psychostimulants have been used in this setting, including methylphenidate, dextroamphetamine, and pemoline (120,121). Psychostimulants pose a threat to the frail elderly with cerebral, psychiatric, and/or cardiac disease. Prudent investigation into non-opioid causes of this complex symptom should be pursued. If there is no contraindication, an empirical trial of a psychostimulant can proceed with the understanding that no firm data exist to support its use.

Nausea is an important complication of opioid therapy (122). One fourth or fewer of patients will have nausea that may recede as therapy continues. Central nervous system disease, intestinal obstruction, and hepatobiliary complications may be confounding factors requiring management. Medical treatment of opioid-induced nausea can be treated with neuroleptics or prokinetic agents. Accurate and frequent vigilance for extrapyramidal symptoms is mandatory. Anticholinergics, antihistamines, and corticosteroids can provoke delirium. Opioid rotation is needed when antiemetics trials are unsuccessful.

Urinary retention is a distressing and potentially life-threatening complication. It is dose related and is more common in men and those receiving infusional opioids. Spinal cord lesions in men and women and prostatic hypertrophy and carcinoma in men are common causes of this complication in advanced disease. Frequent assessment for a palpable bladder is essential and, when present, should be remedied with an indwelling catheter. Cholinergic drugs and alpha-adrenergic blockers are available, but delirium for the former and hypotension for the latter may eclipse their utility.

Myoclonus is a relatively rare but disturbing symptom and may reflect opioid toxicities in the presence of acute medical complications. Clonazepam or phenobarbital in small doses can be useful. In refractory myoclonus, opioid dosing can be diminished if pain relief is adequate; if not, opioid rotation should occur.

Pain management in the elderly with cancer will not succeed when attention to opioid toxicity is lax. When toxicities are appreciated and given attention, a few simple maneuvers can prevent and alleviate suffering. Vanegas et al. (123) published a comprehensive review of opioid side effects.

Pain management guidelines

There are still a large number of barriers to effective pain treatment (124). The publication of pain management guidelines by professional societies attempts to overcome barriers to accurate pain assessment and treatment. Doctors, nurses, patients, and their families can easily receive education. There are now a number of valuable resources.

The AGS has issued two clinical practice guidelines: an earlier publication on cancer pain (125), a later one on chronic pain management (126), and a more recent update (127). The latter includes valuable information on non-pharmacologic pain therapies and the importance of

institutional Continuous Quality Improvement initiatives to improve pain management.

The American Society of Clinical Oncology (ASCO) developed curriculum guidelines for pain assessment and treatment (128). ASCO has emphasized clearing the barriers to evaluation and treatment of cancer pain. Special problems in treatment of the elderly are noted. The National Comprehensive Cancer Network developed practice guidelines (129) that include treatment algorithms and tables regarding opioid dosing and toxicities. A detailed table on ancillary approaches, including the use of co-analgesics and non-pharmacological interventions is noteworthy.

There are additional resources. The AHCPR (now the AHRQ) publication from 1994 has a valuable section on the elderly (81). The Oncology Nursing Society (130), the American Pain Society (131), and the Cancer Pain Section of the American Society of Anesthesiologists (132) have also made valuable contributions.

Patient-family education and caregiver empowerment is a profitable route to overcome barriers. The AHRQ and the ACS provide lucid and easy-to-understand facts about cancer pain. L'Association Internationale Ensemble Contre la Doleur, (The International Association Against Pain) has sponsored programs to encourage patients and families to ask for and expect pain relief from their clinical team when hospitalized.

The Joint Commission on Accreditation of Healthcare Organizations has developed standards that create new expectations for program accreditation (133). This comprehensive initiative underscores the need to recognize adequate pain management as a right, mandate clinical competencies, and institute patient and family education. Standard feasibility studies are currently activated so that nationwide compliance scoring will begin in 2001. Governmental recognition and support of these diversified initiatives are a requirement for their success.

The Council of Europe based in Strasbourg, France, recognizes that all patients should be legally entitled to palliative care and urges physicians to provide adequate pain relief for the terminally ill (134).

Consumer support is a necessary part of transforming pain initiatives into a public health movement. Five components are suggested to achieve this aim: enlist high-profile opinion leaders, challenge commonly held misperceptions, unite legislators and policymakers with clinicians and the public, showcase the results of good practice, and involve consumers and caregivers (135).

There is now abundant literature proving that cancer pain in the elderly can be treated successfully. The unification of the clinical forces in oncology, pain medicine, palliative care, and geriatrics, with a robust grass roots movement and governmental involvement, will obliterate many barriers to cancer pain relief.

Research initiatives

The elderly are commonly excluded from research studies. Cognitive impairment and active co-morbid illnesses are the usual reasons for exclusion. Ageism also plays a role. New opportunities are developing that include the elderly with cancer pain.

The NCI is sponsoring a study run by the Eastern Cooperative Oncology Group (136). Men with advanced prostate cancer and women with advanced breast cancer and pain are eligible. This randomized pilot study will evaluate the worth of an outpatient educational and behavioral skills training program on pain control. The goals are to improve pain control and quality of life.

The NCIC (National Cancer Institute of Canada) Clinical Trials group developed a randomized, placebo-controlled study for chronic pain in patients with advanced cancer (137). Patients with leukemia, lymphoma, or multiple myeloma on stable doses of opioids for strong pain are eligible. Once randomized, they will receive one of two sustained-release morphine preparations followed by dextromethorphan or placebo. The objective of this project is to determine if pain relief by opioids can be improved by lessening opioid side effects by the NMDA receptor antagonist dextromethorphan.

Radiation therapy plays an important role in palliation from bone metastases. The NCI, the North Central Cancer Treatment Group, and the RTOG are actively recruiting patients with breast and prostate cancer suffering from painful bone metastases (138). This randomized study examines the role of single fraction radiotherapy versus multiple fraction response rate and its duration, quality-of-life parameters, and the prospective incidence of pathologic fractures.

As these and newer, emerging studies mature, valuable information will be available to better assist managing cancer pain in the elderly. Linked with useful assessment strategies for the frail and cognitively impaired elder, the incidence and intensity of cancer pain will diminish while quality of life is sustained.

End-of-life care

A majority of people in the United States die in a health care facility. Studies reveal that end-of-life care is poor.

The Study to Understand Prognoses and Preferences for Outcomes and Risks of Treatments (SUPPORT) that included patients with advanced non–small-cell lung cancer and advanced colorectal cancer clearly demonstrated that pain relief, respect for patient treatment preferences, adherence to advance directives, and other indicators revealed poor outcomes (139). The elderly with progressive advanced cancer are electing the Medicare Hospice Benefit for end-of-life care in increasing numbers. Many more, however, are unaware or choose not to elect this palliative care program. The EPEC project (Educating Physicians at End of Life Care) developed by the American Medical Association has made crucial inroads to improve physician practices in this overlooked area of medical care (140).

Dying becomes a proximate event as advanced cancer progresses and multiple co-morbidities take their toll (Table 20.3). Universally accepted principles of pain management for the imminently dying have been developed (141). Frequent pain assessments, continuation of around-the-clock opioids, ensuring a route of opioid administration, and abstaining from the use of opioid antagonists (142) are necessary to achieve a pain-free death.

When death is imminent, refractory pain is a rare event. Pain is refractory when all interventions fail in the presence of consciousness (143). Sedation is a medically and morally acceptable modality of therapy when precise selection criteria are fulfilled (144). Short-acting benzodiazepines, such as lorazepam or midazolam, and phenobarbital can be given as a continuous infusion. A neuroleptic may be necessary in the presence of delirium. Sedation for intractable pain is not indicative of a failure of palliative care, nor should it ever be associated with physician-assisted suicide and euthanasia (145).

Modern culture is ambivalent about death. Medical education views death as a failure and not a necessary

Table 20.6. *Findings in the imminently dying cancer patient*

Progression of metastatic disease
Worsening Karnofsky Performance Status (KPS) score
Increase in symptom number and intensity
Increasing periods of lethargy
Diminished intake of food and fluid
Confusion
Findings of anticipatory bereavement
Frequent fluctuations in vital signs
A recent flurry of:
   laboratory tests
   consultations
   ER visits

segment of life. Daniel Callahan identifies the harmful character of the "technologic imperative" and states that "we can change the way people are cared for at the end of life. It is not ... death that people seem to fear most ... but a life poorly lived" (146).

The SUPPORT study clearly demonstrates the rigidly reflexive use of advanced life support when palliative care would be indicated. The concepts and components of a "good death" are found in a text by Byock (147) and a study by Steinhauser et al. (148). The Greek philosopher Heraclitus said, "For when is death not within ourselves? Living and dead are the same, and so are awake and asleep, young and old" (149). Today's research imperative is to focus on care of the elderly at the end of life so the burden of suffering is ameliorated and that death is peaceful.

Selected resources

American Academy of Hospice and Palliative Medicine
4700 W. Lake Ave.
Glenview, IL 60025-1485
Phone: 847-375-4712
http://www.aahpm.org/

American Alliance of Cancer Pain Initiatives
C/O The Resource Center for State Cancer Pain Initiatives
1300 University Ave., Room 4720
Madison, WI 53706
Phone: 608-265-4013
http://www.fhcrc.org/cipr/aacpi/

American Cancer Society
Phone: 1-800-ACS-2345.
http://www.cancer.org

The American Geriatrics Society
The Empire State Building
350 Fifth Avenue, Suite 801
New York, NY 10118
Phone: 212-308-1414
http://www.americangeriatrics.org/

American Society of Clinical Oncology
225 Reinekers Lane, Suite 650
Alexandria, VA 22314
Phone: 703-299-0150
http://www.asco.org/

Beth Israel Medical Center
Department of Pain Medicine and Palliative Care

First Avenue at 16th Street
New York, NY 10003
Phone: 212-844-8970
http://www.stoppain.org/

British Society of Gerontology
http://www.soc.surrey.ac.uk/bsg/
E-mail: bsg@soc.surrey.ac.uk

Cancer Care, Inc.
275 7th Ave
New York, NY 10001
Phone: 212-302-2400
http://www.cancercare.org/

The Cochrane Pain, Palliative Care and Supportive Care (PaPaS) Collaborative Review Group
http://www.jr2.ox.ac.uk/Cochrane/
c/o Frances Fairman (Review Group Coordinator)
Pain, Palliative & Supportive Care CRG
Pain Relief Unit
The Churchill Hospital
Oxford OX3 7LJ UK
Phone: +44-1865-225762

European Association of Palliative Care
Instituto Nazionale Dei Tumori
Via Venezian 1
20133 Milano
ITALY
Phone: +39-02-2390792
http://www.eapcnet.org/

The Growth House
Phone: 415-255-9045
http://www.growthhouse.org/

Hospice and Palliative Nurses Association
211 N. Whitfield St., Suite 375
Pittsburgh, PA 15206
http://www.hpna.org/

International Association of Gerontology
c/o Centre for Ageing Studies
Mark Oliphant Building
Laffer Drive
Bedford Park SA 5042
Australia
Phone: +61-8-8201-7552
http://www.cas.flinders.edu.au/iag/iag.html

International Association of Gerontology, European Region
P.O. Box 9191 - 28080 Madrid (Spain)
Phone: 34-91-334-50-56
http://www.eriag.org/

International Association for the Study of Pain
IASP Secretariat
909 NE 43rd St., Suite 306
Seattle, WA 98105-6020 USA
Phone: 206-547-6409
http://www.halcyon.com/iasp/
The John A. Hartford Foundation Institute for Geriatric
    Nursing

L'Association Internationale Ensemble Contre la Doleur
http://www.douleur.ch/
E-mail: weibel@swisscancer.ch

Last Acts
c/o Robert Wood Johnson Foundation
PO Box 2316
Princeton, NJ 08543-2316
Phone: 609-452-8701
http://www.lastacts.org/

Mayday Pain Resource Center
http://www.cityofhope.org/mayday/Default.htm

National Hospice and Palliative Care Organization
1700 Diagonal Road, Suite 300
Alexandria, VA 22314
Phone: 800-658-8898
http://www.nhpco.org

The National Institute on Aging
Public Information Office
National Institutes of Health
Building 31, Room 5C27
31 Center Drive MSC 2292
Bethesda, MD 20892-2292
Phone: 1-800-222-2225
http://www.nih.gov/nia/

The New York State Partnership for Long-Term Care
Office of Continuing Care
NYS Department of Health
161 Delaware Avenue
Delmar, NY 12054
Phone: 518-473-8083
http://www.nyspltc.org

University of Wisconsin Pain and Policy Studies Group
1900 University Avenue
Madison, WI 53705-4013
Phone: 608-263-7662
http://www.medsch.wisc.edu/painpolicy/

References

1. Murray A. The sharpest pain. The New York Times, November 1, 1998, p. 15.
2. Chapman CR. Suffering: the contributions of persistent pain. Lancet 353(9171):2233–7, 1999.
3. U.S. Bureau of the Census. Current Population Reports, 25-1104. Washington, DC: United States Government Printing Office, 1993.
4. Yancik R, Ries LA. Aging and cancer in America: demographic and epidemiologic perspectives. Hematol Clin North Am 14(1):17–23, 2000.
5. Landis SH, Murray T, Bolden S, et al. Cancer statistics. CA Cancer J Clin 49(1):8–31, 1999.
6. Yancik R, Ries LA. Cancer in older persons. Magnitude of the problem–how do we apply what we know? Cancer 74 (7 Suppl):1995—2003, 1994.
7. Stanta G, Campagner L, Cavallieri F, et al. Cancer of the oldest old. What we have learned from autopsy studies. Clin Geriatr Med 13(1):55–68, 1997.
8. Ershsler WB. A gerontologist's perspective on cancer biology and treatment. Cancer Control 1(2):103–107, 1994.
9. Campisi J. Aging and cancer: the double-edged sword of replicative senscense. J Am Geriatr Soc 45(4):482–8, 1997.
10. Campisi J, Demre GP, Hara E. (1996). Control of replicative senescence. In: Schneider F, Rowe J, eds. Handbook of the biology of aging. New York: Academic Press, 1996:121–49.
11. Wang E. Senescent human fibroblasts resist programmed cell death, and failure to suppress bcl2 is involved. Cancer Res 55(1):2284–92, 1995.
12. Lupu R, Cardillo M, Harris L, et al. Interaction between erbB receptors and heregulin in breast cancer tumor progression and drug resistance. Semin Cancer Biol 6(3):135–45, 1995.
13. Meyerson M. Role of telomerase in normal and cancer cell. J Clin Oncol 18(13):2626–34, 2000.
14. Turner NJ, Haward RA, Mulley GP, et al. Cancer in old age–is it inadequately investigated and treated? BMJ 319(7205):309–12, 1999.
15. Balducci L, Mowrey K, Parker M. Pharmacology of antineoplastic agents in older patients. In: Balducci L, Lyman GH, Ehrsler WB, eds. Geriatric oncology. Philadelphia: JB Lippincott, 1992:169–80.
16. Ries LA. Ovarian cancer. Survival and treatment differences by age. Cancer 71(2 Suppl):524–9, 1993.
17. Olmi P, Ausili-Cefaro G. Radiotherapy in the elderly: a multicentric prospective study on 2060 patients referred to 37 Italian radiation therapy centers. Rays 22(1 Suppl):53–6, 1997.

18. Wetle T. Age as a risk factor for inadequate treatment. JAMA 258(4):516, 1987.

19. Weinrich SP, Weinrich MC. Cancer knowledge among elderly individuals. Cancer Nurs 9(6):301–7, 1986.

20. Fletcher A. Screening for cancer of the cervix in elderly women. Lancet 335(8681):97–9, 1990.

21. de Rijke JM, Schouten LJ, Schouten HC, et al. Age-specific differences in the diagnostics and treatment of cancer patients aged 50 years and older in the province of Limburg, the Netherlands. Ann Oncol 7(7):677–85, 1996.

22. Deyo R, Applegate WB, Kramer A, et al. The future of geriatric assessment. J Am Geriatr Soc 39(Suppl):S1–S59, 1991.

23. World Health Organization. Cancer pain relief: with a guide to opioid availability, 2nd ed. Geneva: World Heath Organization, 1996.

24. Extermann M, Aapro M. Assessment of the older cancer patient. Hematol Oncol Clin North Am 14(1):63–77, 2000.

25. Overcash J. The case for a geriatric oncology program in a cancer center. In: Balducci L, Lyman GH, Ehrsler WB, eds. Comprehensive geriatric oncology, 2nd ed. Amsterdam: Harwood Academic Publishers, 1998:813–24.

26. Kane R, Kane R. Long-term care. In: Cassel C, ed. Geriatric medicine. New York: Springer-Verlag, 1996:81–107.

27. Carcagno GJ, Kemper P. The evaluation of the national long term care demonstration. 1. An overview of the channeling demonstration and its evaluation. Health Serv Res 23(1):1–22, 1988.

28. Ferrell BA, Ferrell BR, Osterweil D. Pain in the nursing home. J Am Geriatr Soc 38(4):409–14, 1990.

29. Roy R, Michael T. A survey of chronic pain in an elderly population. Can Fam Physician 32:513–6, 1986.

30. Ferrell BA. Pain evaluation and management in the nursing home. Ann Intern Med 123(9):681–7, 1995.

31. Ferrell BA, Ferrell BR, Rivera L. Pain in cognitively impaired nursing home patients. J Pain Symptom Manage 10(8):591–8, 1995.

32. Stein W. Pain in the nursing home. Clin Geriatr Med 17(3):575–94, 2001.

33. Murray MA. Strategies to improve cancer pain in long-term care. Ann Long-Term Care Clin Care Aging 10(3):55–60, 2002.

34. Ouslander JG, Osterweil D, Morley JE. Medical care in the nursing home. New York: McGraw-Hill, 1991.

35. McDonald M. Assessment and management of pain in the cognitively impaired elderly. Geriatr Nurs 20(5):249–53, 1999.

36. Douzjian M, Wilson C, Schultz M, et al. A program to use pain control medication to reduce psychotropic drug use in residents with difficult behavior. Ann Long-Term Care Clin Care Aging 6:174–9, 1998.

37. Feldr KS. Improving assessment and treatment of of pain in cognitively-impaired nursing home residents. Ann Long-Term Care Clin Care Aging 8(9):36–42, 200.

38. Lefebvre-Chapiro S. The Doloplus® 2 scale: evaluating pain in the elderly. Eur J Palliat Care 8(5):191–4, 2001.

39. de Wit R, van Dam F, Abu-Saad HH, et al. Empirical comparison of commonly used measures to evaluate pain treatment in cancer patients with chronic pain. J Clin Oncol 17(4):1280, 1999.

40. Wynne CF, Ling SM, Remsburg R. Comparisons of pain assessment instruments in cognitively intact and cognitively impaired nursing home residents. Geriatr Nurs 21(1):20–3, 2000.

41. Bernabei R, Gambassi G, Lapane K, et al. Management of pain in elderly patients with cancer. SAGE study group. Systematic assessment of geriatric drug use via epidemiology. JAMA 279(23):1877–82, 1998.

42. Feinsod FM, Prochoda KP, Anneberg AL, et al. The medical director's role in pain management for residents of long-term care facilities. Ann Long-Term Care Clin Care Aging 8(10):43–8, 2000.

43. Emanuel EJ, Fairclough DL, Slutsman J, et al. Assistance from family members, friends, paid care givers and volunteers in the care of terminally ill patients. N Engl J Med 341(13):956–63, 1999.

44. Levine C. The loneliness of the long-term care giver. N Engl J Med 340(20):1587–90, 1999.

45. Kelsall DC, Shallop JK, Burnelli T. Cochlear implantation in the elderly. Am J Otol 16(5):609–15, 1995.

46. Zhang K, Nguyen TH, Crandall A, et al. Genetic and macular studies of macular degeneration: recent developments. Surv Ophthalmol 40(1):51–61, 1995.

47. National Institute on Aging. Progress report on Alzheimer's disease, 1998. Bethesda: U.S. Department of Health and Human Services, Public Health Service, National Institutes of Health, National Institute on Aging, 1998.

48. Sengstaken EA, King SA. The problems of pain and its detection in geriatric nursing home residents. J Am Geriatr Soc 41(5):541–4, 1993.

49. Folstein MF, Folstein SE, McHugh PR. A mini-mental state: a practical method for grading the cognitive state of patients for the clinician. J Psychiat Res 12(3):189–98, 1975.

50. Matthews HP, Korbey J, Wilkinson DG, et al. Donepezil in Alzheimer's disease: eighteen month results from Southampton Memory Clinic. Int J Geriatr Psychiatry 15(8):713–20, 2000.

51. Adams T, Page S. New pharmacological treatments for Alzheimer's disease: implications for dementia care nursing. J Adv Nurs 31(5):1183–8, 2000.

52. Alexopoulos GS, Meyers BS, Young RC, et al. The course of geriatric depression with "reversible dementia": a controlled study. Am J Psychiatry 150(11):1693–9, 1993.

53. Inouye SK, van Dyck CH, Alessi CA, et al. Clarifying confusion: the confusion assessment method. A new method for detection of delirium. Ann Intern Med 113(12):941–8, 1990.

54. Weinrich S, Sarna L. Delirium in the older person with cancer. Cancer 74(7 Suppl):2079–91, 1994.

55. Francis J. Delirium in older patients. J Am Geriatr Soc 40(8):829–38, 1992.

56. Cole MG, Primeau FJ. Prognosis of delirium in elderly hospital patients. CMAJ 149(1):41–6, 1993.

57. Fainsinger R, Bruera E. Treatment of delirium in a terminally ill patient. J Pain Symptom Manage 7(1):54–6, 1992.

58. Ferrell BA. Special considerations in the management of pain in the older person. A paper presented as part of the symposium, The Management of Pain and End-Of-Life Issues in Older People: Annual Scientific Meeting of the American Geriatrics Society, May 21, 1999, Philadelphia.

59. DeFlorio M, Massie MJ. Review of depression in cancer: gender differences. Depression 3:66, 1990.

60. American Pain Society. Principles of analgesic use in the treatment of acute pain and cancer pain, 2nd ed. Clin Pharm 9(8):601–12, 1990.

61. Yeasavage J. The Geriatric Depression scale (short-form). Available from: http://www.qlmed.org/Gds.

62. Louhivuori KA, Hakama M. Risk of suicide among cancer patients. Am J Epidemiol 109(1):59–65, 1979.

63. Salzman C. Practical considerations on the pharmacological treatment of depression and anxiety in the elderly. J Clin Psychiatry 51(Suppl):40–3, 1990.

64. Bruera E, Brenneis C, Paterson AH, et al. Use of methylphenidate as an adjuvant to narcotic analgesics in patients with advanced cancer. J Pain Symptom Manage 4(1):3–6, 1989.

65. Myers JK, Weissman MM, Tischler GL. Six-month prevalence of psychiatric disorders in three communities 1980 to 1982. Arch Gen Psychiatry 41(10):959–67, 1984.

66. Moore RA. The diagnosis of alcoholism in a psychiatric hospital: a trial of the Michigan Alcoholism Screening Test (MAST). Am J Psychiatry 128(12):1565–9, 1972.

67. Gambert SR. The elderly. In: Lowinson JH, Ruiz P, Millman RB, Langrod R, eds. Substance abuse: a comprehensive textbook. Baltimore: Williams and Wilkins, 1997:692–9.

68. Pascarelli EF. Drug abuse in the elderly. In: Lowinson JH, Ruiz P, Millman R, et al., eds. Baltimore: Williams and Wilkins, 1997.

69. Moss JH, Lanctot KL. Iatrogenic benzodiazepine withdrawal delirium in hospitalized patients. J Am Geriatr Soc 46(8):1020–2, 1998.

70. Abrams WB, Beers MH, Berkow R, et al, eds. Clinical pharmacology. In: Merck manual of geriatrics, 2nd ed. Whitehouse Station, NJ: Merck Research Laboratories, 1995:255–76.

71. Beers MH, Ouslander JG, Fingold SF, et al. Inappropriate medication prescribing in skilled nursing facilities. Ann Intern Med 117(8):684–9, 1992.

72. Cusack BJ. Polypharmacy and clinical pharmacology. In: Geriatrics review syllabus: a core curriculum in geriatric medicine. New York: American Geriatrics Society, 1989:127–35.

73. Stewart RB, Caranasos GJ. Medication compliance in the elderly. Med Clin North Am 73(6):1551–63, 1989.

74. Rochon PA, Gurwitz JH. Optimising drug treatment for elderly people: the prescribing cascade. BMJ 315(7115):1096–9, 1997.

75. Cleeland CS, Gonin R, Hatfield AK, et al. Pain and its treatment in outpatients with metastatic cancer. N Engl J Med 330(9):592–6, 1994.

76. Redelmeier DA, Tan SH, Booth GL. The treatment of unrelated disorders in patients with chronic medical diseases. N Engl J Med 338(21):1516–20, 1998.

77. Soumerai SB, Ross-Degnan D. Inadequate prescription-drug coverage for Medicare enrollees–a call to action. N Engl J Med 340(9):722–8, 1999.

78. Morrison RS, Wallenstein S, Natale DK, et al. "We don't carry that" failure of pharmacies in predominantly non-white neighborhoods to stock opioid analgesics. N Engl J Med 342(14):1023–6, 2000.

79. Sheehan DC, Forman WB. Symptomatic management of the older person with cancer. Clin Geriatr Med 13(1):203–19, 1997.

80. Rochon PA, Gurwitz JH. (1999). Prescribing for seniors: neither too much nor too little. JAMA 282(2):113–5, 1999.

81. The Agency for Healthcare Policy and Research. Management of cancer pain: adults. Oncol Nurs Forum 21(6):1070–85, 1994.

82. Kalbakis K, Kandylis N, Stavrakakis J, et al. First line chemotherapy with 5-fluorouracil (5-FU), leucovorin (LV) and irinotecan (CPT-11) in advanced colorectal cancer (CRC): a multicenter phase II study. Proc Ann Meeting Am Soc Clin Oncol (18):A989, 1999.

83. Pignon JP, Bourhis J, Domenge C, et al. Chemotherapy added to loco regional treatment for head and neck squamous-cell carcinoma: three meta-analyses of updated individual data. MACH-NC collaborative group: meta-analyses of chemotherapy of head and neck cancer. Lancet 355(9208):949–55, 2000.

84. Auclerc G, Antoine EC, Cajfinger F, et al. Management of advanced prostate cancer. Oncologist 5(1):36–44, 2000.

85. Santen RJ, Harvey HA. Use of aromatose inhibitors in breast carcinoma. Endocr Relat Cancer 6(1):75–92, 1999.

86. Bilodeau BA, Fessele KL. Non-Hodgkin's lymphoma. Semin Oncol Nurs 14(4):273–83, 1998.

87. Kalil N, Cheson BD. Management of chronic lymphocytic leukaemia. Drugs Aging 16(1):9–27, 2000.

88. Burris HA III, Moore MJ, Andersen J, et al. Improvements in survival and clinical benefit with gemcitabine as first-line therapy for patients with advanced pancreas cancer: a randomized trial. J Clin Oncol 15(6):2403–13, 1997.

89. Osoba D, Tannock IF, Ernst DS, et al. Health-related quality of life in men with metastatic prostate cancer treated with prednisone alone or mitoxantrone and prednisone. J Clin Oncol 17(6):1654–63, 1999.

90. Janjan NA, Payne R, Gillis T, et al. Presenting symptoms in patients referred to a multidisciplinary clinic for bone metastases. J Pain Symptom Manage 16(3):171–8, 1998.

91. Jeremic B, Shibamoto Y, Acimovic L, et al. Accelerated hyperfractionated radiation therapy and concurrent 5-fluorouracil/cisplatin chemotherapy for locoregional squamous cell carcinoma of the thoracic esophagus: a phase II study. Int J Radiat Oncol Biol Phys 40(5):1061–6, 1998.

92. Mertens WC, Filipczak LA, Ben-Josef E, et al. Systemic bone-seeking radionuclides for palliation of painful osseous metastases: current concepts. CA: Cancer J Clin 48(6):321–74, 1998.

93. Giammarile F, Mognetti T, Blondet C, et al. Bone pain palliation with 85Sr therapy. J Nucl Med 40(4):585–90, 1999.

94. Serafini AN, Houston SJ, Resche I, et al. Palliation of pain associated with metastatic bone cancer using samarium-153 lexidronam: a double-blind placebo-controlled clinical trial. J Clin Oncol 16(4):1574–81, 1998.

95. Han SH, Zonneberg BA, de Klerk JM, et al. 1999. 186Re-etidronate in breast cancer patients with metastatic bone pain. J Nucl Med 40(4):639–642.

96. Srivastava SC, Atkins HL, Krishnamurthy GT, et al. Treatment of metastatic bone pain with tin-117m stannic diethylenetriaminepentaacetic acid: a phase I/II study. Clin Cancer Res 4(1):61–8, 1998.

97. Cleary JF. Cancer pain management. Cancer Control 7(2):120–31, 2000.

98. Portenoy RK, Payne R, Coluzzi P, et al. Oral transmucosal fentanyl citrate (OTFC) for the treatment of breakthrough pain in cancer patients: a controlled dose titration study. Pain 79(2-3):303–12, 1999.

99. Lipman AG. New and alternative noninvasive opioid dosage forms and routes of administration. Principles and Practice of Supportive Oncology Updates 3(1):1–8, 2000.

100. Ahmedzai S, Brooks D. Transdermal fentanyl versus sustained-release oral morphine in cancer pain: preference, efficacy and quality of life The TTS-Fentanyl Comparative Trial Group. J Pain Symptom Manage 13(5):254–61, 1997.

101. Allen L. Suppositories as drug delivery systems. J Pharm Care Pain Symptom Control 5:17–26, 1997.

102. Mercadante S, Fulfaro F. Alternatives to oral opioids for cancer pain. Oncology 13(2):215–20, 2000.

103. Nelson KA, Glare PA, Walsh D, et al. A prospective, within-patient cross-over study of continuous intravenous and subcutaneous morphine for chronic cancer pain. J Pain Symptom Manage 13(5):262–7, 1997.

104. Stevens RA, Ghazi SM. Routes of opioid analgesic therapy in the management of cancer pain. Cancer Control 7(2):132–41, 2000.

105. Striebel HW, Oelmann T, Spies C, et al. Patient-controlled intranasal analgesia: a method for noninvasive, postoperative pain management. Anesth Analg 83(3):548–51, 1996.

106. Chandler S. Nebulized opioids to treat dyspnea. Am J Hospice Palliat Care 16(1):418–22, 1999.

106. Krajnik M, Zylicz Z, Finlay I, et al. Potential uses of topical opioids in palliative care B report of 6 cases Pain 80(1–2):121–5, 1999.

108. Seamans DP, Wong GY, Wilson JL. Interventional pain therapy for intractable abdominal cancer pain. J Clin Oncol 18(7):1598–600, 2000.

109. Eisenach JC, DuPen S, Dubois M, et al. Epidural clonidine analgesia for intractable cancer pain. The epidural clonidine study group. Pain 61(3):391–9, 1995.

110. Hogan Q, Haddox JD, Abram S, et al. Epidural opiates and local anesthetics for the management of cancer pain. Pain 46(3):271–9, 1991.

111. Jenkins CA, Bruera E. Nonsteroidal anti-inflammatory drugs in adjuvant analgesics in cancer patients. Palliat Med 13(3):183–6, 1999.

112. Portenoy RK. Pain in oncologic and AIDS patients, 3rd ed. Newtown, PA: Handbooks in Healthcare Co, 2000.

113. Brennan MJ. Physiatric approaches to pain management. In: Portenoy RK, Kanner R, eds. Pain management: theory and practice. Philadelphia: FA Davis, 1996:312–22.

114. Puchalski CM. Taking a spiritual history: FICA. Spirituality and Medicine Connection 3:1, 1999.

115. Richardson MA, Sanders T, Palmer JL, et al. Complementary/alternative medicine use in a comprehensive cancer center and the implications for oncology. J Clin Oncol 18(13):2505–14, 2000.

116. Cherny N, Ripamonti C, Pereira J, et al. Strategies to manage the adverse effects of oral morphine: an evidence-based report. J Clin Oncol 19(9):2452–554, 2001.

117. Sykes NP. Current approaches to the management of constipation. Cancer Surv 21:137–46, 1994.

118. Bruera E, Macmillan K, Hanson J, et al. The cognitive effects of the administration of narcotic analgesics in patients with cancer pain. Pain 39(1):13–16, 1989.

119. Portenoy RK. Management of common opioid side effects during long-term therapy of cancer pain. Ann Acad Med Singapore 23(2):160–70, 1994.

120. Bruera E, Fainsinger R, MacEachern T, et al. The use of methylphenidate in patients with incident cancer pain receiving regular opiates. A preliminary report. Pain 50(1):75–7, 1992.

121. Forrest WH Jr, Brown BW Jr, Brown CR, et al. Dextroamphetamine with morphine for the treatment of postoperative pain. N Engl J Med 296(13):712–5, 1977.

122. Campora E, Merlini L, Pace M, et al. The incidence of narcotic-induced emesis. J Pain Symptom Manage 6(7):428–30, 1991.

123. Vanegas G, Ripamonti C, Sbanotto A, et al. Side effects of morphine administration in cancer patients. Cancer Nurs 21(4):289–97, 1998.

124. Pargeon KL, Hailey BJ. Barriers to effective cancer pain management: a review of the literature. J Pain Symptom Manage 18(5):358–68, 1999.

125. American Geriatrics Society Clinical Practice Committee. Management of cancer pain in older patients. J Am Geriatr Soc 45(10):1273–6, 1997.

126. American Geriatrics Society. The management of chronic pain in older persons: AGS panel on chronic pain in older persons. J Am Geriatr Soc 46(5):635–51, 1998.

127. Gloth FM. Pain management in older adults: prevention and treatment. J Am Geriatr Soc 49:188–99, 2001.

128. The Ad Hoc Committee on Cancer Pain of the American Society of Clinical Oncology. Cancer Pain Assessment and Treatment Curriculum Guidelines. J Clin Oncol 10(12):1976–82, 1992.

129. Payne R. Practice guidelines for cancer pain therapy. Issues pertinent to revision of national guidelines. Oncology 12(11A):169–75, 1998.

130. Oncology Nursing Society. Cancer pain management. Oncol Nurs Forum 25(5):817–8, 1998.

131. American Pain Society Quality of Care Committee. Quality improvement guidelines for the treatment of acute pain and cancer pain. JAMA 274(23):1874–80, 1995.

132. American Society of Anesthesiologists Task Force on Pain Management, Cancer Pain Section. Practice guidelines for cancer pain management. Anesthesiology 84(5):1243–57, 1996.

133. Phillips DM. JCAHO pain management standards are unveiled. Joint Commission on Accreditation of Healthcare Organizations. JAMA 284(4):428–9, 2000.

134. Educator with a vision. BMJ 319(7203):146, 1999.

135. Glajchen M. (1997). Creating a consumer demand for pain relief: a role for state cancer pain initiatives. APS Bulletin 7(4):6–7, 1997.

136. National Cancer Institute, Eastern Cooperative Oncology Group. Pain control with recurrent or metastatic breast or prostate cancer. A clinical trial registered at: www.clinicaltrials.gov. Accessed September 19, 2000.

137. National Cancer Institute of Canada Clinical Trials Group. Treatment for chronic pain in patients with advanced cancer. A clinical trial registered at: www.clinicaltrials.gov. Accessed September 19, 2000.

138. National Cancer Institute, North Central Cancer Treatment Group, Radiation Therapy Oncology Group. Radiation therapy in treating patients with bone metastases from breast or prostate cancer: A clinical trial registered at: www.clinicaltrials.gov. Accessed September 19, 2000.

139. The SUPPORT Principal Investigators. A controlled trial to improve care for seriously ill hospitalized patients. The study to understand prognoses and preferences for outcomes and risks of treatments (SUPPORT). JAMA 274(20):1591–8, 1995.

140. American Medical Association. The EPEC (Educating Participants at the End of Life) participant's handbook. Available at: http://www.ama-assn.org/ethic/epec/handbook.htm. Accessed September 4, 2000.

141. Nelson KA, Walsh D, Behrens C, et al. The dying cancer patient. Semin Oncol 27(1):84–9, 2000.

142. Manfredi PL, Ribeiro S, Chandler SW, et al. Inappropriate use of naloxone in cancer patients with pain. J Pain Symptom Manage 11(2):131–4, 1996.

143. Cherny NI, Portenoy RK. Sedation in the management of refractory symptoms: guidelines for evaluation and treatment. J Palliat Care 10(2):31–8, 1994.

144. Wein S. Sedation in the imminently dying patient. Oncology 14(4):585–92, 2000.

145. Portenoy RK. The Wein article reviewed. Oncology 14(4):592–7, 2000.

146. Callahan D. Death and the research imperative. N Engl J Med 342(9):654–6, 2000.

147. Byock I. Dying well: peace and possibilities at the end of life. New York: Riverhead Books, 1998.

148. Steinhauser KE, Clipp EC, McNeilly M, et al. Ann Intern Med 132(10):825–32, 2000.

149. Bartlett J, ed. Familiar quotations, 16th ed. Boston: Little, Brown and Co, 1992:62.

SECTION VII   DIFFICULT PAIN PROBLEMS

21 Cancer pain and depression

MARJANEH ROUHANI
Behavioral Health Care

JAHANDAR SAIFOLLAHI
Michigan State University School of Medicine

WILLIAM S. BREITBART
Memorial Sloan-Kettering Cancer Center

Introduction

Effective management of pain in patients with advanced cancer may benefit from a multidisciplinary approach, enlisting expertise from a wide variety of clinical specialties including neurology, neurosurgery, anesthesiology, and rehabilitation medicine (1–3). The use of psychiatric interventions in the treatment of cancer patients with pain and depression has now also become an integral part of such a comprehensive approach (1–5). This chapter reviews the assessment and management of depression in the patient with cancer pain.

Multidimensional concept of pain in cancer

Pain, especially in advanced cancer, is not a purely nociceptive or physical experience, but involves complex aspects of human functioning including personality, affect, cognition, behavior, and social relations (6). A more enlightened description of the pain resulting from a terminal illness coined by Cecily Saunders (7) is "total pain," a label that attempts to describe the all-encompassing nature of this type of pain. It is important to note that the use of analgesic drugs alone does not always lead to pain relief (8). Syrjala and Chapko (9) demonstrated that psychological factors play a modest but important role in pain intensity. As the interactions of cognitive, emotional, socioenvironmental, and nociceptive aspects of pain are inseparable, the multidimensional nature of pain demands for a multimodal intervention (3). The challenge of untangling and addressing both the physical and psychological issues involved in pain is essential to developing rational and effective management strategies. Psychosocial therapies directed primarily at psychological variables have a profound impact on nociception, whereas somatic therapies directed at nociception have beneficial effects on the psychological aspects of pain. Ideally such somatic and psychosocial therapies are used simultaneously in the multidisciplinary approach to pain management in the terminally ill (4).

Psychological factors in pain experience

The patient with cancer faces many stressors during the course of illness, including dependency, disability, and fear of painful death. Such fears are universal; however, the level of depression is variable and depends on medical factors, social supports, coping capacities, and personality. Pain has profound effects on depression in cancer patients, and psychological factors such as anxiety, depression, and the meaning of pain can intensify cancer pain experience. Daut and Cleeland (10) showed that cancer patients who attribute a new pain to an unrelated benign cause report less interference with their activity and pleasure than cancer patients who believe their pain represents progression of disease. Spiegel and Bloom (11) found that women with metastatic breast cancer experience more intense pain if they believe their pain represents spread of their cancer, and if they are depressed. Beliefs about the meaning of pain and the presence of a mood disturbance are better predictors of level of pain than is the site of metastasis.

In an attempt to define the potential relationships between pain and psychosocial variables, Padilla et al. (12) found that there were pain-related quality of life variables in three domains: 1) physical well-being; 2) psychological well-being consisting of affective factors, cognitive factors, spiritual factors, communication, coping, and meaning of pain or cancer; and 3) interpersonal well-being focusing on social support or role functioning. The perception of marked impairment in activities of daily living has been shown to be associated with increased pain intensity (13). Measures of emotional disturbance have been reported to be predictors of pain in late stages of cancer, and cancer patients with less anxiety and depression are less likely to report pain (14,15). Patients who report negative thoughts about their personal or social competence report increased pain intensity and emotional distress (13). In a prospective study of cancer patients it was found that maladaptive coping strategies, lower levels of self-efficacy, and distress specific to the treatment or disease progression were modest but significant predictors of reports of pain intensity (9).

Psychological variables—such as the amount of control people believe they have over pain, emotional associations and memories of pain, fear of death, depression, anxiety, and hopelessness—contribute to the experience of pain in people with cancer and can increase suffering. Pain appears to have a profound impact on levels of emotional distress and disability. In addition to being significantly more distressed and depressed, those with pain were twice as likely to have suicidal ideation (40%) as those without pain (20%). HIV-infected patients with pain were more functionally impaired. Such functional interference was highly correlated to levels of pain intensity and depression. Those who believed that pain represented a threat to their health reported more intense pain than those who did not see pain as a threat. Patients with pain were more likely to be unemployed or disabled, and they reported less social support. Singer and colleagues (16) also reported an association among the frequency of multiple pains, increased disability, and higher levels of depression.

All too frequently, however, psychological variables are proposed to explain continued pain or lack of response to therapy when in fact medical factors have not been adequately appreciated. Often, the psychiatrist is the last physician to consult on a cancer patient with pain. In that role, one must be vigilant that an accurate pain diagnosis is made and be able to assess the adequacy of the medical analgesic management provided. Depression in terminally ill patients with pain must initially be assumed to be the consequence of uncontrolled pain. Personality factors may be quite distorted by the presence of pain, and relief of pain often results in the disappearance of a perceived psychiatric disorder (17,18).

Psychiatric disorders and pain in cancer/prevalence of depression

There is an increased frequency of psychiatric disorders found in cancer patients with pain. In the Psychosocial Collaborative Oncology Group Study (19) on the prevalence of psychiatric disorders in cancer patients, of the patients who received a psychiatric diagnosis, 39% reported significant pain, whereas only 19% of patients without a psychiatric diagnosis had significant pain. The psychiatric disorders seen in cancer patients with pain include primarily adjustment disorder with depressed or anxious mood (69%) and major depression (15%) (20,21).

Epidural spinal cord compression (ESCC) is a common neurological complication of systemic cancer that occurs in 5%–10% of patients with cancer and can often present with severe pain. These patients are routinely treated with a combination of high-dose dexamethasone and radiotherapy. Patients who receive this high-dose regimen are exposed to as much as 96 mg a day of dexamethasone for up to a week and continue on a tapering course for up to 3 or 4 weeks. Stiefel and colleagues (22) described the psychiatric complications seen in cancer patients undergoing such treatment for epidural spinal cord compression. A total of 22% of patients with ESCC had a major depressive syndrome diagnosed as compared to 4% in the comparison group. Also, delirium was much more common in the dexamethasone treated patients with ESCC, with 24% diagnosed with delirium during the course of treatment as compared to only 10% in the comparison group.

Cancer patients with advanced disease are a particularly vulnerable group. The incidence of pain, depression, and delirium increases with greater debilitation and advanced stages of illness (23). Approximately 25% of all cancer patients experience severe depressive symptoms, with the prevalence increases to 77% in those with advanced illness. The prevalence of organic mental disorders (delirium) among cancer patients requiring psychiatric consultation has been found to range from 25% to 40%, and to be as high as 85% during the terminal stages of illness (24). Opioid analgesics, such as morphine sulfate, can cause confusional states, particularly in the elderly and terminally ill (25).

Assessment of depression in cancer pain

Diagnosing depression may be challenging in cancer patients, as the physical symptoms resulting from cancer overlap with the physical symptoms associated with depression. To overcome this challenge, clinicians have used different diagnostic classification systems. This has led, in turn, to widely varying rates of detection of depression in cancer patients. In addition, unrelieved pain was cited as an important reason why cancer patients seek to hasten their death (26). This poses another challenge in diagnosing depression in the setting of uncontrolled pain.

Table 21.1 lists the Diagnostic and Statistical Manual (DSM-IV) criteria for a diagnosis of major depressive syndrome (27). Kathol and colleagues (28) found as much as a 13% difference in rates of major depression when utilizing criteria of the DSM-III (38%), DSM-III-R (29%), and Research Diagnostic Criteria (RDC) (25%). Many individuals with symptoms of depression do not meet the criteria for major depression or dysthymia and suffer in silence. It is important to appreciate that one could hardly move through a life-threatening illness without suffering from one or more of the symptoms that, if combined, would render a diagnosis of a major depressive disorder.

Five different approaches to the diagnosis of major depression in cancer patients have been described (29,30): 1) an inclusive approach, which includes all symptoms whether or not they may be secondary to illness or treatment; 2) an exclusive approach, which deletes and disregards all physical symptoms from consideration, not allowing them to contribute to a diagnosis of major depressive syndrome; 3) an etiologic approach, whereby the clinician attempts to determine if the physical symptom is due to cancer illness or treatment (and so does not include it) or due to a depressive disorder (in which case it is included as a criterion symptom); 4) a high diagnostic threshold approach, which requires that patients have seven DSM-IV criteria symptoms for major depression; and (5) a substitutive approach, in which physical symptoms of an uncertain etiology are replaced by other non-somatic symptoms. The latter approach is best exemplified by the Endicott Substitution Criteria (31) (Table 21.2), which includes replacing 1) change in

Table 21.2. *Endicott substitution criteria*

Physical/somatic symptom	Psychological symptom substitute
Change in appetite, weight	Tearfulness
	Depressed appearance
Sleep disturbance	Social withdrawal
	Decreased talkativeness
Fatigue	Brooding, self-pity
Loss of energy	Pessimism
Diminished ability to think for concentrate	Lack of reactivity
Indecisiveness	

appetite or weight *with* tearfulness, depressed appearance; 2) sleep disturbance *with* social withdrawal or decreased talkativeness; 3) fatigue or loss of energy *with* brooding, self-pity, or pessimism; and 4) diminished ability to think or concentrate or indecisiveness *with* lack of reactivity.

Chochinov and colleagues (32) studied the prevalence of depression in a terminally ill cancer population and compared low versus high diagnostic thresholds, as well as Endicott Substitution Criteria. Interestingly, identical prevalence rates of 9.2% for major depression and 3.8% for minor depression (total = 13%) were found using RDC high threshold criteria and high threshold Endicott criteria. In another study, Chochinov and colleagues (33) reported that a single item screening measure (i.e., asking, in effect, "Are you depressed?") was as accurate a diagnostic strategy as the use of a structured clinical interview for depression.

Table 21.3 lists a number of available assessment methods for depression, including diagnostic classifica-

Table 21.1. *DSM-IV criteria for major depressive syndrome*

A. At least five of the following symptoms have been persistent for 2 weeks or more:
   1. Depressed mood, dysphoria, loss of interest or pleasure, or anhedonia (at least one symptom must be from this group)
   2. Physical/somatic symptoms: sleep disorder, appetite or weight change, or fatigue or loss of energy
   3. Psychological/cognitive symptoms: worthlessness/guilt, indecisiveness/poor concentration, or thoughts of death/suicidal ideation
B. The symptoms do not meet criteria for a mixed episode.
C. The symptoms cause clinically significant social or occupational impairment.
D. The symptoms are not due to the direct physiological effects of a substance or a general medical condition.
E. The symptoms are not better accounted for by bereavement.

Table 21.3. *Research assessment methods for depression in cancer patients*

Diagnostic Classification Systems
   Diagnostic and Statistical Manual DSM-III, III-R, IV
Endicott Substitution Criteria
   Research Diagnostic Criteria (RDC)

Structured Diagnostic Interviews
   Schedule for Affective Disorders and Schizophrenia (SADS)
   Diagnostic Interview Schedule (DIS)
   Structured Clinical Interview for DSM-III-R (SCID)

Screening Instruments-self report
   General Health Questionnaire-30
   Hospital Anxiety and Depression Scale (HADS)
   Beck Depression Inventory (BDI)
   Rotterdam Symptom Checklist (RSCL)
   Carroll Depression Rating Scale (CDRS)

tion systems, structured diagnostic interviews, and screening instruments. Unfortunately, few studies of depression in terminally ill or advanced cancer patients have used such research assessment methods to date. Additionally, further work is necessary in adapting to the limitations of such methods in their application to populations with advanced cancer. Several options have been proposed for handling the issue of confounding somatic symptoms (30). The DSM-IV recommends that symptoms should be excluded from consideration if they are caused directly by a medical condition. In practice, however, this discrimination can be a difficult one to make. Technically, it also makes the standard for fulfilling diagnostic criteria more stringent (33). For example, when all symptoms are included, a diagnosis of major depression requires that five of nine criterion symptoms be present. If four symptoms are then excluded because of possible confounding with medical illness, then a patient must have all five of the remaining symptoms before the diagnostic criteria for major depression are met. This is a very strict standard that would identify only the most severely depressed patients.

Cassem (34) pointed out that the risks of failing to treat depression because of false-negative diagnoses are more harmful, on balance, than are the risks of initiating unnecessary therapy based on a false-positive diagnosis. Hence, he suggested that it would be better for clinicians to err on the side of caution, and include somatic symptoms in their diagnostic assessments of the medically ill. When this approach is used, however, there is the possibility that the prevalence rates of depressive disorders among medical patients will be exaggerated.

Assessment procedures for depression include criterion-based diagnostic systems, diagnostic interviews, and self-report measures.

Criterion-based diagnostic systems

Criterion-based diagnostic systems include approaches such as DSM-IV or its predecessors (DSM III; DSM-III-R), and the RDC (35). These systems are based on the assumption that depression is a distinct syndromal disorder characterized by a constellation of symptoms, which have a certain minimal level of severity and duration and are associated with impairment in functional and social roles.

Diagnostic interviews

For research purposes, diagnostic assessments are usually conducted using structured interviews such as the

Diagnostic Interview Schedule (DIS) (36), the Structured Clinical Interview for DSM-III-R (SCID) (37), or the Schedule for Affective Disorders and Schizophrenia (SADS) (38). These interviews differ with respect to their degree of structure and in the formats with which the interviewer codes the patient's verbal responses. The DIS is highly structured and can be used by lay interviewers in epidemiological studies. The SCID and SADS are semistructured and are intended for use by clinicians. With the DIS and the SCID, the interviewer is required to code specific symptoms as being either present or absent, whereas with the SADS, the interviewer rates the severity of symptoms on ordinal scales. All of these interview protocols have been subjected to extensive checks of their reliability and validity.

If administered in their entirety, these interviews cover a broad range of common mental disorders. However, they can be very time consuming, which is a serious limitation to their use in palliative care settings. More commonly, investigators administer only the modules within an interview that address the problem of depression. For example, Chochinov and colleagues administered the depression module of the SADS to patients with advanced cancer in an inpatient palliative care unit (31). They found that the inter-rater reliability for the RDC diagnoses of major or minor depression was kappa = 0.76, which reflects substantial agreement that is comparable to the levels found in studies of the general population or psychiatric patients.

Spitzer and colleagues (39) developed a brief screening protocol for use by primary care clinicians that would seem to have good applicability to palliative care. The Primary Care Evaluation of Mental Disorders (PRIME-MD) uses a two-stage approach to review the DSM-IV criteria for major depression, minor depression, and dysthymia. In addition, it addresses the common anxiety syndromes of panic disorder and generalized anxiety disorder, and provides a brief screen for alcohol abuse. In the first stage, the patient completes a one-page self-report checklist that covers only the most central symptoms of each disorder, using a simple "yes/no" response format. Using a structured interview guide, the clinician follows up on those symptoms acknowledged on the checklist (ensuring that they meet DSM-IV severity and duration criteria) and probes the remaining symptoms required to make a diagnosis. Spitzer and colleagues found that the PRIME-MD shows good concordance with independent diagnoses made by mental health professionals, and can be completed within 20 minutes with 95% of patients. Thus, its brevity and comprehensiveness suggest that the PRIME-MD would be a suitable choice for both research and clinical use in cancer, although the self-report component would have to be replaced with an interview administration for the most severely compromised patients.

Sometimes investigators have constructed their own semistructured interviews for use in cancer patients, modifying the diagnostic criteria to account for the unique circumstances of this group of patients (23,40). This approach has some disadvantages, however. The purpose of structured interviews is to enhance the reliability of clinical diagnostic assessments. When well tested, psychometrically sound protocols are already widely available, new interviews must be tested rigorously for their reliability in order to support claims for improvement over existing measures. This has seldom been done in cancer-care research. Hence an expert panel on the neuropsychiatric aspects of advanced cancer has recommended the use of existing validated tools in prevalence and intervention research (41).

Self-report measures

In primary care settings, non-psychiatric clinicians fail to identify depressive disorders in 46% to 67% of the patients who qualify for a diagnosis based on structured interview assessments (39,42). This low rate suggests

that any methods than can increase the accuracy of identification would be welcome additions to clinical care. Accordingly, a considerable body of research has examined the extent to which self-report measures can assist in this process.

Among the measures that have been used in this context are the 11-item short form of the Beck Depression Inventory (BDI-SF) (43); the 14-item Hospital Anxiety and Depression Scale, (HADS) (44); the 60-item General Health Questionnaire (GHQ) (45); the 8-item psychological symptoms subscale of the Rotterdam Symptom Checklist (RSCL) (46); and the 11-item short form of the Carroll Depression Rating Scale (CDRS) (47). Golden and colleagues (48) validated CDRS for use in cancer patients. Although many other self-report measures of depressive symptoms are available in the literature, the advantages of these particular scales is that they have been developed or adapted for use with medical populations, and have been tested in various groups of patients with cancer. Hence, information is available regarding the optimal cut-off scores for maximizing their concordance with the criterion standard of structured interview diagnoses administered by mental health professionals.

Table 21.4 provides an overview of studies with cancer patients that have used self-report measures to determine the sensitivity (proportion of clinically diagnosed patients who score above the optimal cut-off on the ques-

Table 21.4. *Screening for depressive disorders in patients with cancer: Sensitivity and specificity of common self-report measures*

Measure/study	Patients	N	Criterion standard diagnosis	Cut-off score	Sensitivity	Specificity
HADS Hopwood et al. (49)	Advanced breast cancer	81	DSM-III (depression or anxiety disorders)	≥ 18	.75	.74
Razavi et al. (52)	Mixed inpatients	210	Endicott criteria (major depression)	≥ 19	.70	.74
			DSM-III (major depression or adjustment disorder)	≥ 13	.75	.75
Razavi et al. (51)	Lymphoma outpatients	117	DSM-III-R (depression, anxiety or adjustment disorders)	≥ 10	.84	.66
RSCL Hopwood et al. (49)				≥ 11	.75	.80
CDRS Golden et al. (48)	Gynecological cancer	65	DSM-III (major depression)	≥ 3	.87	.62
GHQ Hardman et al. (50)	Oncology inpatients	126	ICD (depression or anxiety disorders)	≥ 11	.79	.66
BDI-SF Chochinov et al. (33)	Mixed palliative care inpatients	197	RDC (major or minor depression)	≥ 8	.79	.71
VAS (100 mm) Chochinov et al. (33)	Mixed palliative care inpatients	197	RDC (major or minor depression)	≥ 55mm	.72	.50

Abbreviations: HADS, Hospital Anxiety and Depression Scale; RSCL, Rotterdam Symptom Checklist; CDRS, Carroll Depression Rating Scale; BDI-SF, Beck Depression Inventory–Short form; VAS, visual analog scale.

tionnaire) and specificity (proportion of non-depressed patients who score below the cut-off). There are two main findings from these studies.

First, even those that have used the same screening questionnaire (i.e., the HADS) have identified optimal cut-off scores that vary over a wide range. The discrepancies appear to be related to the characteristics of the patients, the type and stage of disease, and more important, to the range of depressive syndromes that are included in the criterion-standard diagnosis. For example, studies that include adjustment disorders identify much lower cut-off scores than those that screen only for the more severe major depressive episodes.

Second, none of the available questionnaires provides perfect concordance with structured interviews. Although some studies have reported marginally higher sensitivities associated with certain questionnaires, the trade-off is a lower degree of specificity (32,48–52). In fact, the receiver operating characteristics of each of the questionnaires appear to be roughly comparable, indicating similar empirical performance for screening depressed patients. Therefore, considerations such as a scale's brevity, simplicity, and specific item content should factor into decisions about which ones to select for screening purposes. The average sensitivity (0.78) and specificity (0.71) values translate into estimates that about 22% of depressed patients will *not* score above the cut-off on any particular scale, and the false-positive rate will be in the range of 29% of patients screened. Whether or not these error rates are acceptable depends on the purpose for which the screening is being done. For clinical purposes, a high false-positive rate is not necessarily a problem if screen-positive patients receive a follow-up interview to confirm the diagnosis. A high false-negative rate, on the other hand, presents a greater difficulty because a significant number of depressed patients will not be identified.

There are many reasons to explain the lack of concordance between questionnaire assessments of depression and criterion-based diagnostic systems (53). With questionnaires, for example, different patients can achieve similar summary scores from strongly endorsing only a few items, or from weakly endorsing many items. The content of the specific items in a questionnaire is also important. With some, it could be possible for a patient to score above the scale cut-off without endorsing any individual symptoms that would actually contribute to the diagnosis of depression in a criterion-based system. Finally, most depression rating scales are also correlated highly with measures of anxiety as well as with depression. For these reasons, some investigators caution that the most common

self-report measures of depression should really be used as indices of general distress. Distress in this sense may overlap with the construct of depression as a syndromal disorder; but it is not equivalent (53).

In patients with advanced cancer, questionnaires can also pose a burden for patients whose medical circumstances make it difficult for them to read. For this reason, visual analog scales have come into common use in cancer patient settings (54). Chochinov and colleagues described the screening characteristics of a 100-mm visual analog scale of depressed mood (anchored at the endpoints with the descriptors 0 = "worst possible mood" and 1 = "best possible mood"), while using the Memorial Pain Assessment Card (32,55). The patients composed a mixed group of inpatients with advanced cancer, and the criterion standard diagnoses were major and minor depressive episodes defined according to structured interviews. They found that the optimal cut-off score (55 mm) provided less accurate screening than the Beck Depression Inventory–Short Form. Thus, visual analog scales seem to provide a rather crude substitute for a careful diagnostic interview.

In addition, Chochinov and colleagues (32) also examined a brief interview-based screening for depression, which consisted simply of two questions addressing the core criterion symptoms of depressed mood and less of interest or pleasure in activities. They found that this method was actually quite accurate in identifying patients who qualified for a diagnosis based on the administration of a full interview that covered all of the criterion symptoms of depression. Hence, they recommended that this type of brief screening should be incorporated more routinely into clinical contacts.

In summary, the limitations of assessments with the self-report measures of depression should be recognized. Self-report and visual analog scales can provide gross assessments when direct interviews are not feasible. They are useful in providing additional information for difficult cases, in quantifying the severity of a depressive syndrome, and in monitoring change over time. However, diagnostic interviews remain extremely valuable for direct psychiatric assessments of patients with cancer.

Differentiating major depression from mood disorders caused by cancer and uncontrolled pain

The question of causality in the diagnosis of depression in cancer patients is almost inevitable. How is a medical condition determined to cause a depression? A causal relation is postulated if the clinician demonstrates the presence of a medical condition known to cause depression, and if symptoms improve as the medical condition is treated. There are two core criterion symptoms for major depression in the DSM-IV—depressed mood and anhedonia (Table 21.1). To qualify for the diagnosis, one of these core symptoms must be present, along with at least four other symptoms from the criterion list. In cases where the depressive syndrome is clearly caused by the direct physiological effect of a medication or other psychoactive substance, or by metabolic or neurochemical disturbances created by the disease process, the diagnosis of mood disorder resulting from the general medical condition would be more appropriately applied. However, these diagnoses are very general and require only that dysphoric mood or decreased interest or pleasure is present. In addition, DSM-IV may restrict the use of the diagnosis of major depression in cancer patients because of unclear relationship between depression and cancer. Several authors (34,56,57) credited Munroe (58) with the development of the concept of secondary depression. The RDC defined secondary depression as "a depression occurring in a person who has a preexisting nonaffective psychiatric disorder or a life-threatening medical illness that precedes and parallels the symptoms of depression" (59). The RDC, outlined by Spitzer et al. (35), contained criteria independent of etiology and based on a temporal distinction between primary and secondary depression. This group also proposed the category minor depression, defined as "nonpsychotic episodes of illness in which the most prominent disturbance is a relatively sustained mood of depression without the full depressive syndrome, although some associated features must be present" (35).

Patients with depression resulting from medical illness as compared to major depression present with older age at onset. They are more likely to respond to electroconvulsive therapy, more likely to be improved at discharge, more likely to show "organic" features in the mental status examination, more likely to have much lower incidence of family history of alcoholism and depression (19% of medically ill vs. 36% of psychiatrically ill), and less likely to have suicidal thoughts and commit suicide (10% death by suicide in medically ill sample vs. 45% in psychiatrically ill group).

The core DSM-IV criterion symptom of loss of interest or pleasure in activities merits some discussion when applied to patients with cancer. Ultimately, all patients with advanced cancer will experience a functional decline that restricts their physical ability to participate in activities. Disengagement from areas of interest would be common among individuals who refocus their priorities into areas of deeper significance. When anhedonia is

pervasive, however, and extends to a loss of interest or pleasure in almost all activities, including the social comforts of interaction with family and friends, then most authors consider it to be a valid criterion for the assessment of depression (60,61).

Other depressive disorders

In addition to major depression, there are other diagnoses that have depressed mood as a central presenting feature. Minor depression as described in the RDC is similar to major depression, but requires fewer symptoms to qualify for a diagnosis (two to four symptoms in total). Like major depression, minor depression is considered to be an episodic disorder. Dysthymia, in contrast, is defined as a chronic condition characterized by low-grade depressive symptoms that persist for at least 2 years. Adjustment disorder with depressed mood, on the other hand, describes a relatively short-lived maladaptive reaction to stress. This diagnosis requires that a patient's depressive response to the stressor must be "in excess of a normal and expectable reaction." The diagnosis of adjustment disorder is a controversial one in cancer care (62). It requires a subjective judgment as to what is a "normal and expectable response" to catastrophic medical circumstances. If applied loosely, it risks overpathologizing the experience of some patients by applying a potentially stigmatizing psychiatric label on what may be a normal display of grief.

Cancer pain and suicide

Uncontrolled pain is a major factor in suicide and suicidal ideation in cancer patients (63). The public perceives cancer as an extremely painful disease compared with other medical conditions. In Wisconsin, a study revealed that 69% of the public agreed that cancer pain could cause a person to consider suicide (64). The majority of suicides observed among patients with cancer had severe pain, which was often inadequately controlled or tolerated poorly (65). Although relatively few cancer patients commit suicide, they are at increased risk (64). Patients with advanced cancer are at highest risk and are the most likely to have the complications of pain, depression, delirium, and deficit symptoms. Psychiatric disorders are frequently present in hospitalized cancer patients who attempt suicide. A review of the psychiatric consultation data at Memorial Sloan-Kettering Cancer Center showed that one third of cancer patients who were seen for evaluation of suicide risk received a diagnosis of major depression; approximately

20% met criteria for delirium, and more than 50% were diagnosed with an adjustment disorder (63).

Thoughts of suicide probably occur quite frequently, particularly in the setting of advanced cancer (66), and seem to act as a steam valve for feelings often expressed by patients as "If it gets too bad, I always have a way out." It has been our experience working with terminally ill pain patients that once a trusting and safe relationship develops, patients almost universally reveal that they have had occasionally persistent thoughts of suicide as a means of escaping the threat of being overwhelmed by pain. Recent published reports, however, suggest that suicidal ideation is relatively infrequent in cancer and is limited to those who are significantly depressed. Silberfarb et al. (67) found that only 3 of 146 breast cancer patients had suicidal thoughts, whereas none of the 100 cancer patients interviewed in a Finnish study expressed suicidal thoughts (68). A study conducted at St. Boniface Hospice in Winnipeg, Canada, demonstrated that only 10 of 44 terminally ill cancer patients were suicidal or desired an early death, and all 10 were suffering from clinical depression (69). At Memorial Sloan-Kettering Cancer Center (MSKCC), suicide risk evaluation accounted for 8.6% of psychiatric consultations, usually requested by staff in response to patients verbalizing suicidal wishes (63). In the 71 cancer patients who had suicidal ideation with serious intent, significant pain was a factor in only 30% of cases. In striking contrast, virtually all 71 suicidal cancer patients had a psychiatric disorder (mood disturbance or organic mental disorder) at the time of evaluation (63).

Pain plays an important role in vulnerability to suicide, however. Pain has adverse effects on patients' quality of life and sense of control and impairs the family's ability to provide support. Factors other than pain, such as mood disturbance, delirium, loss of control, and hopelessness, contribute to cancer suicide risk (65).

Inadequate pain management: assessment issues in the treatment of pain

Recent studies suggest that cancer pain is still being undertreated (54). Although it is acknowledged that opioid analgesics are underused, it is also clear from our work and the work of others that adjuvant agents such as the antidepressants are also dramatically underused

Inadequate management of pain is often due the inability to properly assess pain in all its dimensions (1,4,70). All too frequently, psychological variables are proposed to explain continued pain or lack of response to therapy,

when in fact medical factors have not been adequately appreciated. Other causes of inadequate pain management include lack of knowledge of current pharmacotherapeutic or psychotherapeutic approaches, focus on prolonging life rather than alleviating suffering, lack of communication between doctor and patient, limited expectations of patients to achieve pain relief, limited capacity of patients impaired by organic mental disorders to communicate, poor opioid availability, doctors' fear of causing respiratory depression, and, most important, doctors' fear of amplifying addiction and substance abuse. In advanced cancer, several factors have been noted to predict the undermanagement of pain, including a discrepancy between physician and patient in judging the severity of pain, the presence of pain that physicians did not attribute to cancer, better performance status, age ≥70 years, and female sex (71).

Fear of addiction affects both patient adherence to therapy and physician management and can lead to undermedication of pain in cancer patients (3,70,72). Studies of the patterns of chronic opioid analgesic use in patients with cancer have demonstrated that, although tolerance and physical dependence commonly occur, addiction is rare and almost never occurs in an individual without a history of drug abuse before cancer illness (73). Escalation of opioid analgesic use by cancer patients is usually due to progression of cancer.

Addiction is a behavioral pattern of compulsive drug abuse characterized by craving for the drug and overwhelming involvement in obtaining and using it for effects other than pain relief. The management of pain in the cancer patient with an active addiction is challenging, particularly if the addiction includes opioids or is accompanied by a co-morbid psychiatric disorder. Specialized substance abuse consultation services may be helpful in the team approach to these patients.

Persistent cancer pain is often ascribed to a psychological cause when it does not respond to treatment attempts. In our clinical experience we have noted that patients who report their pain as "severe" are quite likely to be viewed as having a psychological contribution to their complaints. Staff members' ability to empathize with a patient's pain complaint may be limited by the intensity of the pain complaint. Grossman et al. (74) found that although there is a high degree of concordance between patient and caregiver ratings of patient pain intensity at the low and moderate levels, this concordance breaks down at high levels. Thus, a clinician's ability to assess a patient's level of pain becomes unreliable once a patient's report of pain intensity rises above 7 on a visual analog rating scale of 0 to 10. Physicians must be educated as to the limitations of their ability to objectively assess the severity of a subjective pain experience. Additionally, patient education is often a useful intervention in such cases. Patients are more likely to be believed and adequately treated if they are taught to request pain relief in a non-hysterical, business-like fashion.

Management of depression in patients with cancer pain

General principles

The relationship with the primary medical caregiver is the most important component of psychotherapeutic support for many patients with a serious illness. Optimally, these relationships are based on mutual trust, respect, and sensitivity. The ability to acknowledge patients as "whole persons" and respond to them on the basis of their own individual personal style and needs tends to work best. Perhaps, more than any other clinical setting, maintaining ongoing contact with the depressed terminally ill patient is of critical importance. This not only ensures that patients will be continually re-evaluated, but also provides reassurance to patients that they will not be abandoned, and care will be forthcoming and available throughout their terminal course.

Supportive psychotherapy with medically ill patients consists of active listening with supportive verbal interventions and occasional interpretations (75). Despite the seriousness of the patient's plight, it is not necessary for the clinician to appear overly solemn or emotionally restrained. Often it is only the psychotherapist, of all the patient's caregivers, who is comfortable enough to converse lightheartedly and allow the patient to talk about their life and experiences, rather than focus solely on impending death. The dying patient who wishes to talk or ask questions about death should be allowed to do so freely, with the therapist maintaining an interested, interactive stance.

Depression in patients with cancer pain is optimally managed using a combination of psychotherapy and antidepressant medication (76). For patients with cancer suffering from major depression, adjustment disorder, or dysthymia, there are a variety of psychosocial interventions with proven efficacy. These include individual psychotherapy, group psychotherapy, hypnotherapy, psychoeducation, relaxation training and biofeedback, and self-help groups (77). Psychotherapeutic interventions, either in the form of individual or group counseling, have

been shown to effectively reduce psychological distress and depressive symptoms in patients with cancer pain (62,78,79). Cognitive-behavioral interventions, such as relaxation and distraction with pleasant imagery, have also been shown to decrease depressive symptoms in patients with mild to moderate levels of depression (80).

Psychopharmacological interventions (i.e., antidepressant medications), however, are the mainstay of management in the treatment of patients with cancer pain with severe depressive symptoms who meet criteria for a major depressive episode (81). The efficacy of antidepressants in the treatment of depression in cancer patients has been well established (82–85).

Nonpharmacologic treatment of depression in cancer pain patients

Psychosocial therapies

The goals of psychotherapy with cancer patients with pain are to provide support, knowledge, and skills. By using short-term supportive psychotherapy focused on the crisis created by the medical illness, the therapist provides emotional support, continuity, and information and assists in adaptation. The therapist has a role in emphasizing past strengths, supporting previously successful coping strategies, and teaching new coping skills such as relaxation, cognitive coping, use of analgesics, self-observation, documentation, assertiveness, and communication skills. Communication skills are of paramount importance for both patient and family, particularly around pain and analgesic issues. The patient and family are the unit of concern, and need a more general, long-term, supportive relationship within the health care system, in addition to specific psychological approaches dealing with pain and dying that a psychiatrist, psychologist, social worker, chaplain, or nurse can provide.

As noted, supportive psychotherapy with the dying patient can be extremely positive. The dying patient also may benefit from pastoral counseling. If a chaplaincy service is available, it should be offered to the patient and family. As the dying process progresses, psychotherapy with the individual patient may become limited by cognitive and speech deficits. It is at this point that the focus of supportive psychotherapeutic interventions shifts primarily to the family. In our experience, a common issue for family members is the level of alertness of the patient. Attempts to control pain are often accompanied by sedation that can limit communication between patient and family. This can sometimes become a source of conflict, with family members disagreeing among themselves or with the patient about what constitutes an appropriate balance between comfort and alertness. It can be helpful for the physician to clarify the patient's preferences, as they relate to these issues, early so that conflict can be avoided and work related to bereavement can begin.

Group interventions with individual patients (even in advanced stages of disease), spouses, couples, and families are a powerful means of sharing experiences and identifying successful coping strategies. The limitations of using group interventions for patients with advanced disease are primarily pragmatic. The patient must be physically comfortable enough to participate and have the cognitive capacity to be aware of group discussion. It is often helpful for family members to attend support groups during the terminal phases of the patient's illness.

Psychotherapeutic interventions that have multiple foci may be most useful. Based on a prospective study of cancer pain, cognitive behavioral and psychoeducational techniques designed to increase support, self-efficacy, and provide education may prove helpful in assisting patients in dealing with increased pain (86). Results of an evaluation of patients with cancer pain indicate that psychological and social variables are significant predictors of pain. More specifically, distress specific to the illness, self-efficacy, and coping styles were predictors of increased pain.

Using psychotherapy to diminish symptoms of anxiety and depression, factors that can intensify pain, empirically has beneficial effects on cancer pain experience. Spiegel and Bloom, (78) in a controlled randomized prospective study, demonstrated the effect of both supportive group therapy for metastatic breast cancer patients in general and, in particular, the effect of hypnotic pain control exercises. Their support group focused not on interpersonal processes or self-exploration, but rather on a series of themes related to the practical and existential problems of living with cancer. Patients were divided into two treatment groups and a control group. The treatment patients experienced significantly less pain than the control patients. Those in the group that combined a self-hypnosis exercise group showed a slight increase, and the control group showed a large increase in pain.

Whereas psychotherapy in the cancer pain setting is primarily non-analytical and focuses on current issues, exploration of reactions to cancer often involve insights into earlier more pervasive life issues. Some patients choose to continue a more exploratory psychotherapy during extended illness-free periods or survivorship.

Psychological interventions for depression in cancer pain patients Over the past 30 years, numerous studies have compared the relative effectiveness of psychotherapy, pharmacotherapy and concurrent therapeutic approaches in the treatment of common psychiatric disorders, such as depression and anxiety. Generally, these studies have demonstrated that the combined approach is somewhat more effective in treating the disorder in question, as well as prevention relapse.

In numerous trials, psychotherapy has been shown to be effective. Most studies show large treatment effects (Table 21.5) (87–92). Two studies suggest an effect of psychotherapy on survival or tumor growth (93,94). Two studies reported low treatment effects, including a cognitive behavioral psychotherapeutic approach designed to raise self-esteem and fighting spirit (95) and a study of relaxation (96). Holland and colleagues (80) reported high treatment effects for both drug and relaxation therapy, with drug effects surpassing relaxation alone. Overall, there is sufficient evidence to credit counseling interventions with a positive effect on depression (87,97,98).

Pharmacological treatment of depression in patients with cancer pain

Pharmacotherapy is the mainstay for treating cancer patients meeting diagnosis criteria for major depression (81). Factors such as prognosis and the timeframe for treatment may play an important role in determining the type of pharmacotherapy for depression. A depressed patient with several months of life expectancy can afford to wait the 2 to 4 weeks it may take to respond to a tricyclic antidepressant. The depressed dying patient with less than 3 weeks to live may do best with a rapid-acting psychostimulant. Patients who are within hours to days of death and in distress are likely to benefit most from the use of sedatives or opioid analgesic infusions.

Antidepressant medications

The efficacy of antidepressants in the treatment of depression in cancer patients has been well established (81–85,99). However, antidepressants are prescribed for the treatment of depression in only 1% to 3% of hospitalized cancer patients and only 5% of terminally ill cancer patients. A survey of antidepressant prescribing in the terminally ill found that out of 1046 cancer patients, only 10% received antidepressants, 76% of whom did not receive them until the last 2 weeks of life (100).

Table 21.5. *Randomized controlled trials in psychological counseling interventions for depression in cancer patients (96)*

Study	Sample	Type of intervention
McArdle et al., 1996 (90)	272 preoperative women with breast cancer	• Breast nurse support: explained routine surgery, wounds, symptoms, prosthesis, exercise for arm, other treatments, gave correct information, allowed expression of feelings, concerns, reassured feelings and concerns were understandable for 20–30 minutes • Volunteer support information, counseling and group meetings, telephone contact
Burton et al., 1995	200 women awaiting mastectomy for breast cancer	• Preoperative interview: discovery of lump, referral to surgeon, beliefs about cause, initial response to need for surgery, need for information, worries about body image, partner's response, social support, life events, regrets, optimism about future, anxiety and depression, psychiatric history, concerns with outcome. Summary of concerns and coping processes used for 45–60 minutes • Psychotherapeutic intervention: contextualized illness and surgery in life situation, explored feelings for 30 min • CHAT: hobbies, holidays, other items of interest for 30 minutes
Linn et al., 1982 (91)	120 men with end-stage cancer, three cancer sites	• Develop trusting relationship, maintain hope, reduce denial, emphasize control over environment and independence, life review to develop sense of meaning, self-esteem, and life satisfaction
Moorey et al., 1993 (95)	134 patients with cancer (cerebral, non-melanoma skin cancer excluded) or cancer recurrence	• Cognitive behavioral therapy for 1 hour × 8 weeks
Edgar et al., 1992 (89)	205, 80% women with breast cancer	• Five sessions of coping skills based psychosocial intervention including problem solving, goal setting, time management, cognitive reappraisal of negative thought, relaxation supplemented by a use of resources workshop
Greer et al., 1992 (88)	156 patients with cancer, primarily women, 4–12 weeks after diagnosis	• Adjuvant psychological therapy for patients and families • Focus on personal meaning of cancer, effect on coping strategies and present problems • Cognitive and behavioral techniques
Cain et al., 1986 (92)	80 women with gynecological cancer	• Discussions on what is cancer and its causes, body image and sexuality, relaxation, diet, exercise, relating to caregivers, friends and family, and goal setting • Attended to fear, anxiety, despair, guilt, self-esteem, anger, alienation and change • Using open discussion, accurate information, expression of fears, relaxation techniques, problem solving, communication techniques, short and long term goal setting
Decker et al., 1992 (191)	82 newly diagnosed outpatients, curative or palliative radiotherapy treatment, 52 men and 30 women (breast 29/82)	• Relaxation training with tape and written instructions six 1 h sessions • Cue controlled relaxation in session 4 with progressive muscle relaxation, coping with tension using cue controlled response • Discussions of concerns related to radiation treatment, affects and sensations
Holland et al., 1991 (80)	Any cancer patient with a score of 6 or more on RDS, or 25 or more on HADS	• Alprazolam X 10 d • Instruction in progressive muscle relaxation with practice TID
Bridge et al., 1988 (96)	154 women with stage I and II breast cancer after 1st session of radiotherapy	• Relaxation techniques in 1 hr session and tape for practice • Imagery group 1 hr session and tape for practice

Adapted from Sellick SM, Crooks DL. Depression and cancer: an appraisal of the literature for prevalence, detection, and practice guideline development for psychological interventions. Psychooncology 8(4):315–33, 1999.

Table 21.6 outlines the antidepressant medications used in cancer patients. There are a number of controlled studies (Table 21.7) of antidepressant drug treatment for depressive disorders in cancer patients in general, but fewer that focus on the terminally ill (87,91,92). To date, imipramine (84,101), mianserin (85), trimipramine (101), alprazolam (80,102), fluoxetine, and desipramine (103) have been studied and shown effective in controlled trials. All of these studies treated cancer patients with depressive symptoms of a certain threshold of severity based on

Table 21.6. *Antidepressant medications used in advanced cancer patients*[a]

Drug	Therapeutic daily dosage mg (PO)
Second-generation antidepressants	
Serotonin selective reuptake inhibitors	
Fluoxetine	10–40
Paroxetine	10–40
Citalopram	20–40
Fluvoxamine	50–300
Sertraline	50–200
Serotonin/norepinephrine reuptake inhibitor	
Venlafaxine	37.5–225
5-HT2 antagonists/serotonin and norepinephrine reuptake inhibitors	
Nefazodone	100–500
Trazodone	150–300
Norepinephrine/dopamine reuptake inhibitor	
Buproprion	200–450
α-2 antagonist/5-HT2 antagonist	
Mirtazapine	7.5–30
Tricyclic antidepressants	
Secondary amine	
Desipramine	25–125
Nortriptyline	25–125
Tertiary amine	
Amitriptyline	25–125
Doxepin	25–125
Imipramine	25–125
Clomipramine	25–125
Heterocyclic antidepressants	
Maprotiline	50–75
Amoxapine	100–150
Psychostimulants	
Dextroamphetamine	5–30
Methylphenidate	5–30
Pemoline	37.5–150
Monoamine oxidase inhibitors	
Isocarboxazid	20–40
Phenelzine	30–60
Tranylcypromine	20–40
Lithium carbonate	600–1200
Benzodiazepines	
Alprazolam	0.75–6.00

[a] Adapted from Massie MJ, Holland JC. Depression and the cancer patient. J Clin Psychiatry 51:12–7, 1990.

observer-rated or self-report measures of depression, distress, or anxiety. None used structured diagnostic interviews to establish DM-III, DSM-III-R, or RDC diagnoses of major depression. Of the two controlled trials of traditional antidepressants in advanced cancer, one study of nortriptyline (104) was not completed because of high attrition rates resulting from drug side effects and disease progression, and another study of alprazolam (102) contained a sample of only 20 patients. Traditional antidepressants such as the tricyclics and tetracyclic drugs have apparently limited roles in the treatment of depression in terminally ill cancer patients because of their unfavorable side effect profiles and the long duration of time required before onset of antidepressant effects.

Several antineoplastic agents use the hepatic cytochrome P450 system, especially the 3A4 isoenzyme. This may be significant in the selection of an antidepressant. For example, nefazodone and fluvoxamine inhibit the 3A4 isoenzyme. Thus, their use requires careful monitoring for increased toxicity if the patient is receiving a chemotherapy regimen that is metabolized through the same isoenzyme. Drug interactions can also be mediated through competition for protein binding. Highly protein-bound antidepressants can displace the chemotherapeutic agent and leave patients vulnerable to serious toxicity. Venlafaxine is the least protein bound (Table 21.8) (5).

Second-generation antidepressants

Selective serotonin re-uptake inhibitors Selective serotonin reuptake inhibitors (SSRIs) are commonly the first line of treatment because of their safety and low side effect profile. They also may be effective as adjunct analgesic drugs, especially for neuropathic pain. It is good practice "to start low and go slow" in cancer patients to reduce gastrointestinal side effects of nausea and transient weight loss. Short-term addition initially of a benzodiazepine helps to prevent anxiety and jitteriness. The SSRIs are safe with chemotherapeutic agents. However, they should be avoided in patients receiving procarbazine for management of some hematological malignancies, because it is a monoamine oxidase inhibitor.

The SSRIs have been found to be as effective in the treatment of depression as the tricyclics (105,106) and have a number of features that may be particularly advantageous for cancer patients. The SSRIs have a very low affinity for adrenergic, cholinergic, and histamine receptors, thus accounting for negligible orthostatic hypotension, urinary retention, memory impairment, sedation, or reduced awareness. They have not been found to cause

Table 21.7. *Controlled clinical trials of antidepressants for depression in cancer patients*

Study	Comments	Drugs	Outcome
Holland et al. (1998) (103)	Multicenter women w/ cancer N = 40 6-week trial	Fluoxetine vs. desipramine vs. placebo	Fluoxetine and desipramine both improve depression, anxiety, and QOL
Van Heeringen & Zivkov (1996)	Women w/ breast cancer N = 55 6-week trial	Mianserin vs. placebo	Mianserin effective in ↓ depression Superior to placebo
Razavi et al. (1996) (193)	Mixed cancer population N = 91 5-week trial	Fluoxetine vs. placebo	No significant differences between fluoxetine and placebo
Costa et al. (1985) (85)	Women w/ cancer N = 73 4-week trial	Mianserin vs. placebo	Mianserin safe and effective ↓ depression, ↑ QOL
Evans et al. (1988) (101)	Women w/ cancer N = 40	Imipramine vs. control	Imipramine improves depression and QOL
Rifkin et al. (1985) (83)	Mixed medical illness cancer N = 42	Trimipramine vs. placebo	Trimipramine superior to placebo
Purohit et al. (1978) (84)	Mixed cancer patients N = 39	Imipramine vs. control	Imipramine improves depressive symptoms

Abbreviation: QOL, quality of life.

clinically significant alterations in cardiac conduction and are generally favorably tolerated along with a wider margin of safety than the tricyclic antidepressants in the event of an overdose. They do not therefore require therapeutic drug level monitoring.

Most of the side effects of SSRIs result from their selective central and peripheral serotonin reuptake properties. Side effects include diarrhea, nausea, vomiting, insomnia, headaches, and sexual dysfunction. Some patients may experience anxiety, tremor, restlessness, and akathisia (the latter is relatively rare, but it can be problematic for the terminally ill patient with Parkinson's disease) (99). These side effects tend to be dose related and may be problematic for patients with advanced disease.

Five SSRIs are available in the United States, including sertraline, fluoxetine, paroxetine, citalopram, and fluvoxamine. With the exception of fluoxetine, whose elimination half-life is 2 to 4 days, the SSRIs have an elimination half-life of about 24 hours. Fluoxetine is the only SSRI with a potent active metabolite, norfluoxetine, whose elimination half-life is 7 to 14 days. Fluoxetine and norfluoxetine do not reach a steady state for 5 to 6 weeks, compared with 4 to 14 days for paroxetine, fluvoxamine, and sertraline. These differences are important, especially for the terminally ill patient in whom a switch from an SSRI to another antidepressant is being considered. If a switch to a monamine oxidase inhibitor is required, the washout period for fluoxetine will be at least 5 weeks, given the potential drug interactions between these two agents. Paroxetine, fluvoxamine, and sertraline require considerably shorter washout periods (10–14 days) under similar circumstances. Since fluoxetine entered the market, there have been several reports of significant drug-drug interactions (100). Until it has been studied further in cancer, fluoxetine should be used cautiously in the debilitated patient. All the SSRIs have

Table 21.8. *Protein binding and CP450 isoenzyme profile of commonly used antidepressants in cancer patients*

Drug	Protein binding	1A2 inhibition	2C9 inhibition	2D6 inhibition	3A4 inhibition
Bupropion	80				
Citalopram	80	+	+	+	
Fluoxetine	94		+++	+++	++
Fluvoxamine	77	+++	+++		+++
Mirtazapine	85				
Nefazodone	99				+++
Paroxetine	95			+++	
Sertraline	98	++			++
Venlafaxine	27				

Adapted from Newport JD, Nemeroff CB. Treatment of depression in the cancer patient. Clin Geriatr 7:40–55, 1999.

the ability to inhibit the hepatic isoenzyme P450 11D6, with sertraline and fluvoxamine being least potent in this regard. Because SSRIs are dependent on hepatic metabolism, this ability becomes significant with respect to dose/plasma level ratios and drug interactions. For the elderly patient with advanced disease, the dose response curve for sertraline appears to be relatively linear. With the other drugs, particularly paroxetine (most potent inhibitor of cytochrome P450 11D6), small dosage increases can result in dramatic elevations in plasma levels. Paroxetine and fluoxetine inhibit the hepatic enzymes responsible for their own clearance (108). These medications should be co-administered cautiously with other drugs that are dependent on this enzyme system for their catabolism (e.g., tricyclics, phenothiazines, type IC antiarrhythmics, quinidine). Fluvoxamine has been shown in some instances to elevate the blood levels of propranolol and warfarin by as much as twofold and should thus not be prescribed together with these agents.

For cancer patients, SSRIs, can be started at approximately half the usual starting dose used in an otherwise healthy patient. Titration of fluoxetine can begin with 5 mg (available in liquid form) given once daily (preferably in the morning). The usual effective range is 10 to 40 mg per day. Given the long half-life of fluoxetine, some patients may only require this drug every second day. Paroxetine can be started at 10 mg once daily (either morning or evening) and has a therapeutic range of 10 to 40 mg per day. Fluvoxamine, which tends to be somewhat more sedating, can be started at 25 mg (in the evenings) and has a therapeutic range of 50 to 300 mg. Sertraline can be initiated at 50 mg, morning or evening, and titrated within a range of 50 to 200 mg per day. If patients experience activating effects on SSRIs, they should not be given at bedtime but rather moved earlier into the day. Gastrointestinal upset can be reduced by ensuring the patient not taking the medication on an empty stomach.

Serotonin-norepinephrine reuptake inhibitor (SNRI)

Venlafaxine (Effexor) is the only antidepressant in this class. It is a potent inhibitor of neuronal serotonin and norepinephrine reuptake and appears to have no significant affinity for muscarinic, histamine, or alpha$_1$-adrenergic receptors. Some patients may experience a modest sustained increase in blood pressure, especially at doses above the recommended initiating dose. Compared with the SSRIs, its protein binding (< 35%) is very low. Few protein binding-induced drug interactions are thus expected. Like other antidepressants, venlafaxine should

not be used in patients receiving monamine oxidase inhibitors. Its side effect profile tends to be generally well tolerated, with few discontinuations. Although there are currently no data addressing its use in the depressed cancer patients, its pharmacokinetic properties and side effect profile suggest it may have a role to play.

Nefazodone and trazodone are chemically related antidepressants. Nefazodone is much less sedating than trazodone but more likely to cause gastrointestinal activation. Nefazodone can be started at 50 mg at bedtime and titrated within a range of 100 to 500 mg per day. Nefazodone usually does not impair sexual function side. It does not have any clinical significant interactions with lorazepam but increases the serum levels of alprazolam and triazolam. Nefazodone has been demonstrated to potentiate opioid analgesics in an animal model (109).

Other atypical antidepressants

If given in sufficient doses (100–300 mg/day), trazodone can be an effective antidepressant. Although its anticholinergic profile is almost negligible, it has considerable affinity for alpha$_1$-adrenoceptors and may thus predispose patients to orthostatic hypotension and its problematic sequelae (i.e., falls, fractures, and head injuries). Trazodone is very sedating and in low doses (100 mg qhs) is helpful in the treatment of the depressed cancer patient with insomnia. It is highly serotonergic, and its use should be considered when the patient requires adjunct analgesic effect in addition to antidepressant effects. Trazodone has little effect on cardiac conduction but can cause arrhythmias in patients with premorbid cardiac disease (110). Trazodone has also been associated with priapism and should thus be used with caution in male patients (111). Trazodone is used alone or in combination with SSRIs. Sedation and weight gain are favorable side effect profiles in patients with insomnia and anorexia. Lack of anticholinergic side effects is helpful in patients prone to delirium and cognitive dysfunction.

Bupropion is a relatively new drug in the United States, and there has not been much experience with its use in the cancer setting. At present, it is not the first drug of choice for depressed patients with cancer. However, one might consider prescribing bupropion if patients have a poor response to a reasonable trial of other antidepressants. Bupropion may have a role in the treatment of the psychomotor retarded depressed cancer patient, as it has energizing effects similar to the stimulant drugs (112). Because of the increased incidence of seizures, however, bupropion should be used cautiously in patients with disorders of the central nervous system. The dopaminergic profile of bupropion may be used to counteract the sexual dysfunction caused by other medications.

Mirtazapine is the 6-aza analog of the tetracyclic antidepressant mianserin. Mirtazapine enhances central noradrenergic and serotonergic activity with blockade of central presynaptic alpha-2 inhibitory receptors and postsynaptic serotonin 5-hydroxytryptamine (5-HT)-2 and 5-HT-3 receptors. Although mirtazapine compares favorably with amitriptyline and trazodone, further studies are needed to compare its clinical efficacy with SSRIs. The drug mainly affects serotonin (5-HT) receptors of the 5-HT2 and 5-HT-3 subtypes, possessing low affinity for 5-HT1A, 5-HT1B, and 5-HT1C receptors. Mirtazapine improves appetite, resulting in weight gain, which is desirable in cancer patients. In addition, the marked sedative effect of this medication proves quite useful in patients with sleeping difficulties.

Tricyclic antidepressants

The use of tricyclic antidepressants (TCAs) in depressed cancer patients requires a careful risk–benefit ratio analysis. Although nearly 70% of patients treated with a tricyclic for nonpsychotic depression can anticipate a positive response, their side effect profile can be troublesome for cancer patients (113). Their multiple pharmacodynamic actions accounting for these side effects include blockade of muscarinic cholinergic receptors, alphaadrenoceptors, and H_1-histamine receptors. The tertiary amines (amitriptyline, doxepin, and imipramine) have a greater propensity to cause side effects than do secondary amines (nortriptyline, desipramine) (108,113). The secondary amines are thus often a preferable choice in the cancer setting.

The anticholinergic side effects of TCAs can include constipation, dry mouth, and urinary retention. To avoid exacerbating symptoms associated with genitourinary outlet obstruction, decreased gastric motility, or stomatitis, less anticholinergic tricyclics, such as desipramine or nortriptyline, are reasonable choices. Those patients who are receiving medication with anticholinergic properties (such as diphenylhydramine or a phenothiazine) are at risk for developing an anticholinergic delirium. Antidepressants with potent anticholinergic properties should be avoided in these patients. The anticholinergic actions of TCAs can also cause serious tachycardia. Their quinidine like effects can lead to arrhythmias by delaying the conduction through the His-Purkinje system. These effects are associated with nonspecific ST-T changes and T waves on the electrocardiograph. TCAs should be avoided in cancer patients with preexisting conduction defects or second- or third-degree heart block.

$Alpha_1$-blockade is associated with postural hypotension and dizziness. This can be of particular concern for the frail, volume-depleted patient who is at risk for falls and subsequent fractures. Nortriptyline and protriptyline are the TCAs least associated with $alpha_1$-blockade. H_1-histamine receptor blockage is associated with sedation and drowsiness. For dying patients already exposed to a variety of sedating agents (e.g., opioids, antiemetics, anxiolytics, neuroleptics), TCAs such as amitriptyline and doxepin are the most likely to accentuate the overall cumulative sedating effects of these medications.

Tricyclic antidepressants should be started at low doses (10–25 mg qhs) and increased in 10- to 25-mg increments every 2 to 4 days, until a therapeutic dose is attained or side effects become a dose-limiting factor. Both depression and pain in cancer patients respond at significantly lower doses of TCAs (25–125 mg) than are necessary in the physically well (150–300 g). To minimize TCA toxicity, plasma levels must be carefully monitored during titration, as well as during steady state.

The choice of TCA depends on a variety of factors, including the nature of the underlying medical condition, the characteristics of the depressive episode, past responses to antidepressant therapy, and the specific drug side effect profile. For depressed cancer patients, the choice of TCA often is made on the basis of a side effect profile, which will be least incompatible with the patients' overall medical condition. Most TCAs are available as rectal suppositories for patients who are no longer able to take medication orally. Outside of the United States, certain TCAs are given as intravenous infusion. Amitriptyline, imipramine, and doxepin are available intramuscularly.

Therapeutic response to TCAs, as with all antidepressants, has a latency time of 3 to 6 weeks. Thus for patients with advanced cancer, psychostimulants may offer a more viable, rapid response alternative.

Many antidepressants have analgesic properties. There is no definite indication that any one drug is more effective than the others, although the most experience has been accrued with amitriptyline.

Heterocyclic antidepressants

The heterocyclic antidepressants have side effect profiles that are similar to the TCAs. Maprotiline should be avoided in patients with brain tumors and in those who are at risk for seizures, as the incidence of seizures is increased with this medication (114). Amoxapine has mild dopamine-blocking activity. Hence, patients who are taking other dopamine blockers (e.g., antiemetics) have an increased risk of developing extrapyramidal symptoms and dyskinesias. Mianserin (not available in the United States) is a serotonergic antidepressant with adjuvant analgesic properties that is used widely in Europe and Latin America. Costa and colleagues (85) showed mianserin to be a safe and effective drug for the treatment of depression in cancer.

Psychostimulants

Psychostimulants currently approved for use in cancer patients include methylphenidate, dextroamphetamine, pemoline, and mazindol. They have been shown to be rapidly effective antidepressants, especially in the cancer setting (Table 21.9) (115–125). Psychostimulants are also useful in diminishing excessive sedation secondary to opioid analgesics. Bruera et al. (126–128) demonstrated that a regimen of 10 mg methylphenidate with breakfast and 5 mg with lunch significantly decreased sedation and potentiated the analgesic effect of an opioid in patients with cancer pain. Dextroamphetamine has also been reported to have additive analgesic effects when used with morphine in postoperative pain (129). Several investigators have demonstrated the efficacy of methylphenidate in the treatment of depression in advanced cancer patients, reporting rapid onset of action (1–3 days) and response rates as high as 85% (117,118). Bruera and colleagues (116) studied mazindol's effects on depression in advanced cancer patients using a double-blind design. The chewable form of pemoline is espe-

cially favorable in those, who can no longer tolerate oral route but can utilize buccal absorption (115).

The psychostimulants are most helpful in the treatment of depression in the cancer setting, especially those with dysphoric mood associated with severe psychomotor slowing and even mild cognitive impairment. Psychostimulants have been shown to improve attention, concentration, and overall performance on neuropsychological testing in the medically ill (130). In relatively low doses, psychostimulants stimulate appetite, promote a sense of well-being, and improve feelings of weakness and fatigue in cancer patients. Treatment with dextroamphetamine or methylphenidate usually begins with a dose of 2.5 mg at 8:00 AM and at noon. The dosage is slowly increased over several days until a desired effect is achieved or side effects (overstimulation, anxiety, insomnia, paranoia, and confusion) intervene. Typically a dose greater than 30 mg per day is not necessary, although occasionally patients require up to 60 mg per day. Patients usually are maintained on methylphenidate for 1 to 2 months, and approximately two thirds will be able to be withdrawn from methylphenidate without a recurrence of depressive symptoms. If symptoms do recur patients can be maintained on a psychostimulant for up to 1 year without significant abuse problems. Tolerance can develop, and adjustment of dose may be necessary. Common side effects of stimulants include nervousness, overstimulation, mild increase in blood pressure and pulse rate, and tremor. More rare side effects include dyskinesias or motor tics, as well as a paranoid psychosis or exacerbation of an underlying and unrecognized confusional state.

Table 21.9. *Clinical trials of psychostimulants in cancer patients*

Study	Comments	Drugs	Outcome
Meyers et al. (1998)	Brain tumor $N = 30$	Methylphenidate	↑ mood ↑ cognition ↑ function
Olin & Masand (1996) (118)	Mixed cancer $N = 59$ Chart review	Dextroamphetamine methylphenidate	↓ depression ↑ appetite
Breitbart & Mermelstein (1992) (115)	Case reports $N = 4$	Pemoline	↑ mood ↑ appetite ↑ energy
Bruera et al. (1992) (128)	Cancer pain $N = 20$ Opioid infusion	Methylphenidate vs. placebo	↑ cognition ↓ sedation
Fernandez et al. (1986)	Mixed cancer $N = 30$	Methylphenidate (up to 80 mg)	Rapid onset ↓ depression
Bruera et al. (1986) (116)	Double blind crossover study $N = 24$	Mazindol	↓ pain ↓ appetite No effect on mood
Joshi et al. (1982)	Terminally ill	Amphetamine	↑ comfort

Pemoline is a unique psychostimulant chemically unrelated to amphetamine. There are several advantages for using pemoline in cancer patients. Pemoline does not have any abuse potential and does not require special prescriptions. In addition, pemoline is available in chewable tablet form with good absorption through the buccal mucosa and is very useful in cancer patients with difficulty swallowing or intestinal obstruction. Pemoline is as effective as methylphenidate and dextroamphetamine in the treatment of depression in cancer patients (115). However, it is better tolerated because of its mild sympathomimetic effects. Pemoline can be started at a dose of 18.75 mg in the morning and at noon, and increased gradually over days. Typically patients require 75 mg a day or less. Pemoline should be used with caution in patients with liver impairment, and liver function tests should be monitored periodically with longer term treatment (131). See Table 21.9 for clinical trials of psychostimulants in cancer patients.

Monoamine oxidase inhibitors

In general, monoamine oxidase inhibitors (MAOIs) are rarely used in the cancer setting. Patients who receive MAOIs must avoid foods rich in tyramine, sympathomimetic drugs (amphetamines, methylphenidate), and medications containing phenylpropanolamine and pseudoephedrine. The combination of these agents with MAOIs may cause hypertensive crisis. MAOIs in combination with opioid analgesics have also been reported to be associated with myoclonus and delirium and must therefore be used together cautiously (132). The use of meperidine while taking MAOIs is absolutely contraindicated and can lead to hyperpyrexia, cardiovascular collapses, and death. MAOIs can also cause considerable orthostatic hypotension. Avoiding these adverse interactions can be particularly problematic for patients with cancer. It is not surprising that MAOIs tend to be reserved in this patient population for those who have shown past preferential responses to them. Among the MAOI drugs available, phenelzine has been shown to have adjuvant analgesic properties in patients with atypical facial pain and migraine (133,134).

The new reversible inhibitors of monoamine oxidase-A (RIMAs) may reduce some of the problems associated with the older MAOIs. There are no studies on the role of RIMAs in depressed cancer patients, but there are interesting theoretical reasons to suggest they may eventually have a larger role to play than the non-selective MAOIs. RIMAs selectively inhibit MAO-A enzyme, therefore leaving MAO-B enzyme available to deal with any tyramine challenge. Moclobemide, a RIMA recently introduced onto the Canadian market, appears to be loosely bound to the MAO-A receptor and is thus relatively easily displaced by tyramine from its binding site. It has a very short half-life, which further reduces the possibility of any prolonged adverse effects (e.g., hypertensive crisis). Dietary restrictions avoidant of tyramine-containing foods are thus not required. The side-effect profile of moclobemide is far more favorable than non-selective MAOIs and tends to be well tolerated. Agents such as meperidine, procarbazine, dextromethorphan, or other ephedrine-containing agents, are still best avoided. Although RIMAs may offer some advantages in the depressed cancer patients over tranylcypromine and isocarboxazid, they will likely remain a second-line choice to other available non-MAOI antidepressants.

Lithium carbonate

Patients who have been receiving lithium carbonate before a cancer illness should be maintained on it throughout their cancer treatment, although close monitoring is necessary in the preoperative and postoperative periods, when fluids and salt may be restricted (135). Maintenance doses of lithium may require reduction in seriously ill patients. Lithium should be prescribed with caution for patients receiving cis-platinum because of the potential nephrotoxicity of both drugs. Several authors have reported possible beneficial effects from the use of lithium in neutropenic cancer patients. However, the functional capabilities of these leukocytes have not been determined. The stimulation effect appears to be transient; no mood changes were noted in these patients (136).

Benzodiazepines and other anxiolytics

The triazolobenzodiazepine alprazolam has been shown to be a mildly effective antidepressant as well as an anxiolytic. Alprazolam is particularly useful in cancer patients who have mixed symptoms of anxiety and depression. Starting dose is 0.25 mg three times a day, and effective doses are usually in the range of 4 to 6 mg daily.

Benzodiazepines have not been thought to have direct analgesic properties, although they are potent anxiolytics and anticonvulsants (137). Some authors have suggested that their anticonvulsant properties make certain benzodiazepine drugs useful in the management of neuropathic pain. Both alprazolam, a unique benzodiazepine with mild antidepressant properties, and clonazepam may be useful in neuropathic pain (138,139). With the use of midazolam by patient-controlled dosage, there was no reduction in the use of postoperative morphine requirements or in the patient's perception of pain (140).

Hydroxyzine is a mild anxiolytic with sedating and analgesic properties that are useful in the anxious cancer patient with pain (141). This antihistamine has antiemetic activity as well.

Electroconvulsive therapy

Occasionally, it is necessary to consider electroconvulsive therapy (ECT) for depressed cancer patients who have depression with psychotic features or in whom treatment with antidepressants poses unacceptable side effects. The safe effective use of ECT in the medically ill has been reviewed by others (81).

Summary

The management of depression associated with cancer pain can be a challenging task for clinicians. A thorough assessment and familiarity with both the pharmacological and nonpharmacological modalities help to distinguish between the distress of unrelieved pain and the depression and provide the tools needed to address depression when it occurs.

References

1. Foley KM. The treatment of cancer pain. N Engl J Med 313(2):84–95, 1985.
2. Foley KM. Pain syndromes in patients with cancer. In: Bonica JJ, Ventafridda V, Jones LE, Loeser JD, eds. Advances in pain research and therapy, vol 2. New York: Raven Press, 1975:59–75.
3. Breitbart W, Holland JC. Psychiatric aspects of cancer pain. In: Foley KM, ed. Advances in pain research and therapy, vol 16. New York: Raven Press, Ltd., 1990:73–87.
4. Breitbart W. Psychiatric management of cancer pain. Cancer 63:2336–42, 1989.
5. Massie MJ, Holland JC. The cancer patient with pain: psychiatric complications and their management. Med Clin North Am 71(2):243–58, 1987.
6. Stiefel F. Psychosocial aspects of cancer pain (see comments). Support Care Cancer 1(3):130–4, 1993.
7. Saunders CM. The management of terminal illness. London: Hospital Medicine Publications, 1967.
8. Hanks GW. Opioid-responsive and opioid-non-responsive pain in cancer. Br Med Bull 47(3):718–31, 1991.
9. Syrjala KL, Chapko ME. Evidence for a biopsychosocial model of cancer treatment-related pain. Pain 61(1):69–79, 1995.
10. Daut RL, Cleeland CS. The prevalence and severity of pain in cancer. Cancer 50(9):1913–18, 1982.
11. Spiegel D, Bloom JR. Pain in metastatic breast cancer. Cancer 52(2):341–5, 1983.
12. Padilla GV, Ferrell B, Grant MM, Rhiner M. Defining the content domain of quality of life for cancer patients with pain. Cancer Nurs 13(2):108–15, 1990.
13. Payne D, Jacobsen P, Breitbart W, et al. Negative thoughts related to pain are associated with greater pain, distress, and disability in AIDS pain. Miami: American Pain Society, 1994.
14. McKegney FP, Bailey LR, Yates JW. Prediction and management of pain in patients with advanced cancer. Gen Hosp Psychiatry 3(2):95–101, 1981.
15. Bond MR, Pearson IB. Psychological aspects of pain in women with advanced cancer of the cervix. J Psychosom Res 13(1):13–9, 1969.
16. Singer EJ, Zorilla C, Fahy-Chandon B, et al. Painful symptoms reported by ambulatory HIV-infected men in a longitudinal study. Pain 54(1):15–9, 1993.
17. Marks RM, Sachar EJ. Undertreatment of medical inpatients with narcotic analgesics. Ann Intern Med 78(2):173–81, 1973.
18. Cleeland CS, Tearnan BH. Behavioral control of cancer pain. In: Holzman D, Turk D, eds. Pain management. New York: Pergamon Press, 1986:193–212.
19. Derogatis LR, Morrow GR, Fetting J, et al. The prevalence of psychiatric disorders among cancer patients. JAMA 249(6):751–7, 1983.
20. Ahles TA, Blanchard EB, Ruckdeschel JC. The multidimensional nature of cancer-related pain. Pain 17(3):277–88, 1983.
21. Woodforde JM, Fielding JR. Pain and cancer. J Psychosom Res 14(4):365–70, 1970.
22. Stiefel FC, Breitbart WS, Holland JC. Corticosteroids in cancer: neuropsychiatric complications. Cancer Invest 7(5):479–91, 1989.
23. Bukberg J, Penman D, Holland JC. Depression in hospitalized cancer patients. Psychosom Med 46(3):199–212, 1984.
24. Massie MJ, Holland J, Glass E. Delirium in terminally ill cancer patients. Am J Psychiatry 140(8):1048–50, 1983.
25. Bruera E, Macmillan K, Hanson J, MacDonald RN. The cognitive effects of the administration of narcotic analgesics in patients with cancer pain. Pain 39(1):13–6, 1989.
26. Sullivan M, Rapp S, Fitzgibbon D, Chapman CR. Pain and the choice to hasten death in patients with painful metastatic cancer. J Palliat Care 13(3):18–28, 1997.
27. American Psychiatric Association. Diagnostic statistical manual of mental disorders, 4th ed. Washington DC: American Psychiatric Association, 1994
28. Kathol RG, Mutgi A, Williams J, et al. Diagnosis of major depression in cancer patients according to four sets of criteria. Am J Psychiatry 147(8):1021–4, 1990.
29. Cohen-Cole S, McDaniel S, et al. Diagnostic assessment of depression in the medically ill. In: Stoudemier A, ed. Principles of medical psychiatry. New York: Oxford University Press, 1995.
30. Cohen-Cole SA, Stoudemire A. Major depression and physical illness. Special considerations in diagnosis and biologic treatment. Psychiatr Clin North Am 10(1):1–17, 1987.

31. Endicott J. Measurement of depression in patients with cancer. Cancer 53(10 Suppl):2243–9, 1984.

32. Chochinov HM, Wilson KG, Enns M, Lander S. Prevalence of depression in the terminally ill: effects of diagnostic criteria and symptom threshold judgments. Am J Psychiatry 151(4):537–40, 1994.

33. Chochinov HM, Wilson KG, Enns M, Lander S. "Are you depressed?" Screening for depression in the terminally ill (see comments). Am J Psychiatry 154(5):674–6, 1997.

34. Cassem EH. Depression and anxiety secondary to medical illness. Psychiatr Clin North Am 13(4):597–612, 1990.

35. Spitzer RL, Endicott J, Robins E. Research diagnostic criteria: rationale and reliability. Arch Gen Psychiatry 35(6):773–82, 1978.

36. Robins LN, Helzer JE, Croughan J, Ratcliff KS. National Institute of Mental Health Diagnostic Interview Schedule. Its history, characteristics, and validity. Arch Gen Psychiatry 38(4):381–9, 1981.

37. Spitzer RL, Williams JBW, Gibbon M, First MB. Structured Clinical Interview for DSM-III-R. Washington DC: American Psychiatric Press, 1990.

38. Endicott J, Spitzer RL. A diagnostic interview: the schedule for affective disorders and schizophrenia. Arch Gen Psychiatry 35(7):837–44, 1978.

39. Spitzer RL, Williams JB, Kroenke K, et al. Utility of a new procedure for diagnosing mental disorders in primary care. The PRIME-MD 1000 study (see comments). JAMA 272(22):1749–56, 1994.

40. Power D, Kelly S, Gilsenan J, et al. Suitable screening tests for cognitive impairment and depression in the terminally ill–a prospective prevalence study. Palliat Med 7(3):213–8, 1993.

41. Breitbart W, Bruera E, Chochinov H, Lynch M. Neuropsychiatric syndromes and psychological symptoms in patients with advanced cancer. J Pain Symptom Manage 10(2):131–41, 1995.

42. Wells KB, Hays RD, Burnam MA, et al. Detection of depressive disorder for patients receiving prepaid or fee-for-service care. Results from the Medical Outcomes Study (see comments). JAMA 262(23):3298–302, 1989.

43. Beck AT, Beck RW. Screening depressed patients in family practice. A rapid technique. Postgrad Med 52(6):81–5, 1972.

44. Zigmond AS, Snaith RP. The hospital anxiety and depression scale. Acta Psychiatr Scand 67(6):361–70, 1983.

45. Goldberg DP. Manual of the general health questionnaire. Windsor, England: NFER Publishing Co., 1978.

46. de Haes JC, van Knippenberg FC, Neijt JP. Measuring psychological and physical distress in cancer patients: structure and application of the Rotterdam Symptom Checklist. Br J Cancer 62(6):1034–8, 1990.

47. Carroll BJ, Feinberg M, Smouse PE, et al. The Carroll rating scale for depression. I. Development, reliability and validation. Br J Psychiatry 138:194–200, 1981.

48. Golden RN, McCartney CF, Haggerty JJ Jr, et al. The detection of depression by patient self-report in women with gynecologic cancer. Int J Psychiatry Med 21(1):17–27, 1991.

49. Hopwood P, Howell A, Maguire P. Screening for psychiatric morbidity in patients with advanced breast cancer: validation of two self-report questionnaires. Br J Cancer 64(2):353–6, 1991.

50. Hardman A, Maguire P, Crowther D. The recognition of psychiatric morbidity on a medical oncology ward. J Psychosom Res 33(2):235–9, 1989.

51. Razavi D, Delvaux N, Bredart A, et al. Screening for psychiatric disorders in a lymphoma out-patient population. Eur J Cancer 11(72):1869–72, 1992.

52. Razavi D, Delvaux N, Farvacques C, Robaye E. Screening for adjustment disorders and major depressive disorders in cancer in-patients (see comments). Br J Psychiatry 156:79–83, 1990.

53. Fechner-Bates S, Coyne JC, Schwenk TL. The relationship of self-reported distress to depressive disorders and other psychopathology. J Consult Clin Psychol 62(3):550–9, 1994.

54. Bruera E, Kuehn N, Miller MJ, et al. The Edmonton Symptom Assessment System (ESAS): a simple method for the assessment of palliative care patients. J Palliat Care 7(2):6–9, 1991.

55. Fishman B, Pasternak S, Wallenstein SL, et al. The Memorial Pain Assessment Card. A valid instrument for the evaluation of cancer pain. Cancer 60(5):1151–8, 1987.

56. Black DW, Winokur G, Nasrallah A. Treatment and outcome in secondary depression: a naturalistic study of 1087 patients. J Clin Psychiatry 48(11):438–41, 1987.

57. Winokur G. The concept of secondary depression and its relationship to comorbidity. Psychiatr Clin North Am 13(4):567–83, 1990.

58. Munroe A. Some familial and social factors in depressive illness. Br J Psychiatry 112:429–41, 1966.

59. Feighner JP, Robins E, Guze SB, et al. Diagnostic criteria for use in psychiatric research. Arch Gen Psychiatry 26(1):57–63, 1972.

60. Passik SD, Breitbart WS. Depression in patients with pancreatic carcinoma. Diagnostic and treatment issues. Cancer 78(3 Suppl):615–26, 1996.

61. Lynch ME. The assessment and prevalence of affective disorders in advanced cancer. J Palliat Care 11(1):10–8, 1995.

62. Massie MJ. Depression. In: Holland JC, Rowland JH, eds. Handbook of psychooncology: psychological care of the patient with cancer. New York: Oxford University Press, 1989:283–90.

63. Breitbart W. Suicide in cancer patients. Oncology 1(2):49–55, 1987.

64. Levin DN, Cleeland CS, Dar R. Public attitudes toward cancer pain. Cancer 56(9):2337–9, 1985.

65. Bolund C. Suicide and cancer. II: Medical and cancer care factors in suicide by cancer patients in Sweden. J Psychosoc Oncol 3:17–30, 1985.

66. Massie MJ, Gagnon P, Holland JC. Depression and suicide in patients with cancer. J Pain Symptom Manage 9(5):325–40, 1994.

67. Silberfarb PM, Maurer LH, Crouthamel CS. Psychosocial aspects of neoplastic disease: I. Functional status of breast

cancer patients during different treatment regimens. Am J Psychiatry 137(4):450–5, 1980.

68. Achte KA, Vauhkonen ML. (Cancer and the psyche). Nord Psykiatr Tidsskr 25(3):199–212, 1971.

69. Brown JH, Henteleff P, Barakat S, Rowe CJ. Is it normal for terminally ill patients to desire death? Am J Psychiatry 143(2):208–11, 1986.

70. Twycross R., ed. Symptom control in far advanced cancer: pain relief. London: Pitman Brooks, 1983.

71. Cleeland CS, Gonin R, Hatfield AK, et al. Pain and its treatment in outpatients with metastatic cancer (see comments). N Engl J Med 330(9):592–6, 1994.

72. Charap AD. The knowledge, attitudes, and experience of medical personnel treating pain in the terminally ill. Mt Sinai J Med 45(4):561–80, 1978.

73. Kanner RM, Foley KM. Patterns of narcotic drug use in a cancer pain clinic. Ann N Y Acad Sci 362:161–72, 1981.

74. Grossman SA, Sheidler VR, Swedeen K, et al. Correlation of patient and caregiver ratings of cancer pain. J Pain Symptom Manage 6(2):53–7, 1991.

75. Cassem NH. The dying patient. In: Hackett TP, Cassem NH, eds. Massachusetts General Hospital handbook of general hospital psychiatry. Littleton, MA: PSG Publishing Co. Inc., 1987:332–52.

76. Maguire P, Hopwood P, Tarrier N, Howell T. Treatment of depression in cancer patients. Acta Psychiatr Scand Suppl 320:81–4, 1985.

77. Newport DJ, Nemeroff CB. Assessment and treatment of depression in the cancer patient. J Psychosom Res 45(3):215–37, 1998.

78. Spiegel D, Bloom JR. Group therapy and hypnosis reduce metastatic breast carcinoma pain. Psychosom Med 45(4):333–9, 1983.

79. Spiegel D, Wissler T. Using family consultation as psychiatric aftercare for schizophrenic patients. Hosp Commun Psychiatry 38(10):1096–9, 1987.

80. Holland JC, Morrow GR, Schmale A, et al. A randomized clinical trial of alprazolam versus progressive muscle relaxation in cancer patients with anxiety and depressive symptoms. J Clin Oncol 9(6):1004–11, 1991.

81. Massie MJ, Holland JC. Depression and the cancer patient. J Clin Psychiatry 51(Suppl):12–7; discussion 18–9, 1990.

82. Popkin MK, Callies AL, Mackenzie TB. The outcome of antidepressant use in the medically ill. Arch Gen Psychiatry 42(12):1160–3, 1985.

83. Rifkin A, Reardon G, Siris S, et al. Trimipramine in physical illness with depression. J Clin Psychiatry 46(2 Pt 2):4–8, 1985.

84. Purohit DR, Navlakha PL, Modi RS, Eshpumiyani R. The role antidepressants in hospitalised cancer patients. (a pilot study). J Assoc Physicians India 26(4):245–8, 1978.

85. Costa D, Mogos I, Toma T. Efficacy and safety of mianserin in the treatment of depression of women with cancer. Acta Psychiatr Scand Suppl 320:85–92, 1985.

86. Syrjala KL, Cummings C, Donaldson GW. Hypnosis or cognitive behavioral training for the reduction of pain and nausea during cancer treatment: a controlled clinical trial (see comments). Pain 48(2):137–46, 1992.

87. Sellick SM, Crooks DL. Depression and cancer: an appraisal of the literature for prevalence, detection, and practice guideline development for psychological interventions. Psychooncology 8(4):315–33, 1999.

88. Greer S, Moorey S, Baruch JD, et al. Adjuvant psychological therapy for patients with cancer: a prospective randomised trial (see comments). BMJ 304(6828):675–80, 1992.

89. Edgar L, Rosberger Z, Nowlis D. Coping with cancer during the first year after diagnosis. Assessment and intervention. Cancer 69(3):817–28, 1992.

90. McArdle JM, George WD, McArdle CS, et al. Psychological support for patients undergoing breast cancer surgery: a randomised study (see comments). BMJ 312(7034):813–6, 1996.

91. Linn MW, Linn BS, Harris R. Effects of counseling for late stage cancer patients. Cancer 49(5):1048–55, 1982.

92. Cain EN, Kohorn EI, Quinlan DM, et al. Psychosocial benefits of a cancer support group. Cancer 57(1):183–9, 1986.

93. Spiegel D. Cancer and depression. Br J Psychiatry Suppl 30:109–16, 1996.

94. de Vries MJ, Schilder JN, Mulder CL, et al. Phase II study of psychotherapeutic intervention in advanced cancer. Psychooncology 6(2):129–37, 1997.

95. Moorey S, Greer S, Watson M, et al. Adjuvant psychological therapy for patients with cancer: outcomes at one year. Psychooncology 3:39–46, 1993.

96. Bridge LR, Benson P, Pietroni PC, Priest RG. Relaxation and imagery in the treatment of breast cancer. BMJ 297(6657):1169–72, 1988.

97. Fawzy FI, Fawzy NW, Arndt LA, Pasnau RO. Critical review of psychosocial interventions in cancer care. Arch Gen Psychiatry 52(2):100–13, 1995.

98. Meyer TJ, Mark MM. Effects of psychosocial interventions with adult cancer patients: a meta-analysis of randomized experiments (see comments). Health Psychol 14(2):101–8, 1995.

99. Preskorn SH, Burke M. Somatic therapy for major depressive disorder: selection of an antidepressant (see comments). J Clin Psychiatry 53(Suppl):5–18, 1992.

100. Lloyd-Williams M, Friedman T, Rudd N. A survey of antidepressant prescribing in the terminally ill. Palliat Med 13(3):243–8, 1999.

101. Evans DL, McCartney CF, Haggerty JJ Jr, et al. Treatment of depression in cancer patients is associated with better life adaptation: a pilot study. Psychosom Med 50(1):73–6, 1988.

102. Carroll B. Alprazolam, promising in treatment of depression in cancer patients. Psychiatric Times (May):46, 47, 1990.

103. Holland JC, Romano SJ, Heiligenstein JH, et al. A controlled trial of fluoxetine and desipramine in depressed women with advanced cancer. Psychooncology 7(4):291–300, 1998.

104. Lansky SB, List MA, Herrmann CA, et al. Absence of major depressive disorder in female cancer patients. J Clin Oncol 3(11):1553–60, 1985.

105. Mendels J. Clinical experience with serotonin reuptake inhibiting antidepressants. J Clin Psychiatry 48(Suppl):26–30, 1987.

106. Glassman AH. The newer antidepressant drugs and their cardiovascular effects. Psychopharmacol Bull 20(2):272–9, 1984.

107. Ciraulo DA, Shader RI. Fluoxetine drug-drug interactions. I. Antidepressants and antipsychotics. J Clin Psychopharmacol 10(1):48–50, 1990.

108. Preskorn SH. Recent pharmacologic advances in antidepressant therapy for the elderly. Am J Med 94(5A):2S–12S, 1993.

109. Pick CG, Paul D, Eison MS, Pasternak GW. Potentiation of opioid analgesia by the antidepressant nefazodone. Eur J Pharmacol 211(3):375–81, 1992.

110. Rudorfer MV, Potter WZ. Antidepressants. A comparative review of the clinical pharmacology and therapeutic use of the "newer" versus the "older" drugs. Drugs 37(5):713–38, 1989.

111. Scher M, Krieger JN, Juergens S. Trazodone and priapism. Am J Psychiatry 140(10):1362–3, 1983.

112. Shopsin B. Bupropion: a new clinical profile in the psychobiology of depression. J Clin Psychiatry 44(5 Pt 2):140–2, 1983.

113. Davis JM, Glassman AH. Antidepressant drugs. In: Kaplan HI, Sadock BJ, eds. Comprehensive textbook of psychiatry. Baltimore: Williams and Wilkins, 1989.

114. Lloyd AH. Practical considerations in the use of maprotiline (Ludiomil) in general practice. J Int Med Res 5(Suppl 4):122–38, 1977.

115. Breitbart W, Mermelstein H. Pemoline. An alternative psychostimulant for the management of depressive disorders in cancer patients. Psychosomatics 33(3):352–6, 1992.

116. Bruera E, Carraro S, Roca E, et al. Double-blind evaluation of the effects of mazindol on pain, depression, anxiety, appetite, and activity in terminal cancer patients. Cancer Treat Rep 70(2):295–8, 1986.

117. Fernandez F, Adams F, Holmes VF, et al. Methylphenidate for depressive disorders in cancer patients. An alternative to standard antidepressants. Psychosomatics 28(9):455–61, 1987.

118. Olin J, Masand P. Psychostimulants for depression in hospitalized cancer patients. Psychosomatics 37(1):57–62, 1996.

119. Kaufmann MW, Murray GB, Cassem NH. Use of psychostimulants in medically ill depressed patients. Psychosomatics 23(8):817–9, 1982.

120. Katon W, Raskind M. Treatment of depression in the medically ill elderly with methylphenidate. Am J Psychiatry 137(8):963–5, 1980.

121. Fisch RZ. Methylphenidate for medical in-patients. Int J Psychiatry Med 15(1):75–9, 1985.

122. Chiarello RJ, Cole JO. The use of psychostimulants in general psychiatry. A reconsideration. Arch Gen Psychiatry 44(3):286–95, 1987.

123. Burns MM, Eisendrath SJ. Dextroamphetamine treatment for depression in terminally ill patients. Psychosomatics 35(1):80–3, 1994.

124. Satel SL, Nelson JC. Stimulants in the treatment of depression: a critical overview. J Clin Psychiatry 50(7):241–9, 1989.

125. Woods SW, Tesar GE, Murray GB, Cassem NH. Psychostimulant treatment of depressive disorders secondary to medical illness. J Clin Psychiatry 47(1):12–5, 1986.

126. Bruera E, Chadwick S, Brenneis C, et al. Methylphenidate associated with narcotics for the treatment of cancer pain. Cancer Treat Rep 71(1):67–70, 1987.

127. Bruera E, Brenneis C, Paterson AH, MacDonald RN. Use of methylphenidate as an adjuvant to narcotic analgesics in patients with advanced cancer. J Pain Symptom Manage 4(1):3–6, 1989.

128. Bruera E, Fainsinger R, MacEachern T, Hanson J. The use of methylphenidate in patients with incident cancer pain receiving regular opiates. A preliminary report. Pain 50(1):75–7, 1992.

129. Forrest WH Jr, Brown BW Jr, Brown CR, et al. Dextroamphetamine with morphine for the treatment of postoperative pain. N Engl J Med 296(13):712–5, 1977.

130. Fernandez F, Adams F, Levy JK, et al. Cognitive impairment due to AIDS-related complex and its response to psychostimulants. Psychosomatics 29(1):38–46, 1988.

131. Nehra A, Mullick F, Ishak KG, Zimmerman HJ. Pemoline-associated hepatic injury. Gastroenterology 99(5):1517–9, 1990.

132. Breitbart WS. Psychiatric complications of cancer. In: Brain MC, ed. Current therapy in hematology oncology, vol 3. Toronto and Philadelphia: BC Decker Inc., 1988:268–74.

133. Lascelles RG. Atypical facial pain and depression. Br J Psychiatry 112(488):651–9, 1966.

134. Anthony M, Lance JW. Monoamine oxidase inhibition in the treatment of migraine. Arch Neurol 21(3):263–8, 1969.

135. Greenberg DB, Younger J, Kaufman SD. Management of lithium in patients with cancer. Psychosomatics 34(5):388–94, 1993.

136. Stein RS, Flexner JH, Graber SE. Lithium and granulocytopenia during induction therapy of acute myelogenous leukemia: update of an ongoing trial. Adv Exp Med Biol 127:187–97, 1980.

137. Coda BA, Mackie A, Hill HF. Influence of alprazolam on opioid analgesia and side effects during steady-state morphine infusions. Pain 50(3):309–16, 1992.

138. Caccia MR. Clonazepam in facial neuralgia and cluster headache. Clinical and electrophysiological study. Eur Neurol 13(6):560–3, 1975.

139. Swerdlow M, Cundill JG. Anticonvulsant drugs used in the treatment of lancinating pain. A comparison. Anaesthesia 36(12):1129–32, 1981.

140. Egan KJ, Ready LB, Nessly M, Greer BE. Self-administration of midazolam for postoperative anxiety: a double blinded study. Pain 49(1):3–8, 1992.

141. Rumore MM, Schlichting DA. Clinical efficacy of antihistaminics as analgesics. Pain 25(1):7–22, 1986.

22 Neuropathic pain

CHRISTOPHER J. WATLING AND DWIGHT E. MOULIN
University of Western Ontario

Introduction

Neuropathic pain occurs frequently in patients with cancer, both from direct tumor infiltration of neural structures and as a consequence of treatment of the neoplasm. Management of neuropathic pain presents a number of challenges. Such pain is often more resistant to conventional analgesic approaches than is nociceptive pain. Many of these patients will have mixed pain problems, where neuropathic pain is combined with elements of somatic or visceral nociceptive pain. Neuropathic pain also may signal progressive and often incurable disease, adding a significant suffering component to the pain problem.

Successful management of neuropathic cancer pain requires an understanding of the pathophysiologic processes that generate this type of pain and of the distinctive clinical features that identify it. In addition, a knowledge of the various clinical neuropathic pain syndromes that occur in the cancer patient and of the range of available treatments is essential.

Pathophysiology

Neuropathic pain occurs as a result of aberrant somatosensory processing in the nervous system, and as such may be sustained by peripheral mechanisms, central mechanisms, or both. Pain after peripheral nerve injury may occur through a variety of mechanisms. When a nerve is compressed or distended, nerve trunk pain may occur as a result of activation of the nervi nervorum, the normal nociceptive afferents that innervate the nerve sheaths themselves (1). Damage to primary nociceptive afferents may result in spontaneous ectopic activity, perhaps secondary to focal demyelination with exposure of sodium channels (2). Regenerating afferents may form neuromas, where sodium channels accumulate and spontaneous

activity occurs (3). The dorsal root ganglion may represent an additional site of ectopic activity (3). Damaged peripheral receptors may also become sensitized to circulating catecholamines. In cases of sympathetically maintained pain, there may be aberrant sympathetic-sensory coupling, such that efferent activity in sympathetic nerves provides ongoing activation of injured and sensitized sensory afferents (3).

Often, however, neuropathic pain fails to respond to procedures that interrupt sensory transmission pathways at the level of the primary sensory afferent or the dorsal horn (2), suggesting that central generators may also be involved. Peripheral nerve injury can evoke numerous changes in the central nervous system, which contribute to persisting pain. Central neurons may become sensitized and fire spontaneously or in response to low-threshold or non-noxious stimuli. Sensitization of second-order spinal cord neurons may explain the presence of pain outside the distribution of the injured nerve (4). A "wind-up" phenomenon may be observed whereby repetitive C-fiber input leads to an increased central response to subsequent C-fiber stimuli; this phenomenon results in part from the action of excitatory amino acids on N-methyl-D-aspartate (NMDA) receptors (5).

The multitude of potential mechanisms for neuropathic pain may explain interindividual variations in response to treatment. Even for a given individual, more than one mechanism may be at work. Also, as injury in one part of the nervous system can trigger dysfunction at other levels of the nervous system, the mechanism of pain generation for any one individual may change over time, further complicating attempts at management (6).

Clinical features of neuropathic pain

Neuropathic pain generally has distinctive characteristics that differentiate it from nociceptive pain and can be elicited by a thorough pain history. Individuals typically describe constant, dysesthetic pain, which is burning, throbbing, or pressure-like. Very often, paroxysmal pain, described as stabbing or electrical in quality, is superimposed on the underlying constant pain. These paroxysmal pains may occur spontaneously or may be provoked by movement or tactile stimulation. Patients may also report allodynia, which refers to pain provoked by a normally non-painful stimulus (7). Allodynia may occur with normally innocuous light touch, warm or cool stimuli; a characteristic complaint is that the touch of clothing or bed sheets against the affected part is exquisitely painful (6). Often, patients will have difficulty describing neuropathic pain, as its sensations are unfamiliar and beyond the realm of pain that has previously been experienced.

A careful neurologic examination is essential in cancer patients with suspected neuropathic pain. Often, examination will reveal motor or sensory deficits that allow accurate localization of the lesion responsible for the pain syndrome. For example, the combination of intrinsic hand muscle weakness and sensory loss along the medial arm and forearm suggests a Pancoast's syndrome resulting from invasion of the lower brachial plexus by an apical lung tumor. The finding of a band of sensory loss in a cancer patient with neuropathic chest and trunk pain points to involvement of a thoracic nerve root or an intercostal nerve.

The physical signs specific to neuropathic pain may involve raised thresholds for sensory stimuli, exaggerated responses to various sensory stimuli, or combinations of these phenomena. Hyperalgesia, characterized by a painful sensation of abnormal severity in response to a noxious stimulus such as a pinprick (7), may be observed, sometimes in areas where the individual paradoxically describes numbness. Repeated mechanical stimulation may produce pain of explosive onset and unusual severity, or pain that radiates outside the territory of the injured nerve (6), reflecting temporal and spatial summation of the stimulus. Some individuals also experience after-sensations, where sensation persists even after a stimulus is removed. Recognition of these characteristic clinical features facilitates the identification of pain as neuropathic, which has significant treatment implications.

Specific neuropathic pain syndromes in the cancer patient

Several neuropathic cancer pain syndromes have been described (Table 22.1). Neuropathic pain may be the result of direct tumor involvement or may occur as a

Table 22.1. *Neuropathic pain syndromes in patients with cancer*

Pain syndromes resulting from direct tumor involvement
Epidural spinal cord compression
Leptomeningeal metastases
Malignant brachial plexopathy
Malignant lumbosacral plexopathy
Cranial neuralgias
Intercostal neuralgia
Paraneoplastic syndromes
Paraneoplastic peripheral neuropathy
Pain syndromes resulting from cancer surgery
Postmastectomy pain
Postthoracotomy pain
Postradical neck dissection pain
Postamputation phantom and/or stump pain
Pain syndromes resulting from radiation therapy
Radiation plexopathy
Radiation myelopathy
Radiation-induced peripheral nerve tumors
Pain syndromes resulting from chemotherapy
Painful peripheral neuropathy
Herpes zoster and postherpetic neuralgia

result of cancer treatment, including surgery, radiation treatment, and chemotherapy. Some of the more common neuropathic pain syndromes are described next.

Pain syndromes caused by direct tumor involvement

Epidural spinal cord compression
Spinal cord compression is a relatively common complication of cancer. The vertebral bodies are the most common sites of bone metastases, and cord compression most often results from direct tumor spread from an involved vertebral body into the epidural space. As such, all patients with vertebral metastases are at risk for epidural spinal cord compression (8).

Epidural spinal cord compression is heralded by pain in more than 90% of cases (9). Pain may be localized at the site of bone involvement or may be radicular as a result of nerve root compression. Pain may be accompanied by symptoms and signs of neurologic compromise, including motor, sensory, and autonomic dysfunction, and these features may progress rapidly.

Treatment of epidural spinal cord compression generally consists of immediate administration of corticosteroids followed promptly by radiotherapy. Steroids dramatically relieve the pain of epidural cord compression, in most patients (8), and may result in transient improvements in neurologic function. Radiotherapy may preserve or improve neurologic function by inducing tumor shrinkage, and will effectively relieve pain in many patients. In some cases, surgical decompression may be the preferred method of treatment. Possible indications for choosing surgery over radiation as initial therapy include lack of diagnosis, spinal instability, and tumors that are relatively radioresistant (10). Early recognition of this potentially devastating syndrome is critical, as neurologic outcome is primarily determined by the degree of pretreatment impairment (11). A high level of clinical suspicion, therefore, is required when evaluating a cancer patient with back or radicular pain.

Leptomeningeal metastases

Leptomeningeal carcinomatosis occurs in approximately 5% of patients with cancer, with cancers of the breast and lung and melanomas representing the most common primary sites (12). Pain is a frequent presenting symptom, and may manifest as headache, neck or back pain, or radicular pain (13,14). Neurologic manifestations of leptomeningeal metastases are protean, however, and diagnosis requires a high level of clinical suspicion. The presence of symptoms and signs representing involvement of multiple levels within the neuraxis may be an important diagnostic clue (12). Treatment may involve focal radiation to symptomatic areas and intrathecal chemotherapy, although outcomes are often disappointing in spite of aggressive therapy (15).

Malignant plexopathy

The brachial plexus may be invaded by tumor in cases of apical lung neoplasms (Pancoast's syndrome) or from axillary lymph node involvement in breast cancer or lymphoma (16). Pain is generally the primary symptom of neoplastic brachial plexus involvement, and usually begins as a deep, aching pain in the shoulder with radiation to the medial arm and hand (9). Neurologic symptoms and signs reflect involvement of the C8 and T1 nerve roots and may include paresthesias and sensory loss in the medial hand and arm and intrinsic hand muscle weakness. Extension of tumor into the epidural space may occur, placing the individual at risk for spinal cord compression. Epidural extension may be heralded by rapidly increasing pain, signs of diffuse plexus involvement, or the development of a Horner syndrome. As pain generally precedes the development of other neurologic symptoms and signs, however, a high index of suspicion is required for early diagnosis (17). Routine chest radiographs may reveal evidence of an apical lung mass, but diagnosis often requires computed tomography (CT) or magnetic resonance imaging (MRI) scanning through the

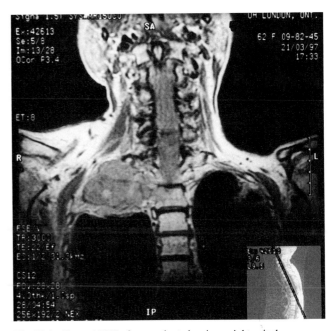

Fig. 22.1. Coronal MRI of upper chest showing a right apical (Pancoast) tumor invading the lower brachial plexus.

brachial plexus (Fig. 22.1). Radiation therapy provides pain relief in about half of the cases, but generally does not result in improved neurologic function (18). Pain from neoplastic brachial plexopathy often proves difficult to manage and may become disabling if not treated aggressively (9).

Malignant lumbosacral plexopathy most often results from direct extension of abdominal or pelvic neoplasms, although it may also occur secondary to lymph node metastases from extraabdominal tumors. The most common primary tumors are colorectal tumors, sarcomas, genitourinary and breast tumors, and lymphomas (19). As with brachial plexopathy, pain is the most common presenting symptom and may precede other neurologic symptoms and signs by weeks to months (19). Pain, typically dull and aching, is located in the low back or buttock region and may radiate into the leg. The neurologic examination may initially be normal, but with time characteristic signs develop that include weakness and sensory loss in the distribution of more than one nerve root along with reflex asymmetry. CT or MRI of the abdomen and pelvis will usually demonstrate the extent of tumor (Fig. 22.2). MRI of the spine should also be considered in selected patients, as epidural extension of tumor may occur (19). Again, the response to radiation treatment may be disappointing, and an aggressive pain management strategy may be required.

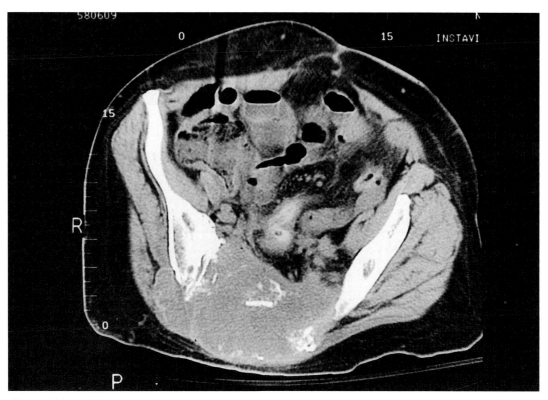

Fig. 22.2. A CT scan of the pelvis showing a large metastatic tumor mass involving the right hemipelvis with destruction of the sacrum. The patient presented with a lumbosacral plexopathy.

Pain syndromes related to cancer treatment

Postmastectomy pain syndrome

Postmastectomy pain syndrome may occur after any surgical procedure on the breast, including lumpectomy, mastectomy, and axillary node dissection (20). Pain affects 4%–20% of women after such procedures (21), and occurs because of injury to the intercostobrachial nerve, a cutaneous branch of T1–T2. Affected individuals typically describe aching or burning pain in the axilla, medial upper arm, and/or anterior chest wall, often with superimposed shock-like pains and allodynia. Pain can begin immediately after surgery, or after a pain-free interval, and may persist for years. Unlike postthoracotomy pain, the postmastectomy pain syndrome is rarely an indicator of recurrent tumor (20).

Postthoracotomy pain

After thoracotomy, some individuals experience persistent neuropathic pain at the site of the incision secondary to surgical injury to the intercostal nerves (8). In many patients, however, the appearance of postthoracotomy pain is more ominous, signaling tumor recurrence. Kanner et al. (22) described three patterns of pain after thoracotomy. In the first group, immediate postoperative pain diminished within 2 months of surgery, then recurred at some later point. This pattern was always associated with recurrent tumor. In the second group, postoperative pain was persistent and gradually increased over time; again, tumor recurrence was found in most cases. In the third group, postoperative pain was stable or decreased over time; tumor recurrence was unlikely. Patients presenting with postthoracotomy pain therefore require careful evaluation for recurrent tumor, preferably with a CT scan of the chest (23).

Postradical neck dissection syndrome

A neuropathic pain syndrome may occur after radical neck dissection secondary to damage to the superficial cervical plexus. Patients may report continuous burning dysesthesias, lancinating pain, and/or allodynia in the anterolateral neck, shoulder, jaw, and ear (24). Many of these patients may also have a myofascial component to their pain (24). Patients developing pain after radical neck dissection require careful evaluation to exclude recurrent tumor (20).

Phantom limb and stump pain

After limb amputation, patients commonly experience both painful and non-painful phantom sensations.

Phantom breast pain has also been described after mastectomy (25). Phantom pain after limb amputation may follow a characteristic "spike" pattern, with an initial increase in pain intensity after surgery followed by a gradual decline (26). Late appearance of severe phantom pain may signal tumor recurrence and requires thorough evaluation (27). Persisting stump pain after limb amputation may be a result of neuroma formation at the surgical site or other local factors including poor wound healing, poor prosthesis fit, or tumor recurrence (26).

Postradiation pain syndromes

Brachial plexopathy may appear months to years after radiation to the plexus and is more likely when the radiation dose exceeds 6000 cGy. In contrast to malignant plexopathy, radiation plexopathy is less often painful, and the pain that does occur is rarely severe; however, distinguishing radiation plexopathy from recurrent tumor may be difficult. The early assertion that radiation-induced brachial plexopathy preferentially involves the upper trunk of the brachial plexus (16) has not been supported by further studies (28–30). Both neoplastic and radiation-induced brachial plexopathy tend to manifest as lower trunk or diffuse involvement of the brachial plexus. Therefore, the distribution of upper extremity weakness and sensory loss cannot reliably differentiate neoplastic from radiation-induced brachial plexopathy. The presence of myokymia on electromyography argues in favor of radiation plexopathy, whereas more severe pain, a Horner's syndrome, and the presence of a discrete mass on CT or MRI point to tumor recurrence.

Less commonly, radiation plexopathy may affect the lumbosacral plexus. Again, the risk is greatest with higher radiation doses, but rare examples of plexopathy at relatively low radiation doses are described (31). Radiation plexopathy most often presents with indolent weakness of one or both legs. Pain is uncommon at onset, but ultimately affects up to 50% of individuals with radiation-induced lumbosacral plexopathy, although rarely to the degree that is seen with malignant plexus invasion (31).

Radiation myelopathy is an uncommon, dose-dependent complication of radiation therapy. Pain is uncommon, but may include focal spine pain, radicular pain, or burning dysesthesias below the level of the lesion (32). This syndrome must be differentiated from epidural spinal cord compression and leptomeningeal metastases.

Pain syndromes resulting from chemotherapy

Several chemotherapeutic agents may produce a painful peripheral neuropathy, generally associated with distal sensory loss and weakness. Offending agents include vincristine and other vinca alkaloids, cis-platinum, VP-16, procarbazine, paclitaxel, and suramin (32). Symptoms usually resolve partially or completely when the drug is discontinued, but on occasion neuropathic pain may persist.

Herpes zoster infection and postherpetic neuralgia

Herpes zoster is much more common in patients who are immunocompromised by malignancy or its treatment. Pain, itching, or paresthesias in the involved dermatome may precede the appearance of the typical vesicular rash by up to several days. Although pain typically diminishes after the rash resolves, neuropathic pain may persist in some patients. Postherpetic neuralgia consists of constant burning pain in the involved dermatome, often with superimposed lancinating pains and allodynia. This pain is often severe and debilitating and may persist for years (33). Postherpetic neuralgia is more frequent with increasing age and may occur more frequently in the cancer population (34).

Antiviral agents such as acyclovir, famcyclovir, and valacyclovir may reduce the duration of the rash and alleviate pain during the acute illness (35). The effect of these interventions on the subsequent development of postherpetic neuralgia remains uncertain, although recent meta-analyses have suggested that initial treatment with acyclovir may reduce the incidence of residual pain at 6 months (36,37), whereas famcyclovir and valacyclovir may reduce the duration but not the incidence of postherpetic neuralgia (38).

Management of neuropathic cancer pain

Successful management of neuropathic cancer pain begins with a thorough evaluation of the pain complaint to establish an accurate diagnosis. It is particularly important to identify those pain-producing lesions that may respond to antineoplastic treatment so that such treatment may be initiated in a timely manner. For example, urgent decompressive surgery or radiation may protect neurologic function and relieve pain in epidural spinal cord compression, and focal radiotherapy may also be effective in radicular pain from leptomeningeal metastases. In one study, a comprehensive evaluation by a neurology-based cancer pain service resulted in the identification of new pathology in 64% of cases, whereas 18% of patients were referred for further antineoplastic therapy to treat their pain (39).

Pharmacologic approaches

Pharmacologic treatment represents the mainstay of neuropathic cancer pain management. Numerous medica-

Table 22.2. *Pharmacological agents for the treatment of neuropathic pain*

Antidepressants
    Tricyclics (amitriptyline, nortriptyline, desipramine,
        imipramine)
    SSRIs (paroxetine, citalopram)
    Others (venlafaxine)
Anticonvulsants
    Carbamazepine
    Phenytoin
    Gabapentin
    Lamotrigine
Local anesthetics
    Lidocaine
    Mexiletine
Topical agents
    Capsaicin
    EMLA cream
    Topical lidocaine
Opioids
    Morphine
    Hydromorphone
    Oxycodone
    Fentanyl
    Methadone
    Tramadol
NMDA antagonists
    Ketamine

Abbreviation: SSRIs, selective serotonin reuptake inhibitors.

tions have shown efficacy in the management of neuropathic pain (Table 22.2). Many of these drugs are considered adjuvant analgesics; that is, the drugs were designed for indications other than pain but can be analgesic in certain circumstances. Few of these drugs have been specifically evaluated in cancer patients with neuropathic pain. Their potential usefulness is often extrapolated from studies in patients with chronic nonmalignant neuropathic pain.

Antidepressants
The tricyclic antidepressants are well established for the treatment of neuropathic pain (40). Randomized controlled trials have established the analgesic efficacy of various tricyclic antidepressants in both painful diabetic neuropathy (41–44) and postherpetic neuralgia (45,46). Tricyclic antidepressants may be effective both for sustained, burning pain and for lancinating pain (44). Although the analgesic effect of the tricyclic antidepressants does not appear to be mediated by mood elevation (44–46), some cancer patients undoubtedly also benefit from the ameliorating effects of these drugs on depression, sleep, and appetite.

The selective serotonin reuptake inhibitors, although generally better tolerated than the tricyclic antidepressants, have proved disappointing in the management of neuropathic pain. Although small, randomized, controlled trials have shown modest efficacy for paroxetine and citalopram in the treatment of painful diabetic neuropathy (47,48), another study showed no analgesic efficacy for fluoxetine (43). Venlafaxine is a novel antidepressant that, like the tricyclics, inhibits the neuronal reuptake of both serotonin and norepinephrine, but that has a more favorable side-effect profile. Experimental and anecdotal evidence suggests that venlafaxine may prove useful as an analgesic (49,50), but evidence from randomized controlled trials is lacking. The role of these newer antidepressants in managing neuropathic pain remains poorly defined, and the older tricyclic antidepressants should still be considered first-line therapy.

Anticonvulsants
Several of the anticonvulsant drugs have demonstrated efficacy in the management of neuropathic pain. Carbamazepine has shown benefit in the treatment of painful diabetic neuropathy and trigeminal neuralgia (51,52). Phenytoin, whose mechanism of action is similar to that of carbamazepine, demonstrated efficacy in diabetic neuropathy pain (53). These drugs may be particularly useful in the management of paroxysmal, lancinating pain, although burning, dysesthetic pain may also respond. Clonazepam and valproic acid have also been advocated for the management of neuropathic pain, but evidence supporting their efficacy is lacking (54–56).

Gabapentin is a newer anticonvulsant that has been shown to be effective in the treatment of postherpetic neuralgia and painful diabetic neuropathy in recent randomized placebo-controlled trials (57,58). A randomized double-blind study showed the efficacy of gabapentin to be comparable but not superior to amitriptyline for painful diabetic neuropathy (59). A recent unblinded evaluation of gabapentin in neuropathic cancer pain supports its potential usefulness in this patient population (60).

Lamotrigine is a novel anticonvulsant drug whose mechanism of action involves both blockage of voltage-sensitive sodium channels and inhibition of glutamate and aspartate release. Several case series suggest that this drug may be effective in managing neuropathic pain of both central and peripheral origin (61–63). Lamotrigine was effective in treating painful diabetic neuropathy in an open trial (64) and also was analgesic in small randomized controlled trials in refractory trigeminal neuralgia

(65) and HIV-associated painful neuropathy (66). A larger randomized controlled trial of lamotrigine for neuropathic pain of various etiologies, however, failed to demonstrate an analgesic effect (67). Nonetheless, lamotrigine may represent a useful addition to the list of pharmacologic options for neuropathic pain.

Systemically administered local anesthetics

Lidocaine and mexiletine are local anesthetic drugs that block sodium channels and can suppress ectopic neural activity at concentrations that do not block nerve conduction (68). Intravenous lidocaine was shown to be effective in a small randomized study of patients with painful diabetic neuropathy (69). Another small randomized study of patients with chronic neuropathic pain of various etiologies also showed a benefit from intravenous lidocaine and suggested that response to lidocaine was predictive of subsequent response to oral mexiletine (70). Lidocaine was superior to placebo, but inferior to morphine, in a study of postherpetic neuralgia (71). Two randomized, double-blind studies of intravenous lidocaine for neuropathic pain in cancer patients, however, showed no benefit (72,73).

Oral mexiletine was superior to placebo in small, randomized, double-blind studies of pain resulting from peripheral nerve damage of mixed origin (74) and diabetic neuropathy (75). In one study of central neuropathic pain secondary to spinal cord injury, however, mexiletine was ineffective (76). The use of mexiletine may be limited by its potential cardiotoxic and gastrointestinal side effects. Another oral local anesthetic, tocainide, was found to be effective in a small study of trigeminal neuralgia (77), but with its potential for causing even more serious toxicity than mexiletine, its use cannot be recommended.

A recent review concludes that the evidence for the effectiveness of oral mexiletine in neuropathic pain is not compelling, and that cancer pain in particular has not been convincingly shown to respond to systemically administered local anesthetics (78). Still, there may be a subgroup of patients with refractory neuropathic cancer pain for whom this approach may be of benefit.

Topical agents

Capsaicin desensitizes small unmyelinated nociceptors by depleting substance P. Results of randomized trials of repeated applications of topical capsaicin for painful peripheral neuropathy have been mixed; one study showed a very modest benefit in painful diabetic neuropathy (79), but another showed no benefit in painful polyneuropathy of mixed origin (80). The use of topical local anesthetics is perhaps more promising. Topical lidocaine has been shown to produce significant pain relief without clinically significant serum levels in patients with postherpetic neuralgia (81,82), and open studies have indicated similar efficacy for EMLA (eutectic mixture of local anesthetics) cream in postherpetic neuralgia (83,84). The absence of systemic side effects when local anesthetics are administered topically may be a significant advantage in many patients.

NMDA antagonists

Repetitive C-fiber input results in an increased response to further C-fiber stimuli. This central sensitization, termed "wind up," may account for the hyperalgesia and allodynia so characteristic of neuropathic pain and is mediated by NMDA receptors (5). NMDA-receptor antagonists therefore may be of use in the management of neuropathic pain.

One such agent is ketamine. Intravenous ketamine was shown to provide superior analgesia to placebo in studies of chronic posttraumatic neuropathic pain (85) and of an experimental pain model using intradermal capsaicin (86). Successful treatment of neuropathic pain has also been reported with ketamine administered orally (87) or by continuous subcutaneous infusion (88). Unfortunately, ketamine produces a high incidence of severe, psychomimetic side effects, although these may be limited by concurrent use of haloperidol or midazolam (87,88).

Dextromethorphan is a potent NMDA antagonist with a long safety record as an antitussive, making it an attractive candidate as an analgesic. Controlled studies of low-dose dextromethorphan in cancer pain (5) and nonmalignant neuropathic pain (89) showed no benefit, however. High-dose dextromethorphan was shown to be analgesic in diabetic neuropathy but not in postherpetic neuralgia (90).

Although ketamine and dextromethorphan have been the most widely studied of the NMDA antagonists, a number of other agents are also being investigated. For example, a recent open trial of single dose intravenous magnesium sulfate in cancer-related neuropathic pain suggested that a useful analgesic effect may be obtained in some individuals (91); magnesium is known to block the NMDA receptor. A small case series suggested a dramatic benefit from amantadine in patients with chronic neuropathic pain and postulated that the benefit of amantadine was mediated through its inhibition of the NMDA receptor (92). This class of drugs certainly merits further study, although it cannot yet be recommended for routine use in neuropathic cancer pain.

Opioids

The analgesic efficacy of opioids in neuropathic pain remains a subject of controversy. Arner and Meyerson (93) found that infusions of morphine were ineffective in relieving neuropathic pain, although these results may be confounded by selection bias, small sample size, and lack of individual drug titration (94). Subsequently, however, evidence has accumulated to suggest that opioids may indeed be effective in neuropathic pain. Randomized controlled trials in postherpetic neuralgia have demonstrated analgesic benefit from morphine (71) and oxycodone (95). Intravenous fentanyl was shown to provide superior analgesia to both diazepam (active placebo) and saline (inert placebo) in a randomized study of patients with non-malignant neuropathic pain (96), and a subsequent open prospective study of transdermal fentanyl showed that a minority of patients achieved sustained pain relief (97). A retrospective analysis of individually titrated opioid infusions in patients with neuropathic pain indicated that reasonable pain relief could be achieved, but that the opioid dose-response curve was shifted to the right in many patients with neuropathic pain (98). Taken together, these data suggest that although neuropathic pain may be less opioid responsive than nociceptive pain, effective pain relief may be achieved in some individuals when the principle of titrating the dose to analgesia or side effects is followed. The potential for intolerable opioid side effects may be higher in patients with neuropathic pain because of the relatively higher opioid doses required to achieve adequate analgesia.

Recently, there has been renewed interest in the use of methadone in pain management. Methadone has high affinity for both mu and delta opioid receptors, but also acts as an NMDA receptor antagonist, suggesting that it may be of particular value in the management of neuropathic pain (99). Randomized studies are lacking, but a number of reports suggest promising results with methadone in neuropathic pain (100–102). Use of methadone is complicated, however, by large interindividual variations in its pharmacokinetics (99).

Another opioid of particular interest is tramadol, which may produce additional analgesic effects through its inhibition of serotonin and norepinephrine reuptake (103). A randomized study of individuals with painful peripheral neuropathy showed that tramadol relieved both spontaneous pain and allodynia more effectively than placebo (104).

Anesthetic techniques

Peripheral nerve blocks may be beneficial in patients with segmental pain involving the thorax or abdomen, where interruption of involved motor or sensory fibers can be achieved without producing significant disability. An individual with somatic and neuropathic pain from a rib metastasis, for example, can be treated first with a local anesthetic block to localize the lesion, followed by a neurolytic block using phenol, alcohol, or cryoanalgesia.

For patients with advanced disease who have severe intractable pain or unacceptable side effects from systemic opioid administration, continuous epidural or intrathecal infusion of morphine and/or bupivicaine maybe beneficial. Both agents provide selective analgesia at the spinal level. Morphine acts directly on opioid receptors in the spinal cord and bupivicaine provides conduction block along nerve roots. A combined infusion of morphine and bupivicaine can provide excellent pain relief allowing for a marked reduction in systemic opioid dose and therefore fewer opioid-related side effects (105). That an epidural or intrathecal catheter can be implanted in the home is another major advantage of this technique (106).

For pain in advanced cancer involving several spinal segments, injection of a neurolytic agent into the subarachnoid space may be another option. Subarachnoid neurolysis is best suited for patients with advanced, terminal disease where loss of bladder function is no longer an issue. Phenol 5% in glycerin is the preferred neurolytic agent; it has both local anesthetic and neurolytic properties and is painless to inject (107). Subarachnoid phenol effectively produces a chemical dorsal rhizotomy. The results of subarachnoid phenol neurolysis for malignant neuropathic pain are difficult to interpret, as most reported patients are being treated for somatic as well as neuropathic pain. Good pain relief, however, has been reported in about 50% of patients undergoing phenol neurolysis, with complication rates in the range of 1%–14% (108). Bowel and bladder dysfunction and lower extremity weakness are the main potential complications. In patients where this treatment modality fails to provide pain relief, there may be a central pain generator that has become independent of the peripheral nerve lesion.

Neurosurgical approaches

Neuroablative procedures provide pain relief by modifying pain pathways and may be of use in selected individuals whose pain is refractory to pharmacotherapy. In general, however, nociceptive pain responds more reliably than neuropathic pain to such procedures. Many individuals with neuropathic cancer pain will have abnormalities in central somatosensory processing, sometimes extending to thalamic and cortical levels, rendering ineffective procedures such as neurectomy, cordotomy, and rhizotomy (109).

Cordotomy is the most widely used of the neuroablative procedures. The procedure, which may be performed percutaneously at the cervical level, interrupts the ascending lateral spinothalamic tract. It is most useful in the management of intractable, unilateral lower extremity pain, although relief of upper extremity pain may also be achievable (110). In a recent series, unilateral percutaneous cordotomy provided pain relief in more than 85% of patients, and 50% of patients with bilateral or midline pain experienced relief after bilateral cordotomies. Complications included urinary retention, hemiparesis, and the development of mirror-image pain (111). The risk of serious adverse effects, such as bladder and sexual dysfunction and respiratory compromise, is significantly increased with bilateral cordotomies (112). Nociceptive pain is said to be more reliably responsive to cordotomy than is neuropathic or deafferentation pain (112), although interpretation of study results is difficult, as most have not specified the mechanism of pain in their reported cases.

Conclusion

Cancer and its treatment may injure the nervous system in many ways, triggering a variety of pathological processes at both peripheral and central levels. As such, neuropathic cancer pain is a heterogeneous disorder, requiring individualized assessment and management.

Effective management of neuropathic cancer pain begins with an accurate pain diagnosis and an understanding of the physical, psychosocial, and emotional factors affecting the pain experience. Identifying those neuropathic pain syndromes that may respond to primary antineoplastic therapy is important. Many individuals with neuropathic cancer pain, however, have advanced disease and are not candidates for further antineoplastic therapy, whereas others have pain syndromes that either fail to respond to antineoplastic treatment or are actually caused by such treatment. Individualized analgesic pharmacotherapy is therefore the cornerstone of neuropathic pain management. Numerous agents may be effective, but successful treatment often entails a frustrating trial and error process. The individual differences in responsivity to treatment may reflect the variety of different pathophysiological processes at play. Fortunately, the therapeutic armamentarium is expanding, as newer anticonvulsants such as gabapentin and lamotrigine join

well-established adjuvant analgesics such as tricyclic antidepressants and carbamazepine, and as increasing evidence supports the use of opioids in neuropathic pain. Future developments may see a better defined role for newer agents such as the NMDA antagonists, and for older agents with previously unrecognized potential, such as methadone.

In spite of these many treatment options, however, managing neuropathic cancer pain remains a difficult challenge. Current treatments often provide incomplete relief, sometimes at the expense of side effects that have a significant negative impact on quality of life. Improvements in the future will depend on research that improves our understanding of the mechanisms behind this complex problem, and of the means by which these pain-generating processes can be modified.

References

1. Asbury AK, Fields HL. Pain due to peripheral nerve damage: an hypothesis. Neurology 34:1587–90, 1984.
2. Elliott KJ. Taxonomy and mechanisms of neuropathic pain. Semin Neurol 14(3):195–205, 1994.
3. Devor M. The pathophysiology of damaged peripheral nerves. In: Wall PD, Melzack R, eds. Textbook of pain. Edinburgh: Churchill Livingstone, 1994:79–100.
4. Bennett GJ, Xie YK. A peripheral mononeuropathy in rat. Pain 33:87–108, 1988.
5. Mercadante S, Casuccio A, Genovese G. Ineffectiveness of dextromethorphan in cancer pain. J Pain Symptom Manage 16(5):317–22, 1998.
6. Bennett GJ. Neuropathic pain. In: Wall PD, Melzack R, eds. Textbook of pain. Edinburgh: Churchill Livingstone, 1994:201–24.
7. Mersky H, ed. Classification of chronic pain: description of chronic pain syndromes and definition of pain terms. Pain (Suppl) 3:S1, 1986.
8. Kelly JB, Payne R. Pain syndromes in the cancer patient. Neurol Clin 9(4):937–53, 1991.
9. Posner JB. Neurologic complications of cancer. Philadelphia: FA Davis Company, 1995:111–42.
10. Bates T. A review of local radiotherapy in the treatment of bone metastases and cord compression. Int J Radiat Oncol Biol Phys 23:217–21, 1992.
11. Faul CM, Flickinger JC. The use of radiation in the management of spinal metastases. J Neurooncol 23:149–61, 1995.
12. Grossman SA, Krabak MJ. Leptomeningeal carcinomatosis. Cancer Treat Rev 25:103–19, 1999.
13. Wolfgang G, Marcus D, Ulrike S. LC: clinical syndrome in different primaries. J Neurooncol 38:103–10, 1998.
14. Little JR, Dale AJD, Okazaki H, et al. Meningeal carcinomatosis–clinical manifestations. Arch Neurol 30:138–43, 1974.

15. Grant R, Naylor B, Greenberg HS, et al. Clinical outcome in aggressively treated meningeal carcinomatosis. Arch Neurol 51:457–61, 1994.

16. Kori SH, Foley KM, Posner JB. Brachial plexus lesions in patients with cancer: 100 cases. Neurology 31:45–50, 1981.

17. Patt RB. Classification of cancer pain and cancer pain syndromes. In: Patt RB, ed. Cancer pain. Philadelphia: Lippincott-Raven, 1993:13.

18. Ampil FL. Radiotherapy for carcinomatous brachial plexopathy: a clinical study of 23 cases. Cancer 56:2185–8, 1985.

19. Jaeckle KA, Young DF, Foley KM. The natural history of lumbosacral plexopathy in cancer. Neurology 35:8–15, 1985.

20. Portenoy RK. Cancer pain—epidemiology and syndromes. Cancer 63:2298–307, 1989.

21. Stevens PE, Dibble SL, Miaskowski C. Prevalence, characteristics, and impact of postmastectomy pain syndrome: an investigation of women's experiences. Pain 61:61–8, 1995.

22. Kanner R, Martini N, Foley KM. Nature and incidence of post-thoracotomy pain. Proc Am Soc Clin Oncol 1:152, 1982.

23. Foley KM. Pain syndromes in patients with cancer. In: Portenoy RK, Kanner RM, eds. Pain management—theory and practice. Philadelphia: FA Davis, 1996:207.

24. Sist T, Miner M, Lema M. Characteristics of postradical neck pain syndrome: a report of 25 cases. J Pain Symptom Manage 18(2):95–102, 1999.

25. Kroner K, Krebs B, Skov J, et al. Immediate and long-term phantom breast pain syndrome after mastectomy: incidence, clinical characteristics, relationship to premastectomy breast pain. Pain 36:327–35, 1989.

26. Weinstein SM. Phantom limb pain and related disorders. Neurol Clin 16(4):919–35, 1998.

27. Sugarbaker PH, Weiss CM, Davidson DD, et al. Increasing phantom limb pain as a symptom of cancer recurrence. Cancer 54:373–5, 1984.

28. Lederman RJ, Wilbourne AJ. Brachial plexopathy: recurrent cancer or radiation? Neurology 34:1331–35, 1984.

29. Harper CM, Thomas JE, Cascino TL, et al. Distinction between neoplastic and radiation-induced brachial plexopathy, with emphasis on the role of EMG. Neurology 39:502–6, 1989.

30. Thyagarajan D, Cascino T, Harms G. Magnetic resonance imaging in brachial plexopathy of cancer. Neurology 45:421–7, 1995.

31. Thomas JE, Cascino TL, Earle JD. Differential diagnosis between radiation and tumor plexopathy of the pelvis. Neurology 35:1–7, 1985.

32. Hammack JE. Neurologic pain syndromes in cancer patients. In: Samuels MA, Feske S, eds. Office practice of neurology. New York: Churchill Livingstone, 1996:934–44.

33. Kost RG, Straus SE. Postherpetic neuralgia–pathogenesis, treatment, and prevention. N Engl J Med 335(1):32–42, 1996.

34. Rusthoven JJ, Ahlgren P, Elhakim T, et al. Risk factors for varicella zoster disseminated infection among adult cancer patients with localized zoster. Cancer 62:1641–6, 1988.

35. Wood MJ. Current experience with antiviral therapy for acute herpes zoster. Ann Neurol 35:S65–S68, 1994.

36. Jackson JL, Gibbons R, Meyer G, et al. The effect of treating herpes zoster with oral acyclovir in preventing postherpetic neuralgia. A meta-analysis. Arch Intern Med 157(8):909–12, 1997.

37. Wood MJ, Kay R, Dworkin RH, et al. Oral acyclovir therapy accelerates pain resolution in patients with herpes zoster: a meta-analysis of placebo-controlled trials. Clin Infect Dis 22(2):341–7, 1996.

38. Alper BS, Lewis PR. Does treatment of acute herpes zoster prevent or shorten postherpetic neuralgia? J Fam Pract 49(3):255–64, 2000.

39. Gonzales GR, Elliott KJ, Portenoy RK, Foley KM. The impact of a comprehensive evaluation in the management of cancer pain. Pain 47:141–4, 1991.

40. Watson CPN, Watt-Watson JH. Treatment of neuropathic pain: focus on antidepressants, opioids, and gabapentin. Pain Res Manage 4(4):168–78, 1999.

41. Kvinesdal B, Molin J, Froland A, Gram LF. Imipramine treatment of painful diabetic neuropathy. JAMA 251(13):1727–30, 1984.

42. Gomez-Perez FJ, Rull JA, Dies H, et al. Nortiptyline and fluphenazine in the symptomatic treatment of diabetic neuropathy. A double-blind cross-over study. Pain 23:395–400, 1985.

43. Max MB, Lynch SA, Muir J, et al. Effects of desipramine, amitriptyline, and fluoxetine on pain in diabetic neuropathy. N Engl J Med 326:1250–6, 1992.

44. Max MB, Culnane M, Schafer SC, et al. Amitriptyline relieves diabetic neuropathy pain in patients with normal or depressed mood. Neurology 37:589–96, 1987.

45. Watson CP, Evans RJ, Reed K, et al. Amitriptyline versus placebo in postherpetic neuralgia. Neurology 32:671–3, 1982.

46. Kishore-Kumar R, Max MB, Schafer SC, et al. Desipramine relieves postherpetic neuralgia. Clin Pharmacol Ther 47:305–12, 1990.

47. Sindrup SH, Gram LF, Brosen K, et al. The selective serotonin reuptake inhibitor paroxetine is effective in the treatment of diabetic neuropathy symptoms. Pain 42:135–44, 1990.

48. Sindrup SH, Bjerre U, Dejgaard A, et al. The selective serotonin reuptake inhibitor citalopram relieves the symptoms of diabetic neuropathy. Clin Pharmacol Ther 52:547–52, 1992.

49. Lang E, Hord AH, Denson D. Venlafaxine hydrochloride (Effexor™) relieves thermal hyperalgesia in rats with an experimental mononeuropathy. Pain 68:151–5, 1996.

50. Taylor K, Rowbotham MC. Venlafaxine hydrochloride and chronic pain. West J Med 165:147–8, 1996.

51. Rull J, Quibrera R, Gonzalez-Millan H, et al. Symptomatic treatment of peripheral diabetic neuropathy with carbamazepine: double-blind crossover study. Diabetologia 5:215–20, 1969.

52. Campbell FG, Graham JG, Zilkha KJ. Clinical trial of carbamazepine (Tegretol) in trigeminal neuralgia. J Neurol Neurosurg Psychiatry 29:265–7, 1966.

53. Chadda VS, Mathur MS. Double blind study of the effects of diphenylhydantoin sodium on diabetic neuropathy. J Assoc Physicians India 26:403–6, 1978.

54. Drewes AM, Andreasen A, Poulsen LH. Valproate for treatment of chronic central pain after spinal cord injury. A double-blind cross-over study. Paraplegia 32(8):565–9, 1994.

55. Wiffen P, McQuay H, Carroll D, et al. Anticonvulsant drugs for acute and chronic pain. Cochrane Database Syst Rev 2:CD001133, 2000.

56. Reddy S, Patt RB. The benzodiazepines as adjuvant analgesics. J Pain Symptom Manage 9(8):510–4, 1994.

57. Rowbotham M, Harden N, Stacey B, et al. Gabapentin for the treatment of postherpetic neuralgia. A randomized controlled trial. JAMA 280(21):1837–42, 1998.

58. Backonja M, Beydoun A, Edwards K, et al. Gabapentin for the symptomatic treatment of painful neuropathy in patients with diabetes mellitus. JAMA 280(21):1831–6, 1998.

59. Morello CM, Leckband SG, Stoner CP, et al. Randomized double-blind study comparing the efficacy of gabapentin with amitriptyline on diabetic peripheral neuropathy pain. Arch Intern Med 159:1931–7, 1999.

60. Caraceni A, Zecca E, Martini C, et al. Gabapentin as an adjuvant to opioid analgesia for neuropathic cancer pain. J Pain Symptom Manage 17(6):441–5, 1999.

61. Canavero S, Bonicalzi V. Lamotrigine control of central pain. Pain 68:179–81, 1996.

62. Carrieri PB, Bonuso S, Bruno R, et al. Efficacy of lamotrigine on sensory symptoms and pain in peripheral neuropathies. J Pain Symptom Manage 18(3):154–6, 1999.

63. Devulder J, De Laat M. Lamotrigine in the treatment of chronic refractory neuropathic pain. J Pain Symptom Manage 19(5):398–403, 2000.

64. Eisenberg E, Alon N, Ishay A, et al. Lamotrigine in the treatment of painful diabetic neuropathy. Eur J Neurol 5:167–73, 1998.

65. Zakrzewska JM, Chaudry Z, Nurmikko TJ, et al. Lamotrigine (Lamictal) in refractory trigeminal neuralgia: results from a double-blind placebo controlled crossover trial. Pain 73:223–30, 1997.

66. Simpson DM, Olney R, McArthur JC, et al. A placebo-controlled trial of lamotrigine for painful HIV-associated neuropathy. Neurology 54:2115–19, 2000.

67. McCleane G. 200 mg daily of lamotrigine has no analgesic effect in neuropathic pain: a randomised, double-blind, placebo controlled trial. Pain 83:105–7, 1999.

68. Devor M, Wall PD, Catalan N. Systemic lidocaine silences ectopic neuroma and DRG discharge without blocking nerve conduction. Pain 48(2):261–8, 1992.

69. Kastrup J, Petersen P, Dejgard A, et al. Intravenous lidocaine infusion–a new treatment of chronic painful diabetic neuropathy? Pain 28:69–75, 1987.

70. Galer BS, Harle J, Rowbotham MC. Response to intravenous lidocaine infusion predicts subsequent response to oral mexiletine: a prospective study. J Pain Symptom Manage 12(3):161–7, 1996.

71. Rowbotham MC, Reisner-Keller LA, Fields HL. Both intravenous lidocaine and morphine reduce the pain of postherpetic neuralgia. Neurology 41:1024–8, 1991.

72. Bruera E, Ripamonti C, Brenneis C, et al. A randomized double-blind crossover trial of intravenous lidocaine in the treatment of neuropathic cancer pain. J Pain Symptom Manage 7(3):138–40, 1992.

73. Ellemann K, Sjogren P, Banning A-M, et al. Trial of intravenous lidocaine on painful neuropathy in cancer patients. Clin J Pain 5:291–4, 1989.

74. Chabal C, Jacobson L, Mariano A, et al. The use of oral mexiletine for the treatment of pain after peripheral nerve injury. Anesthesiology 77:513–17, 1992.

75. Dejgard A, Petersen P, Kastrup J. Mexiletine for treatment of chronic painful diabetic neuropathy. Lancet 1:9–11, 1988.

76. Chiou-Tan FY, Tuel SM, Johnson JC, et al. Effect of mexiletine on spinal cord injury dysesthetic pain. Am J Phys Med Rehabil 75:84–7, 1996.

77. Lindstrom P, Lindblom U. The analgesic effect of tocainide in trigeminal neuralgia. Pain 28:45–50, 1987.

78. Kalso E, Tramer MR, McQuay HJ, et al. Systemic local anaesthetic-type drugs in chronic pain: a systematic review. Eur J Pain 2:3–14, 1998.

79. The Capsaicin Study Group. Treatment of painful diabetic neuropathy with topical capsaicin. A multicenter, double-blind, vehicle-controlled study. Arch Intern Med 151:2225–9, 1991.

80. Low PA, Opfer-Gehrking TL, Dyck PJ, et al. Double-blind, placebo-controlled study of the application of capsaicin cream in chronic distal painful polyneuropathy. Pain 62:163–8, 1995.

81. Rowbotham MC, Davies PS, Verkempinck C, et al. Lidocaine patch: double-blind controlled study of a new treatment method for post-herpetic neuralgia. Pain 65:39–44, 1996.

82. Galer BS, Rowbotham MC, Perander J, et al. Topical lidocaine patch relieves postherpetic neuralgia more effectively than a vehicle topical patch: results of an enriched enrollment study. Pain 80:533–8, 1999.

83. Stow PJ, Glynn CJ, Minor B. EMLA cream in the treatment of post-herpetic neuralgia. Efficacy and pharmacokinetic profile. Pain 39:301–5, 1989.

84. Attal N, Brasseur L, Chauvin M, et al. Effects of single and repeated applications of a eutectic mixture of local anaesthetics (EMLA) cream on spontaneous and evoked pain in post-herpetic neuralgia. Pain 81:203–9, 1999.

85. Max MB, Byas-Smith MG, Gracely RH, et al. Intravenous infusion of the NMDA antagonist, ketamine, in chronic post-traumatic pain with allodynia: a double-blind comparison to alfentanil and placebo. Clin Neuropharmacol 18:360–8, 1995.

86. Park KM, Max MB, Robinovitz E, et al. Effects of intravenous ketamine, alfentanil, or placebo on pain, pinprick hyperalgesia, and allodynia produced by intradermal capsaicin in human subjects. Pain 63:163–72, 1995.

87. Fisher K, Hagen NA. Analgesic effect of oral ketamine in chronic neuropathic pain of spinal origin: a case report. J Pain Symptom Manage 18(1):61–6, 1999.

88. Mercadante S. Ketamine in cancer pain: an update. Palliat Med 10:225–30, 1996.

89. McQuay HJ, Carroll D, Jadad AR, et al. Dextromethorphan for the treatment of neuropathic pain: a double-blind randomised controlled crossover trial with integral n-of-1 design. Pain 59:127–33, 1994.

90. Nelson KA, Park KM, Robinovitz E, et al. High-dose dextromethorphan versus placebo in painful diabetic neuropathy and postherpetic neuralgia. Neurology 48:1212–18, 1997.

91. Crosby V, Wilcock A, Corcoran R. The safety and efficacy of a single dose (500 mg or 1 g) of intravenous magnesium sulfate in neuropathic pain poorly responsive to strong opioid analgesics in patients with cancer. J Pain Symptom Manage 19(1):35–9, 2000.

92. Eisenberg E, Pud D. Can patients with chronic neuropathic pain be cured by acute administration of the NMDA receptor antagonist amantadine? Pain 74:337–9, 1998.

93. Arner S, Meyerson BA. Lack of analgesic effect of opioids on neuropathic and idiopathic forms of pain. Pain 33:11–23, 1988.

94. Dellemijn P. Are opioids effective in relieving neuropathic pain? Pain 80:453–62, 1999.

95. Watson CPN, Babul N. Efficacy of oxycodone in neuropathic pain: a randomized trial in postherpetic neuralgia. Neurology 50(6):1837–41, 1998.

96. Dellemijn PLI, Vanneste JAL. Randomised double-blind active-placebo-controlled crossover trial of intravenous fentanyl in neuropathic pain. Lancet 349:753–8, 1997.

97. Dellemijn PLI, van Duijn H, Vanneste JAL. Prolonged treatment with transdermal fentanyl in neuropathic pain. J Pain Symptom Manage 16(4):220–9, 1998.

98. Portenoy RK, Foley KM, Inturrisi CE. The nature of opioid responsiveness and its implications for neuropathic pain: new hypotheses derived from studies of opioid infusions. Pain 43:273–86, 1990.

99. Bruera E, Neumann CM. Role of methadone in the management of pain in cancer patients. Oncology 13(9):275–82, 1999.

100. Makin MK, Ellershaw JE. Methadone can be used to manage neuropathic pain related to cancer. BMJ 317:81, 1998.

101. Vigano A, Fan D, Bruera E. Individualized use of methadone and opioid rotation in the comprehensive management of cancer pain associated with poor prognostic indicators. Pain 67:115–19, 1996.

102. Gagnon B, Bruera E. Differences in the ratios of morphine to methadone in patients with neuropathic pain versus non-neuropathic pain. J Pain Symptom Manage 18(2):120–25, 1999.

103. Raffa RB, Friderichs E, Reimann W, et al. Opioid and non-opioid components independently contribute to the mechanism of action of tramadol, an atypical opioid analgesic. J Pharmacol Exp Ther 260:275–85, 1992.

104. Sindrup SH, Andersen G, Madsen C, et al. Tramadol relieves pain and allodynia in polyneuropathy: a randomised, double-blind, controlled trial. Pain 83:85–90, 1999.

105. van Dongen RT, Crul BJ, van Egmond J. Intrathecal coadministration of bupivacaine diminishes morphine dose progression during long-term intrathecal infusion in cancer patients. Clin J Pain 15(3):166–72, 1999.

106. Mercadante S. Intrathecal morphine and bupivacaine in advanced cancer pain patients implanted at home. J Pain Symptom Manage 9(3):201–7, 1994.

107. Cousins MJ. Chronic pain and neurolytic neural blockade. In: Cousins MJ, Bridenbaugh PO, eds. Neural blockade in clinical anesthesia and management of pain, 2nd ed. Philadelphia: JB Lippincott, 1988:1053–84.

108. Swerdlow M. Subarachnoid and extradural neurolytic blocks. In: Bonica JJ, Ventafridda V, eds. Advances in pain research and therapy vol. 2. New York: Raven Press, 1979:325–37.

109. Moulin DE. Neuropathic cancer pain: syndromes and clinical controversies. In: Bruera E, Portenoy RK, eds. Topics in palliative care. vol. 2. New York: Oxford University Press, 1998:7–29.

110. Ischia S, Ischia A, Luzani A, et al. Results up to death in the treatment of persistent cervico-thoracic (Pancoast) and thoracic malignant pain by unilateral percutaneous cervical cordotomy. Pain 21:339–55, 1985.

111. Sanders M, Zuurmond W. Safety of unilateral and bilateral percutaneous cervical cordotomy in 80 terminally ill cancer patients. J Clin Oncol 13:1509–2, 1995.

112. Sundaresan N, DiGiacinto GV, Hughes JEO. Neurosurgery in the treatment of cancer pain. Cancer 63:2365–77, 1989.

23 Breakthrough pain

PERRY G. FINE
University of Utah School of Medicine

Introduction

During the 1970s and 1980s, when it became increasingly clear that intense pain had long been an underrecognized and poorly treated manifestation of cancer, it became apparent that cancer patients commonly experience intermittent exacerbations of severe pain against a background of continuous, or baseline, pain (1,2). On the heels of the World Health Organization analgesic ladder approach to general pain control, this recognition led to treatment guidelines and patient care manuals recommending management of these episodic pains as routine practice (3–9).

The term *breakthrough pain* (BTP) can be found in the pain management literature starting about a decade ago (10–14). An operational definition was offered at that time by Portenoy and Hagen (15), who suggested that "breakthrough pain … refers generally to a transitory exacerbation of pain that occurs on a background of otherwise stable pain in a patient receiving chronic opioid therapy." This definition seems to have gained widespread acceptance, with only minimal (published) debate as to its overall accuracy or utility (16).

Evidence that BTP, at the very least, has become recognized as an important aspect of overall cancer care can be found on two fronts. First, a growing number of review articles and practice recommendation guidelines on this subject have been published in recent years. They affirm the view that BTP needs to be evaluated and treated as part of the overall cancer pain management plan (17–29). In addition, reports of analgesic clinical trials for the management of cancer pain have begun to routinely incorporate a treatment arm for BTP in the methodology (30–37).

Incidence and prevalence of breakthrough pain

There are few studies that give comprehensive epidemiological details of BTP in various populations of patients

with cancer. The first published prospective evaluation of BTP was carried out at Memorial Sloan-Kettering Cancer Center (15). In this survey, 63% of patients with otherwise well-controlled baseline pain experienced BTP. Demographically, patients of both genders, representing all age groups and a heterogeneous representation of tumor types, using a wide dose range of opioid analgesic use characterized this study group. Descriptive analysis of BTPs in this report disclosed that 33% were of somatic etiology, 20% were visceral in nature, 27% were neuropathic, and 20% were mixed. A follow-up study in the same institution a decade later, structured to further delineate the characteristics and impact of BTP on inpatients with cancer, found that 51.2% of the 164 patients who met study criteria experienced BTP during the preceding day (31).

The prevalence of BTP in patients with far-advanced disease appears to be somewhat higher than that reported in earlier stages of disease. In a relatively small study of home-based hospice patients (with a life expectancy that was found to be less than 30 days, on average), 86% of patients who had well-controlled baseline pain experienced BTP on a regular and recurring basis; 75% of the patients in this group had metastatic cancer (38). A more recent study of hospice patients, almost all with cancer diagnoses, revealed a similar prevalence rate (89%) of BTP, corroborating the conclusion that BTP is common in patients with far-advanced disease (39).

Another perspective on the epidemiology of BTP is the commonplace lack of recognition, evaluation, and treatment of this type of pain. Several studies have reported figures that specifically address BTP and give insight into the prevalence of this problem of non-identification and poor treatment. An evaluation of pharmacological management of cancer pain in rural Minnesota determined that about three fourths of the surveyed patients taking analgesics for pain were using an opioid analgesic (40). Only one in five patients who were using around-the-clock medications for continuous analgesia were using medications specifically for BTP. This 20% utilization rate of BTP medications suggests undertreatment based on previously cited prevalence data. It is suggested that these discrepancies represent gaps in information and education, both on the part of the public and the medical profession.

Another record review of practice patterns evaluated pain management documentation in a cancer outpatient treatment facility (41). The authors point out that pain severity ratings and opioid doses were either not documented in two thirds of cases, or when documented, occurred in less than 25% of a given patient's visits in half of those cases. Medication use for BTP was never mentioned in just over 70% of cases, and only one out of four physicians documented pain severity in more than 15% of visits. Opioid dose was recorded more than 30% of the time by only 25% of physicians. The authors concluded that these deficiencies are responsible for negative quality of life outcomes in overall cancer treatment. Zeppetella et al. (39) found that at the time of hospice admission, of 218 patients with BTP, only 64% had strong opioid analgesics available to them for pain control, and of these, less than half had access to rescue doses for BTP.

Finally, a performance-based testing program was instituted to evaluate the skills of house staff (resident physicians) in assessing and managing cancer pain (42). Opioid analgesics were prescribed by almost all resident physicians (98%); however, only 18% of these physicians-in-training prescribed for regular use, and the majority (88%) did not prescribe for BTP. Results of this study suggest that training and mentoring in contemporary approaches to cancer pain management strategies are inadequate. This finding illuminates a major reason behind the prevalence of poorly controlled BTP pain in community settings.

Characteristics of breakthrough pain

The same studies that evaluated prevalence of BTP have also provided insight into the incidence and other characteristics of BTP in cancer patients at various stages of disease. The first prospective evaluation from the Memorial Sloan-Kettering Cancer Center led to the identification of three different types of BTP: incident pain (related to an activity, action, or event), spontaneous pain (no evident precipitating event), and end-of-dose failure (reduction in analgesic blood levels of around-the-clock medication resulting in a "breaking through" baseline pain) (15). This differentiating terminology seems to have broad application, as it has been adopted by most subsequent authors in their descriptions of BTP and in daily clinical practice. The importance of this nomenclature is that recognition and identification of subsets of BTP lead to different treatment strategies.

Incident pain is generally predictable, and so pretreatment in anticipation of an inciting event can prevent serious pain from developing. End-of-dose failure can be recognized by patients or their caregivers keeping diaries, associating time of pain to time of last dose or regularly scheduled medication. Once this pattern is recognized, either an increase in the around-the-clock analgesic dose can ensue, or the interval between regularly scheduled doses can be shortened. The choice depends on factors such as convenience and side effects, most notably excessive sedation. Spontaneous pains are more challenging. Often times these are neuropathic or visceral in origin, such as gastrointestinal or urinary bladder cramps, which are highly unpredictable, excruciating, disabling, and evanescent. As a result, they are very difficult to treat at the time of occurrence other than by implementing prophylactic measures through disease-modifying therapies or use of pain-modulating and -attenuating drugs. These medications include anticholinergics, muscle relaxants, antiepileptics, local anesthetics, and various classes of antidepressants (43).

The time from BTP onset to maximal pain and the duration of BTPs are quite variable. Almost half of all BTP episodes in one inpatient cancer pain study were of very rapid onset, with the duration varying from seconds to hours (15). Similar to these data, patients in a home hospice setting were found to have an average of three episodes of BTP each day, with a mean pain intensity of 7 on a 10-point scale, compared to baseline pain scores averaging 3 out of 10 (38). In this population, BTPs lasted an average of 52 minutes, and the range of time to relief, either spontaneously or after commencing a variety of pharmacological or non-pharmacological interventions, was 5 to 60 minutes. Another survey of cancer patients found a high correlation between the occurrence of breakthrough pain and the presence of pain-related functional impairment, depressed mood, and anxiety (31). An important finding from this study is that BTP is an independent contributor to impaired functioning and psychological distress, signaling the need to actively prevent and treat its occurrence.

Management of breakthrough pain

The few studies that have evaluated the means by which patients manage to control BTPs suggest that use of a so-called rescue dose of an opioid analgesic is the most common method (15,38). Other methods that patients commonly apply in an effort to relieve BTP, either alone or while awaiting the onset of pharmacologically induced relief when it is available, are changing position, applying heat or cold, squeezing or massaging the painful area, ingesting an antacid, and applying cognitive/behavioral skills such as imaging or relaxation. The efficacy of these maneuvers for the relief of BTP is not well studied, but it appears that they are only of modest benefit.

Patients who have intravenous access devices and patient-controlled analgesia pumps can immediately respond to acute exacerbations of pain by self-administration of an intravenous dose of opioid analgesic. Similar approaches have been used with neuraxial drug delivery systems. However, it is impractical to apply these interventional approaches in the vast majority of patients with cancer who experience BTP. Therefore, the mainstay of pharmacological therapy has been immediate release, relatively short-acting orally administered opioid analgesics, such as oxycodone, morphine, and hydrocodone. Because enteral absorption is not always an option, sublingual morphine administration has become an increasingly common approach to BTP treatment (44). Based on a critical review of available literature, there is doubt as to whether this route offers any particular pharmacokinetic advantage to the oral route in terms of speed of onset or peak effects (45).

During this last decade, newfound understanding of the prevalence, severity, and consequences of inadequate approaches to the management of BTP have led to intensely focused pharmacologic research in this area. Spurred by a case report of a patient with excruciating and debilitating breakthrough pain resulting from an apical lung tumor whose symptoms were finally brought under control with oral transmucosal fentanyl citrate (OTFC) (14), this novel approach to noninvasive, rapid onset, short-duration potent opioid analgesia has subsequently undergone extensive evaluation (46).

In an open label study of cancer patients experiencing episodes of BTP on a daily basis, it was found that OTFC provided onset of meaningful pain relief within 10 minutes, with concomitant improvements in sense of well-being and perceived activity level (47). Pharmacokinetic studies soon revealed the pharmacologically important differences in transmucosal uptake of OTFC, as differentiated from the much slower and lower blood levels achieved by gastrointestinal absorption of fentanyl. Because some of the dissolving fentanyl lozenge

becomes mixed with saliva and are swallowed, subjecting the drug to both gastric degradation and first-pass hepatic metabolism, the overall bioavailability of OTFC is 50% (48).

The efficacy and safety of OTFC for the treatment of BTP in cancer have been borne out in several controlled clinical trials. A randomized, double-blind, placebo-controlled trial (RCT) of OTFC in 89 opioid-tolerant patients resulted in significant improvements in pain intensity compared with placebo (49). In another RCT, 62 adult cancer patients received either 200 µg or 400 µg OTFC with the option to increase the dose until adequate pain relief was obtained. The effective dose was then used for 2 subsequent days. The majority of patients found a dose of OTFC that more effectively and rapidly relieved BTP than previously used opioid formulations (50). A multicenter open-label study evaluated the long-term safety of OTFC for cancer BTP in a total of 155 patients (51). A total of 41,766 units of OTFC were used (dose range 200–1600 µg) over the evaluation period that lasted more than a year. There were no reported serious adverse events or safety concerns, and about 92% of BTP episodes were successfully treated.

Of interest, the effective dose of OTFC does not directly correlate with patients' baseline opioid analgesic doses (52). Rapid tissue absorption with a steep plasma uptake concentration curve and mirrored central nervous system exposure, owing to the lipophilic nature of fentanyl, may account for this observation. In spite of this rapid flux phenomenon, tolerance to the therapeutic effects of OTFC does not appear to be consequential. Long-term use of OTFC has been reported to be continually effective and preferred by cancer patients who had experiences with other options for BTP control (51,53).

The clinical trials with OTFC represent the only group of well-controlled studies ever performed to evaluate treatment outcomes of BTP. The U.S. Food and Drug Administration approved OTFC (Actiq™) for the treatment of BTP in opioid-tolerant cancer patients in November, 1998. In the United States, it is available in doses of 200, 400, 600, 800, 1200, and 1600 µg. Each dose is individually sealed in child-resistant foil pouches that require scissors to open. The dose units are raspberry flavored and appear opaque white with "Rx" molded onto the handle. Several review articles have discussed the development, clinical trials outcomes, and indications for this novel analgesic (46,54,55).

The oral transmucosal route is the first and only well-studied, regulator body approved and proprietarily available approach to noninvasive rapid drug delivery for the management of BTP. Other methods are still in the experimental phase, with little published data to determine whether they hold promise. As of yet unpublished investigations have explored the use of intranasal fentanyl and ophthalmic drops of sufentanil for control of episodic pain. It remains to be determined whether the advent of noninvasive drug delivery for the treatment of BTP will meaningfully improve the quality of life of patients with advanced cancer.

References

1. Bonica JJ. Cancer pain. In: Bonica, JJ, ed. The management of pain, 2nd ed., vol. 1. Philadelphia: Lee and Febiger, 1990:400–14.

2. Bonica JJ. Treatment of cancer pain: current status and future needs. In: Fields HL, Dubner R, Cervero F, Jones LE, eds. Advances in pain research and therapy, vol. 9. New York: Raven Press, 1985:589–616.

3. World Health Organization. Cancer Pain relief. Geneva: World Health Organization, 1986.

4. Ventafridda V, Tamburini M, Caraceni A, et al. A validation study of the WHO methods for cancer pain relief. Cancer 59:850–6, 1987.

5. Jacox A, Carr DB, Payne R, et al. Management of cancer pain. Clinical Practice Guideline No. 9. AHCPR Publication No. 94-0592. Rockville, MD: Agency for Health Care Policy and Research, 1994.

6. American Pain Society. Principles of analgesic use in the treatment of acute pain and cancer pain, 4th ed. Glenview, IL: American Pain Society, 1999.

7. Storey P. Primer of palliative care. Gainesville, FL: Academy of Hospice Physicians, 1994.

8. Fine PG. The hospice companion: processes to optimize care during the last phase of life. Scottsdale, AZ: VistaCare, Inc., 1998.

9. Wrede-Seaman L. Symptom management algorithms: a handbook for palliative care, 2nd ed. Yakima, WA: Intellicard, 1999.

10. Portenoy RK, Hagan NA. Breakthrough pain: definition and management. Oncology 3(Suppl): 25–9, 1989.

11. Swanson G, Smith J, Bulich R, et al. Patient-controlled analgesia for chronic cancer pain in the ambulatory setting: a report of 117 patients. J Clin Oncol 7(12):1903–8, 1989.

12. Wagner JC, Souders GD, Coffman LK, et al. Management of chronic cancer pain using a computerized ambulatory patient-controlled analgesia pump. Hosp Pharm 24:639–44, 1989.

13. Portenoy RK, Maldonado M, Fitzmartin R, et al. Oral controlled-release morphine sulfate: analgesic efficacy and side effects of a 100 mg tablet in cancer pain patients. Cancer 63(11): 2284–8, 1989.

14. Ashburn MA, Fine PG, Stanley TH. Oral transmucosal fentanyl citrate for the treatment of breakthrough cancer pain: a case report. Anesthesiology 71(4): 615–7, 1989.

15. Portenoy RK, Hagen NA. Breakthrough pain: definition, prevalence and characteristics. Pain 41:273–81, 1990.

16. Mercadante S. What is the definition of breakthrough pain? Pain 45:107, 1991.

17. Payne R. Transdermal fentanyl: suggested recommendations for clinical use. J Pain Symptom Manage 7(3 Suppl.):40–4, 1992.

18. McQuay HJ, Jadad AR. Incident pain. Cancer Surv 21:17–24, 1994.

19. Hammack JE, Loprinzi CL. Use of orally administered opioids for cancer-related pain. Mayo Clin Proc 69:384–90, 1994.

20. Payne R. Factors influencing quality of life in cancer patients: the role of transdermal fentanyl in the management of pain. Semin Oncol 25(3 Suppl.):47–53, 1998.

21. Cleary JF, Coluzzi PH, Fine PG, et al. Cancer pain management: update on breakthrough pain. In: Portenoy RK, ed. Supplement to seminars in oncology, vol. 24, no. 5, suppl 16. Philadelphia: WB Saunders 1997:1–42.

22. McCaffery M, McKitrick LF. Planning for breakthrough pain. Am J Nurs 96(6):24, 1996.

23. Mercadante S, Arcuri E. Breakthrough pain in cancer patients: pathophysiology and treatment. Cancer Treat Rev 24:425–32, 1998.

24. Coluzzi PH. Cancer pain management: newer perspectives on opioids and episodic pain. Am J Hosp Palliat Care 15:13–22, 1998.

25. Patt RB, Ellison NM. Breakthough pain in cancer patients: characteristics, prevalence, and treatment. Oncology 12:1035–46, 1998.

26. Evans N, Palmer A. Controlling breakthrough pain in palliative care. Nursing Standard 13(7):53–4, 1998.

27. The Steering Committee on Clinical Practice Guidelines for the Care and Treatment of Breast Cancer. The management of chronic pain in patients with breast cancer. Can Med Assoc J 158(3 Suppl.):71–81, 1998.

28. Scholz M. An effective way to manage breakthrough pain. RN 62(5):102, 1999.

29. Levy MH. Pain control in patients with cancer. Oncology 13(5 Suppl):9–14, 1999.

30. Moulin DE, Kreeft JH, Murray-Parsons N, Bouquillan AI. Comparison of continuous and intravenous hyrdomorphone infusions for management of cancer pain. Lancet 337:465–8, 1991.

31. Portenoy RK, Payne D, Jacobsen P. Breakthrough pain: characteristics and impact in patients with cancer pain. Pain 81:129–34, 1999.

32. Deschamps M, Band PR, Hislop TG, et al. The evaluation of analgesic effects in cancer patients exemplified by a double-blind, crossover study of immediate-release versus controlled release morphine. J Pain Symptom Manage 7(7):384–92, 1992.

33. Walsh TD, MacDonald N, Bruera E, et al. A controlled study of sustained-release morphine sulfate tablets in chronic pain from advanced cancer. Am J Clin Oncol 15:268–72, 1992.

34. Arkinstall W, Sandler A, Goughnour B. Efficacy of controlled-release codeine in chronic non-malignant pain: a ran-

domized, placebo-controlled clinical trial. Pain 62:169–78, 1995.

35. Wong JO, Chiu GL, Tsao CJ, et al. Comparison of oral-controlled-release morphine with transdermal fentanyl in terminal cancer pain. Acta Anaesthesiol Sin 35:25–32, 1997.

36. Hagen N, Babul N. Comparative clinical efficacy and safety of a novel controlled-release oxycodone formulation and controlled-release hydromorphone in the treatment of cancer pain. Cancer 79:1428–37, 1997.

37. Rosenbluth RJ, Reder RF, Slagle NS, et al. Long-term administration of controlled-release oxycodone tablets for the treatment of cancer pain. Cancer Invest 16:562–71, 1998.

38. Fine PG, Busch MA. Characteristics of breakthrough pain by hospice patients and their caregivers. J Pain Symptom Manage 16(3):179–83, 1998.

39. Zeppetella G, O'Doherty CA, Collins S. Prevalence and characteristics of breakthrough pain in cancer patients admitted to hospice. J Pain Sympom Manage 20(2):87–92, 2000.

40. Lichtblau L, Belgrade M, Auld R, et al. Pharmacological management of cancer pain in rural Minnesota. J Pain Symptom Manage 12(5):283–9, 1996.

41. Weber M, Huber C. Documentation of severe pain, opioid doses and opioid-related side effects in outpatients with cancer: a retrospective study. J Pain Symptom Manage 17(1): 49–54, 1999.

42. Sloan PA, Donnelly MB, Schwartz, et al. Cancer pain assessment and management by housestaff. Pain 67:475–81, 1996.

43. Paice J, Fine PG. Pain at the end of life. In: Ferrell RB, Coyle N, eds. The textbook of palliative nursing. New York: Oxford University Press, 2001:76–90.

44. Robison JM, Wilkie DJ, Campbell B. Sublingual and oral morphine administration. Nurs Clin North Am 30:725–43, 1995.

45. Coluzzi PH. Sublingual morphine: efficacy reviewed. J Pain Symptom Manage 16:184–92, 1998.

46. Fine PG, Streisand J. A review of oral transmuscosal fentanyl citrate: potent, rapid and noninvasive opioid analgesia. J Palliat Med 1:55–64, 1998.

47. Fine PG, Marcus M, De Boer J, et al. An open label study of oral transmucosal fentanyl citrate (OTFC) for the treatment of breakthrough cancer pain. Pain 45:149–53, 1991.

48. Streisand JB, Varvel JR, Stanski DR, et al. Absorption and bioavailability of oral transmucosal fentanyl citrate. Anesthesiology 75:223–9, 1991.

49. Farrar JT, Cleary J, Rauck R, et al. Oral transmucosal fentanyl citrate: randomized, double-blinded, placebo-controlled trial for the treatment of breakthrough pain in cancer patients. J Natl Cancer Inst 90(8):611–6, 1998.

50. Christie J, Simmonds M, Patt R. Dose-titration, multicenter study of oral transmucosal fentanyl for persistent pain. J Clin Oncol 16(10):328–45, 1998.

51. Payne R, Coluzzi P, Hart L, et al. Long-term safety of oral transmucosal fentanyl citrate for breakthrough cancer pain. J Pain Symptom Manage 22(1):575–83, 2001.

52. Portenoy RK, Payne R, Coluzzi P, et al. Oral transmucosal fentanyl citrate (OTFC) for the treatment of breakthrough pain in cancer patients: a controlled dose titration study. Pain 79:303–12, 1999.

53. Patt RB: Long-term safety and efficacy of oral transmucosal fentanyl citrate (OTFC, Actiq™) for treatment of breakthrough cancer pain [abstract]. 23rd Annual Scientific Meeting, American Pain Society, 1997, New Orleans.

54. Rhiner M, Coluzzi PH. Managing breakthrough pain. New method expands treatment options. Adv Nurse Pract 6:41–3, 1998.

55. Pasero C, McCaffery M. Managing breakthrough pain with OTFC. Am J Nurs 99(4):20, 1999.

24 Bone pain

EDUARDO D. BRUERA AND CATHERINE SWEENEY
The University of Texas M. D. Anderson Cancer Center

Introduction

The skeleton is one of the most common sites of tumor metastases. Metastatic cancer invades bone in 60%–84% of cases (1). Up to 80% of all bone metastases are related to cancer of the breast, prostate, lung, thyroid, and kidney. Multiple myeloma is also commonly associated with skeletal disease. Approximately 70% of patients with bone metastases develop pain (2,3). In addition to pain, metastatic bone disease results in immobility, frequent hospital admissions, pathological fractures, metabolic complications such as hypercalcemia, neurological abnormalities, and bone marrow infiltration and suppression. These devastating symptoms can have a prolonged effect and also have major psychosocial implications. Detection of bone metastases may be the first indicator that cancer has not been cured; bone is the first site of recurrence in up to 40% of women with breast cancer. Patients suffering from bone metastases secondary to breast cancer survive an average of 34 months, with a range of 1 to 90 months (4).

This chapter primarily discusses pain associated with bone metastases. In addition, some of the recent developments in the prevention and management of osteolysis are addressed.

Pathophysiology of bone pain

The invasion of bone by tumor is well understood; however, the mechanisms of nociception are not well known. The three main mechanisms by which the skeleton is affected by cancer are primary bone cancer, direct invasion from adjacent primary tumors, and bone metastases. The last is by far the most common mechanism; primary tumors of bone are much less common. Figure 24.1 summarizes the four sequential steps in the development of a painful bone metastasis.

Arrest of the metastatic cell in the bone marrow

Primary tumors such as lung or breast will grow and invade adjacent normal tissues. As part of their growth, these tumors will penetrate to the blood and lymphatic vessels, and cells will be carried to different areas. Although the likelihood of a certain tumor invading bone as compared to other organs can be associated with the anatomical location of the tumor (for example, colon cancer drainage into the portal systems makes it more likely to metastasize into the liver), metastatic sites cannot be predicted from anatomic considerations alone. A number of animal and human tumor models show clear preference for metastases to one or two specific organs, which might be explained by organ tropism (5). Although tumor cells disseminate to all organs, they can adhere to the endothelial surface of the bone marrow in some patients, probably because of the presence of organ-specific endothelial determinants such as glycoproteins, or because of the presence of local growth factors, cytokines, or hormones present in the bone or bone marrow (5–8).

Extravasation and growth in the interstitium

Once the tumor cell has been arrested in the bone marrow, it proceeds to extravasate and grow in the interstitium before causing direct bone destruction. This local growth is conditioned by mechanical processes, local enzymes, growth factors and host response. Although the invasive behavior of cancer in soft tissues can largely be explained on a purely mechanical basis, this mechanical theory cannot explain the invasion or destruction of calcified tissue. Therefore in addition to the simple increased tumor size resulting from cell division, a number of products of malignant cells directly or indirectly cause resorption of bone, allowing tumor cells to grow into the

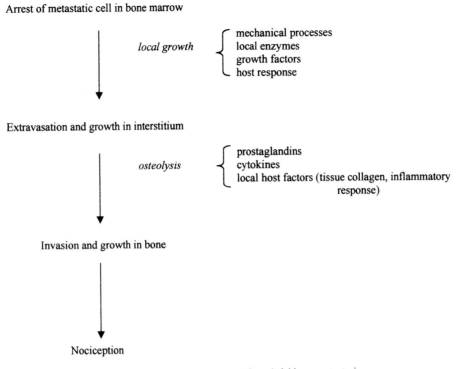

Arrest of metastatic cell in bone marrow

local growth { mechanical processes
local enzymes
growth factors
host response

Extravasation and growth in interstitium

osteolysis { prostaglandins
cytokines
local host factors (tissue collagen, inflammatory
response)

Invasion and growth in bone

Nociception

Fig. 24.1. Steps in the development of a painful bone metastasis.

reabsorbed space. Prostaglandins and cytokines, mainly in breast or renal cancer, probably play a major role in osteolysis. In some cases, specific factors capable of stimulating the osteoclast have been described. Finally, the local host environment affects the ability of tumor cells to invade. Tissues rich in collagen resist invasion because they act as a strong mechanical barrier. On the other hand, the inflammatory response of the host might aid tumor cell invasion by providing leukocytes with a large content of proteolytic enzymes, which can destroy host tissues (9).

Invasion and growth in the bone

Because the process of bone metastases almost always starts in the bone marrow, bones more frequently involved are those with a high proportion of red marrow such as the axial skeleton (10). Bone metastases are usually multiple at the time of diagnosis with the exception of renal carcinoma or neuroblastoma, in which up to 10% of patients may have a single site of bone involvement (5–8). Metastatic cancer growth in the bone results in a combination of bone destruction and bone formation. In patients with radiographic appearance of lytic skeletal metastases, bone destruction predominates, resulting in

the net loss of bone. In patients with blastic metastases, excessive amounts of bone formation develop with less bone destruction. Whereas lytic metastases tend to be highly cellular, sclerotic metastases are relatively acellular and contain large islands of intramembranous new bone formation in the fibrous stroma (for example, metastatic prostatic carcinoma). Although the initial process of bone destruction is mediated by osteoclasts, during the late stages of the metastatic process; the osteoclasts disappear, but osteolysis continues. This is probably due to tumor growth action (6). Osteosclerosis is mediated by osteoblasts, possibly stimulated by factors derived from the bone stroma.

Nociception

Although the mechanisms for the invasion and growth of metastatic cancer in bone have been well elucidated in recent years, the cause of bone pain is not well understood. Between one fourth and one third of fully developed bone metastases will not cause any pain (3,6). The presence or absence of pain has not been correlated with type of tumor, location of the metastases, size of the metastases, gender, and age of patients (11). Moreover, some patients present with multiple metastases, but only some of them are painful. There is limited knowledge of the events by which bone metastases give rise to pain sensation. Many nerves are found in the periosteum, and others enter bones via the blood vessels. Increased bone marrow pressure has been associated with pain in osteoarthritis (12), but distention or distortion of the periosteum can also account for the pain in some tumors (13). Among the potential chemical mediators and modulations of nociception, histamine, 5-hydroxytryptamine, substance P, and a number of cytokines have been found in bone tumors. Many of these chemicals are capable of causing hyperalgesia when injected intradermally, and they might be able to sensitize pain nerve endings to various other mediators (13).

Clinical features

Autopsy studies suggest that the skeleton is the third most common site of cancer metastases, surpassed only by lung and liver. Pathological fractures have been reported to occur in 8%–30% of patients with bone metastases. Among patients treated surgically for bone metastases, the main source is breast, accounting for approximately 50% of total cases. Proximal parts of long bones are generally involved before the distal parts, and the bones that are fractured more often are femur (50%), humerus (15%), or both (6,14). Other tumors capable of causing pathological fractures are kidney (10%), lung (10%), and thyroid (5%). Cord compression occurs in approximately 5% of patients. The most common primary tumors associated with this complication are breast (20%–30%) and lung (15%). Metastases from the prostate account for a fairly small percentage of the operative cases, partly because they most often occur in the lumbar spine where they are not likely to cause spinal cord compression and partly because they tend to be osteoblastic with a relatively low incidence of fracture (14).

Hypercalcemia occurs in approximately 10% of patients with malignancy and even more commonly in those with metastatic bone disease (15). When present, hypercalcemia causes significant cognitive impairment that makes the assessment and management of the pain syndrome more difficult.

The diagnosis of bone metastases is usually very simple, even in patients with unknown primary tumor. Bone scans are highly sensitive for the detection of bone metastases but are relatively non-specific (16). The false-negative rate for bone scans is approximately 8%; the false-positive rate may be as high as 40%–50% when only a few positive lesions are observed. Therefore,

abnormal observations in the bone scan should be confirmed radiologically (6,16). Radiography is specific but quite insensitive. At least 50% of the bone must be destroyed in the beam axis of the x-ray before lesions involving the medulla can be seen radiographically. In contrast, lesions that involve the cortex are detected when they are much smaller (2,3).

Computed tomography (CT) or magnetic resonance imaging (MRI) give additional information, especially for lesions on the spine or when the possibility of spinal cord involvement is suspected, or in direct involvement by tumors of the head and neck or intrathoracic malignancies (16).

Another dimension of skeletal complication in malignancy exists in women who have been treated for breast cancer. This group has an increased risk of osteoporosis because of premature menopause induced by chemotherapy (17), and some chemotherapeutic agents are known to adversely affect bone formation (18). This increased risk of skeletal complications exists even in the absence of metastatic disease. Women with treated breast cancer without evidence of metastatic disease have been shown to have a five times higher risk of vertebral fracture than normal, and the risk was found to be 20 times higher in women with soft-tissue metastases without evidence of bone metastases (19).

Pain syndromes

Table 24.1 summarizes the most frequent syndromes associated with bone involvement by cancer.

Continuous bone pain

Continuous bone pain is the most frequent presentation of pain. Pain is usually well localized to one or more specific bone areas and can be pinpointed by the patient with relative ease. It usually has a gradual onset over a period of weeks or months, becoming progressively more severe in intensity. It can be dull in character and/or have a deep boring sensation that aches or burns and may be accompanied by episodes of stabbing discomfort (20,21). Pain usually increases with pressure on

Table 24.1. *Bone pain syndromes*

- Continuous bone pain
- Incident pain
- Mixed bone and neuropathic pain
- Mixed bone and visceral pain

the area of involvement, which may account for it worsening at night when the patient is lying down. Because of the higher prevalence of axial skeletal metastases, this pain is more likely to involve pelvis, rib cage, lumbar, dorsal, or cervical spine.

Incident pain

Patients with incident pain have mild or no pain while resting but suffer severe exacerbation when they perform the pain-causing maneuver (moving, standing, walking, etc.). Bone metastases are the most frequent cause of incident pain. Recent data suggest that episodes of incident pain occur in almost two thirds of patients with cancer pain, with a frequency range from just a few to several hundred per day, suggesting that incident pain is a serious management problem (20,22,23). Incident pain responds less well to opioids than continuous pain (20), because movement-related pain is repetitive and unpredictable, and doses of opioids required to control it may produce unacceptable side effects when the patient is at rest (24,25).

Mixed bone and neuropathic pain

In addition to either continuous or incident somatic bone pain, these patients present evidence of involvement of areas of the central or peripheral nervous system. Most frequently, these patients present evidence of neuropathic pain as a result of involvement of the spinal cord, nerve routes, or peripheral nerves. The typical "burning" or "tingling" nature of the pain, the radiation following nerve distribution, and the presence of sensory or motor deficits are indicators of mixed bone/neurpoathic pain syndromes. Pain related to spinal cord compression from collapse of a vertebral body is typically exacerbated by coughing, sneezing, and straining and becomes worse on straight leg raising. The location of the tumor frequently facilitates the diagnosis (22).

Mixed bone and visceral pain

These patients present with simultaneous metastatic locations in bone as well as in different intra-abdominal or intrathoracic organs. In our experience, the most frequent associations are the presence of metastatic bone pain with intra-abdominal tumor or liver metastases. The diagnosis of visceral pain is usually relatively easy to make, and some patients may require specific analgesic techniques aimed to control the visceral component and,

therefore, inadequate diagnosis of the pain syndrome will have prognostic and therapeutic implications (22).

Treatment

Table 24.2 summarizes some of the available treatment modalities for bone pain. Time to pain relief and other beneficial effects vary with different types of treatment. This may influence the choice of treatment in an individual patient; for example, if life expectancy is very short it may not be appropriate to commence treatment with bisphosphonates, radiotherapy, or radioisotopes. Table 24.3 shows expected time to first pain relief with various modalities of treatment.

A recent study looking at risks of complications from bone metastases in breast cancer found that patients with metastatic disease confined to the skeleton are most likely to develop pathological fractures, to require radiotherapy to painful osseous deposits, and to develop spinal cord compression (26). This is at least in part due to the increased survival in this group compared to those with both osseous and extraosseous metastases. Median survival for patients with bone and liver metastases was 5.5 months. In a placebo-controlled study in 382 patients with bone metastases from breast cancer treated with intravenous pamidronate, statistically significant reductions in the need for radiotherapy and surgery to bone and in the occurrence of non-vertebral fractures was seen after 6, 9, and 12 months of treatment, respectively (27). By identifying those most at risk of skeletal complications and looking at time to benefit from specific treatments, studies such as these may improve cost–benefit analysis by helping to target those most likely to benefit from a particular treatment approach.

Patients with bone involvement frequently require multimodal therapy consisting of the management of the primary cancer, analgesics, and/or measures to prevent further osteolysis and/or fractures. The role of some of these interventions is described next.

Table 24.2. *Treatment modalities for bone pain*

- Opioid analgesics
- Non-steroidal anti-inflammatory drugs
- Corticosteroids
- Bisphosphonates
- Radiation therapy
- Radioisotopes
- Orthopedic surgery
- Hormones—chemotherapy
- Other treatments

Table 24.3. *Time to expected first improvement in pain with various treatments*

Treatment	Approximate time to first relief
Bisphosphonates	1 week
Calcitonin	1–7 days
External beam radiotherapy	2–3 weeks
Hemibody radiation	2–3 days
Radioisotopes	1–3 weeks
Hormonal treatments	2–8 weeks

Opioid analgesics

Bone pain usually responds well to opioids (28,29), and they remain the mainstay treatment for symptom control of both isolated bone involvement areas and for diffuse bone pain (30). Table 24.4 summarizes general principles of opioid use for bone pain. A regular around-the-clock dosing of an opioid is advised, as most patients experience continuous pain. In addition a breakthrough or rescue dose should be prescribed for breakthrough pain on an as-needed basis. The dose can then be titrated to achieve adequate pain control. A majority of patients will likely require a strong opioid agonist such as morphine, hydromorphone, oxycodone, fentanyl, or methadone. At the same time, measures to prevent common side effects such as constipation and nausea should be implemented. In addition, knowledge of common neuropsychiatric side effects such as opioid-induced delirium, hallucinations, myoclonus, and excessive sedation, and their management strategies is essential (31). With regard to route of administration, the oral route is preferred, although on occasion, an alternative route is required. The subcutaneous route has been shown to be as effective as the intravenous route and more convenient. Other options include rectal and transdermal formulations.

With regard to incident pain, titration of opioids may prove difficult, and these individuals may require short-acting breakthrough or rescue doses of analgesics to provide pain relief that breaks through the chronic daily pain (20,32). It is usually advised to take these breakthrough

Table 24.4. *Opioids for bone pain*

- Regular administration
- Consider adjuvants (bisphosphonates, non-steroidal anti-inflammatory drugs, corticosteroids)
- Prevent side effects (nausea, constipation, sedation)
- Less effective for incidental-neuropathic bone pain

or rescue doses before an activity that may elicit pain. Unfortunately, most patients with incidental pain find limited benefit from currently available breakthrough analgesics, as the duration of pain is shorter than the latency for analgesia (33). Newer, highly liposoluble opioids such as transmucosal fentanyl could prove particularly useful in the management of incidental bone pain (34,35). In cases where severe sedation arises as a symptom of dose-limiting opioid toxicity during the intervals between incident pain, the addition of a psychostimulant could be considered. This may allow patients to tolerate a higher dose of opioids by reducing sedation and, thereby, improving analgesia (33).

Non-steroidal anti-inflammatory drugs

Although these medications are advised as the first-line approach for the management of mild to moderate cancer pain by the World Health Organization (36), strong methodologically sound studies have yet to establish evidence-based support in favor of non-steroidal anti-inflammatory drugs (NSAIDs) in cancer pain (37). Moreover, the use of NSAIDs carries the risk of the development of adverse reactions, particularly gastrointestinal, renal, and hematological. NSAIDs may cause renal insufficiency by impairing intrarenal blood flow via inhibition of prostacyclin, a renovasodilator. Thus, renal impairment can result in opioid metabolite accumulation giving rise to various neuropsychiatric toxicities (38,39).

Most NSAIDs are inhibitors of both cyclo-oxygenase-1 (COX-1) and cyclo-oxygenase-2 (COX-2). COX-1 is associated with production of prostaglandins, which are believed to protect gastrointestinal mucosa (40). In animal models, NSAID-induced gastrointestinal (GI) tract toxicity has been isolated to inhibition of COX-1 activity (41,42). The new NSAIDs, which are selective COX-2 inhibitors, have improved safety profiles with respect to adverse GI effects. Their use has been shown to result in less gastroduodenal ulcers and upper GI tract bleeding than other NSAIDs, which are not selective COX-2 inhibitors (43–45). Both celecoxib and rofecoxib are approved by the U.S. Food and Drug Administration, celecoxib for the treatment of rheumatoid arthritis and osteoarthritis and rofecoxib for use in acute pain and osteoarthritis. In the absence of long-term safety data from prospective trials, the COX-2 inhibitors still carry the standard NSAID class warnings regarding upper GI side effects. Renal complications of COX-2 inhibitors appear to be similar to those of other NSAIDs (46).

Adjuvant analgesics

Corticosteroids

Corticosteroids appear to be effective in reducing bone pain from a variety of solid tumors. Apart from their adjuvant analgesic properties, corticosteroids have various other potential benefits for patients with advanced disease including improvement in appetite, decrease in nausea, and improvement in the sensation of well-being (47). The ideal type of corticosteroid and optimal dose has not been well established, and dose recommendations are mainly based on uncontrolled anecdotal reports and clinical experience. Recommended corticosteroids and doses are 4 to 8 mg of dexamethasone orally or subcutaneously two to three times per day, 20 to 40 mg of prednisone orally two to three times per day, or 16 to 32 mg of methylprednisolone orally two to three times per day (48). Dexamethasone appears to be preferred because of ease of administration on a twice daily basis, in addition to its minimal to absent mineralocorticoid effects. If effectiveness is demonstrated, the corticosteroid dose should be gradually tapered to the lowest possible effective dose or, if possible, be discontinued so as to avoid long-term adverse effects (42). Corticosteroids have also been found to be beneficial in the treatment of spinal cord compression and should be initiated early when spinal cord compression is suspected (49). In patients with relatively long expected survival, maintenance therapy with corticosteroids should be carefully weighted against the potential side effects including immunosuppression, avascular necrosis, edema, hyperglycemia, proximal myopathy, and neuropsychiatric side effects (50). With regard to the latter, delirium has been found to be more common than mood disorders in cancer patients making use of dexamethasone (51). As steroid myopathy can contribute further to decreased ambulation and immobility, this side effect, in particular, should be observed more closely. If it arises, consideration can be given to discontinuing the corticosteroid, which often results in complete reversibility of the problem (52). Another option for those who are benefiting from the use of a corticosteroid is to change to a nonfluorinated steroid such as methylprednisolone or prednisone (53).

Bisphosphonates

Bisphosphonates are an important component in the treatment of painful skeletal metastases. They are analogs of pyrophosphate, a natural inhibitor of the formation of cal-

Table 24.5. *Clinical effects of bisphosphonates*

	Level of evidence
Analgesia	I
Prevention of osteolysis	I
Prevention of bone metastasis	II
Improved survival	II

cium phosphate crystals. After systemic administration, these drugs have a complex effect on the function and differentiation of osteoclasts. Evidence is emerging that bisphosphonates may have direct antitumor effects in addition to their effect on osteoclasts (54,55). In vitro they inhibit breast and prostate tumor cell invasion (56) and also inhibit the proteolytic activity of matrix metalloproteinases in tumor cells. The mechanism for this appears to involve the chelation of zinc by the phosphonate group (54). In addition bisphosphonates may have an apoptotic effect on macrophages and tumor cells (55).

There are many bisphosphonates. All are capable of treating disorders of bone resorption such as osteolytic metastases and osteoporosis; however, traditionally some have been researched and used for treatment of certain conditions more than others. Clodronate and pamidronate have been studied most extensively in malignant disease, particularly in multiple myeloma and breast cancer. Studies have also been conducted with other solid tumors including lung, gastrointestinal, and prostatic cancer (2). Table 24.5 summarizes some of the clinical effects of these drugs. Bisphosphonates are currently used for three main indications in the treatment of metastatic bone disease: to treat bone pain, to prevent skeletal complications, and to treat hypercalcemia.

A recent review of phase III trials of a number of bisphosphonates in the treatment of painful metastatic bone disease reported strong evidence from numerous double-blind crossover trials for analgesic effects for these drugs (57). Therefore, bisphosphonates are a valuable analgesic treatment for most patients with painful metastatic bone disease. Clodronate probably has a shorter duration of analgesic effects as compared to pamidronate. However, one of its main advantages is that it can be delivered in relatively small volumes subcutaneously with excellent local tolerance (58,59). Subcutaneous administration can be particularly useful for patients in rural areas, at home, or in continuing care facilities, or for those patients in whom intravenous access becomes difficult because of poor veins (57).

A recent systematic review has addressed the role of bisphosphonates in the prevention of osteolysis (60). The author identified 18 randomized controlled trials providing level 1 evidence for the use of bisphosphonates to reduce both skeletal events and pain in multiple myeloma and breast cancer. Long-term follow-up (24 months) results from two prospective, multicenter, randomized, double-blind, placebo-controlled trials have been published. Pamidronate as a supplement to antineoplastic therapy has been shown on long-term follow-up evaluation in breast cancer patients with skeletal metastases to be superior to antineoplastic therapy alone in palliating symptoms and in preventing non-vertebral pathological fractures, hypercalcemia, and skeletal complications such as the need for surgery or radiotherapy. It was also found to delay the median time to first skeletal complication from 7 months in the placebo group to 12.7 months in the pamidronate group (61).

Studies of oral clodronate in breast cancer patients has shown it to be effective in reducing the rate of morbid skeletal events (62), to significantly lengthen the time to first skeletal event (63), and to reduce the number of new skeletal metastases (64–67). Conflicting evidence exists regarding clodronate and its effect on nonosseous metastases. Three studies have looked at oral clodronate 1600 mg daily in women with breast cancer. Diel et al. (65) conducted a randomized controlled trial of oral clodronate over 2 years in women with breast cancer who had tumor cells detected in their bone marrow and found a significantly lower incidence of both osseous and visceral metastases in the treated group. Longer term follow-up evaluation at a median time of 53 months showed that the prophylactic effect on bone metastases was still seen but was weakened, and the effect on visceral metastases was no longer seen (66). The analysis of a larger multicenter, placebo-controlled, double-blind study of all women with primary breast cancer demonstrated a significant reduction in the incidence of bone metastases, but no statistical difference in the number of visceral metastases in the treated group (67). A randomized controlled study in Finland of node-positive, breast cancer patients indicated no significant difference between those who were treated with oral clodronate and control subjects in the incidence of bony metastases, an increase in the number of visceral metastases, and a deterioration in the overall survival (68). There were methodological differences in the groups, which may in part explain the dramatically different findings. Diel et al. studied patients with tumor cells in their bone marrow (patients with distant metastases were excluded). It is possible that this group may benefit most from prophylaxis. The multicenter study was by far the largest and the only placebo-controlled study of the three. Clodronate has been extensively studied and has been used for many years, and there has not been previous evidence that clodronate can adversely affect metastatic disease or survival in cancer patients. Further studies are required to clarify this issue.

Bisphosphonates have poor intestinal absorption (<5%) and a short half-life. When taken orally, they must be taken with water at least 2 hours before and 2 hours after ingestion of food. They localize selectively to bone and are retained very well there. They are generally well tolerated. The more common side effects are nausea, vomiting, fever, and elevation of serum creatinine. Nausea and vomiting are more common in first-generation bisphosphonates (etidronate and clodronate) and less common in newer drugs such as pamidronate and ibandronate. Hypocalcemia may occur with intravenous administration of bisphosphonates for bone pain, especially in patients who are normocalcemic before treatment (69,70). Esophageal erosions and ulceration are a rare but potentially serious complication of oral bisphosphonate administration, and for this reason it is recommended that tablets are taken with about 200 ml of water when the patient is upright and that the patient remains upright for at least 30 minutes afterward. Caution is advised in patients with upper gastrointestinal problems, and bisphosphonates are contraindicated in those with achalasia or strictures, which cause delayed esophageal emptying. Patients should be advised to discontinue the drug and seek medical advice if esophageal symptoms develop.

Newer bisphosphonates include alendronate, ibandronate, risedronate, and zoledrolate. There is preliminary evidence that some of the newer bisphosphonates retain their effects on hypercalcemia and pain and require much lower dosages. Ibandronate and zoledronate have been used in the treatment of hypercalcemia of malignancy; the effective doses for intravenous use appear to be as low as 2 to 4 mg and 1 to 2 mg, respectively (71). Zoledronate in doses of 4 to 8 mg has been shown to be superior to pamidronate 80 mg in reducing cancer hypercalcemia (72). Oral risedronate 5 mg daily has been shown to actually increase bone mass (73). An intermittent regimen of oral risedronate 30 mg/day for 2 out of 12 weeks gave similar results (74). There is recent evidence that oral ibandronate has potent effects on reducing the rate of bone resorption in patients with metastatic bone disease (75).

There is a lack of direct comparative evidence between different bisphosphonates in metastatic bone disease. At present intravenous pamidronate is the only bisphosphonate approved for use in bone metastases in the United States.

The idea of oral or even transdermal administration, especially for the newer more potent bisphosphonates, is appealing. Compared with the intravenous route for the treatment of bone metastases, the effects of oral administration have been marginal, and there have not been many well-designed, placebo-controlled studies of oral bisphosphonates (76). Further trials with the specific endpoints of effects on bone pain and skeletal complications in patients with metastatic osseous disease are needed to accurately assess their effectiveness. The new bisphosphonates offer possible advantages in terms of side effects, administration routes, and regimens, but more research is required to assess their clinical benefits.

The American Society of Clinical Oncology Bisphosphonates Expert Panel has issued guidelines on the role of bisphosphonates in breast cancer based on currently available information (77). The following summarizes their findings and guidelines:

- Bisphosphonates have not had an impact on overall survival in breast cancer.
- Benefits have been reduction in skeletal complications (pathologic fractures, radiation, spinal cord compression, hypercalcemia, and surgery for fracture or impending fracture).
- Intravenous pamidronate 90 mg over 1 to 2 hours every 3 to 4 weeks is recommended in patients who have evidence of lytic destruction of bone on plain radiographs and who are concurrently receiving systemic hormonal or chemotherapy.
- Start bisphosphonates in women with an abnormal bone scan and an abnormal CT or MRI scan showing bone destruction and localized pain, but normal plain radiograph is considered reasonable.
- Bisphosphonates are not recommended in patients with an asymptomatic abnormal bone scan and normal radiographs.
- Intravenous pamidronate is recommended in women with pain caused by osteolytic metastases to relieve pain when used concurrently with systemic chemotherapy and/or hormonal therapy.
- Oral bisphosphonates can be used for prevention of osteoporosis in premenopausal women with treatment-induced menopause.
- Use of bisphosphonates is not currently recommended in patients without evidence of bony metastases. This includes patients with extraskeletal metastases and those with high risk for future bony metastasis.

The expert panel advised that future research is warranted to identify clinical predictors of when to start and stop therapy, to integrate their use with other treatments for bone metastases, to identify their role in the adjuvant setting in preventing bone metastases, and to better determine their cost–benefit consequences.

Many areas in which the use of bisphosphonates are not currently recommended are due to lack of evidence rather than proven lack of effect. There are many questions related to bisphosphonate use, which need to be answered with further research:

- Do bisphosphonates have a real preventative effect on the formation of new skeletal or visceral metastases? If so, in which group should we use them for prophylaxis?
- Do bisphosphonates have an antitumor effect in humans?
- Are the newer bisphosphonates more clinically effective or safer in the treatment of painful metastatic bone disease?
- Is oral or transdermal administration of newer bisphosphonates as effective as the intravenous route? If so, are intermittent oral regimes as beneficial as a regular daily dose?

If direct antitumor effects of bisphosphonates are confirmed in vivo, bisphosphonates may have a role, not only by helping to manage and prevent complications of preexisting painful skeletal metastases, but also in preventing new metastases by modifying the natural history of cancer in some patients.

Calcitonin

Salmon calcitonin is used in the management of benign bone pain in Paget's disease and osteoporosis. A number of studies have shown it to have use in metastatic bone pain (78–80). Some studies have shown benefit occurring within a few days of initiation of subcutaneous calcitonin (78,81) and even as early as 12 hours (80). It is cheaper than bisphosphonates and comes in subcutaneous and nasal preparations; however, it has a more troublesome side effect profile and appears to be less potent than bisphosphonates, and the latter have generally superseded its use. Because of its rapid onset of action it may have an advantage in individual patients with severe acute bone pain or in those with a very short survival time.

Radioisotopes/radiopharmaceuticals

Bone seeking radioisotopes are administered parenterally, and all bony metastatic sites are targeted at once, unlike external beam radiotherapy. Table 24.6 compares various

Table 24.6. *Comparison of radioisotopes*

Radioisotope	Status	Half-life (days)	Response rate (%) (days)	Time to response (months)	Duration of effect	Hematological toxicity
[89]Sr	Licensed	50.5	60–80	10–20	2–12	Moderate
[153]Sm EDTMP	Licensed	1.95	70–75	5–10	2–6	Mild/moderate
[186]Re HEDP	Clinical trials	3.8	60–75	5–10	1–4	Mild/moderate

radioisotopes. Bone-seeking radioisotopes such as strontium-89 have been found to be effective in randomized controlled trials (89,90). The disadvantages of strontium therapy include potential for severe hematological toxicity, delay in pain relief, and high cost. There is substantial evidence that samarium-153 EDTMP has a therapeutic benefit comparable to strontium-89 (91,92), and it is now licensed for use in the United States. 186 Re-1,1-hydroxyethylidene diphosphonate (HDEP) is not yet licensed for use in the United States, and clinical experience with this agent is limited. A recent open clinical trial in 60 patients looked at the short- and long-term effects of the treatment of painful bony metastases. It was found it to give relief of pain in patients with a variety of tumors. A total of 80% of individuals treated had prompt relief of pain (clinically evident pain relief in first week), 31% experienced complete relief, 34% partial relief, and 14% minimal relief of pain. It was effective against both advanced and relatively early stages of metastatic disease. Transient World Health Organization grade 1–2 hematological toxicity was seen with complete recovery. The duration of pain relief lasted from 3 weeks to 12 months and correlated positively with the degree of response. There was also an indication that [186]Re-HEDP may slow the progression of metastatic bone disease (93). Further research is required to look at this potential effect. Radioisotopes should show selective uptake in metastases rather than normal bone, and they should be cleared quickly from normal bone and soft tissues. Generally, radioisotopes could be considered in patients with refractory multifocal pain caused by metastatic disease. Eligible patients should have life expectancy longer than 3 months, sufficient bone marrow reserve, and no further chemotherapy planned. Absolute platelet count less than $60,000 \times 10^6$ or a recent rapid fall in platelet count or a white cell count of less than 2.5×10^6 are contraindications to the use of radioisotopes owing to the risks of further bone marrow suppression after treatment. Patients with advanced prostate cancer may have subclinical disseminated intravascular coagulation, and it is advisable to screen for this with blood tests before initiating therapy (94).

The slow onset of effect makes this modality inappropriate as single therapy for patients with severe cancer pain. Clinical experience in the setting of palliative care in hospice does not seem to mirror the positive effects reported in the literature. Although it may be well tolerated in the short term, data concerning long-term toxicity are very limited. At present there is insufficient evidence to support the use of radiopharmaceutical therapy in patients with multiple painless skeletal metastases or those with prostate cancer and a rising prostate-specific antigen as evidence of treatment failure, but with no bone scan evidence of metastases (94). Trials are underway in this area. Radioisotopes are an expensive treatment option when compared, for example, to bisphosphonates, and they must prove themselves to be cost effective. There are also ongoing trials to compare radiopharmaceuticals with bisphosphonates and to determine if cisplatin as a radiosensitizer can improve effectiveness of radiopharmaceuticals.

Radiotherapy

External beam radiation directed at the site of pain is well established and the treatment of choice for local bone pain resulting from metastatic disease (82). Pain relief usually occurs in 2 to 4 weeks. It is not suitable where there are multiple painful metastatic sites; in these patients, hemibody wide-field irradiation may be useful. The upper body or lower body may be irradiated (usually in a single fraction of 6 Gy for upper body and 8 Gy for lower body), and pain relief often occurs within 1 to 2 days, which is considerably earlier than in those who have external beam radiotherapy to a local lesion. In one series 73% of those treated with a single dose of hemibody irradiation experienced pain relief (83). The side effect profile is more troublesome than with external beam radiation; the majority of patients develop a period of bone marrow suppression, and there is a risk of potentially fatal radiation pneumonitis in those who have upper hemibody irradiation. The other radiation treatment modality that is useful for patients with bone pain from multiple metastatic sites is administration of bone-seeking radioisotopes.

There is some evidence that radiotherapy to individual bony sites in brief courses for pain relief offers significant cost advantage over narcotic analgesics (84). Traditionally, radiation has been administered in multiple fractions over several days and weeks, although current evidence indicates that single fractions are as effective as multiple fractions when pain relief is the goal (85–87).

Two recent large prospective randomized trials compared single fraction and multiple fraction radiotherapy for local metastatic skeletal pain (85,86). Their findings are summarized in Table 24.7.

The Bone Pain Trial Working Party study randomized 761 patients to receive either single fraction 8 Gy or a multifraction schedule of either 20 Gy in 5 fractions or 30 Gy in 10 fractions. Patients were monitored for 12 months. Overall survival was the same in both groups, with 44% of patients alive at the end of the 12-month study period. No statistical difference was observed between the groups in time to first improvement of pain, time to complete pain relief, time to first increase in pain, or in class of analgesics used. A total of 78% experienced pain relief in both groups, with complete pain relief in 57% of the single fraction group and 58% of the multifraction group (difference in proportions = −1%, 95% CI = −9% to 6%). Retreatment was twice as common in the single fraction group. This was thought to reflect a greater willingness to retreat with radiotherapy after single fraction rather than a greater need. No significant difference was seen in the incidence of nausea, vomiting, pathological fracture, or spinal cord compression (85).

The Dutch Bone Metastasis Study randomized 1171 patients to receive either single fraction with 8 Gy or multiple fraction with 4 Gy × 6 fractions. Median survival was 7 months; overall pain response rate was 71%, with a complete response rate of 35%. There were no significant differences for these parameters between the two groups. The two treatment schedules were thought to be equivalent in terms of palliation rate. No significant differences were found in time to response, mean pain scores, time to progression of pain to original level, side effects (nausea, vomiting, tiredness, itching, and painful skin), percentage of patients using pain medication (including strong opioids), or quality of life. Incidence of spinal cord compression was similar; however, significantly more patients in the single fraction group experienced pathological fractures—4% vs. 2% in the multiple fraction treatment group. There were significantly more retreatments in the single fraction group (25%) than in the multifraction group (7%). Retreatment appeared to depend on preceding pain score ($p < 0.0001$)—the higher the original pain score the higher the chance of retreatment. Retreatments were done at a lower pain score and earlier in the single fraction group indicating that physicians were more willing to retreat this group. There was no indication that treatment effects depend on tumor type or localization of bone metastases. The equality of single and multiple fraction treatment was also seen in long-term survivors (86). The authors pointed out that there may be a group of patients in whom single fraction treatment is not the best approach and indicated that further analysis of their data was needed to look at this area.

A smaller prospective, non-randomized study of 205 patients with a variety of primary tumors found that aggres-

Table 24.7. *Summary of two large trials comparing single fraction and multiple fraction radiotherapy*

	BPTWP ($n = 761$)		DBMS ($n = 1171$)	
	Single fraction	Multiple fraction	Single fraction	Multiple fraction
Overall response rate (%)	78	78	72	69
Complete response rate (%)	57	58	37	33
Retreatment rate (%)	23[a]	10[a]	25[b]	07[b]
Survival, time to response, class of analgesics	NSD	NSD		
Nausea, vomiting	NSD	NSD		
Spinal cord compression	NSD	NSD		
Pathological fracture rate	NSD	4% single fraction vs. 2% multiple fraction ($p < 0.05$)		

Abbreviations: BPTWP, Bone Pain Trial Working Party; DBMS, Dutch Bone Metastasis Group; NSD, no significant difference.
[a] $p < 0.001$
[b] $p < 0.0001$

sive protracted radiotherapy treatment offered advantages in patients in whom the expected life span was not short (88).

When convenience for the patient and the economic benefit are taken into account, single fraction radiotherapy has many advantages and is preferable to multiple fraction radiotherapy for the majority of patients with uncomplicated metastatic bone pain.

Orthopedic surgery

The possible direct consequences of not managing bone metastases adequately are fracture, pain, and neurological deficits. Pathological fractures of bone will generally not heal by themselves because of excessive osteoclastic activity in the area of the metastasis. This situation is further complicated because patients are often undernourished and their overall physical condition is compromised by their primary disease. Current techniques for surgical management of pathological fractures are extremely effective in alleviating pain and allowing patients to resume mobility, often without the need for external support. Table 24.8 outlines the percentage of patients getting good or excellent pain relief from various procedures. Improvement in pain and mobility significantly improves the quality of the remaining months or years of these individuals. Long-term survival of patients after the first pathological fracture from malignancy has more than tripled for most cancers in the last 25 years. Surgical techniques for stabilizing pathological or impending fractures must be individualized for the area of involvement, the particular qualities of the bone involved, and the potential for involvement of adjacent soft tissue structures (95).

Many factors must be taken into account when considering the suitability of an individual patient for surgery. Fitness for surgery, the degree of pain or functional loss, the potential benefits to be gained, and the potential risks of surgery need to be taken into account. An expected survival of only weeks to months is not necessarily a contraindication to surgery (10). Even in bedridden terminally ill patients, orthopedic procedures may improve some degree of function and ease the nursing care of the patient. In many cases, particularly in those involved in pathological fractures of the hips and lower extremities, surgery offers the only definite therapy to control pain and improve mobility. Quality of life is much better without the fear of fracture or pain, and surgery should be considered even if life expectancy is short.

Orthopedic surgical interventions are useful in three main areas:

* Prevention and treatment of long bone fractures
* Reconstruction of major joints
* Reconstruction/stabilization of the spine with or without decompression

Prophylactic stabilization or fixation is recommended where there is a high risk of pathological fracture. It is much easier to treat an impending fracture than a complete fracture of a long bone. Lesions in long bones that involve at least 50% of the cortex have at least a 50% chance of fracture if not reinforced (96). Fracture is more imminent if the lesion is purely lytic and exceeds 5 cm in length. Purely blastic lesions have a much lower risk of fracture and rarely require prophylactic fixation (10). Pain on weight bearing may be a warning of impending fracture.

Upper and lower limb long bone fractures such as those of the femoral shaft, tibia, humerus, radius, and ulna require an intramedullary rod. These act as load-sharing devices distributing stresses along the bone in a graduated fashion. Plate and screw fixation is not suitable for these bones, as it results in excessive stress being applied to the area of bone where it is fixated. If the bone in this area is weakened by a metastatic lesion, another pathological fracture is likely to develop. Because it is not a main structural member, the fibula generally does not require an intramedullary rod. Fixation devices for lower extremity long bone such as femur must be able to withstand weight-bearing stresses. Those used in upper limbs are often subjected to forces inherent with lifting and pulling in addition to heavy compressive forces, particularly in patients who require crutches or other devices to assist them in walking. The efficacy of subsequent irradiation is improved by debulking as much tumor tissue as possible by curettage at the time of surgery. Defects may be filled with methylmethacrylate.

Occasionally it is necessary to replace an entire joint or one component of a joint. Proximal femoral lesions involving the head, neck, and/or intertrochanteric regions may require replacement prostheses. Prostheses are also required for lesions in the proximal humerus affecting

Table 24.8. *Percentage of patients experiencing good or excellent pain relief with various orthopedic procedures for metastatic bone disease*[95]

Procedure	Pain relief (%)
Internal fixation of long bone fracture	96
Acetabular joint reconstruction	84
Decompression and stabilization of vertebra	88

the articular cartilage or when fractures occur through the anatomical neck of the humerus. In the knee if there is destruction of articular cartilage that prevents painless articulation, a total knee replacement is indicated.

Most spinal metastases can be managed conservatively. Surgical intervention is required in those presenting with progressive neurological compromise or spinal instability. Stability of the spine can be assessed using the Kostuik classification system. The vertebra is divided into six columns: right and left anterior and posterior vertebral body columns and right and left posterior columns, which include the pedicles. These can be best assessed on the axial view of a CT scan. Destruction of two columns is considered stable; three or more is considered unstable and fracture is likely. If the spine is stable and the patient's pain is due to bone destruction alone or compression from tumor alone, external beam irradiation will often be effective. If the tumor is not radiosensitive or if there is compression as a result of tumor and debris such as bone, disk, or ligamentous material, a surgical approach may be required. Mechanical instability, neural compression caused by tumor growth, and progressing neurological deficit during or after radiotherapy are indications for surgery to decompress and stabilize the spinal column. Techniques for vertebral stabilization have improved and include anterior and posterior approaches and endoscopic techniques. Most vertebral lesions that require decompression and stabilization originate in the vertebral body and are best managed by an anterior approach. Decompression and stability can be achieved satisfactorily in this way. This approach is superior to a posterior approach in terms of improvement in neurological function (97). Less frequently, tumor destruction posteriorly (e.g., of pedicles) necessitates the use of a posterior in addition to an anterior approach. Percutaneous vertebroplasty (methylmethacrylate cement injection) is another technique that has been used for spinal stabilization, but its use seems to be limited in patients with vertebral compression fractures related to malignancy (98).

External beam irradiation is given to almost all patients after surgery. This helps achieve pain control and inhibits local disease progression. It may be commenced 2 weeks after surgery if the wound is healed, and there is no other local complication.

Rehabilitation is important in patients who have had surgery for a pathological fracture. In more advanced cancer patients, rehabilitation aims to relieve discomfort and improve quality of life by reducing physical dependence. This differs from rehabilitation in other areas where the goals are the return of the individual to a higher level of functioning such as return to work. The need and motivation for rehabilitation in the terminally ill patient are high (99). Those cancer patients who have required surgical treatment of a fracture are particularly in need of rehabilitation and, if possible, mobilization, in order to improve level of functioning and prevent muscle wasting caused by immobility. Physical therapy is especially important in patients with paraplegia to help them gain control and independence and to try to prevent complications such as pressure sores and phlebitis.

Hormonal therapy and chemotherapy

Antineoplastic interventions are of great importance in the management of metastatic bone pain. In some cases, such as prostate and breast cancer, simple hormonal interventions are capable of achieving pain relief in 60%–80% of patients with minimal cost and toxicity. It is important to remember that even in the most successful cases of pain improvement with hormonal and/or chemotherapy, analgesia will occur after a minimum of 2 to 8 weeks. Therefore, a plan for appropriate analgesic therapy needs to be in place for at least this period of time. Medical oncologists need to effectively manage pain with the previously mentioned techniques while antineoplastic interventions are being considered and administered.

Other treatments

Anesthesiological techniques such as nerve blocks or intraspinal infusion of opioids and local anesthetics can be effective in patients who have not improved with other treatments. The main limitation of these interventions is their high cost and need for specialized services for the maintenance of treatments.

Neurosurgical procedures such as percutaneous cordotomy can be useful for unilateral pain syndromes below the waist. Analgesia has been reported to be prompt and occur in the great majority of patients with this technique.

Future research

The pathophysiology of bone pain is not well understood. The potential role of different tumor, endothelial, and host humoral factors needs to be adequately established. By increasing our knowledge on the role of different factors on the production of nociception at the bone level, it will be possible in the future to develop specific analgesic techniques. Bone pain syndromes have not been appropriately characterized. A better definition of the clinical presentation of different bone pain syndromes will allow researchers and clinicians to better express the characteristics of patient populations and to evaluate therapeutic techniques. The role of the newer COX-2 NSAIDs should be established in bone pain. Although these agents have in their favor the great difference in effects between the COX-2 (pathological) and COX-1 (physiological) pathways, their effectiveness in cancer bone pain may be limited because of their relatively limited effects on central nervous system cyclo-oxygenase. The role of bisphosphonates needs to be better clarified. However, the currently available agents and those that are in development hold the most promise for the management of bone pain. Finally, the role of more traditional interventions such as chemotherapy, hormonal therapy, and even radiation therapy needs to be better characterized in clinical trials that provide for adequate blinding. These trials will hopefully better illustrate the real potential of these agents in cancer-related bone pain.

References

1. Galasko CSB. Skeletal metastases. Clin Orthoped 210:18–30, 1986.
2. Pereira J. Management of bone pain. In: Portenoy R, Bruera E, eds. Topics in palliative care, vol. 3. New York, Oxford: Oxford University Press, 1998:79–116.
3. Lote K, Walloe A, Bjersand A. Bone metastases: prognosis diagnosis and treatment. Acta Radiol Oncol 25:227–32, 1986.
4. Koenders PG, Beex LV, Kloppenborg PWC, et al. Human breast cancer: survival from metastases. Breast Cancer Res Treat 21:173–80, 1992.
5. Liotta LA, Stetler-Stevenson WGD. Principles and practice of oncology. Philadelphia: Lippincott, 1989:98–115.
6. Nilsen OS, Munro AJ, Tannock F. Bone metastases: pathophysiology and management policy. J Clin Oncol 25:227–32, 1986.
7. Berretoni BA, Carter JR. Mechanisms of cancer metastases to bone. J Bone Joint Surg 68A:308–12, 1986.
8. Carter RL. Patterns and mechanisms of bone metastases. J R Soc Med Suppl (9) 78:2–6, 1985.
9. Mundy GR, Raisz LG, Cooper RA, et al. Evidence for the secretion of an osteoclast stimulating factor in myeloma. N Engl J Med 291:1041–6, 1974.
10. Frassica FJ, Frassica DA, Lietman SA, et al. Surgical palliation of malignant bone pain. In: Portenoy R, Bruera E, eds. Topics in palliative care. vol 3. New York, Oxford: Oxford University Press, 1998:139–62.
11. Front D, Schneck SO, Frankel A, Robinson E. Bone metastases and bone pain in breast cancer. Are they closely associated? JAMA 242:1747–8, 1979.
12. Hungerford DS. Bone marrow pressure and intramedullary venography, In: Owen R, Goodfellow J, Bullogh P, eds. Scientific foundations of orthopaedics and traumatology. London: Haineman, 1980:357–61.
13. Bennett A. The role of biochemical mediators in peripheral nociception and bone pain. Cancer Surv 7:55–67, 1988.
14. Albright JA, Gillespie TE, Butaud TR. Treatment of bone metastases. Semin Oncol 17:418–34, 1980.
15. Morton AR, Ritch PS. Hypercalcemia. In: Berger AM, Portenoy RK, Weissman DE, eds. Principles and practice of supportive oncology. Philadelphia, New York: Lippincott, 1998:411–25.
16. Healley JH. Metastatic cancer to the bone. In: DeVita VT, Hellman S, Rosenberg SA, eds. Cancer principles and practice of oncology. Philadelphia, New York: Lippincott, 1997:2570–86.
17. Koyama H, Wada T, Nishizawa Y, et al. Cyclophosphamide induced ovarian failure and its therapeutic significance in patients with breast cancer. Cancer 39:1403–9, 1977.
18. Friedlender GE, Tross RB, Doganis AC, et al. Effects of chemotherapeutic agents on bone. Short-term methotrexate and doxorubecin treatment in a rat model [abstract]. J Bone Joint Surg 66A:602–7, 1984.
19. Kanis JA, McCloskey EV, Powles T, et al. A high incidence of vertebral fracture in women with breast cancer. Br J Cancer 78(7–8):1179–81, 1999.
20. Portenoy RK, Hagen N. Breakthrough pain. Definition, prevalence and characteristics. Pain 41:273–83, 1990.
21. Coleman RE. Skeletal complications of malignancy. Cancer Suppl 80 (8):1588–94, 1997.
22. Bruera E, Macmillan K, Hanson J, Macdonald RN. The Edmonton staging system for cancer pain: preliminary report. Pain 37:203–9, 1989.
23. Cleeland C, Portenoy RK, Bruera E, et al. Systematic approaches to cancer pain management [abstract]. Proc Am Pain Soc 81:130, 1991.
24. Hanks GW, Justins DM. Cancer pain: management. Lancet 339:1031–6, 1992.
25. O'Neill WM, Justins DM, Hanks GW. Pain associated with malignant disease. Curr Opin Anaesthesiol 6:845–51, 1993.
26. Plunkett TA, Smith P, Rubens RD. Risks of complications from bone metastases in breast cancer. Eur J Cancer 36:476–82, 2000.
27. Hortobagyi GN, Theriault RL, Porter L, et al. Efficacy of pamidronate in reducing skeletal complications in patients with breast cancer and lytic bone metastases. N Engl J Med 335:1785–91, 1996.
28. Campa JA, Payne R. The management of intractable bone pain: a clinician's perspective. Semin Nucl Med 22:3–10, 1992.
29. Hanks GW. Pharmacological treatment of bone pain. Cancer Surv 7:87–101, 1998.
30. Pereira J. The management of bone pain. In: Portenoy RK, Bruera E, eds. Topics in palliative care, vol. 3. New York, Oxford: Oxford University Press, 1998:79–116.
31. Pereira J, Bruera E. Emerging neuropsychiatric toxicities of opioids. J Pharm Care Pain Symptom Control 5(4):3–29, 1997.

32. Payne R. Mechanisms and management of bone pain. Cancer Suppl 80(8):1608–13, 1997.

33. Bruera E, Fainsinger R, MacEachern T, Hanson J. The use of methylphenidate in patients with incident cancer pain receiving regular opiates. A preliminary report. Pain 50:75–7, 1992.

34. Coluzzi P. A titration study of oral transmucosal fentanyl citrate for breakthrough pain in cancer patients. Proceedings of A.S.C.O. [abstract #143]. 16:41a, 1997.

35. Lyss AP. Long-term use of oral transmucosal fentanyl citrate (OTFC) for breakthrough pain in cancer patients. Proceedings of A.S.C.O. [abstract #144] 16:41a, 1997.

36. Foley K. The treatment of cancer pain. N Engl J Med 313:84–95, 1985.

37. Eisenberg E, Berkey CS, Carr DB, et al. Efficacy and safety of nonsteroidal anti-inflammatory drugs for cancer pain: a meta-analysis. J Clin Oncol 12:2756–65, 1994.

38. Stiefel F, Morant R. Case report: morphine intoxication during acute reversible renal insufficiency. J Palliat Care 7:45–7, 1991.

39. Fainsinger RL, Miller MJ, Bruera E. Letter to the Editor: Morphine intoxication during acute reversible renal insufficiency. J Palliat Care, 8(2):52–3, 1992.

40. Cryer B. Nonsteroidal anti-inflammatory drugs and gastrointestinal disease. In: Feldman M, Scharschmidt BF, Sleisenger MH, eds. Sleisenger and Fordtran's gastrointestinal and liver disease, 6th ed. Philadelphia: WB Saunders, 1998:343–57.

41. Chan C, Boyce S, Brideau C, et al. Pharmacology of a selective cyclooxygenase-2 inhibitor. L-745, 337: a novel non-steroidal anti-inflammatory agent with an ulcerogenic sparing effect in rat and nonhuman primate stomach. J Pharmacol Exp Ther 274:1531–7, 1995.

42. Masferrer J, Zweifel B, Manning PT, et al. Selective inhibition of inducible cyclooxygenase 2 in vivo is anti-inflammatory and non-ulcerogenic. Proc Natl Acad Sci USA 91:3228–32, 1994.

43. Simon LS, Weaver AL, Graham DY, et al. Anti-inflammatory and upper gastrointestinal effects of celecobix in rheumatoid arthritis: a randomized controlled trial. 282:1921–8, 1999.

44. Langman MJ, Jensen DM, Watson DJ, et al. Adverse upper gastrointestinal effects of rofecoxib compared with NSAIDs. 282:1929–33, 1999.

45. Hawkey C, Laine L, Simon T, et al. Comparison of the effect of rofecoxib, ibuprofen and placebo on the gastroduodenal mucosa of patients with osteoarthritis: a randomized double-blind, placebo-controlled trial. The Rofecoxib Osteoarthritis Endoscopy Multinational Study Group. Arthritis Rheum 43(2):370–7, 2000.

46. Swan SK, Rudy DW, Lasseter KC, et al. Effect of cyclooxygenase-2 inhibition on renal function in elderly persons receiving a low-salt diet. A randomized controlled trial. Ann Intern Med 133(1):1–9, 2000.

47. Ettinger AB, Portenoy RK. The use of corticosteroids in the treatment of symptoms associated with cancer. J Pain Symptom Manage 3:99–103, 1988.

48. Levy M. Pharmacological treatment of cancer pain. N Engl J Med 335:1124–32, 1996.

49. Grant R, Papadopoulos SM, Sandler HM, Greenberg HS. Metastatic epidural spinal cord compression: current concepts and treatment. J Nucl Oncol 19:79–92, 1994.

50. Twycross R. The risks and benefits of corticosteroids in advanced cancer. Drug Safety 11:163–78, 1994.

51. Stiefel FC, Breitbard WS, Holland JC. Corticosteroids in cancer: neuropsychiatric complications. Cancer Invest 7(5):479–91, 1989.

52. Vincent FM. The neuropsychiatric complications of corticosteroid therapy. Compr Ther 21(9):524–8, 1995.

53. Dropcho EJ, Twycross RG, Trueman T. Steroid-induced weakness in patients with primary brain tumors. Postgrad Med J 59:702–6, 1983.

54. Boissier S, Ferras M, Peyruchaud O, et al. Bisphosphonates inhibit breast and prostate carcinoma cell invasion, an early event in the formation of bone metastases. 60(11):2949–54, 2000.

55. Diel IJ. Antitumor effects of bisphosphonates: first evidence and possible mechanisms. Drugs 59(3):391–9, 2000.

56. Boissier S, Magnetto S, Frappart L, et al. Bisphosphonates inhibit prostate and breast carcinoma cell adhesion to unmineralized and mineralized bone extracellular matrices. Cancer Res 57(18):3890–4, 1997.

57. Fulfaro F, Casuccio A, Ticozzi C, Ripamonti C. The role of bisphosphonates in the treatment of painful metastatic bone disease: a review of phase III trials. Pain 78(3):157–69, 1998.

58. Walker P, Watanabe S, Lawlor P, et al. Subcutaneous clodronate: a study evaluating efficacy in hypercalcemia of malignancy and local toxicity. Ann Oncol 8:915–6, 1997.

59. Walker P, Bruera E. The role of bisphosphonates in the prevention of osteolysis in palliative care patients. 12th International Congress on Care of the Terminally Ill. J Palliat Care 14:120, 1998.

60. Bloomfield DJ. Should bisphosphonates be part of the standard therapy of patients with multiple myeloma or bone metastases from other cancers? An evidence-based review. J Clin Oncol 16:1218–25, 1998.

61. Lipton A, Theriault RL, Hortobagyi GN, et al. Pamidronate prevents skeletal complications and is effective palliating treatment in women with breast carcinoma and osteolytic bone metastases: long term follow-up of two randomized, placebo-controlled trials. Cancer 88(5):1082–90, 2000.

62. Patterson AH, Powles TJ, Kanis JA, et al. Double-blind controlled trial of oral clodronate in patients with bone metastases from breast cancer. J Clin Oncol 11:59–65, 1993.

63. Kristensen B, Ejlertsen B, Groenvold M, et al. Oral clodronate in breast cancer patients with bone metastases: a randomized study. J Intern Med 246(1):67–74, 1999.

64. Kanis JA, Powles T, Patterson AH, et al. Clodronate decreases the frequency of skeletal metastases in women with breast cancer. Bone 19(6):663–7, 1996.

65. Diel IJ, Solomayer EF, Costa SD, et al. Reduction in new metastases in breast cancer with adjuvant clodronate treatment. N Engl J Med 339(6):357–63, 1998.

66. Diel IJ, Solomayer E, Gollan C, et al. Bisphosphonates in the reduction of metastases in breast cancer-results of the extended follow-up of the first study population [abstract]. Proc Am Soc Clin Oncol 19:82, 2000.

67. Powles TJ, Pattison AH, Nevantaus A, et al. Adjuvant clodronate reduces the incidence of bone metastases in patients with primary operable breast cancer [abstract]. Proc Am Soc Clin Oncol 17:468, 1998.

68. Saarto T, Blomqvist C, Virkkunen P, et al. No reduction of bone metastases with adjuvant clodronate treatment in node positive breast cancer patients [abstract]. Proc Am Soc Clin Oncol 18:489, 1999.

69. McIntyre E, Bruera E. Case report. Symptomatic hypocalcemia after intravenous pamidronate. J Palliat Care 12(1):46–7, 1996.

70. Purohit OP, Anthony C, Radstone CR, et al. High-dose intravenous pamidronate for metastatic bone pain, Br J Cancer 70(3):554–8, 1994.

71. Gatti D, Adami S. New bisphosphonates in the treatment of bone diseases. Drugs Aging 15(4):285–96, 1999.

72. Major P, Lortholary A, Hon J, et al. Zoledronic acid is superior to pamidronate in the treatment of tumor-induced hypercalcemia: a pooled analysis [abstract]. Proc Am Soc Clin Oncol 19:604, 2000.

73. Mortensen L, Charles P, Bekker PJ, et al. Risedronate increases bone mass in an early postmenopausal population: two years of treatment plus one year of follow up. J Clin Endocrinol Metab 83(2):396–402, 1998.

74. Delmas PD, Balena R, Confravreux E. Bisphosphonate risedronate prevents bone loss in women with artificial menopause due to chemotherapy of breast cancer: a double-blind placebo controlled study. J Clin Oncol 15(3):955–62, 1997.

75. Coleman RE, Purohit OP, Black C, et al. Double-blind, randomized placebo-controlled, dose-finding study of oral ibandronate in patients with metastatic bone disease. Ann Oncol 10(3):311–6, 1999.

76. Major PP, Lipton A, Berenson J, Hortobagyi G. Oral bisphosphonates: a review of clinical use in patients with bone metastases. Cancer 88(1):6–14, 2000.

77. Hillner BE, Ingle JN, Berenson JR, et al. American Society of Clinical Oncology guideline on the role of bisphosphonates in breast cancer. American Society of Clinical Oncology Bisphosphonates Expert Panel. J Clin Oncol 18(6):1378–91, 2000.

78. Schiraldi GF, Soresi E, Locicero S, et al. Salmon calcitonin in cancer pain: comparison between two different treatment schedules. Int J Clin Pharmacol Ther Toxicol 25(4):229–32, 1987.

79. Quadt C, Geyer J, Weiner N, et al. Effects of salmon calcitonin on bone metastases in breast cancer patients. Eur J Pharmacol 183:1702, 1990.

80. Mystakidou K, Befon S, Hondros K. Continuous subcutaneous administration of high-dose salmon calcitonin in bone metastasis: pain control and beta-endorphin plasma levels. J Pain Symptom Manage 18(5):323–30, 1999.

81. Kreeger L, Hutton-Potts J. The use of calcitonin in the treatment of metastatic bone pain. J Pain Symptom Manage 17(1):2–5, 1999.

82. Hoskin PJ. Radiotherapy for bone pain. Pain 63:137–9, 1995.

83. Salazar OM, Rubin P, Hendrickson FR, et al. Single-dose half-body irradiation for palliation of multiple bone metastases from solid tumors. Final Radiation Therapy Oncology Group report. Cancer 58(1):29–36, 1986.

84. Macklis RM, Cornelli H, Lasher J. Brief courses of palliative radiotherapy for metastatic bone pain: a pilot cost-minimization comparison with narcotic analgesics. Am J Clin Oncol 21(6):617–22, 1998.

85. Bone Pain Trial Working Party. 8 Gy single fraction radiotherapy for the treatment of metastatic skeletal pain: randomised comparison with a multifraction schedule over 12 months of patient follow-up. Radiother Oncol 52(2):111–21, 1999.

86. Steenland E, Leer JW, van Houwelingen H, et al. The effect of a single fraction compared to multiple fractions on painful bone metastases: a global analysis of the Dutch Bone Metastasis Study. Radiother Oncol 52(2):101–9, 1999.

87. McQuay HJ, Carroll D, Moore RA. Radiotherapy for painful bone metastases: a systematic review. Clin Oncol 9:150–4, 1997.

88. Arcangeli G, Giovinazzo G, Saracino B, et al. Radiation therapy in the management of symptomatic bone metastases: the effect of total dose and histology on pain relief and response duration. Int J Radiat Oncol Biol Phys 42(5): 1119–26, 1998.

89. Lewington VJ, McEwan AJB, Ackery DM, et al. A prospective, randomized double-blind crossover study to examine the efficacy of strontium-89 in pain palliation in patients with advanced prostate cancer metastatic to bone. Eur J Cancer 27:954–8, 1991.

90. Quilty PM, Kirk D, Bolger JJ, et al. A comparison of the palliative effects of strontium-89 and external beam radiotherapy in metastatic prostate cancer. Radiother Oncol 31:33–40, 1994.

91. Serafini AN, Houston SJ, Resche I, et al. Palliation of pain associated with metastatic bone cancer using samarium-153 lexidronam: a double-blind placebo-controlled cinical trial. J Clin Oncol 16(4):1574–81, 1998.

92. Tian JH, Zhang JM, Hou QT, et al. Multicenter trial on the efficacy and toxicity of single-dose samarium-153-ethylene diamine tetramethylene phosphonate as a palliative treatment for painful skeletal metastases in China. Eur J Nucl Med 26(1):2–7, 1999.

93. Sciuto R, Tofani A, Festa A, et al. Short- and long-term effects of 186Re-1,1-hydroxyethylidene diphosphonate in the treatment of painful bone metastases. J Nucl Med 41(4):647–54, 2000.

94. McEwan AJB. Use of radionuclides for the palliation of bone metastases. Semin Radiat Oncol 10(2):103–14, 2000.

95. Harrington KD. Orthopedic surgical management of skeletal complications of malignancy. Cancer 15;80 (8 Suppl):1614–27, 1997.

96. Fidler M. Prophylactic internal fixation of secondary neoplastic deposits in long bones. Br Med J 1(849):341–3, 1973.
97. Harrington KD. Anterior decompression and stabilization of
the spine as a treatment for vertebral collapse and spinal cord
compression from metastatic malignancy. Clin Orthop
233:177–97, 1988.

98. Barr JD, Barr MS, Lemley TJ, McCann RM. Percutaneous
vertebroplasty for pain relief and spinal stabilization. Spine
15;25(8):923–8, 2000.
99. Wallson KA, Burger C, Smith RA, Baugher RJ. Comparing
the quality of death for hospice and non-hospice cancer
patients. Med Care 26:177–82, 1988.

SECTION VIII   SPECIAL TOPICS

25 Pain in medical illness: ethical foundations

PAULINE LESAGE
Beth Israel Medical Center

RUSSELL K. PORTENOY
Albert Einstein College of Medicine

"No moral impulse seems more deeply embedded than the need to relieve suffering ... it has become a foundation stone for the practice of medicine, and it is at the core of the social and welfare programmes of all civilized nations."

Daniel Callahan (1)

Introduction

By introducing major modifications in the historical concepts underlying medical treatments, science and technology have created a certain "chaos" in the care of seriously ill patients. What might have been considered good medical practice for advanced disease before the "biological revolution" is now questioned. Where to draw the line? Where to set limits? Many variables now must be considered in the management of patients with advanced illnesses, including the recognition of ethics as a foundation for clinical practice, the acknowledgment of new rights, and social changes related to health care. Ethical and legal considerations now must constantly inform decision making. Medicine has been caught in a difficult dilemma: Not only does it have to consider its own complexities, but it also has to face a much different social context than existed just a short time ago.

Numerous ethical guidelines and recommendations have been proposed by diverse authorities to help clinicians in their decision making. Recommendations can be found in reports of special presidential or national commissions (2,3), in major congressional reports (4), in policy statements of national organizations (5,6), in guidelines from bioethics institute (7), and in professional journals (8). There is now a body of literature, policy, and law that present an agreed upon set of principles and values, as well as recommendations, for clinical practice.

Nevertheless, medicine's appropriation of these guidelines is lagging behind, as demonstrated by numerous studies on medical practices. The Study to Understand Prognoses and Preferences for Outcomes and Risks of Treatment (SUPPORT) documented serious problems with terminal care: patients experienced considerable pain, communication between physicians and patients was poor, and physicians misunderstood patient's preferences regarding cardiopulmonary resuscitation (9). Other studies have confirmed these deficiencies (10–12).

With the aging of society and the increased prevalence of cancer and other devastating diseases such as AIDS, the goals of medicine need to be refocused. It is essential to reaffirm traditional responsibilities for relieving pain and symptoms, to respond to patients' concerns, to guide their decision-making process, and to respect their informed choices. The need to address these considerations while striving to optimize the technical aspects of care with more humanistic aspects has become a fundamental challenge in the practice of medicine (13–15).

Ethical principles

Ethics is a generic term for different ways to examine moral life. Among many other considerations, bioethics involves practical reasoning about individual patients, balancing their values, hopes, and beliefs with values and principles of medicine and society (16). The most common approach to the resolution of difficult ethical questions is organized around basic principles (17). Ethical principles are general guides that may be applied to the resolution of a particular moral situation and constitute the underlying moral justification for an action. These basic principles—autonomy, beneficence, non-maleficence, and justice (16,18)—must be balanced through case-by-case analyses. None is absolute, and they may compete in the moral resolution of any issue.

Autonomy recognizes the right and ability of an individual to decide for himself or herself based on his or her values and beliefs. It is an affirmation of the person's inviolability. It implies that, with rare exceptions, treatments cannot be imposed against the wishes of the individual and that the choices of individuals must be respected even if they differ from the recommended course of care. Patient's decisions must be informed and free, never coerced. Respect for autonomy implies that the professional must tell the truth, exchange accurate information, and restrain from undue influence. Informed consent is a direct application of the autonomy principle.

Beneficence implies positive acts to maximize the benefits of care. It requires a thoughtful balancing of benefits and harms. It is the most commonly used principle in the application of care. Examples of this principle include delivering effective and beneficial treatment for pain or other symptoms, providing sensitive support, and meeting the obligation to warn against potential dangers.

The principle of *nonmaleficence* supposes that "one ought not to inflict harm deliberately." It is an application of Hippocrates' adage: "Do no harm." It also includes the moral requirement of serving the well-being of patients, following standards of care, and performing risk–benefit assessments. The notion of "harm" interpreted in its broad sense should include physical and mental anguish (suffering). The principle of nonmaleficence supports several moral rules such as "do not kill," and "do not cause pain," etc. Violation of this principle may include offering information in an insensitive way, continuing aggressive therapy despite the likelihood of unsatisfactory results, providing unwanted sedation, and withholding or withdrawing treatment without consent.

Justice implies fairness in the application of care and allocation of resources. It implies that patients receive care to which they are entitled medically and legally. Justice can be translated into "give to each equally" or "to each according to need" or "to each his due." The principle of justice supposes societal considerations and a sense of a common good. The right to health care is an example of this principle.

The basic ethical principles have generated other important principles of care. For example, the *"principle of double effect,"* which is central to many decisions in palliative care, is derived from the principle of nonmaleficence. It has been invoked to support statements that an act potentially having a foreseen harmful effect (such as death) does not always fall under moral prohibitions (such as the rule against killing). It is considered when obligations or values conflict and cannot be realized simultaneously (18). According to double effect, there is a moral difference between the intended effects of a person's action and the unintentional, but foreseen, effects of the action. The desirable effect (good) is linked to an undesirable effect (bad); the good effect is direct and intended, whereas the undesirable effect is indirect and not intended. The principle of double effect has been widely used in moral writings and is particularly useful in end-of-life decision making (see later).

In the administration of medical care, legal requirements cannot be ignored. Some situations that are defensible under ethical principles may not be acceptable under legal provisions. Because law is based on societal values and represents a societal consensus on particular issues, it is not as universal and justified as ethics. Legal provisions impose limits and sanctions on policies, behaviors, and issues of a determined society. The law provides a framework to guide decisions, practices, and requirements that need to be fulfilled to avoid liability. Health care systems and practices in most countries rely on different legal systems: common or civil law, criminal law, statutory law, and regulatory, and disciplinary law.

Clinical decision making

With modern medicine offering countless new technologies and treatments, health care decision making can become a difficult and complex task. The best treatment decisions have been described by medical ethicists as a "combination of medical, emotional, aesthetic, religious, philosophical, social, interpersonal and personal judgments" (16). Considering the complexity involved, patients must take an active role by bringing their histories, values, philosophies, and emotional needs to the decision-making process.

Goals of care

To optimize decision making, the goals of care need to be defined. The determination of goals must consider the stage of the disease (prognosis) and related uncertainty, the possible treatment options, and the personal values, hopes, and understanding of the patient or decision maker. The goals of care are dynamic, not static. They can change rapidly and are sometimes contradictory. They should be realistic. Withholding or withdrawing disease-modifying treatments may be an acceptable alternative in advanced disease, but less so in the early phase of an incurable disease. Continual reassessment of goals is essential to ensure quality of care in accordance with patient wishes.

Confusion about goals can derive in part from a false dichotomy: medical care can either cure disease or alleviate suffering. With the advent of palliative medicine over the last three decades, this distinction is no longer defensible (19,20). In reality, numerous goals are possible, and more than one can be pursued within the context of current realities (21). These may include avoidance of premature death, maintenance or improvement in function, relief of suffering, maintenance of quality of life, and preparation for a good death. Each of these goals may be valid and each must be discussed according to individual circumstances.

In clarifying goals, health care professionals have the difficult task of determining the benefits or harms of procedures or treatments. This is a direct application of the proportionality principle. The latter states that "a medical treatment is ethically mandatory to the extent that it is likely to confer greater benefits than burdens upon the patient" (2,16). Finding the appropriate therapy and avoiding futile treatment are overriding goals of medicine. This task is based on an understanding of futility, informed consent, and decision making in the setting of impaired patient judgment.

Futility

It has long been recognized that the medical profession has no obligation to provide futile medical treatment. Hippocrates advised physicians to "refuse to treat those who are overmastered by their diseases, realizing that in such cases medicine is powerless" (22). This statement may be well understood but does not often simplify the interpretation of medical futility. Futility is a complex, ambiguous, controversial, and subjective concept. Many definitions have been proposed (23–28), and terminology is diverse. It has been equated with "impossible," "rare," "unusual," "hopeless," "nonbeneficial," "inappropriate," and "unreasonable" care. Usually it is defined according to the goals of a specific therapy, its probability of success (quantitative aspect), and the quality of the expected result (qualitative aspect). A treatment is not futile if there is "a real chance of achieving some desirable end, whether that end is cure of the patient, patient comfort, patient dignity, or even comfort to the family" (23).

Defining futility is replete with ambiguity. Are all goals of a treatment acceptable and valuable? What constitutes a desirable end? For some, a treatment is not futile unless it is unlikely to produce any physiologic effect on the body (25). Considering that health care has been defined as a state of physical, mental, and social well-being (29), this view may be too limiting.

If futility is defined in terms of a likelihood of success, what probability of success is acceptable? Considering the uncertainties inherent in medical practice, defining futility based on probability alone cannot be acceptable. This is particularly true given the larger variation in the extent to which patients and physicians are willing to pursue treatments perceived to have a likelihood of failure. In one study, for example, physicians were asked to define "futility" in terms of the likelihood of therapeutic success; the specified likelihood varied between 0% and 60% (median 5%) (30).

The quality of the result adds some insight to the definition of futility because it provides an additional dimension. The overall beneficence of the therapy does not only relate to its effectiveness. This implies the acknowledgment that the goal of a medical treatment is not merely "to cause an effect on some portion of the patient's anatomy, physiology, or chemistry, but to benefit the patient as a whole" (24). Nonetheless, the range of benefits that should be considered is not always clear. If they address quality of life, the complexity of the analysis is great.

The definition of futility cannot be based uniquely on medical criteria (physiologic futility) but also must refer to a "reasonable confidence (quantitative aspect) of providing the sorts of benefits (qualitative) that physicians and patients legitimately expect of the medical enterprise" (31). Given the serious ambiguities that threaten its legitimacy and its highly subjective nature, the concept of futility should be used with caution as a rationale to limit therapy, or adjust the goals of care. It should be evaluated in a broader context and consider the motives underlying demands for "futile" or "unreasonable" treatments, or the desire to withhold treatment based on a futility rationale. Many factors must be weighed, including medical uncertainty, anguish of the family facing an eventual separation, the fear of death or the unknown, denial, and the health care professional's attitude of "doing everything that is possible."

Futility is rarely unequivocal or absolute. The issue often is raised in the face of conflicts over treatment, and there may be misunderstanding among team members, family, and patient. Resolving conflict through better communication and objective information often will eliminate the specific issue of futility. As stated by Younger (32), "when therapeutic innovation becomes technological imperative and hope turns into pathological denial, patients and their families suffer unnecessarily. The concept of futility may provide a much needed corrective, but will better fulfill its promise if those applying it also give attention to the social, psychological, and institutional problems that fostered demands for futile care in the first place."

Informed consent

Katz noted that "the practice of silence was a part of a long and venerable tradition (of medicine) that desired not to be dismissed lightly" (33). Hippocrates, in the Decorum, wrote: "Perform (these duties) calmly and adroitly concealing most things from the patient while you are attending to him (. .) revealing nothing of the patient's future or present condition" (34). This historical trend began to change in some cultures during the second half of the 20th century. The theory of informed consent emerged in medicine from a changing perspective about the nature of the doctor-patient relationship, in ethics as the principle of autonomy, and in law as the right to self-determination. Informed consent implies that decisions about medical care are made in a collaborative manner between patient and physician and thus are resolved through good communication. Informed consent is an expression of trust shaped in the doctor–patient partnership.

Although consent is well accepted in principle, it may be difficult to achieve because of the problems inherent in medical communication, such as the use of technical language; focus on medical uncertainties; the failure to adapt to patient limitations, fears, and culture; limits of patient's understanding; and distraction or the effects of medication or illness. Skillful physician communication is essential to the practice of informed consent and truthtelling is critical to the patients' ability to make reasonable medical decisions. Choices made on the basis of emotion and/or insufficient information can compromise informed consent. Truth telling is particularly challenging in the context of advanced illness because data are often lacking, and the desire to support hope may blur information. Although a decision sometimes is made to limit information for therapeutic purposes (therapeutic privilege), it should be an exception and openly acknowledged when it occurs.

Legal requirements for consent may vary with the legal system of different countries. Generally, in routine practice, informed consent must be obtained before a treatment can be administered (33). This usually implies that a competent patient or proxy receives appropriate information (disclosure), can make a well-considered decision (is informed), and subsequently can express that consent (consent) without coercion (35). The information provided has to be understood and sufficient for the patient to make the best decision possible under the circumstances.

For a patient to be adequately informed, information must be given about the nature and purpose of the proposed treatment or procedure, its risks and benefits, and any available alternatives (35). "Risk" is the element of information most difficult to qualify and to explain. Communications about risk must be consistent with the standard of disclosure (which can vary among different legal systems) and take into account the nature of the risk, its magnitude, and its probability. Serious and frequent risks must be disclosed; remote risks need not be disclosed, unless important and grave. In common law, the legally accepted standard for information is based on conventional professional practice and what any reasonable person would want to know in the same circumstances (35).

To be valid, consent to care must be given by a competent patient or his or her designee. The determination of capacity is a matter of clinical judgment, and there is no consensus on a set of criteria for its evaluation (35,36). Most argue that capacity requires the ability to understand the information, evaluate the options in accordance with the patient's own values, and communicate choices. Although distinct from an assessment of capacity, mental status evaluation is often used as a screening tool. Capacity may fluctuate over time, and it is important to remember that consent is specific to a particular decision and is not necessarily final. Capacity warrants constant re-evaluation.

When a patient is determined to lack capacity to decide, the evaluation that justifies this determination should be recorded in the medical record. Responsible health care providers should be made aware of and become familiar with the person who will make health care decisions for the person.

Decision making for the incompetent

If the patient lacks capacity, someone must be designated to make decisions on the patient's behalf (35,36). This person can be a "guardian" if appointed by the court (rarely the case for terminally ill patients), a "health care agent" designated by written proxy appointed through advance care planning (specifically a living will or durable power of attorney for health care), or a "surrogate" chosen from eligible individuals in a manner that varies with state laws.

Decisions made by third parties must conform to a legal standard, either "best interest" or "substituted judgment" (35). In the "best interest" standard, the decision is made in accordance with what is seen as most beneficial for the patient. This is a direct application of the principle of beneficence and proportionality: maximize benefit and avoid harm. The "substituted judgment" standard aims to implement the subjective preferences of the patient. It takes into consideration the patient's past behavior, statements, or choices. Laws may vary concerning the level of evidence required to state that the patient had a specific preference. They may vary according to the type of decision made (e.g., higher standard for withdrawal of nutrition). Substituted judgment may be preferable, but is applicable only when patients have expressed their wishes. This criterion is applied to the case of advance directives.

Advance directives

Advance directives are oral or written instructions specifying the wishes of a person concerning medical treatment in anticipation of future incapacity (37). They may also provide for designation of a health care agent to make decisions under the same circumstances. They constitute a direct application of the autonomy principle and represent a form of consent. Advance directives can take different forms, including personal letters and medical directives.

The most common types of advance directive are the living will and the durable power of attorney for health care (the person given the power of attorney is known as the health care proxy). These directives can be general or specific. A living will is a legal document that specifies the treatments that would be acceptable or unacceptable to a patient in case of incapacity. Usually, it takes the form of a directive to limit life-sustaining treatment in the face of a life-threatening illness. Durable power of attorney is a document appointing a health care agent or proxy to make decisions according to the incapacitated patient's preference.

In the United States, living wills and laws appointing a health care proxy generally are accepted but vary across states (38). For the most part, they are statutory documents created by state legislatures. They also constitute advisory documents and, for that reason, can act as evidence of the patient's expressed wishes and be binding beyond the state borders. Physicians following directives in living wills are granted immunity against allegations based on the type of care rendered to an incompetent patient.

Ethics of pain and suffering

The relief of pain and suffering has always been a moral responsibility of physicians (22,39). Nowadays, the accessibility, availability, and effectiveness of various methods of pain control make this duty even more compelling. Knowledge in the use of analgesics is mandatory, and not relieving pain optimally is tantamount to moral (40) and legal malpractice (41–43). In principle, physicians are in strong agreement with ethical recommendations regarding pain control (44). Solomon and colleagues (44) showed that 87% of physicians and nurses believed that it is possible to prevent dying patients from feeling much pain, and 81% reported that the most common form of drug abuse in the care of the dying is underuse of opioids (44). Unfortunately, this acceptance of the need for optimal pain control often is not translated into practice (19,40,41,44).

Many factors contribute to the undertreatment of pain. These include deficient skills and outdated attitudes on the part of health care professionals, patient underreporting and poor treatment adherence, and system-wide impediments to optimal analgesic therapy (19). Among other factors, undertreatment of cancer pain has been associated with minority status, female sex, and history of substance abuse (10).

Opioids are sometimes withheld in the setting of advanced medical illness because of fears of hastening death. This attitude requires careful analysis from the ethical and legal perspectives, as well as the medical perspective. Medically, it is now widely accepted that properly administered opioid therapy will rarely, if ever, cause respiratory depression or hasten death. As Twycross observed: "These views stem from ignorance about and misunderstanding of the correct use of morphine in cancer patients with pain. Indeed patients who are truly sentenced to a "kind of living death" are the ones who are not prescribed an adequate analgesic regimen" (45). If doses of an opioid sufficient to relieve pain were to hasten death, as an unintended effect, it may be ethically justifiable according to the principle of double effect, if the conditions discussed next are met. In the setting of pain in advanced medical illness, physicians' concerns about the risks of opioid therapy sometimes relate to inadequate appreciation of both medical and ethical considerations.

Authoritative bodies, such as the U.S. President's Commission for the Study of Ethical Problems in Medicine (2), the Law Reform Commission of Canada (3), and the House of Lords in England (46) have stated that the provision of necessary pain relief is not a matter of potential legal liability. In some locales, legislation has been proposed to protect health care professionals from legal liability if they substantially comply with accepted guidelines for treatment of pain (47). The U.S. Supreme Court strongly affirmed the physicians' obligation to provide adequate pain relief at the end of life, even if it may unintentionally accelerate death, acknowledging, therefore, a right to pain control and relief of suffering (48). The use of analgesics, even if this might hasten death, is considered a standard of good medical practice, and not subject to liability if applied in good faith. Conversely, courts have recognized that improper pain management is a breach of good medical practice and is unacceptable (42,43).

Sedation in terminal illness

Another set of issues related to pain in those with advanced illness concerns the use of sedation to treat refractory symptoms. Good palliative medicine can alleviate suffering caused by pain and other symptoms in most cases (29,49–52). When suffering cannot be managed at the end of life, sedation may represent an option. Sedation at the end-of-life may be controversial, however, and possibly unacceptable to some patients, families, and health care providers (29,53).

Although the definition of "terminal sedation" has been debated (54,55), the vast majority of experts in palliative care define it as a clinical intervention in patients who are perceived to be near death (53,54,56), by which unconsciousness is induced as a mean to relieve symptoms that cannot be otherwise satisfactorily. It is considered an exceptional therapeutic measure with specific indications intended to alleviate suffering in the imminently dying.

Although it must be acknowledged that sedation for intractable symptoms could possibly accelerate the dying process, it may be ethically justifiable under the principle of double effect (57). The approach has been accepted directly by various medical societies and ethicists (15,58–60), and indirectly by the U.S. Supreme Court (48). There is little disagreement among palliative care professionals about the necessity of using sedation to achieve symptom control in some dying patients. However, variability in the use of terminal sedation highlights the uncertainty surrounding this practice (53,61–63).

Some have considered sedation in the imminently dying as a form of "euthanasia in disguise" (64). This reasoning fails to note the fundamental differences between the two practices (55,65). Their intent is differ-

ent (death is the unintended, although foreseen, result in sedation, as opposed to the intended result in assisted suicide and euthanasia) and they diverge in their actions undertaken (a sedative dose is not a killing dose). The option of sedation recognizes the right to be relieved of suffering, not the right to die. To be legally acceptable, sedation should be carried out in a manner consistent with the intent of alleviating suffering. The action should reflect the purpose.

The literature shows a lack of consensus with regard to medications, dosages, and routes used to induce sedation (53,54). Benzodiazepines and barbiturates, or a combination of these agents, are the most widely used drugs, but the approach has also been implemented using opioids, neuroleptics, ketamine, propofol, and others. Whatever the agent selected, dose titration to achieve relief is required before continuing maintenance therapy at the lowest dosage possible.

Because of the serious implications of sedation in the imminently dying, its implementation should follow guidelines based on compassion, consideration, and trust (66). When presented as a therapeutic option, sedation may be perceived by the patient or family as a sign of disease severity as well as suffering. Sedation should be implemented only after clarification of the medical condition, a thorough discussion with the patient and family has taken place, consent has been obtained, and the goals of care have been clearly established. Once sedation has been activated, ongoing information should be provided to family and staff, questions should be answered, and ethical and legal implications should be clarified (66).

Other end-of-life issues

Withholding/withdrawing therapy

In a course of a chronic illness, there may come a point beyond which a treatment becomes futile or disproportionate. At this time, withholding or withdrawing a therapy may be considered (2,67). These practices imply that the patient does without a medical intervention that might have been expected to extend life in some circumstances (reference 2, p. 2, note 1), but now is perceived as futile or averse. Withholding occurs when a treatment is not provided; withdrawing is defined as ending treatment that has no demonstrated value. Both practices relate to the proportionality of treatment and are applied in the context of an incurable or irreversible condition. Refusing the medical intervention, or withdrawing one that has been applied, allows the disease to take its natural course; if death occurs, it is the result of the underlying disease. Although health care professionals often believe that there is a distinction between withholding and withdrawal (44)—there may be a tacit belief that once a treatment is started, it cannot be stopped—this assumption has no ethical, legal, or medical basis, and the distinction is more psychologically compelling than logically sound (7,68).

Withholding and withdrawing therapies have been well accepted as part of good medical practice by various authoritative bodies (2,13,69). They have received legal acknowledgment in the United States (70,71). Many institutions have drafted policies addressing these issues.

Although the withholding and withdrawing of therapies have been described mainly in situations related to technical interventions (e.g., ventilator support, hemodialysis), the reasoning also applies to chemotherapy, artificial hydration and nutrition, and any therapy offered at the end of life to delay death (72). In this regard, withholding and withdrawal of treatment must be clearly distinguished from physician-assisted suicide (PAS) and euthanasia (see later).

Do-not-resuscitate order

Cardiopulmonary resuscitation was originally developed as a closed-chest massage for victims of sudden cardiac or respiratory arrest. The overall survival rate averages 15% under the best circumstances (good health status and resuscitation started within 5 minutes of arrest) (73). Survival is related to the underlying illness; it is almost never successful in patients with chronic debilitating illnesses (1%–4%) (74).

The medical, ethical, and legal issues involved in resuscitation have been extensively discussed in the literature (75–77). Like any other treatment, physicians have the obligation to clarify the medical indication for the therapy, as well as patients' wishes concerning resuscitation. In practice, discussion and implementation of the do-not-resuscitate (DNR) order seem highly problematic and poorly achieved by medical staff. In the large SUPPORT trial, investigators demonstrated that only 47% of physicians knew when their patients preferred to avoid CPR, and 46% of DNR orders were written within 2 days of death (9). These results failed to improve with an intervention designed to facilitate advance care planning and patient–physician communication (9). The lack of focus on goals of care, poor medical training in communication, residual uncertainties about the success rate of DNR, and misinterpretation of futility all contribute to these difficulties.

The DNR order must be distinguished from other aspects of care offered near the end of life. A patient who has elected a DNR designation can still continue parenteral nutrition and be treated aggressively for an infection or any other condition. These other issues warrant an open discussion with the patient, who must be informed about the various options for treatment. The discussion about resuscitation should be placed into the broader context of life-prolonging therapies. This will prevent a sense of abandonment, which can be implicit in DNR discussions.

Artificial hydration and nutrition

Because of the high symbolic value of nutrition, the question of withholding or withdrawing artificial hydration or alimentation is often difficult to address with the patient and family. It can be perceived as neglect, abandonment, or hastening death. The decision-making process of the patient and family can be helped by an open discussion about the misperceptions, advantages and concerns associated with artificial nutrition. It has been shown by many authors that, with few exceptions, patients with incurable neoplastic disease do not benefit from artificial nutrition (78,79). It also has been documented that, in certain circumstances, artificial fluids and nutrition may worsen edema, ascites, pulmonary and other secretions, and dyspnea (80,81). In case law, artificial nutrition and hydration have been considered a treatment and, as such, governed by the same legal and ethical principles of withholding or withdrawal (82,83).

Discussion surrounding nutrition and hydration must take into account the emotions and religious beliefs attached to this issue. Although the discourse is rarely neutral, it can strive to be explanatory and place these interventions into the context of the overall goals of care.

Ventilator withdrawal

The withdrawal of ventilator support from a patient is clinically and ethically challenging for patients, families, and members of the health care team. The uncertainty of the outcome, as well as the dramatic events surrounding the procedure, contribute to the challenge, especially in the case of immediate extubation (84). The technique for ventilator removal should be addressed with the patient and family, when possible. Terminal weaning to assess the patient's comfort during the procedure, followed by aggressive interventions to prevent symptoms, such as breathlessness and anxiety, are essential (85). It is ethical and legal to use a combination of opioid and anxiolytic therapies to treat these symptoms.

Physician-assisted suicide and euthanasia

Euthanasia and physician-assisted suicide (PAS) have been the subject of intense debate for centuries (86–90). The current debate is framed by the acceptance of withholding and withdrawing life-sustaining therapies, the self-determination movement, the promotion of choice in decision making at the end of life, and changes in social values.

The debate on PAS and euthanasia has been fraught with difficulty, in part because of the use of ambiguous and confusing terms (86,91–93). PAS is best defined as "aiding or helping to bring about death for compassionate reasons" (94). This definition implies that the intention is clear (death of the patient) and the performing agent is the patient, the accessory agent (providing the means) is the physician, and the motive is usually compassion. Although there have been many definitions of euthanasia, or more precisely many categories (active, passive, voluntary, involuntary), it is now well accepted that euthanasia means to "bring or give death for compassionate reasons" (58,94). In this case the intention is similarly clear (death of the patient), the performing agent is the physician or third party, and the motive is usually compassion.

In the clinical setting, a request for PAS or euthanasia should be taken seriously. It is important to clarify the request, assess the underlying motives, re-emphasize the commitment to symptom control and provision of palliative care, and discuss alternatives.

The debate on euthanasia generally has focused on the principle of autonomy, the distinction between killing and letting die, the relief of suffering, and the "slippery slope" argument (89,94–97). Each of these considerations may be framed to support or oppose euthanasia.

Assisted suicide or euthanasia implies the right to be relieved from pain and suffering, as well as the right to die. For many, it is seen as the extrapolation of the principle of autonomy: one can choose the moment and means of one's death. The debate struggles with the appropriateness of limits to autonomy (98,99). The observation that palliative interventions can lead some patients to change their minds about assisted suicide (100) raises fundamental questions about the reality of autonomy when patients (and sometimes physicians) are unsure about the potential for further palliative care, which may relieve suffering without the necessity of death.

Advocates of euthanasia and PAS may draw comparisons to the withholding or withdrawal of treatment, neglecting the distinction between killing and letting die (40,99,101). This is difficult to justify. Although killing and letting die have the same end result (e.g., the death of the patient), they are quite different in their intent (102). Death is the unplanned but foreseen result in withholding and withdrawal of treatment, as opposed to the intended effect in euthanasia and PAS. The latter represents another application of the principle of double effect. Again, intent or purpose is traditionally used by the law to distinguish between two acts that have the same result (48).

Although a patient's request for PAS can be broadly interpreted as a cry for help, each person has a set of personal reasons for the desire to hasten death. Unrelieved pain may not be the major or sole reason for requests for physician-assisted death (91,103–106). In a Dutch study, unrelieved pain was the sole reason for euthanasia requests in 5% of the cases, was part of the problem in 40%, and was not reported at all in the remaining cases (92). Instead, depression, unrelieved psychosocial distress, loss of dignity, loss of control, other quality of life issues, and perceived burden on the family were the most common justifications (91,103). Other studies also highlight the importance of depression (107–109). Physicians, patients, and the public find PAS and euthanasia more acceptable for patients in persistent pain than those who wish to spare their families (107).

The potential for abuse of euthanasia and PAS is expressed by those opposed to these practices (99,101,110,111). Evidence for abuse of euthanasia may be found in Dutch data, which include 0.8% of deaths without explicit and repeated requests from the patient (in half of these cases there may have been previous discussions with the patient about such measures) (112). Data from the United States have shown that 19% of critical care nurses had engaged in some form of euthanasia or PAS, at times without physician supervision or outside the hospital (113). These observations also raise the "slippery slope" argument (95,110,111). If PAS or euthanasia becomes common practice, it may not be possible to limit these practices to terminal illness or to those capable of providing fully informed consent. Determination of guidelines or safeguards remain difficult and somewhat illusory, as the underlying concepts are ill defined (114). What is intolerable pain? What is a terminal condition? Is the consent really informed? In a society that prioritizes cost control, there is even a concern that policy makers or health care professionals would be tempted to shorten a lengthy incurable illness (115). As stated by the New York Task Force on Life and Law "the dangers of a dramatic change in public policy (legalization of PAS and euthanasia) would far outweigh any possible benefits. In light of the pervasive failure of our health care system to treat pain, and diagnose and treat depression, legalizing assisted suicide and euthanasia would be profoundly dangerous for many individuals who are ill and vulnerable. The risks would be most severe for those who are elderly, poor, socially disadvantaged, or without access to medical care" (109).

Over the last two decades, there has been progress in the legal acknowledgment of patients' rights at the end of life. Patients have the right to refuse unwanted treatment or to stop once it has been started (116,117). They have the right to forego life-sustaining therapies (70,118). There is also a recognized right to intensive palliative care and control of pain (48,119). Euthanasia is illegal in all countries except The Netherlands. Assisted suicide was legalized for a time in the Northern Territory of Australia (120) and is currently legal in Oregon. The U.S. Supreme Court ruled that there is no constitutionally guaranteed right to PAS or euthanasia, and, therefore, no constitutional right to die (42,70,121).

Access to palliative care

Most people die after experiencing a protracted, life-threatening illness with a slow decline or unpredictable terminal course. Currently, 9 million people around the world develop cancer. By 2015, this figure is expected to rise to 15 million. The size of the population aged 60 years and over is increasing dramatically and will rise from the present 9.3% to 15% in the year 2030 (122). The need to develop health care resources to meet changing needs is critical. One such need is for access to optimal palliative care at the end of life. Although hospices and palliative care programs have emerged to address this need, most countries do not have access to palliative care services. In the United States, only 15% of all dying patients and 25% to 35% of patients with cancer die in hospice programs, and most referrals to hospice are made very late in the course of terminal illness (123). There are yet very few hospital-based and home-based palliative care programs, and there is substantial evidence that undertreatment of pain and other symptoms continues to be a profound problem, as discussed previously (10,122,124).

Many reasons are proffered to explain the limited access to palliative care at the end of life (125). Frequently, neither the public nor the health care providers acknowledge the importance of end-of-life care. It is often introduced late in the disease and has little impact. Clinicians receive no formal training in palliative medicine and end-of-life

care, lack skills in communication and assessment of the goals of care, and have attitudes and fears that may be barriers to the care of the dying (126,127). Patients' fears, cultural beliefs, denial, or lack of awareness about prognosis also may interfere with the willingness to be referred to hospice or pursue palliative care.

Although there is growing support for access to palliative care, particularly at the end of life, there is still much to do (122). Educating the general public, health care professionals, and policy makers; changing health care systems; and adapting to rapid technological changes remain significant challenges for palliative care. The ability of societies and individuals to pay for optimal palliative care is a great concern. The nature of palliative care, including uncertainties related to prognosis and cost–benefit of interventions, make cost projections difficult (115). In a time of cost control and limited resources, societies are therefore moving slowly to introduce palliative care into health care system. There are numerous challenges in integrating palliative care, and in identifying the funds necessary to optimize treatment and support specialists. It will be regrettable if individuals have to choose PAS or euthanasia to alleviate their suffering because of the unavailability of palliative care (128).

Research

The last set of ethical challenges relates to research. Although there is a well-established consensus about the use of human subjects under certain conditions, research in advanced illness generates intense ethical debate (129,130). Research, in this specific population, is ethically charged with the inherent problems of any research, such as informed consent, the depersonalization issue, the balance between risks and benefits, the vulnerability of subjects, the use of placebo, and the possibility of conflicting loyalties of the physician-researcher. These issues may be amplified by the nature of advanced illness (129).

Patients' vulnerability probably represents the most important concern. Because the very diagnosis of incurable illness carries the burden of fear and despair, patients may agree more readily to unproven interventions. The illusion of a cure may have a greater influence on their participation than in other populations. The nature of the disease, with its high level of disability, fatigue, depression, and perhaps cognitive impairment, may alter the patient's response to proposals that might not be in their best interests.

A prerequisite to research, as well as any treatment, is informed consent. In the context of serious illness, particularly when associated with unrelieved pain, patients' understanding and competence may be altered (131,132). The regulations that govern informed consent for research are more demanding than for usual medical treatments. The subject must be presented with the diagnosis, prognosis, alternative treatments, and the consequences of no treatment. He or she must be told that participation is voluntary, that therapy can be withdrawn at any time, and that access to conventional medical treatments will not be altered by his or her decision to participate or not. In advanced illness, all this information is processed though a filter shaped by the issues inherent in vulnerability. "Selective hearing" is not unusual in this group of patients (133,134). Cognitive impairment can be subtle and go unrecognized unless tested specifically (132).

The clinical instability related to advanced illness adds to the ethical complexity of participation in research. Poor performance status of many medically ill patients is often invoked to deny enrollment in different trials and research protocols. Although such an attitude may conform to the proportionality or beneficence principle, too much emphasis on this aspect may be detrimental over time because it limits the scope of research in a manner that may be excessive.

The use of placebo in palliative care research also is considered controversial, especially in pain research. The Guidelines of the National Council for Hospice and Specialist Palliative Care Services on Research in Palliative Care specify that "giving a placebo is not justified if there is a therapy known to be more effective than a placebo" (135). But what if there is no known effective therapy or the overriding need is to demonstrate the effectiveness of a therapy? Placebo trials can be ethical if a placebo does not replace standard therapy, patients know that they be receiving a placebo, there is uncertainty as to the merits of the treatments being tested in the trial, and patients have access to therapy if distress increases (136).

Research in palliative care has been proven to be beneficial to participating patients, as it has for other patients (137). The need to document practices, to promote good palliative care as evidence based, and to expand the scientific basis of this care are valid reasons to pursue research in these patients (130). It would be unfortunate to jeopardize research for patients with serious illness without careful consideration of the benefits and burdens associated with both the withholding of the option to participate and the granting of this option. Review of research protocols by ethics committees constitutes a warranty of respect for ethical principles and due process.

Conclusion

Medical care is changing significantly. To meet the challenges of the 21st century, some changes in the culture of medicine are necessary. Ethical and legal considerations must be integrated in the clinical decision-making process. By providing an intellectual and pragmatic framework for pursuing the values of autonomy, beneficence and justice, ethics is central to the development of a comprehensive, compassionate and respectful practice of medicine, especially in the management of pain and difficult decisions related to palliative care.

References

1. Callahan C. The troubled dream of life: in search of a peaceful death. New York: Simon and Schuster, 1993:94.
2. President's Commission for the Study of Ethical Problems in Medicine and Biomedical and Behavioral Research. Deciding to Forego Life-Sustaining Treatment: Ethical, Medical, and Legal Issues in Treatment Decisions. Washington, DC: US Government Printing Office, 1983.
3. Commission de reforme du droit du Canada. Euthonasie, aide au suicide et interruption detraitement. Document de travail 28, Ottawa, Ministere des approvisionnements et services, Canada 1982.
4. Life-sustaining technologies and the elderly. Washington, DC: US Congress, Office of Technology Assessment, 1987.
5. Current Opinions of the Council on Ethical and Judicial Affairs of the American Medical Association. Withholding or withdrawing life prolonging treatment. Chicago: American Medical Association, 1992.
6. American Nurses' Association Task Force on the Nurse's Role in End-of-Life Decisions. Position statement on foregoing artificial nutrition and hydration. Washington, DC: American Nurses' Association, 1992.
7. Hastings Center. Guidelines on the termination of life-sustaining treatment and the care of the dying. Bloomington & Indianapolis: Indiana University Press, 1987:6.
8. Wanzer SH, Adelstein SJ, Cranford RE, et al. The physician's responsibility toward hopelessly ill patients. N Engl J Med 310:955–9, 1984.
9. The SUPPORT Principal Investigators for the SUPPORT Project. A controlled trial to improve care for seriously ill hospitalized patients: the Study to Understand Prognoses and Preferences for Outcomes and Risks of Treatments (SUPPORT). JAMA 274:1591–8, 1995.
10. Cleeland CS, Gonin R, Hatfield AK, et al. Pain and its treatment in outpatients with metastatic cancer. N Engl J Med 330:592–6, 1994.
11. Seckler AB, Meier DB, Mulvihill M, Paris BEC. Substituted judgment: how accurate are proxy predictions? Ann Intern Med 115:92–8, 1991.
12. Carver AC, Vickrey BG, Bernat JL, et al. End-of-life care: a survey of US neurologists' attitudes, behavior, and knowledge. Neurology 53:284–93, 1999.

13. American Medical Association Council on Scientific Affairs. Good care of the dying patient. JAMA 275:474–8, 1996.

14. American Board of Internal Medicine End-of-Life Patient Care Project Committee. Caring for the dying: identification and promotion of physician competency. Philadelphia: American Board of Internal Medicine, 1996.

15. American College of Physicians Ethics and Human Rights Committee. Ethics manual. Ann Intern Med 117:946–60, 1992.

16. Jonsen AR, Siegler M, Winsdale WJ. Clinical ethics, 3rd ed. New York: McGraw-Hill, 1992.

17. Pellegrino ED. The metamorphosis of medical ethics. JAMA 269:1158–62, 1993.

18. Beauchamp TL, Childress JF, eds. Principles of biomedical ethics, 4th ed. New York: Oxford University Press, 1994.

19. Portenoy RK. Contemporary diagnosis and management of pain in oncology and AIDS patients, 3rd ed. Newtown, PA: Handbooks in Health Care Co, 2000:43–5.

20. Billings JA. What is palliative care? J Palliat Med 1:73–81, 1998.

21. Cassell EJ. The nature of suffering and the goals of medicine. N Engl J Med 306:639–45, 1982.

22. Hippocrates. The art. In: Reiser SJ, Dyck AJ, Curran WJ, eds. Ethics in medicine: historical perspectives and contemporary concerns. Cambridge, MA: MIT Press, 1977:6–7.

23. Rosner F, Kark PR, Bennett AJ, et al. Medical futility. NYS J Med 92:485–8, 1992.

24. Schneiderman LJ, Jecker NS, Jonsen AR. Medical futility: its meaning and ethical implications. Ann Intern Med 112:949–54, 1990.

25. Truog RD, Brett AS, Frader J. The problem with futility. N Engl J Med 326:1560–3, 1992.

26. Brett AS, McCullough LB. When patients request specific interventions: defining the limits of the physician's obligation. N Engl J Med 315:1347–51, 1986.

27. Cranford R, Gostin L. Futility: a concept in search of a definition. J Med Health Care 20:307, 1992.

28. Swanson JW, McCrary SV. Doing all they can: physicians who deny medical futility. J Law, Med Ethics 22(4):318–26, 1994.

29. World Health Organization. Cancer Pain Relief and Palliative Care. Geneva: World Health Organization, 1996.

30. McCrary SV. Physician's quantitative assessments of medical futility. J Med Ethics 5(2):100, 1994.

31. Brody H. The multiple facets of futility. J Clin Ethics 52:142, 1994.

32. Younger SJ. Futility in clinical practice. J Am Geriatr Soc 42(8):889, 1994.

33. Katz J. Informed consent: ethical and legal issues. In: Arras JD, Steinbock B, eds. Ethical issues in modern medicine. Mountain View, CA: Mayfield Publishing Co, 1995:87–97.

34. Selections from the Hippocratic Corpus "Decorum XVI." In: Reiser SJ, Dick AJ, Curran WJ, eds. Ethics in medicine. Cambridge, MA: MIT Press, 1977.

35. Appelbaum PS, Lidz CW, Meisel A. Informed consent. Legal theory and clinical practice. New York: Oxford University Press, 1987.

36. Neveloff-Dubler N, Farber-Post L. Truth telling and informed consent. In: Holland J, ed. Psycho-oncology. New York: Oxford University Press, 1998.

37. Emanuel LL, Barry MJ, Emanuel EJ, Stoeckle JD. Advance directives: can patients' stated treatment choices be used to infer unstated choices? Medical Care 32(2):95–105, 1994.

38. Annas GJ. The health care proxy and the living will. N Engl J Med 324:1210–3, 1991.

39. Gregory J. On the duties and offices of physicians. London: W Straham, 1772.

40. Pellegrino ED. Doctors must not kill. J Clin Ethics 3:95–107, 1992.

41. Somerville MA. Death of pain: pain, suffering, and ethics. In: Gebhart GF, Hammond DL, Jensen TS, eds. Proceedings of the 7th World Congress on Pain, Progress in Pain Research and Management, vol 2. Seattle: IASP Press, 1994.

42. *State v McAfee,* 259 Ga. 579, 385S.L. 2d 651 (Ga.1989).

43. *Estate of Henry James v Hill Haven Corp.,* Superior Court Div. 89 CVS 64, Hartford County, NC (Jan 15, 1991).

44. Solomon MZ, O'Donnell L, Jennings B, et al. Decisions near the end of life: professional views of life-sustaining treatments. Am J Public Health 83(1):14–24 1993.

45. Twycross RG, Lack SA. Therapeutics in terminal cancer. London: Pitman, 1984:184.

46. *Airedale NHS Trust v Bland* (1993) 1 ALL E.R. 821; (1993) 1 H.L.J. 7.

47. Johnson S. Disciplinary actions and pain relief: analysis of the Pain Relief Act. J Law Med Ethics 24:319–27, 1996.

48. *Vacco v Quill,* 117 S Ct 2293 (1997).

49. Wallston KA, Burger C, Smith RA, Baugher RJ. Comparing the quality of death for hospice and non-hospice cancer patients. Med Care 26:177–82, 1998.

50. Ventafridda V, Ripamonti C, De Conno F, et al. Symptom prevalence and control during cancer patients' last days of life. J Palliat Care 6:7–11, 1990.

51. Byock I. Dying well: prospects for growth at the end of life. New York: Riverhead Books, 1997.

52. Coyle N, Adelhardt J, Foley KM, Portenoy RK. Character of terminal illness in the advanced cancer patient: pain and other symptoms during the last four weeks of life. J Pain Symptom Manage 5:83–93, 1990.

53. Chater S, Viola R, Paterson J, Jarvis V. Sedation for intractable distress in the dying: a survey of experts. Palliat Med 12:255–69, 1998.

54. Cherny NI, Portenoy RK. Sedation in the management of refractory symptoms: guidelines for evaluation and treatment. J Palliat Care 10:31–8, 1994.

55. Mount B. Morphine drips, terminal sedation, and slow euthanasia: definitions and facts, not anecdotes. J Palliat Care 12:31–7, 1996.

56. Quill T, Lo B, Brock D. Palliative options of last resort: a comparison of voluntary stopping eating and drinking, terminal sedation, physician-assisted suicide, and voluntary euthanasia. JAMA 278:2099–104, 1997.

57. Sulmasy DP. The use and abuse of the principle of double effect. Clin Pract 3:86–90, 1996.

58. American Medical Association Council on Ethical and Judicial Affairs. Decisions near the end of life. JAMA 267:2229–33, 1992.

59. Wanzer SH, Federman DD, Adelstein SJ, et al. The physician's responsibility toward hopelessly ill patients–a second look. N Engl J Med 129:844–9, 1989.

60. Byock IR. When suffering persists. J Palliat Care 10:8–13, 1994.

61. Morita T, Inoue S, Chihara S. Sedation for symptom control in Japan: the importance of intermittent use and communication with family members. J Pain Symptom Manage 12:32–8, 1996.

62. Ventafridda V, Ripamonti C, De Conno F, et al. Symptom prevalence and control during cancer patients' last days of life. J Palliat Care 6:7–11, 1990.

63. Fainsinger R, MacEachern T, Hanson J, et al. Symptom control during the last week of life on a palliative care unit. J Palliat Care 7:5–11, 1991.

64. Billings J, Block S. Slow euthanasia. J Palliat Care 12:38–41, 1996.

65. Cavanaugh TA. The ethics of death hastening or death-causing palliative analgesic administration to the terminally ill. J Pain Symptom Manage 12:248–54, 1996.

66. Cherny N, Coyle N, Foley K. Guidelines in the care of the dying cancer patient. Hematol Oncol Clin North Am 1:261–86, 1996.

67. The Hastings Center. Guidelines on the termination of life sustaining treatment in the care of the dying. Briarcliff Manor, NY: The Hastings Center, 1987.

68. Lesage P, Latimer E. Case 2. In: MacDonald N, Boisvert M, Dungeon D, et al, eds. Palliative medicine: a case based manual. New York: Oxford University Press, 1998.

69. AGS Ethics Committee. A position statement from the American Geriatrics Society. J Am Geriatr Soc 43:477–8, 1995.

70. Burt RA. The Supreme Court speaks. Not assisted suicide but a constitutional right to palliative care. N Engl J Med 337:1234, 1997.

71. Meisel A. Legal myths about terminating life support. Arch Intern Med 151:1497–502, 1991.

72. AMA, Statement of Council on Ethical and Judicial Affairs. Withholding or withdrawing life-prolonging medical treatment. JAMA 256:471, 1986.

73. Blackhall LJ. Must we always use CPR? N Engl J Med 317:1281–5, 1987.

74. Faber-Langendorf K. Resuscitation of patients with metastatic cancer: is a transient benefit still futile? Arch Intern Med 151:235–9, 1991.

75. Tomlinson T, Broday H. Futility and the ethics of resuscitation. JAMA 264:1276–80, 1990.

76. Lo B. Unanswered questions about DNR orders. JAMA 265:1874–75, 1991.

77. Council on Ethical and Judicial Affairs, American Medical Association. Guidelines for the appropriate use of do-not-resuscitate orders. JAMA 265:1868–71, 1991.

78. Barber MD, Fearon KC, Delmore G, Loprinzi CL. Current controversies in cancer: should cancer patients with incurable disease receive parenteral or enteral nutritional support? Eur J Cancer 34:279–85, 1998.

79. Torelli GF, Campos AC, Meguid MM. Use of TPN in terminally ill cancer patients. Nutrition 15:665–7, 1999.

80. Zerwekh JV. Do dying patients really need IV fluids? Am J Nurs 97:26–31, 1997.

81. Zerwekh JV. The dehydration question. Nursing 83:47–51, 1983.

82. *Brophy v New England Sinai Hospital* 497 N.E. 2d 626 (Mass. 1986).

83. *Cruzan v Director Missouri Dept. of Health,* United States Supreme Court, no 88-1503, June 25th, 1990.

84. Edwards MJ, Tolle SW. Disconnecting a ventilator at the request of a patient who knows he will then die: the doctor's anguish. Ann Intern Med 117:254–6, 1992.

85. Wilson WC, Smedira NG, Fink C, et al. Ordering and administration of sedatives and analgesics during the withholding and withdrawal of life support from critically ill patients. JAMA 267:949–53, 1992.

86. Kelleher MJ, Chambers D, Corcoran P, et al. Euthanasia and related practices world wide. Crisis 19:109–15, 1998.

87. Gittelman DK. Euthanasia and physician-assisted suicide. South Med J 92:369–74, 1999.

88. Kasting GA. The nonnecessity of euthanasia. In: Humber JD, Almeder RF, Kasting GA, eds. Physician-assisted death. Totowa, NJ: Humana Press, 1993:25–43.

89. Brody H. Assisted death–a compassionate response to a medical failure. N Engl J Med 327:1384–8, 1992.

90. Meir DE, Emmons CA, Wallenstein S, et al. A national survey of physician-assisted suicide and euthanasia in the United States. N Engl J Med 338:1193–1201, 1998.

91. van der Maas PJ, van der Wal G, Averkate I, et al. Euthanasia, physician-assisted suicide, and other practices involving the end of life in the Netherlands, 1990–1995. N Engl J Med 335:1699–1705, 1996.

92. van der Maas PJ, van Delden JJ, Pijnenborg L. Euthanasia and other medical decisions concerning the end of life: an investigation, vol. 2. New York: Elsevier, 1992.

93. Miller IG, Fins JJ, Snyder L, et al. Assisted suicide compared with refusal of treatment: a valid distinction? Ann Intern Med 132:470–5, 2000.

94. Emanuel EJ. Euthanasia: historical, ethical and empiric perspectives. Arch Intern Med 154:1890–1901, 1994.

95. Ryan CJ. Pulling up the runway: the effect of new evidence on euthanasia's slippery slope. J Med Ethics 24:341–4, 1998.

96. Brock DW. Voluntary active euthanasia. Hastings Center Rep 22:11–22, 1992.

97. Cassel C, Meir DE. Morals and moralism in the debate over euthanasia and assisted suicide. N Engl J Med 323:750–2, 1990.

98. Salem T. Physician-assisted suicide: promoting autonomy—or medicalizing suicide. Hastings Center Rep 29.3:30–6, 1999.

99. Callahan D. When self-determination runs amok. Hastings Cent Rep 22:52–5, 1992.

100. Ganzini L, Nelson HD, Schmidt TA, et al. Physicians' experience with the Oregon Death With Dignity Act. N Engl J Med 342:557–604, 2000.

101. Kass LR. Is there a right to die? Hastings Cent Rep 23:34–43, 1993.

102. Miller FG, Fins JJ, Snyder L. Assisted suicide compared with refusal of treatment: a valid distinction? Ann Intern Med 132:470–5, 2000.

103. Back AL, Wallace JI, Starks HE, Pearlman RA. Physician-assisted suicide and euthanasia in Washington State. Patient requests and physician responses. JAMA 275:919–25, 1996.

104. Seale C, Addington-Hall J. Euthanasia: why people want to die earlier. Soc Sci Med 39:647–54, 1994.

105. Foley K. The relationship of pain and symptom management to patient request for physician-assisted suicide. J Pain Symptom Manage 6:289–97, 1991.

106. Emanuel EJ. Ethics of treatment: palliative and terminal care. In: Holland JC, ed. Psycho-oncology. New York: Oxford University Press, 1998.

107. Emanuel EJ, Fairclough DL, Daniels ER, Clarridge BR. Euthanasia and physician-assisted assisted suicide: attitudes and experiences of oncology patients, oncologists, and the public. Lancet 347:1805–10, 1996.

108. Breitbart W, Rosenfeld BD, Passik SD. Interest in physician-assisted suicide among ambulatory HIV-infected patients. Am J Psychiatry 153:238–42, 1996.

109. The New York Task Force on Life and the Law. When death is sought: assisted suicide and euthanasia in the medical context. New York: NYS Task Force on Life and the Law, 1994.

110. Singer PA, Siegler M. Euthanasia–a critique. N Engl J Med 322:1881–3, 1990.

111. Capron AM. Euthanasia in the Netherlands: American observations. Hastings Cent Rep 22:30–3, 1992.

112. van der Maas PJ, van Delden JJM, Pinjnenborg L, Looman CWM. Euthanasia and other medical decisions concerning the end of life. Lancet 338:669–74, 1991.

113. Asch D. The role of critical care nurses in euthanasia and physician-assisted suicide. N Engl J Med 334:1374–9, 1996.

114. Caplan AL, Snyder L, Faber-Langendoen K. The role of guidelines in the practice of physician-assisted suicide. Ann Intern Med 132:476–81, 2000.

115. Emanuel EJ, Emanuel LL. The economics of dying. The illusion of cost savings at the end of life. N Engl J Med 330:540–4, 1994.

116. Glantz LH. Withholding and withdrawing treatment: the role of the criminal law. Law Med Health Care 15:231–41, 1987–1988.

117. Meisel A, Grenvick A, Pinkus RL, Snyder JV. Hospital guidelines for deciding about life-sustaining treatment: dealing with health limbo. Crit Care Med 14:239–46, 1986.

118. Miller DK, Coe RM, Hyers TM. Achieving consensus on withdrawing or withholding care for critically ill patients. J Gen Intern Med 7:475–80, 1992.

119. Alpers A., Lo, B. Futility: not just a medical issue. Law, Medicine of Health Care 20:4:327 (1992).

120. Ryan CJ, Kaye M. Euthanasia in Australia—the Northern Territory Rights of the Terminally Ill Act. N Engl J Med 334:326–8, 1996.

121. Wecht CH. The right to die and physician-assisted suicide. Medical, legal, ethical aspects. Part I, II. Med Law 17:477–91, 581–601, 1998.

122. Stjernsward J. The international hospice movement from the perspective of the World Health Organization. In: Saunders C, Kastenbaum R, eds. Hospice Care on the International Scene. New York: Springer Publishing Co., 1997:9–15.

123. Christakis NA, Escare JJ. Survival of Medicare patients after enrollment in hospice programs. N Engl J Med 335:172–82, 1996.

124. Pargeon KL, Hailey BJ. Barriers to effective cancer pain management: a review of the literature. J Pain Symptom Manage 18:358–68, 1999.

125. Rhymes JA. Barriers to effective palliative care of terminal patients: an international perspective. Clin Geriatr Med 12:407–16, 1996.

126. Von Roenn JH, Cleeland CS, Gonin R, et al. Physician attitudes and practice in cancer pain management. A survey from the Eastern Cooperative Oncology Group. Ann Intern Med 119:121–6, 1993.

127. Meier DE, Morrison RS, Cassel CK. Improving palliative care. Ann Intern Med 127:225–30, 1997.

128. Preston TA. Taking charge of the last stages of life. Final victory. Facing death on your own terms. Forum 2000, Roseville, CA.

129. De Raeve L. Ethical issues in palliative care research. Palliat Med 8:298–305, 1994.

130. Mount BM, Cohen R, MacDonald N, et al. Ethical issues in palliative care research revisited. Palliat Med 9:165–70, 1995.

131. Bruera E, Franco JJ, Maltoni M, et al. Changing pattern of agitated impaired mental status in patients with advanced cancer: association with cognitive monitoring, hydration, and opiate rotation. J Pain Symptom Manage 10:287–91, 1995.

132. Bruera E, Spachynski K, MacEachern T, Hanson J. Cognitive failure in cancer patients in clinical trials [Letter]. Lancet 341:247–8, 1993.

133. Schaeffer MH, Krantz DS, Wichman A, et al. The impact of disease severity on the informed consent process in clinical research. Am J Med 1:261–8, 1996.

134. Markman M. Ethical difficulties with randomized clinical trials involving cancer patients: examples from the field of gynecologic oncology. J Clin Ethics 3:193–5, 1992.

135. Guidelines in Research in Palliative Care. London: The National Council for Hospice and Specialist Palliative Care Services, 1995.

136. Roy DJ, MacDonald, N. Ethical issues in palliative care. In: Doyle D, Hanks GW, MacDonald N, eds. Oxford textbook of palliative medicine, 2nd ed. Oxford: Oxford University Press, 1999:97–105.

137. MacDonald N. Suffering and dying in cancer patients: research frontiers in controlling confusion, cachexia, and dyspnea. West J Med 163:278–86, 1995.

26 Understanding clinical trials in pain research

JOHN T. FARRAR AND SCOTT D. HALPERN
University of Pennsylvania School of Medicine

Introduction

The randomized, controlled trial (RCT) is a modern innovation; the first RCT—the British Medical Research Council's trial of streptomycin for pulmonary tuberculosis—was published in 1948 (1,2). Despite this brief history, the RCT now represents the "gold standard" for evaluating the efficacy of new medical interventions and new applications for existing interventions. Unfortunately, the marked increase in the use of RCTs during the past 50 years (3) has not been accompanied by corresponding advances in overcoming the method's several limitations. Indeed, several potential scientific and ethical difficulties continue to limit the use of RCTs in some clinical contexts and hinder the interpretation of their results in others.

In this chapter, we first discuss the various strengths and limitations common to all RCTs, making special reference to trials of pain management interventions when appropriate. We describe the structure of an RCT, consider how several decisions regarding trial design can influence the trial's results, discuss basic issues in the analysis of trial data, and attempt to guide readers in interpreting a trial's results. Because no research experiment can ever be perfect, we hope this chapter will provide clinicians with sufficient understanding of the proper structure of, and inherent problems with, RCTs to be able to ascertain whether the results of published trials are 1) likely to be valid and 2) likely to apply to their patients.

Anatomy of a trial

Designing and conducting an RCT requires investigators to carefully consider several design issues. The decisions investigators make regarding each component of an RCT can dramatically influence the outcome of the trial. Thus, subtle flaws in a trial's design or conduct may lead inves-

tigators and readers to draw inappropriate conclusions from tarnished data.

It is also important to understand that even a perfectly designed clinical trial is not guaranteed to find the right answer to a research question. Several statistical parameters can be computed to gauge a trial's probability of reaching false-positive and false-negative conclusions, but neither of these probabilities can ever be reduced to zero. Thus, no single trial should ever be considered to provide definitive proof of the efficacy, or lack thereof, of an intervention; replication of the trial's results in other similarly designed trials will always be preferable for clinicians making decisions about patient care.

The question

The single most important step in designing a trial is to clearly and specifically define the research question to be answered. This may seem relatively straightforward, but to reduce an important clinical question to a testable hypothesis is often a tremendous challenge. This challenge typically arises from difficulties in replicating clinical reality in the research setting. At other times, clinically relevant questions may be translated easily into a research question, but answering such questions would require prohibitively large numbers of participants. Finally, ethical concerns may also influence which questions may be studied, and the ways in which trials are designed to answer these questions.

When investigators encounter these problems, they commonly attempt to modify the research question to one that is more readily answerable. However, if we test a different question, we get an answer to a different question; this answer may or may not apply to the original clinical scenario we set out to investigate. Attempting to answer the right question in the setting of an RCT may require compromises in the study design that sacrifice either precision or protection from bias. Such compromises may reduce the value of the knowledge to be gained from the research, and hence alter the risk-benefit calculus necessary to justify the research (4–6). If investigators are not confident, at the outset of the trial, of the clinical importance of answering the proposed question, then alternative, observational research methods should be considered.

The second step in defining the research question is to specifically document the primary outcome to be assessed. This must be done a priori, before the data are collected or analyzed. In order for the probability of finding the correct answer to remain within acceptable limits, both the nature of this outcome and what would be considered a clinically important effect of an intervention on this outcome must be defined. Although multiple outcomes may be tested within a single trial, each should be identified at the outset, and none should subsequently replace the primary outcome after the data have been collected and analyzed (a posteriori).

Randomization

In trials aimed at evaluating new analgesic therapies, patients are randomly assigned to one of two or more treatment groups to ensure that these groups are as similar as possible in all ways other than their assigned treatment. Randomization attempts to reduce the possibility that the results will be influenced, or confounded, by other variables, such as age or disease severity, that are also related to outcome. By minimizing the possibility of confounding, RCTs enable investigators to more confidently attribute observed differences in group outcomes to the assigned treatments.

By contrast, observational studies, such as case-control, cohort, or cross-sectional studies, depend on nature to set up the experiment. As such, there is a substantial possibility that known or unknown biases may affect the results, and even lead to a wrong conclusion.

True randomization requires both a valid means of generating random numbers and a mechanism to protect the integrity of random assignment. In trials with multiple sites, handling the randomization centrally may ensure consistent application of the randomization procedure across sites. Additionally, such central control of the randomization scheme prevents members of the study team, some of whom may not be blinded to a patient's treatment allocation, from influencing the assignment.

When randomization works correctly and when sufficient numbers of patients are enrolled, the distributions of all potential confounding variables (some of which can never be measured or controlled) are likely to be equal across groups. However, in smaller trials, or in large, multicenter trials with few participants from a given center, chance alone may cause significant differences in the distributions of demographic or disease-related characteristics between groups. To avoid the bias that may ensue in such cases, investigators may use block randomization to ensure that selected participant characteristics will be equally distributed. For example, if investigators wished to guarantee an equal sex distribution among two treatment arms at each site, they may randomize by blocks of six participants each, within which three participants would be male and three would be female.

Control group

Three primary types of control groups may be used in trials of pain management interventions: 1) a placebo control, 2) a no-treatment control, or 3) an active control. We discuss the latter two control groups in some detail here and explain why no-treatment control groups are generally not preferred.

Placebo-controlled trials

Pain management trials most commonly include a placebo control group. A placebo is defined as an inactive treatment designed to mimic, as closely as possible, the characteristics of the active treatment except for the specific component being tested. In drug trials, this means an inactive substance is formulated to have similar appearance and route of administration to the active treatment.

There are two primary benefits to using a placebo control group, rather than a no-treatment control group. First, the use of a placebo control allows the specific efficacy of the new intervention to be distinguished from the many nonspecific effects, including the well-known placebo effect (7,8). The magnitude of the total non-specific effects in a given study can be estimated by the mean (or median) response in the placebo control group. Assuming a simple additive model of treatment effects, then placebo control group response can be subtracted from the mean response in the active treatment group to estimate the specific efficacy of the new intervention. Though the extent of non-specific treatment effects, across a broad range of clinical interventions, has recently been questioned, they appear to be real and of particularly large magnitude in studies of the management of pain (9).

The second benefit of using a placebo control group is that it allows the study to be conducted in a double-blind fashion, thereby avoiding the biases that may ensue if patients, investigators, or both knew who was receiving which treatment. We discuss the nature of these biases more fully later. The key point for present purposes is that the potential for avoiding these biases is directly related to the ability to keep both patients and evaluators blind. Because it would be impossible to blind participants or evaluators if one group received a treatment and the other did not, bias is more likely to influence trials using no-treatment controls than those using placebo controls (assuming the placebo is indistinguishable from the active treatment, see later).

There are also costs to using a placebo control. The first and most obvious is that the placebo group patients with pain are not given active treatment despite the existence of known effective interventions. The ethics of placebo-controlled trials in such settings remains a hotly debated topic (10–13), and is considered further at the end of this chapter. The second cost to conducting placebo-controlled trials is that, although they remain the "gold standard" for documenting absolute efficacy, they do not always answer a clinically relevant question. Practicing clinicians, who have several analgesics at their disposal, do not need to know whether another analgesic medication works better than nothing, but rather, how the new analgesic compares to existing standards of care (14).

No-treatment-controlled trials

There are two primary situations in which it may be important to include a control group of participants who receive no intervention (active or inactive). The first situation arises when determining the overall efficacy of a new intervention is critical, but there are practical and/or ethical problems with using a placebo or sham control. For example, it is often difficult to construct an appropriate sham intervention for many trials of surgical interventions. Even if adequate shams could be constructed, some feel that assigning patients to receive an invasive, but non-active, intervention is unethical (15).

The second situation arises when a goal of the trial is to ascertain the magnitude of the placebo effect. To measure the placebo effect properly requires comparison of patients receiving placebo with those receiving no treatment at all. A recent meta-analysis of 114 trials in which both placebo and no-treatment controls were used has shown that in many areas, the placebo effect is far less than might be expected (9). In pain research, however,

these authors found that patients in placebo control groups typically have far more favorable outcomes than those in no-treatment-control groups (9).

Noninferiority and equivalence trials

Given the foregoing concerns about placebo-controlled trials and the inability of no-treatment control groups to maintain blinding, investigators may decide to show that a new drug is either "no worse than" (a noninferiority trial) or "as good as" (an equivalence trial) a treatment that is commonly accepted as effective. Indeed, in evaluating therapeutics for conditions in which the risks of placebo assignment are widely regarded as too great, such as thrombolytic agents for acute myocardial infarction or stroke, active-controlled, noninferiority trials are the standard (16,17).

These trials are presently not considered standard for problems such as hypertension, hyperlipidemia, and pain, because the risks of temporarily foregoing active treatment are not as obvious, and because there are several potential problems with interpreting such studies (10,18–22). The first problem is that equivalence trials essentially aim to confirm the conventional null hypothesis of no treatment difference, which may create inappropriate incentives for conducting "sloppy" research (23). Second, such trials generally require larger numbers of participants, because equivalence or noninferiority must be documented within relatively narrow margins. Third, demonstrating that two treatments are the same does not show that either of them worked. This problem has been referred to as a problem with "assay sensitivity," because such trials require the external assumption that the standard therapy would have proven superior to placebo had a placebo arm been included (10). Because of these concerns, current regulatory guidelines still call for placebo-controlled trials to evaluate treatments for problems such as pain (24). The risks and benefits of this guideline remain hotly debated.

Participant selection

Another critical decision for investigators designing trials, and for clinicians attempting to discern whether a trial's results apply to their patients, regards the selection of study participants. There are two conflicting priorities in the selection of participants: 1) ensuring similarities between participants in the experimental and control groups, and 2) testing a new treatment in a broader sample of patients more likely to reflect all those who could benefit from using the intervention. To meet the first goal, investigators attempt to enroll patients who are relatively homogenous. Strict inclusion and exclusion criteria allow greater confidence that the observed outcomes are attributable to the treatments being compared and limit the amount of statistical noise that might obscure the result.

By contrast, meeting the second goal requires enrolling participants from a more heterogeneous population. Because of the large interpersonal variability inherent in such a population, this approach can substantially increase the number of participants required to ensure that the trial has adequate statistical power to document a treatment difference, if one exists. Despite this disadvantage, enrolling a heterogeneous sample allows subgroup analyses to be conducted, and so potential variations in a treatment's efficacy among higher- and lower-risk patients may be identified. Thus, there are advantages and disadvantages to enrolling more or less homogeneous participants. As a result, early investigations of efficacy are commonly conducted using a select group of participants, whereas later, more definitive trials attempt to enroll more broadly representative patient samples. Physicians should, therefore, consider the composition of a given trial's sample to determine the extent to which the results are generalizable to their own patients.

Blinding

Over the last century, a growing understanding of the variable nature of illness, the ability of the mind to influence the functioning of the body, and the desire to enhance the experimental rigor of clinical trials have increased appreciation of the need for blinding. Again, a goal of clinical trials is to design the experiment such that any changes seen at the end of the trial may be attributed specifically to the treatment being studied. To accommodate this goal, not only must all comparison groups be similar at the start, but participants in all groups must think they are getting the real treatment. If one group knows they are getting a placebo or control medication, the trial may spuriously reveal a benefit in the active treatment group because control participants' beliefs that they are receiving a less effective intervention may, itself, reduce the benefit observed in the control group.

Thus, blinding of the participants is of paramount importance, and investigators must attempt to overcome the myriad ways in which participants may decipher their treatment assignment (that is, unblind themselves). In particular, if a medication has a specific taste, common side effects, or other distinctive traits, it is impor-

tant that the placebo mimic these characteristics as closely as possible. Thus, it is common practice to use saline injections as controls for intravenous medications. Even in evaluating surgical interventions, sham procedures have occasionally been used by making skin incisions (25) or burr holes in the skull (26) to mimic the real surgical procedures.

In addition to creating a suitable placebo, investigators should validate that the blinding was maintained by asking participants what treatment they think they received and why. Such questions should be posed to participants both during the trial, and at the trial's completion (27). If the blinding is successful, the participants' guesses should be no more accurate than chance (e.g., 50% in a typical 2-arm trial). Ideally, all patients will think they received the active medication.

However, ample evidence from many clinical fields suggests that participant blinding is difficult to maintain (27–35). These studies reveal that participants can often predict their receipt of placebo because of the absence of side effects, whereas participants receiving an active intervention may be unblinded by noting adverse effects of the intervention.

When only participants are blinded to the treatment received, the study is termed a single-blind trial. However, double-blind trials, in which investigators attempt to keep both participants and those evaluating the participants' response from knowing the treatment assignments, are generally preferable. Blinding of those who evaluate the participants' outcomes is also critical so as to minimize the chance that evaluators will more favorably rate those known to be receiving the innovative treatment, thereby biasing the trial toward finding a benefit of that treatment. Although evaluator blinding may seem to be of less importance in trials of interventions for pain, in which the participants typically report their perceived symptoms, it remains essential to minimize the possibilities that investigators would impart different levels of enthusiasm, or prescribe different co-interventions, to patients in the different groups.

Sample size

The statistical power of an RCT to show a difference between treatments is determined by 1) the number of participants to be enrolled, 2) the effect size (treatment difference) that is deemed to be clinically important, 3) the variability of the outcomes in the two groups, and 4) the p value (type I error rate, or α) chosen to connote statistical significance (typically set at 0.05). Ultimately, however, the size of the sample to be tested is the variable investigators most commonly adjust to obtain adequate power—that is, an adequate probability of detecting a meaningful treatment difference when one truly exists.

By tradition, researchers consider a study to be adequately powered if it has at least an 80% chance of detecting a clinically significant effect when one exists (that is, if $\beta \leq 0.2$). However, this exact value is arbitrary; higher power will always be preferable. Furthermore, in practice, the power of a particular trial is set by considering both the number of participants that can reasonably be enrolled, and the relative importance of limiting false-negative conclusions (i.e., type II errors) versus limiting false-positive conclusions (i.e., type I errors).

It is a truism that with a sufficiently large sample size, any real difference between groups, no matter how small or clinically irrelevant, can be shown to be statistically significant. The converse is also true: a large, clinically important difference between treatments can fail to reach statistical significance when inadequate numbers of participants are enrolled.

The most common method of calculating the sample size required to achieve 80% (or greater) power is to first determine 1) the size of the effect that would be considered clinically important, 2) the anticipated response in the control group, and 3) the expected variability of the outcomes in both groups. This last determination may be particularly difficult to estimate and should, when possible, be based on evidence from prior studies of similar diseases and/or treatments.

An alternate method of presenting a priori sample-size considerations is to calculate the size of the effect that would need to be present to produce a statistically significant outcome, given a fixed number of participants. Although this approach is rarely preferable to setting the sample size to detect a specified difference, it remains in common use. In such cases, authors should at least present this information in the manuscript to help readers determine whether the trial may be relevant to their clinical practices.

Outcome measurement

Another critical decision to be made in planning an RCT is how to measure the chosen outcome of interest. For example, if investigators are interested in studying the effects of a new antihypertensive agent on systolic and diastolic blood pressure, should they measure these values with a mercury sphygmomanometer or via an arterial line? In addition to *how* the outcome will be measured,

investigators must further consider *when* and *how often* to measure the outcome. Are single readings once each week adequate, or should participants be equipped with ambulatory blood pressure monitors to obtain multiple readings throughout the day? Finally, investigators must consider how to account for other variables that could alter the measurement, such as body position when the blood pressure is assessed.

Regardless of what measurement technique is chosen, it should be characterized by three features. First, the measurement should be *reliable*—if the same measure is used repetitively in the same person under identical conditions without this person's condition changing, then the measure should produce the same results each time. Second, the measure should be *valid*—it should measure exactly what it is intended to measure. Third, the measure should be *responsive*—it should change over time if the condition being measured has truly changed. Although a full discussion of these concepts is beyond the scope of this chapter, the topics are well covered in many textbooks (36).

For present purposes, the critical point is that in evaluating a published trial, readers should be comfortable that the measurement used meets these three criteria in the situation in which it was used. If the outcome measure is not routinely used in clinical practice, its reliability, validity, and responsiveness should be formally tested and documented in the trial report.

It is also important to understand that a more responsive scale is not necessarily a better one. If a measure records changes in values that are too small to be clinically important, it may be overly responsive. For example, the use of visual analog scales in pain studies has been shown to be more responsive than the common integer scales, in part because the 100-mm scale allows a broader range of potential responses. However, changes of less than 10% on a visual analog scale are unlikely to be clinically important. Thus the usual analogue scale is unlikely to provide more valid answers than could be obtained on a numerical rating scale from 0 to 10.

Whereas the criteria of reliability, validity, and responsiveness may be readily appreciated when measuring blood pressure, they are far more difficult when measuring the effects of treatments intended to alleviate symptoms. For example, in pain management, the primary goal is to improve the patient's subjective sense of comfort. For this purpose, investigators might ask a simple question, such as, "Do you feel better, yes or no?" Because such a measure has only two possible responses, it may not provide an adequately responsive measure of pain relief.

To help differentiate the level of response, investigators might ask, "What percentage of pain relief do you get from the treatment?" However, such questions require patients to remember their previous condition. Alternatively, investigators could use a 0 to 10 numerical rating scale at both the beginning and end of the study to measure the change in pain over time. Deciding which measurement is most appropriate for a given clinical situation should be informed by considerations of how much change in the measure would be important to the patient, and the ability of the chosen scale to detect such a change.

Another measurement concern in pain management trials is that a change in pain may be only one component of an overall quality of life. Thus, symptomatic reports may be considered surrogate markers for changes in the broader outcome of quality of life. Conversely, assessing changes in quality of life may be insufficient because they cannot specifically connote changes in pain. Variables related to but not themselves the direct link to the disease are called surrogate markers.

The use of surrogate markers is widespread in clinical trials. For example, investigators routinely monitor changes in serum cholesterol to provide a surrogate measure for the risk of myocardial infarction. However, using a surrogate measure requires making the assumption, that, for example, a reduction in cholesterol will also reduce the risk of myocardial infarction. Alternatively, if the use of an experimental analgesic agent relieves pain but produces substantial side effects, the patient may not consider its use to be advantageous from the perspective of their quality of life. Therefore, if investigators wish to know an intervention's effects on both the level of pain and the overall quality of life, then they must use tools to measure both.

In summary, there is no single measurement strategy that is universally applicable, or always preferable. Investigators and readers should carefully consider what question a trial is specifically attempting to answer, whether this is an appropriate question, and whether the chosen measurement scale is up to the task of answering that question.

Analysis

Investigators planning an RCT should also document a specific analytic strategy before commencing the trial. While different analytic approaches may be possible considering the structure of the data. Each approach will produce an answer to a different research question. Thus, the same data can be used to answer several different questions depending on which analyses are performed.

However, to be valid, the chosen analysis strategy must be appropriate to evaluate the primary research question, in addition to being compatible with the nature of the data collected. The most important considerations in planning and conducting a clinical trial are considered here.

Effect size

The first and most important result of any analysis entails the measure of the effect size. In RCTs, effect sizes are often calculated by determining a summary value for the primary outcome in each group and then calculating the difference between these group values to reveal the treatment effect. There are two primary forms for the summary value of a set of trial data: 1) the central tendency (e.g., mean, median, or mode) of the response among participants, and 2) the proportion of participants who achieve a defined level of response.

For example, in a hypertension trial, investigators could report the mean change in diastolic blood pressure (central tendency), or the proportion of hypertensive patients who achieve diastolic blood pressures below 90 mmHg. If one were interested in the effect of an intervention on hospital length of stay, it might be acceptable to report either the median time spent in the hospital for each group (central tendency), or the proportion of patients in each group who are discharged within 3 days, 4 days, or some other predefined time period. Finally, in trials of pain management, in which the outcome of reported pain symptoms is provided on a numeric scale, investigators might either report the mean response in each group, or the percentage of patients in each group reporting pain reductions of 33% (or 50%) or greater. In each case, the units of these summary values should correspond to the units of the outcome measure.

Choices regarding how to best present the summary measures should reflect the type of information that is most relevant for practicing clinicians. For example, measures of central tendency do not typically account for the variable responses among individuals in a group. When this variability is great, measures of central tendency will have little application to the corresponding clinical situations. Rather, for most health care providers, the question of interest is the probability of a given treatment working for a given patient.

For example, suppose investigators reported that the mean response in the active treatment group was an improvement of 10% on a standard pain scale. This same result could apply to data indicating that 1) every patient in the active treatment group improved by 10% (a unimodal distribution), 2) half of the patients in the treatment group improved by 20% and half had no improvement (a bimodal distribution), or 3) half of the patients in the active treatment group improved by 40%, and half deteriorated by 20% (also a bimodal distribution). Because these three descriptions of the underlying data could yield strikingly different clinical decisions, a central tendency analysis does not produce a unique answer to the critical question. In this case, it may be more useful to present the data by analyzing the proportions of patients in each group who improve or deteriorate by a clinically important amount.

In fact, clinical experience with pain interventions suggests that many medications produce bimodal distributions of response. In patients with cancer-related pain, it is often difficult to discern the predominant type of pain (i.e., somatic nociceptive vs. visceral nociceptive vs. neuropathic). If only one type of pain is likely to be responsive to the therapy, there will be two or more distinct populations in the treatment group. Headache is another area in which investigators now frequently view response as dichotomous, as it is difficult to know the underlying etiology in many headache patients (37–39). Another example is facial neuralgia: anticonvulsant medications work well, but only in some patients (40). A third example involves the use of tricyclic antidepressants used for neuropathic pain. These agents also appear to work well in some patients, but have virtually no effect in others (41).

What is a clinically important difference?

A common concern about presenting the proportion of "responders" is the need to define a level of response to be considered clinically important. Thus, the determination of a clinically important difference (CID) in a patient's symptoms plays a key role in the interpretation of pain studies. Two methods for determining the CID are "expert opinion," and an assessment of how changes in symptom scales correspond to responses to global questions (42–44). Regardless of the method used, however, each requires that a somewhat arbitrary decision be made in defining the scale to be considered the standard.

Two recent reports have used clinical trial data to estimate the CID for measures of pain. These reports demonstrated that a 33% change in the pain intensity score is considered clinically important by a majority of patients (45,46). Although there may be honest disagreement about how to establish a CID, reporting outcomes in this way provide information that can be more readily translated into improved patient care.

Statistical considerations

Statistical significance (P values and confidence intervals)

In addition to the test statistic summarizing the effect size results of statistical analyses generate an accompanying p-value, which documents the probability that this effect size could occur by chance, assuming that the null hypothesis is true. Most commonly, investigators will accept a 1/20 chance of rejecting the null hypothesis when it is, in fact, true (a false-positive conclusion). Thus, the corresponding p value of 0.05 or less is generally used to document statistical significance. However, it is important to recognize that this value is strictly arbitrary, that there are frequent occasions when different levels may be appropriate. In addition to the test this convention implies that apparently significant results still have a 5% chance of having occurred by chance alone.

This traditional method of hypothesis testing, in which p values are reported to quantify the significance of a result, is gradually being replaced by methods to gauge the range of plausible results that are compatible with the data. The most common method for presenting this range is to report a point estimate of the effect size, along with a 95% confidence interval around this estimate. A 95% confidence interval will include the true population value of the effect size 19 times out of 20 (95%). Thus, confidence intervals can help readers determine the uncertainty inherent in any result—the narrower the interval, the more precise the estimate of the true effect, and thus, the more confident readers can be that the reported result is "right."

Multiple comparisons

It is also important to realize that when investigators choose a p value of 0.05 as an acceptable type I (false-positive) error rate, this value will apply only to a single comparison between groups. In most clinical trials, however, performing multiple outcome comparisons can be informative. The greater the number of comparisons, the more likely it is that at least one of them will be spuriously positive by chance alone. If an a priori decision is made to perform multiple comparisons, the p value must be adjusted. Of the several available methods for adjusting this value, the simplest is to divide the p value by the number of comparisons to be performed, and to then use this new p value as the cut-off for statistical significance across all analyses.

A related issue is the distinction between comparisons chosen a priori, and those that investigators choose to conduct post hoc, or after the data has been collected. There are many times when post hoc comparisons can be informative, but the results of such analyses should never be considered conclusive since they were not explicitly planned at the outset. Rather, results of post hoc analyses may be considered exploratory, intended to guide future investigations. Authors can help highlight this distinction by reporting which comparisons were chosen a priori, and which were not.

Evidence from multiple measures

In addition to the reported effect size and statistical significance of the results, corroborative evidence from multiple analyses can be used to support or refute a study's hypothesis. If multiple related measures are obtained, and the analyses of each show similar results, then there it is less likely that any one of the positive results arose by chance. Although there is no specific statistical test to document this phenomenon, showing that multiple related measures all produce similar types of effects lends support to the validity of the conclusions that are drawn.

Evaluating side effects

Evaluating side effects of interventions tested in clinical trials is subject to the same considerations as those used to evaluate measures of efficacy. The major difference is that, in many cases, the side effects to be evaluated are not specified a priori, but are evaluated only when they are observed to occur. Because many common side effects occur spontaneously, independent of the treatment received, it is important to compare their incidence in the active treatment and control groups. Again, with many possible side effects requiring multiple comparisons, the chance that one or more will be observed more commonly in the treatment group is increased. Such differences should not be ignored, but observing them repeatedly in multiple trials can increase one's confidence that they may be specifically attributed to the treatment received.

Publication

Thorough presentation of methods and results

Given that many components of a trial are central to interpreting the results, it is vital that trial reports be accurate, complete, and objective in their presentation of all important aspects of the trial. In particular, the a priori

hypothesis should be clearly stated, and the discovery of other findings properly identified. All randomized participants must be accounted for in the publication, and an intention-to-treat analysis of all participants is typically appropriate, even when some participants drop out early in the study or never receive their assigned intervention. Subsequent subgroup analyses can focus on those who complete the trial, but these should not be considered as the primary result. A careful description of the randomization and blinding procedures is also important to assure readers that the trial was properly conducted. Finally, brief descriptions of the rationale behind the choice of measurement tools and analytic strategies can be helpful.

Negative studies are as important as positive ones

There is now good evidence for a publication bias against negative studies, as authors prefer to write up positive ones and editors prefer to publish the same (47,48). This can lead to difficulties for clinicians who want a true picture of the nature of the evidence for a particular treatment.

Potential limitations of RCTs

There are several issues inherent in the design and conduct of RCTs that may threaten the internal validity of the results, that is, the likelihood that the treatment comparison is free from bias. Even when the comparison is internally valid, the external validity, or generalizability of the results, may be limited. Finally, because the conditions in which trials are conducted only weakly approximate clinical reality, physicians must be cautious in using the results to guide clinical decisions in other populations. We will briefly discuss each of these potential problems below. More detailed discussions of these issues are provided by Feinstein (49) and by Kramer and Shapiro (50).

Underenrollment

Underenrollment occurs when too few research participants are enrolled to provide adequate statistical power to answer the study's primary research questions. The inability to recruit sufficient numbers of eligible patients is the most common cause of insufficient statistical power in RCTs (51–56). Such underenrollment has been attributed to characteristics of 1) clinicians who refer their patients (57–59), 2) patients who choose to be screened (60) or enrolled (61), 3) investigators who design the trials (62), and 4) institutions at which the trials are conducted (62–64).

Among these challenges to adequate participant recruitment, reluctance to enroll in RCTs is likely the most formidable. It has been observed that patients are generally less willing to participate in RCTs than in non-randomized, observational studies (50). In addition to yielding unacceptably high probabilities for type II errors, the resulting underenrollment substantially reduces the trial's precision in quantifying the treatment effect.

Selective enrollment

Even when properly designed and carefully conducted, clinical trials can only provide information specific to the population from which the study participants were drawn. If this population does not include elderly patients, women, or children, for example, then applying the results to these clinical populations requires extrapolation. Although extrapolating results may sometimes be reasonable, it must always be done cautiously because both the beneficial and adverse effects of an intervention can vary across populations.

In addition, participants in RCTs often differ from the general population in ways that may be related to their outcome. Selective enrollment occurs when particular subgroups within the target population enroll in proportions greater or less than their representation in that population (65,66). Causes of selective enrollment include 1) a narrow recruitment strategy, 2) differential access to the study among subgroups of potential participants, 3) different levels of willingness to participate among potential participants, and 4) different levels of clinicians' willingness to refer different types of patients for enrollment. Each of these problems limits the generalizability of the trial's results (49,50,66–68), and hence reduces their applicability to clinical practice.

These limitations may dramatically alter the conclusions to be drawn from the trial if differences between those who enroll and those who do not are related to outcome. Enrolling a selected sample of participants may prohibit the detection of group differences in the absolute or relative risk reduction for having an adverse outcome (or in the absolute or relative enhancement of the probability of responding favorably).

For example, consider a placebo-controlled trial of a novel opiate to treat chronic pain. Patients whose pain is presently well managed on a regimen of other opiates may have different levels of willingness to participate in

such a trial than will those whose pain remains debilitating. Specifically, patients for whom currently available drugs have provided good pain control may be less willing to be taken off their medication and risk being assigned to either another drug that may not work as well, or to placebo. By contrast, those whose pain has not been adequately controlled may be more likely to participate in such a trial because doing so provides an opportunity to receive a promising new drug.

Patients who have not responded well to currently available opiates, however, may also be less likely to respond to the new drug. If so, then the selective enrollment of these patients may reduce the observed efficacy of the drug in the trial, compared to the efficacy that might have been observed among a more representative sample of the population of patients in pain. The results of this comparison of the study drug to placebo would therefore not be generalizable beyond the enrolled sample of patients not responding to standard interventions. If new drug offered a favorable side effect profile, then using the trial's results to support a conclusion that new drug is of limited value would prevent an otherwise useful agent from being added to physicians' pain-treating armamentarium.

Poor participant adherence

In clinical settings, patients often do not adhere to their prescribed treatment regimens. This problem may be even more pronounced in RCTs because many participants will receive a treatment they would not have chosen if given the opportunity (50). If patients believe they are receiving a non-preferred treatment, their enthusiasm for the trial and subsequent adherence to their assigned treatment may wane.

There is accumulating evidence that study participants make concerted efforts to unblind themselves, and that participants who become aware of their treatment assignment may be more likely to drop out of the study. For example, many patients assigned to the placebo groups in both the initial phase II trial of zidovudine (AZT) for AIDS patients (69), and in a randomized trial of vitamin E for patients with Alzheimer's disease (70), appear to have become unblinded, and even to have obtained access to the active agents (71–73). Even more problematically, widespread unblinding in the AIDS Clinical Trials Group 019 study (74) not only allowed approximately 9% of those assigned to the placebo to receive AZT, but contributed to the drop-out rate in the placebo group, being one-third higher than it was in the active treatment group (75).

Participant nonadherence and drop-out can substantially bias the results of a trial (76). Although intention-to-treat analyses may mitigate this bias, if non-adherence or drop-out rates are higher in one group than in the other, such analyses may also prevent a true effect of treatment from being detected. Thus, investigators should make concerted efforts to monitor participant adherence, and to report drop-out rates in their manuscripts. When such problems exist, the results of the trial must be interpreted cautiously.

Ethical issues in pain research

Investigators who conduct clinical pain research must obtain informed consent from participants that meets HIPPA guidelines (77,78). Obtaining adequate informed consent, however, is often difficult due to uncertainties regarding the kind and extent of information patients want when considering whether to enroll in a trial (79). Recently, investigators have begun exploring pain patients' preferences regarding the information about the trial that would be important for them to know in deciding whether participation is in their best interests (79). Further efforts to qualify and quantify not only patients' information needs, but also their preferences for enrolling in different types of trials, may substantially increase both the ability of informed consent to serve its intended purpose of respecting patients' autonomy, and enhance the efficiency of patient recruitment.

Another lingering ethical issue in pain research regards the standard comparison of new pain interventions to placebo. Patients who enroll in such studies must typically forego known effective treatments for their pain for the duration of the trial. Although investigators typically make analgesics available for participants experiencing intolerable pain, the risk of worsened pain while enrolled in the study remains. We have previously briefly discussed the relative merits of active-controlled and placebo-controlled trials. We suggest that the scientific merits of placebo-controlled trials continue to be considered in light of the risks to enrolled patients, as well as the value of the information such trials can provide for guiding clinicians' prescribing practices. Ongoing revisions to the Declaration of Helsinki (80), the most widely cited international doctrine of research ethics, may influence the viability of placebo-controlled pain trials in the future.

Conclusions

In this chapter, several fundamental considerations for investigators planning clinical trials, and for clinicians attempting to discern the applicability of such trials to their practices have been outlined. Special consideration has been considered to the nuances of clinical trials for pain management interventions. In summary, randomized, controlled trials remain the best available means of evaluating novel pain interventions, and for determining how these interventions may be used optimally once they are approved. Despite the strengths of the design, readers of trial reports should be mindful of the many difficulties inherent in extrapolating from the results obtained in a trial setting to the use of these same interventions in clinical practice.

References

1. Medical Research Council. Streptomycin treatment of pulmonary tuberculosis. Br Med J 2:769–82, 1948.
2. Anonymous. Fifty years of randomised controlled trials. BMJ 317, 1998.
3. Peto R, Baigent C. Trials: the next 50 years. BMJ 317:1170–71, 1998.
4. Freedman B. Scientific value and validity as ethical requirements for research: a proposed explication. Irb: a Review of Human Subjects Research. 9(6):7–10, 1987 Nov–Dec.
5. Rutstein DD. The ethical design of human experiments. In: Freund PA, ed. Experimentation with human subjects. New York: George Braziller, 1970:383–401.
6. Emmanuel EJ, Wendler D, Grady C. What makes clinical research ethical? JAMA 283:2701–11, 2000.
7. Chaput de Saintonge DM, Herxheimer A. Harnessing placebo effects in health care. Lancet 344:995–8, 1994.
8. Kleijnen J, de Craen AJM, Everdingen JV, Krol L. Placebo effect in double-blind clinical trials: a review of interactions with medications. Lancet 344:1347–9, 1994.
9. Hrobjartsson A, Gotzsche PC. Is the placebo powerless? An analysis of clinical trials comparing placebo with no treatment. N Engl J Med 344:1594–602, 2001.
10. Temple R, Ellenberg SS. Placebo-controlled trials and active-control trials in the evaluation of new treatments. Part 1. Ethical and scientific issues. Ann Intern Med 133:455–63, 2000.
11. Freedman B, Glass KC, Weijer C. Placebo orthodoxy in clinical research II: ethical, legal, and regulatory myths. J Law Med Ethics 24:252–9, 1996.
12. Freedman B, Weijer C, Glass KC. Placebo orthodoxy in clinical research I: empirical and methodological myths. J Law Med Ethics 24:243–51, 1996.
13. Rothman KJ, Michels KB. The continuing unethical use of placebo controls. N Engl J Med 331:394–8, 1994.
14. Halpern SD, Karlawish JHT. Placebo-controlled trials are unethical in clinical hypertension research. Arch Intern Med 160:3167–8, 2000.
15. Macklin R. The ethical problems with sham surgery in clinical research. N Engl J Med 341:992–6, 1999.

16. Anonymous. A comparison of continuous infusion of alteplase with double-bolus administration for acute myocardial infarction. The Continuous Infusion versus Double-Bolus Administration of Alteplase (COBALT) Investigators. N Engl J Med 337:1124–30, 1997.

17. Anonymous. A comparison of reteplase with alteplase for acute myocardial infarction. The Global Use of Strategies to Open Occluded Coronary Arteries (GUSTO III) Investigators. N Engl J Med 337:1118–23, 1997.

18. Anonymous. Single-bolus tenecteplase compared with front-loaded alteplase in acute myocardial infarction: the ASSENT-2 double-blind randomised trial. Assessment of the Safety and Efficacy of a New Thrombolytic Investigators. Lancet 354:716–22, 1999.

19. Temple RJ. When are clinical trials of a given agent vs. placebo no longer appropriate or feasible? Control Clin Trials 18:613–20, 1997.

20. Temple R. Problems in interpreting active control equivalence trials. Accountability Res 4:267–75, 1996.

21. Jones B, Jarvis P, Lewis JA, Ebbutt AF. Trials to assess equivalence: the importance of rigorous methods. BMJ 313:36–9, 1996.

22. Fleming TR. Design and interpretation of equivalence trials. Am Heart J 139:S171–6, 2000.

23. Ellenberg SS, Temple R. Placebo-controlled trials and active-control trials in the evaluation of new treatments. Part 2. Practical issues and specific cases. Ann Intern Med 133:464–70, 2000.

24. Food and Drug Administration. Guidance for industry: E 10: choice of control group and related issues in clinical trials. Rockville, MD: Department of Health and Human Services, 2001.

25. Cobb LA, Thomas GI, Dillard DH, et al. An evaluation of internal-mammary-artery ligation by double-blind technic. N Engl J Med 260:1115–8, 1959.

26. Freeman TB, Vawter DE, Leaverton PE, et al. Use of placebo surgery in controlled trials of a cellular-based therapy for Parkinson's disease. N Engl J Med 341:988–92, 1999.

27. Morin CM, Colecchi C, Brink D, et al. How "blind" are double-blind placebo-controlled trials of benzodiazepine hypnotics? Sleep 18:240–5, 1995.

28. Karlowski TR, Chalmers TC, Frenkel LD, et al. Ascorbic acid for the common cold: a prophylactic and therapeutic trial. JAMA 231:1038–42, 1975.

29. Howard J, Whittemore AS, Hoover J, Panos M. The Aspirin Myocardial Infarction Study Research Group: how blind was the patient blind in AMIS? Clin Pharmacol Ther 32:543–53, 1982.

30. Brownell KD, Stunkard AJ. The double-blind in danger: untoward consequences of informed consent. Am J Psychiatry 139:1487–89, 1982.

31. Byrington R, Curb DJ, Mattson ME. Assessment of blindness at the conclusion of the beta-blocker heart attack trial. JAMA 253:1733–36, 1985.

32. Rabkin JG, Markowitz JS, Stewart J, et al. How blind is blind? Assessment of patient and doctor medication guesses in a placebo-controlled trial of imipramine and phenelzine. Psychiatry Res 19:75–86, 1986.

33. Moscussi M, Byrne L, Weintraub M, Cox C. Blinding, unblinding and the placebo effect: an analysis of patients' guesses of treatment assignment in a double-blind clinical trial. Clin Pharmacol Ther 41:259–65, 1987.

34. Fisher S, Greenberg RP. How sound is the double-blind design for evaluating psychotropic drugs? J Nerv Ment Dis 181:345–50, 1993.

35. Basoglu M, Marks I, Livanou M, Swinson R. Double-blindness procedures, rater blindness, and ratings of outcome: observations from a controlled trial. Arch Gen Psychiatry 54:744–8, 1997.

36. Streiner DL, Norman GR. Health measurement scales: a practical guide to their development and use. New York: Oxford University Press, 1995.

37. Gerber WD, Diener HC, Scholz E, Niederberger U. Responders and non-responders to metoprolol, propranolol and nifedipine treatment in migraine prophylaxis: a dose-range study based on time-series analysis. Cephalalgia 11:37–45, 1991.

38. Leijon G, Boivie J. Central post-stroke pain—a controlled trial of amitriptyline and carbamazepine. Pain 36:27–36, 1989.

39. Davis CP, Torre PR, Williams C, et al. Ketorolac versus meperidine-plus-promethazine treatment of migraine headache: evaluations by patients. Am J Emerg Med 13:146–50, 1995.

40. Fromm GH, Terrence CF, Maroon JC. Trigeminal neuralgia: current concepts regarding etiology and pathogenesis. Arch Neurol 41:1204–7, 1984.

41. Max MB. Combining opioids with other drugs: challenges in clinical trial design. In: Gebhart GF, Hammond DL, Jensen TS, eds. Progress in pain research and management, vol. 2. Seattle: IASP Press, 1994:569–85.

42. Jaeschke R, Singer J, Guyatt GH. Measurement of health status. Ascertaining the minimal clinically important difference. Control Clin Trials 10:407–15, 1989.

43. Jaeschke R, Guyatt GH, Keller J, Singer J. Interpreting changes in quality-of-life score in N of 1 randomized trials. Control Clin Trials 12:226S–33S, 1991.

44. Todd KH. Clinical versus statistical significance in the assessment of pain relief. Ann Emerg Med 27:439–41, 1996.

45. Farrar JT, Young JP, LaMoreaux L, et al. Clinical importance of changes in chronic pain intensity measured on an 11-point numerical pain rating scale. Pain 94:149–58, 2001.

46. Farrar JT, Portenoy RK, Berlin JA, et al. Defining the clinically important difference in pain outcome measures. Pain 88:287–94, 2000.

47. Begg CB, Berlin JA. Publication bias: a problem in interpreting medical data. J R Statistical Soc A 151:419–63, 1988.

48. Reidenberg MM. Decreasing publication bias. Clin Pharmacol Ther 63:1–3, 1998.

49. Feinstein AR. An additional basic science for clinical medicine. II. The limitations of randomized trials. Ann Intern Med 99:544–50, 1983.

50. Kramer MS, Shapiro SH. Scientific challenges in the application of randomized trials. JAMA 252:2739–45, 1984.

51. Freiman JA, Chalmers TC, Smith H Jr, Kuebler RR. The importance of beta, the type II error and sample size in the design and interpretation of the randomized controlled trial: survey of 71 "negative" trials. N Engl J Med 299:690–4, 1978.

52. Altman DG. Statistics and ethics in medical research III: how large a sample? Br Med J 281:1336–8, 1980.

53. Collins JF, Bingham SF, Weiss DG, et al. Some adaptive strategies for inadequate sample acquisition in Veterans Administration cooperative clinical trials. Control Clin Trials 1:227–48, 1980.

54. Hunningshake DB, Darby CA, Probstfield JL. Recruitment experience in clinical trials: literature summary and annotated bibliography. Control Clin Trials 8:6S–30S, 1987.

55. Meinert CL. Patient recruitment and enrollment. Clinical trials: design, conduct, and analysis. New York: Oxford University Press, 1986:149–58.

56. Nathan RA. How important is patient recruitment in performing clinical trials? J Asthma 36:213–16, 1999.

57. Taylor KM, Margolese RG, Soskolne CI. Physicians' reasons for not entering eligible patients in a randomized clinical trial of adjuvant surgery for breast cancer. N Engl J Med 310:1363–7, 1984.

58. Taylor KM. Physician participation in a randomized clinical trial for ocular melanoma. Ann Ophthalmol 24:337–44, 1992.

59. Taylor KM, Feldstein ML, Skeel RT, et al. Fundamental dilemmas of the randomized clinical trial process: results of a survey of the 1,737 Eastern Cooperative Oncology Group investigators. J Clin Oncol 12:1796–805, 1994.

60. Greenlick MR, Bailey JW, Wild J, Grover J. Characteristics of men most likely to respond to an invitation to be screened. Am J Public Health 69:1011–5, 1979.

61. Barofsky I, Sugarbaker PH. Determinants of patient nonparticipation in randmized clinical trials for the treatment of sarcomas. Cancer Clin Trials 2:137–46, 1979.

62. Collins JF, Williford WO, Weiss DG, et al. Planning patient recruitment: fantasy and reality. Stat Med 3:435–43, 1984.

63. Begg CB, Carbone PP, Elson PJ, Zelen M. Participation of community hospitals in clinical trials. Analysis of five years of experience in the Eastern Cooperative Oncology Group. N Engl J Med 306:1076–80, 1982.

64. Shea S, Bigger T Jr., Campion J, et al. Enrollment in clinical trials: institutional factors affecting enrollment in the Cardiac Arrhythmia Suppression Trial (CAST). Control Clin Trials 13:466–86, 1992.

65. Mant D. Can randomised trials inform clinical decisions about individual patients? Lancet 353:743–6, 1999.

66. Halpern SD, Metzger DS, Berlin JA, Ubel PA. Who will enroll? Predicting participation in a phase II AIDS vaccine trial. J Acq Immun Def Syn 27:281–8, 2001.

67. Guyatt GH. Methodologic problems in clinical trials in heart failure. J Chronic Dis 38:353–63, 1985.

68. Ellenberg JH. Cohort studies: selection bias in observational and experimental studies. Stat Med 13:557–67, 1994.

69. Fischl MA, Richman DD, Grieco MH, et al. The efficacy of azidothymidine (AZT) in the treatment of patients with AIDS and AIDS-related complex: a double-blind, placebo-controlled trial. N Engl J Med 317:185–91, 1987.

70. Sano M, Ernesto C, Thomas RG. A controlled trial of selegiline, alpha-tocopheral, or both as treatment for Alzheimer's disease. N Engl J Med 336:1216–22, 1997.

71. Kodish E, Lantos JD, Siegler M. Ethical considerations in randomized controlled clinical trials. Cancer 65:2400–4, 1990.

72. Epstein S. Impure science: AIDS, activism, and the politics of knowledge. Berkeley: University of California at Berkeley Press, 1996.

73. Karlawish JHT, Whitehouse PJ. Is the placebo control obsolete in a world after donepezil and vitamin E? Arch Neurol 55:1420–24, 1998.

74. Volberding PA, Lagakos SW, Koch MA, et al. Zidovudine in asymptomatic human immunodeficiency virus infection: a controlled trial in persons with fewer than 500 CD4-positive cells per cubic millimeter. N Engl J Med 322:941–9, 1990.

75. Merrigan TC. You can teach an old dog new tricks: how AIDS trials are pioneering new strategies. N Engl J Med 323:1341–43, 1990.

76. Peto R, Collins R, Gray R. Large-scale randomized evidence: large, simple trials and overviews of trials. J Clin Epidemiol 48:23–40, 1995.

77. National Commission for the Protection of Human Subjects of Biomedical and Behavioral Research. The Belmont Report. Ethical principles and guidelines for the protection of human subjects of research. Washington, DC: US Government Printing Office, 1979.

78. World Medical Association. Declaration of Helsinki: recommendations guiding physicians in biomedical research involving human subjects. JAMA 277:925–6, 1997.

79. Casarett D, Karlawish JHT, Sankar P, et al. Obtaining informed consent for clinical pain research: patients' concerns and information needs. Pain 92:223–9, 2001.

80. World Medical Association. International Declaration of Helsinki, 1964. October, 2000. http://www.wma.net/e/policy/17-c_e.html.

27 Legal and regulatory aspects of opioid treatment: the United States experience

JUNE L. DAHL
University of Wisconsin-Madison School of Medicine

Introduction

Pain is the most common and perhaps the most feared symptom of cancer (1–4). About one third of persons with cancer have pain at the time their disease is diagnosed and more than two thirds with advanced disease have pain (4–7). Almost all pain of cancer can be relieved with currently available pharmacological and non-pharmacological therapies (4–8). Unfortunately, studies carried out over the past 20 years reveal that often these therapies are not used appropriately. As a result, persons with cancer, even those at the end of life, suffer needlessly from pain (4,9–13). Therefore, it is not surprising that a recent survey found that the general public fear being in pain at the end of life more than they fear death (14).

The reasons for undertreatment of pain have also been thoroughly documented over the last 20 years. These include lack of knowledge and inappropriate attitudes among health care professionals, and patients and families, as well as barriers in the health care and regulatory systems (15–18).

If the magnitude of the problem and the reasons for undertreatment have been known for so long, why does the problem still exist? There are no simple answers to that question. Possible solutions are complicated by the fact that myths and misperceptions about pain and its management are pervasive among health care professionals, patients, and families. Furthermore, the Herculean task of removing the barriers to effective pain management has been undertaken by a relatively small, but dedicated core of health care professionals who know that pain can and should be managed, that relief of pain is a basic human right. Far too many health care professionals have not been taught how to assess and manage pain; far too many members of the general public view pain as

an inevitable, essentially untreatable, part of cancer; and far too few health care facilities have made pain management a priority.

There is much evidence that the laws and regulations designed to reduce prescription drug diversion and abuse have had a significant impact on the management of cancer pain (4,19–22). This chapter addresses the legal and regulatory barriers in the United States, the evidence for their impact on the medical use of opioids, and the progress that is being made to overcome the identified barriers. There is a brief description of the limitations on the supply and distribution of pain-relieving drugs that are common in other parts of the world, especially in developing countries. The reader is referred to other resources for more details about the challenging subject of opioid availability (23,24).

Opioid analgesics have long been the drugs of choice for the management of moderate to severe pain associated with cancer (4–8,23). Yet, in spite of their documented effectiveness, they are often underused, a factor that has contributed significantly to the undertreatment of cancer pain. Physicians may give inappropriate drugs or inadequate doses at inappropriate dosing intervals (9,17,25), nurses may undermedicate (18), pharmacists may not stock opioids (26,27), and patients may be reluctant to take these drugs (4,15,16). There may be reluctance to prescribe because of lack of knowledge of basic analgesic pharmacology, fear and misunderstanding of tolerance and addiction (4,17,18), and/or concerns that large doses of these drugs may kill patients (28,29).

The history of our attitudes about opioids and other drugs that have the potential to be abused has been well chronicled (30,31). At times there has been an almost hysterical fear of opioids among the general public, as well as an almost puritanical reluctance to use painkillers. There has been, and sometimes still is, apprehension surrounding even the routine use of opioids, a fear that has been termed opiophobia (32). These attitudes have been strengthened by our very real drug abuse problem and by a past history of repressive attitudes among drug control and law enforcement officials. Fortunately, as described later, those attitudes are changing.

Health care professionals fear regulatory scrutiny. Medical decision making about the use of opioids continues to be influenced by regulatory policies or fear of regulators. For example, more than half of Wisconsin physicians who responded to a 1991 survey said that they would occasionally reduce drug dosage or quantity or limit refills because of fears of regulatory scrutiny (33). In a 1993 report, oncologists in the Eastern Cooperative Oncology Group ranked excessive regulation of analgesics among the top four barriers to effective pain management in their settings (17).

The California Department of Consumer Affairs convened a Summit on Effective Pain Management in March of 1994, which was co-sponsored by the California Medical Association and the California medical, nursing, and pharmacy boards. The Summit was called in recognition of the fact that "because of fear of investigation or action by regulatory boards or law enforcement, health care professionals have often been unwilling to prescribe or dispense strong pain medications appropriately" (34). A 1996 report to the Florida legislature from the Florida Pain Commission stated that "hospice workers noted problems with some physicians who still seem reluctant to prescribe appropriately for the terminally ill because of concerns of licensure censure" (35). Nine out of ten respondents to a survey conducted by the Michigan Department of Consumer & Industry Services, Bureau of Health Services said that the requirements of the Michigan Official Prescription Program "may prevent them from providing needed Schedule II medications to patients" (36). In 1997, the New York State Public Health Council established an ad hoc Committee on Pain Management to identify the barriers to effective pain management in the state and recommend ways to overcome those impediments. The Committee, working in conjunction with the Medical Society of the State of New York, surveyed 6000 physicians to assess their fears about possible disciplinary or administrative actions resulting from the use of opioids. A majority indicated that they were very concerned about regulatory investigation. In its final report published in 1998, the Committee wrote: "New York health care practioners may underprescribe pain medication due to fear of unwarranted legal consequences" (37).

In spite of the documented fears of practitioners, there is no evidence that large numbers of physicians or pharmacists are sanctioned for the prescribing or dispensing of opioids to patients in pain. According to the Federation of State Medical Boards, in 1997 about 8% of disciplinary actions against U.S. physicians involved a controlled substances violation. About 12% of those disciplinary actions resulted in license revocation. This is about 0.9% of all disciplinary actions (38). Nevertheless, a few well-publicized cases have cast a pall over the professions involved in the prescribing and dispensing of controlled substances and left them with the perception that regulatory sanctions are very common. Furthermore, the impact of an investigative process on those professionals who are suspected of or charged with a violation of the law and subsequently exonerated is enormous. There is not only the personal angst associated with being investigated by a government agency, but also the potential financial impact, as most professionals retain counsel and probably will need to take time off from their practices to appear at hearings.

It is important to understand what it is about past and current drug laws and regulations that created such fear in health care professionals. Even though the fears appear to be based on perceptions rather than reality, they are still very real. A current continuing education program on controlled substances laws for U.S. pharmacists obviously reinforces the paranoia. It is subtitled: "Adhering to federal and state regulations is crucial to preventing liability; even innocent errors can lead to significant penalties" (39).

Laws and regulations

The laws and regulations that govern the production and distribution of controlled substances generally, and opioid analgesics in particular, are intended to prevent their diversion to the illicit market and to protect the public from the adverse consequences associated with the abuse of these drugs. These are established by international treaties and federal and state laws and regulations.

International drug control

The Single Convention on Narcotic Drugs, adopted in 1961 and amended in 1972, is the international treaty that regulates the production, manufacture, import, export, and distribution of narcotic drugs for medical use (40). Countries that are party to the Single Convention are required to control all aspects of the use of opioids within their territories and all international movement of opioids. Despite the Convention's emphasis on combating illicit drug traffic, the treaty is not intended to reduce the use of opioids needed for legitimate medical purposes. The Single Convention on Narcotic Drugs recognizes the important medical use of opioids to relieve pain and suffering and states that these drugs are indispensable for the public health: "The medical use of narcotic drugs continues to be indispensable for the relief of pain and suffering and adequate provision must be made to ensure the availability of narcotic drugs for such purposes" (23).

The treaty emphasizes the importance of a balanced drug control policy—preventing the diversion and abuse of prescription drugs while ensuring their availability for legitimate medical purposes (23,41). Reports on production, manufacture, imports, exports, and consumption of opioids must be made to the International Narcotics Control Board (INCB) in Vienna, Austria (42). Each country must supply a realistic estimate of the amounts of these drugs it will need to meet the demand for their medical use. The legislative, regulatory, and administrative impediments in various countries that lead to underutilization of opioids in turn lead to low estimates of a nation's need for pain medicines. A joint document prepared by the INCB and the World Health Organization Expert Committee on Pain Relief and Palliative Care recognized that "concern about illicit drug use and its social consequences had curtailed the availability of opioid drugs to patients with cancer pain" (23). The two organizations made specific recommendations to enhance the availability of these drugs to patients in pain: 1) review the administrative practices of opioid drug control with a view to their simplification so as not to impede legitimate use of opioids by patients, and 2) determine the probable needs of the country, based on estimates of present consumption plus the "best guess" of needs for the likely number of cancer patients to be treated (23).

The Pain and Policy Studies Group at the University of Wisconsin-Madison has worked diligently to remove the barriers that prevent access to pain medicines in other countries of the world (43). The World Health Organization has published self-assessment guidelines to encourage governments to achieve better pain management by identifying and overcoming regulatory barriers to opioid availability (44).

Federal laws and regulations

Origins of opioid control

The laws of the United States also recognize that opioids are necessary for the public health. They mandate that there be scientific and medical input into drug control decisions. They guarantee drug availability and place no restrictions on the amount or the length of time that a drug can be prescribed. These very positive aspects of federal law need to be placed in an historical context, however, because only in this way can one understand the origins of many opioid myths and misperceptions that still adversely affect pain management practices.

Opium use gradually increased in the United States over the course of the 19th century (45). Many patent medicines contained opium; by the latter part of the century, opium and morphine "were widely prescribed by physicians to treat pain, cough, diarrhea and dysentery, as well as a host of disorders from anemia and angina to diabetes, tetanus, menstrual and menopausal discomforts, the vomiting of pregnancy and to calm teething babies" (31). Physicians referred to opium and morphine as "God's own medicine." Physicians prescribed these drugs to bring a sense of tranquility and well-being, because there was little that could be done for many illnesses; morphine was even used as a substitute for alcohol (30,31). Not everyone was supportive of these practices; eventually "there was medical consensus that morphine had been overused by physicians, that addiction was a substantial possibility, and that the addition of opioids to patent medicines should be stopped" (30). Dr. Oliver Wendell Holmes, Sr., Dean of the Harvard Medical School, stated that the constant prescription of morphine by physicians in the western United States "had rendered habitual use very prevalent." Interestingly, surveys of users showed they were primarily from the middle to upper middle classes and were using morphine as a "tranquilizer" not because they experienced euphoria from the drug. By the turn of the century there appeared to be a significant population of addicts[1] and that resulted in public and governmental demands to decrease drug availability. An important step toward this goal occurred in 1906 when Congress passed the first Pure Food and Drug Act in spite of vigorous opposition from the patent medicine interests. The Act required that medicines that

---

[1] The term *addict* was never clearly defined in the literature of the time. Still today there is confusion about the meaning of addiction. It is often erroneously used synonymously with tolerance and physical dependence. While there may have been lack of clarity about the meaning of the term at the turn of the century, there is no question that addicts were viewed with contempt (30,31). As late as 1962, the U.S. Supreme Court described a drug addict as "one of the walking dead" and failed to separate the direct effects of opioids from the effects related to the socioeconomic conditions of addicts (31).

contained opioids and certain other drugs be clearly labeled. Later amendments required that the quantity of each drug be stated; eventually standards for purity were established.

Another major step was taken in 1914 when Congress passed the Harrison Act, the first major federal antinarcotic law (46). Its intent was to curb recreational use and non-medical use of opioids. Before the Harrison Act, there were few if any legal controls over the sale and distribution of opium or its derivatives in the United States. The Harrison Act grew out of U.S. obligations under new international treaties aimed at reducing opium traffic throughout the world. It was not intended to regulate medical practice. There was nothing in the Act that prevented the dispensing or distribution of any opioids (narcotics) to a patient by a physician, dentist, or veterinary surgeon in the course of his professional practice so long as they were registered as required by the Act. It was assumed by many physicians that supplying opioids to individuals to maintain an addiction was a legitimate part of medical practice. However, law enforcement officers of the time concluded that such action was illegal under the Harrison Act. The controversy was resolved when the Supreme Court provided a definitive interpretation of the Act in 1919 (47). The Court ruled that it was against the law for physicians to prescribe opioids to maintain an addiction.

In the years that followed there was vigorous prosecution of physicians under this interpretation; some were convicted and sent to prison, others left their practices in disgrace. The addiction problem was blamed on physicians. Indeed physicians awakened rather slowly to the fact that opioids could be addicting. The feeling that physicians contribute significantly to the addiction problem persists to this day and colors physician prescribing and patient acceptance of these pain relievers. Many adhere to the mistaken belief that persons inevitably become addicted if they are given opioids for pain relief.

The Controlled Substances Act
By the late 1960s there were more than 50 federal laws that dealt with substances and drugs that could be abused. The Food Drug and Cosmetic Act of 1962 established the U.S. Food and Drug Administration (FDA) as the agency that approved drugs, including opioids, as safe and effective for medical use. However, the regulation of drugs of abuse was split between two bureaus. The Bureau of Drug Abuse Control, which was part of the FDA, regulated stimulants, depressants, and hallucinogens. The Bureau of Narcotics and Dangerous Drugs in the Department of Justice regulated marijuana,

cocaine, and opioids. In 1970, Congress repealed the multiple federal laws and passed the Controlled Substances Act (CSA) to regulate the manufacturing, distribution, dispensing, and delivery of drugs or substances that are subject to, or have the potential for, abuse or physical or psychological dependence (48). The CSA is sometimes referred to as Title 2 of the Comprehensive Drug Abuse Prevention and Control Act of 1970.

In 1973, the Drug Enforcement Administration (DEA) was created in the Department of Justice. The CSA is administered by the DEA; the CSA empowers the DEA to register all persons, businesses, and institutions conducting any activity that involves controlled substances. The DEA does this by issuing registration numbers that must be renewed every 3 years; however, manufacturers and distributors must register every year. The agency also regulates precursor chemicals that may be used in producing controlled substances, as well as machinery used in manufacturing controlled substances and controlled substances analogs. (See references 39, 49–51 for more complete descriptions of federal controlled substances laws.)

Separate DEA registrations are required for each individual site at which controlled substances are stored or dispensed. Every pharmacy must have its own separate registration and DEA number. If a chain has 100 pharmacies, each operating at a separate street address, there must be 100 separate registrations. Separate registrations are also required for multiple activities even if they occur at the same location. A large health care facility may manufacture, distribute, and dispense controlled substances. Each activity requires a separate registration, and an additional registration is required for research.

When prescribing controlled substances, the following must be included on the prescription order (as noted below, some states require the use of special prescription forms):

- Patient's name and address
- Prescriber's name, address, and DEA registration number
- Prescriber's signature
- Name and quantity of the drug prescribed and directions for use

The CSA classifies medicinal substances into a hierarchy of five schedules based on their medical usefulness and their abuse and dependence-producing potential (Table 27.1). Initially, the CSA gave the FDA the authority to determine whether a drug would be classified as a controlled substance, and if so, in which schedule it would be placed. In 1986, the FDA's authority for sched-

Table 27.1. *Federal schedules for controlled substances*

Schedule			
I	No currently accepted medical use in the United States High potential for abuse	Hallucinogenic substances; heroin and certain other opioids; methaqualone	Available for research, instructional use, and chemical analysis purpose
II	Currently accepted medical use in the United States High potential for abuse Severe liability to cause psychological or physical dependence	Opium, morphine, codeine, hydro-morphone, oxycodone, oxymorphone, methadone, fentanyl, dextroamphetamine, methamphetamine, methylphenidate; amobarbital, pentobarbital, secobarbital	Written prescription required except in emergencies; however, written prescriptions may be transmitted by fax in some instances (see text) No refills
III	Potential for abuse less than for drugs in schedules I and II Abuse may lead to moderate or lower physical and psychological dependence than substances in schedules I or II	Combinations of codeine with aspirin or acetaminophen; certain sedative drugs; dronabinol; buprenorphine	Oral prescription orders allowed Prescription orders valid for 6 months Five refills allowed in 6 months
IV	Lower potential for abuse than drugs in schedule III Limited physical or psychological dependence	Benzodiazepines, phenobarbital, propoxyphene, certain sedative drugs, butorphanol	Same restriction as for schedule III
V	Potential for abuse is less than for drugs in schedule IV	Antitussive, antidiarrheal preparations containing moderate quantities of opioids	May be dispensed without a prescription

uling drugs was assumed by the DEA. The DEA now has primary responsibility for promulgating the regulations that implement, interpret, and enforce the CSA.

Most opioid analgesics are in Schedules II and III. Schedule II drugs include morphine, hydromorphone, methadone, levorphanol, fentanyl, codeine, oxycodone, and combination products with oxycodone and a non-opioid. Federal limitations on prescribing orders for Schedule II drugs include (52):

- Written prescription orders are required except for emergencies; in emergencies oral prescription orders are permitted, but with two restrictions: the amount prescribed and dispensed is limited to the amount adequate to treat the patient during the emergency period, and a written prescription order must be received by the pharmacist within 7 days. Under earlier regulations, the prescription order had to be received within 72 hours.
- Written prescriptions for Schedule II drugs may be transmitted by fax to infusion pharmacies and pharmacies that service long-term care facilities.
- If a pharmacist is unable to supply the full quantity of the written or oral emergency prescription, the remaining portion can be filled within 72 hours.
- No further quantity may be supplied beyond 72 hours without a new prescription.

- A prescription may be filled in partial quantities for patients who are terminally ill or in long-term care facilities; the remainder of the drug must be dispensed within 60 days of the prescription date.
- No refills are allowed

Schedule III and IV analgesics include combination products that contain aspirin or acetaminophen with codeine or propoxyphene, respectively. Benzodiazepines are in Schedule IV. Schedule III and IV drugs are subject to less stringent regulations. Prescription orders are valid for 6 months from the date of issue, and a maximum of five refills is allowed within 6 months of issuance of the prescription. Written prescriptions for drugs in Schedules III, IV, and V may be transmitted by fax, but the written prescription must be presented at the time the drug is dispensed. However, infusion pharmacies and pharmacies that service long-term care facilities can consider the fax as a "written prescription." The abuse potential of Schedule V drugs is considered so low that they may be dispensed without a prescription in many states. Codeine containing cough suppressants and antidiarrheals are in Schedule V.

It is important to emphasize that the federal government does not regulate medical practice—this is a function of the states. However, through the work of various agencies and some policy statements, there is some federal involvement. In 1974, Congress adopted a law to prohibit physicians from prescribing opioids to detoxify or maintain opioid addiction (unless they were operating as part of a separately registered narcotic treatment program). This law does *not* prohibit the prescribing of methadone for pain control. Because of its long duration of action and its relatively low cost, methadone can be very valuable for the management of certain chronic pain problems.

The DEA has declared that the CSA was not intended to interfere with physicians who used opioids to treat intractable pain (52). The DEA reiterated and communicated this policy to U.S. physicians, pharmacists, and mid-level practitioners through a series of manuals. A statement on the use of controlled substances for pain control will be included in revisions of those publications.

State laws and regulations

States have also promulgated laws and regulations to prevent diversion and abuse of controlled substances. The reader is referred to the comprehensive analysis of state laws and regulations published by the Pain and Policy Studies Group at the University of Wisconsin Medical School (43,51). The controlled substances laws in most states are based on a 1970 model law called the Uniform Controlled Substances Act (UCSA). The goal of the UCSA was to establish a uniform national drug control policy that would result in repeal of antiquated state laws. Not all states repealed their old laws and as will be discussed later, some adopted laws and regulations that are more stringent than those in federal law.

For example, some state laws do not explicitly recognize that opioids are essential to the public health; in other words, they do not articulate the importance of balance that is found in federal law. States may limit the quantity of a drug that may be prescribed or dispensed at one time. Some states enforce limits of a 30- or 34-day supply; other states caution against prescribing an *excessive amount,* a term that has no meaning in the modern world of pain management. Some state laws and regulations contain inaccurate or confusing definitions of addiction. Some appear to prohibit the use of opioids for pain control in persons who have a history of substance abuse (51). Furthermore, as discussed later, several states have implemented special programs for monitoring the prescribing and dispensing of controlled substances that require the use of government-issued prescription forms. States that have granted nurse practitioners prescribing authority may or may not allow them to prescribe controlled substances or may prohibit their prescribing of

Schedule II drugs (53). Practitioners must comply with both the federal and state laws that govern their practice.

Multiple copy prescription programs

Certain states have implemented paper-based, government-issued multiple copy prescription programs (MCPPs) as a means of monitoring the prescribing and dispensing of Schedule II controlled substances (50). The first MCPP program, which was adopted in California in 1939, required prescribers to write prescriptions on triplicate forms, one copy stayed with the prescriber, one with the pharmacist, and the third went to a state agency. Between 1943 and 1988, other states adopted MCPPs that required the use of triplicates, duplicates, or single-copy forms.

The year after a triplicate program was introduced in the State of Texas in 1982, there was a dramatic decrease in the prescribing of Schedule II controlled substances (54). Regulators claimed that decrease indicated a drop in inappropriate prescribing, but others asserted that the imposition of triplicates increased fears of government scrutiny of medical practice (55–57). In 1996, Wastila and Bishop (57) reported their analysis of the impact of MCPPs on opioid and non-opioid analgesic use. Their data showed that pain patients in states with MCPPs were less likely to receive a Schedule II opioid and more likely to obtain a prescription for a Schedule III medication. In addition MCPPs were associated with lower rates of use of analgesics as a whole. Unfortunately, there are no published studies of the impact of MCPPs on diversion and abuse of Schedule II opioids in spite of the fact that prevention of diversion is the purpose for which the programs are intended.

The switch to electronic monitoring

Computerized prescription data systems are frequently used for third-party reimbursement and are able to readily identify physicians and patients who prescribe or consume large quantities of drugs. To date, 16 states have implemented electronic prescription monitoring programs, or electronic data transmission (EDT) systems, to track controlled substances (58). Idaho, Kentucky, Michigan and Utah track Schedule II–V; Hawaii, Nevada, Tennessee and Wyoming monitor Schedule II–IV; Rhode Island tracks Schedule II–III; and the others track only Schedule II drugs. EDT systems have one important benefit: they do not require physicians to use special prescription forms for controlled substances, forms that clearly signal that a regulatory agency is scrutinizing their medical practice. However, four states use electronic data transmission systems in conjunction with single-copy serialized forms. In some cases, a single-copy system requires prescribers to buy serialized prescription pads from the state and use these special forms when prescribing controlled substances. Pharmacists enter the information on the prescription into a computer and transmit the information to a state agency. There are no studies of the impact of single-copy systems on physician prescribing, but one policy specialist feels that "they are likely to have the same chilling effect on opioid prescribing as have the MCPPs" (59). There are no studies that document the impact of single-copy systems on diversion and abuse of controlled substances.

Intractable pain treatment laws

Some state legislatures have adopted laws to affirm the appropriateness of using opioids to treat intractable pain. The first Intractable Pain Treatment Act (IPTA) was adopted by Texas in 1989, and a year later California adopted a law modeled on the Texas Act (43,51,60). The passage of these laws, now in place in 11 states, was promoted by persons with chronic non-cancer pain whose physicians were uncertain about the legality of prescribing opioids for extended periods of time for persons who do not have cancer. Protection of physicians who prescribe opioids for pain control is a worthy goal, but unfortunately, some IPTAs create additional barriers. The very term *intractable pain* gives cause for concern. Intractable pain is defined, as "a pain state in which the cause of the pain cannot be removed or otherwise treated and for which in the generally accepted course of medical practice no relief or cure of the cause of the pain is possible or none has been found after reasonable efforts" (60). This term could apply to the person whose cancer has been "cured" but who continues to experience pain caused by conditions resulting from surgery or chemotherapy or radiotherapy. Who defines the meaning of the phrase *the generally accepted course of medical practice?* What constitutes reasonable efforts? How many expensive and invasive procedures must be carried out before it is decided that there have been reasonable efforts?

Some ITPAs do not allow the use of opioids for the treatment of pain patients who have a history of substance abuse; others require a second opinion from a specialist in the organ system believed to be the cause of pain. However, there is no requirement for that specialist to have specific knowledge about pain assessment and management. Joranson (61) drew attention to state pain commissions as vehicles for studying and addressing impediments to effective pain management, such as regulatory barriers. So long as these commissions "are well informed, have adequate support and a balanced agenda," he viewed them as being positive forces for improving the regulatory climate in a state. Pain commissions were formed in Massachusetts, Florida, and several other states in the early to mid 1990s, but are now inactive. Recently, there has been a resurgence of interest in using task forces or commissions to advance pain management efforts. The New Mexico State Senate recently established a study group, as did the Maryland legislature. The Michigan Commission on Death and Dying was effective in bringing regulatory reform in that state: eliminating the requirement for single-copy prescription forms and replacing the term "intractable pain" with the single word "pain" in existing laws and regulations.

Medical board guidelines

Several state medical boards have issued guidelines or statements that address the use of opioids for the treatment of chronic pain (43,51). In California, similar guidelines were issued by the nursing and pharmacy boards (62). These guidelines provide an official statement of a board's policy regarding a particular issue: for example, what constitutes appropriate use of opioids for the management of pain. Now more than half of the states (63) have adopted pain guidelines. Their emphasis varies: some do not state that quality medical practice dictates that persons have access to appropriate and effective pain relief; others do not recognize that opioid analgesics may be essential in the treatment of pain, including chronic pain. Some suggest, as do certain IPTAs, that opioids are the "court of last resort." One requires physicians to demonstrate that "other measures and drugs have been inadequate or not tolerated before beginning treatment with opioids" (64). A few suggest outmoded approaches to therapy such as "consider drug holidays to monitor compliance and continued need (65)."

In 1998, The Federation of State Medical Boards of the United States issued Model Guidelines for the Use of Controlled Substances for the Treatment of Pain (66). The Federation believed that guidelines based on the model would protect "legitimate medical uses of controlled substances while preventing drug diversion and eliminating inappropriate prescribing practices" and has urged state licensing boards to adopt them. Such guidelines are critical in light of the results of a survey of members of state medical boards (67). Only 75% of the respondents agreed that the prescribing of opioids for cancer patients with pain was legal and generally accepted medical practice! If the patient with cancer and pain had a history of substance abuse, the percentage decreased significantly. And yet there is nothing in state or federal laws that prohibits the prescribing of opioids to such persons, and it is clearly accepted medical practice (4). Von Roenn et al. (17) found oncologists were reluctant to prescribe Schedule II opioids to persons with cancer unless those persons had a very short life expectancy. Hyman (68) has suggested that the key to appropriate enforcement of controlled substances laws and regulations by medical boards is to enhance members' level of knowledge about pain and its management. Gilson and Joranson (69) described the implementation of educational programs for state medical board members and staff that have stimulated boards to remove regulatory barriers to effective pain management. They concluded that "these have also brought important, although not profound, improvements in knowledge, attitudes and beliefs of board members" (69)

Codifying the myth of double effect

Myths about opioids provide significant barriers to the effective management of pain. Tolerance and addiction are common concerns, but recently a third myth seems to have taken hold: the myth of double effect, the unproven assumption that opioids shorten life (28,29). This myth is now codified in several state intractable pain treatment acts and appears in guidelines promulgated by certain medical boards (e.g., "a licensed health care provider who administers, prescribes or dispenses medications or procedures to relieve a person's pain or discomfort, even if the medication or procedure may hasten or increase the risk of death) (70,71)." Although such language is intended to provide comfort to prescribers, it may instead reinforce existing paranoia about the risks associated with the prescribing of opioids, especially the very large doses that may be required to provide pain relief at the end of life.

Health care providers' liability for inadequate pain management

Some have suggested that instead of sanctioning health care professionals for overprescribing, they should be sanctioned for underprescribing. Health care facilities as well as health care professionals should be held liable for poor pain management (72). In 1990, a North Carolina long-term care facility was held liable for failure to treat a resident who died in terrible pain because of the decision by the facility and a nurse to withhold pain medication that was ordered by the patient's physician (73). The

Georgia Supreme Court affirmed a patient's right not only to have unwanted medical treated discontinued, but also to receive medication to manage his pain at the time (72). And then in 1999, the Oregon Board of Medical Examiners sanctioned a physician who failed to provide adequate pain relief for his patients (74). This was an astonishing action in view of the Board's long history of sanctioning physicians for overtreatment. In a statement adopted in 1999, the Oregon Board "urges the use of effective pain control for all patients irrespective of the etiology of their pain. The Board will consider clearly documented undertreatment of pain to be a violation equal to overtreatment and will investigate allegations in the same manner (75)." Obviously, they followed through on that commitment. It is hoped that other state medical boards will follow Oregon's lead. Board actions should be balanced so as "to protect legitimate medical use of controlled substances while preventing drug diversion and eliminating inappropriate prescribing practices (66)."

Summary

Recent dramatic advances in the science and medicine of pain have been accompanied by unprecedented changes in laws and regulations that deal with the use of controlled substances for pain control. The Institute of Medicine's Report on Improving Care at the End of Life (21) called attention to the fact that prescription drug laws that are intended to minimize drug addiction and diversion can compromise effective pain management. Both the DEA and state regulatory authorities have publicly acknowledged that opioid analgesics may be essential in the treatment of acute and chronic pain and that laws and regulations may discourage the prescribing and dispensing of these drugs. In the fall of 2001, the DEA and 21 health organizations issued a joint policy statement titled: *Promoting Pain Relief and Preventing Abuse of Pain Medications: A Critical Balancing Act* (76). Many states have taken action to reduce or eliminate regulatory barriers. At the same time other states have established controlled substances monitoring programs with single-copy prescription form requirements that can impact adversely on prescribing practices and ultimately affect the quality of pain management.

The Pain and Policy Studies Group has identified provisions in state laws, regulations, and medical board guidelines that may impede effective pain management and/or contain ambiguous language. Their Guide to Evaluation (43,51) provides the information essential for eliminating remaining barriers and encouraging additional change. It is incumbent on health care professionals who are committed to improving the management of pain to familiarize themselves with the regulations that are operative in their state, to identify barriers, and to engage regulators in dialogue so as to ensure that there is a balanced regulatory climate in the state.

It may be useful to promulgate consensus statements, such as those from the Federation of State Medical Boards (66) and the American Pain Society and American Academy of Pain Medicine (77), to clarify the appropriate role of opioids in pain management. These and the recent consensus statement on definitions related to the use of opioids (78) can be used to educate colleagues, regulators, patients, and families about the meaning of tolerance, physical dependence, and addiction. Prescribers must follow the guidelines for the use of opioids for pain control. Prescribers must document their plan of treatment and regularly assess and document response to the treatment plan. Thorough documentation is critical to protecting a practice from the vagaries of a regulatory challenge.

There is a critical need for research in this arena: Research is needed to provide definitive data to assess the impact of the increased medical use of opioids on their diversion and abuse, the impact of laws and regulations on pain management, as well as the impact of laws and regulations on diversion and abuse of controlled substances. A recent report that the increased medical use of opioid analgesics from 1990 to 1996 did not appear to lead to an increase in drug diversion represents an important beginning (79). Such studies are necessary to ensure that the dialogue between health care professionals and regulators is based on fact and not on unproven assumptions.

In fact, much of our problem arises from misperceptions and inappropriate attitudes of physicians, medical boards, lawmakers, patients, and the public: Reform needs to go beyond revisions in policies written by governmental authorities. It needs to affect our values, "to help establish appropriate pain management as a component of the standard of care" (72). The pain assessment and management standards recently adopted by the Joint Commission on Accreditation of Healthcare Organizations do establish such standards of care (80,81). These will provide critical support to those who are committed to ensuring that all persons with cancer and pain have competent and compassionate care.

References

1. Daut RI, Cleeland CS. The prevalence and severity of pain in cancer. Cancer 50:1913–18, 1982.

2. Cleeland CS. The impact of pain on the patient with cancer. Cancer 54:2635–41, 1984.

3. Levin DN, Cleeland CS, Dar R. Public attitudes toward cancer pain. Cancer 56:2337–39, 1985.

4. Jacox AK, Carr DB, Payne R, et al. Management of cancer pain, clinical practice guideline, No. 9. US Department of Health and Human Services, Public Health Service, AHCPR Publication No. 94-0592. Rockville, MD: Agency for Health Care Policy and Research, 1994.

5. Foley KM. The treatment of cancer pain. N Engl J Med 313:84–95, 1985.

6. Levy MH. Pharmacologic treatment of cancer pain. N Engl J Med 335:1124–32, 1996.

7. Portenoy RK, Lesage P. Management of cancer pain. Lancet 353:1695–1700, 1999.

8. American Pain Society. Principles of analgesic use in the treatment of acute pain and cancer pain, 4th ed. Glenview, IL: American Pain Society, 1999.

9. Cleeland CS, Gonin R, Hatfield AK, et al. Pain and its treatment in outpatients with metastatic cancer. N Engl J Med 330:592–6, 1994.

10. SUPPORT Study Principle Investigators. A controlled trial to improve care for seriously ill, hospitalized patients: a study to understand prognoses and preferences for outcomes and risks of treatments. JAMA 274:1591–8, 1995.

11. Lynn J, Teno JM, Phillips RS, et al. Perceptions by family members of the dying experience in older and seriously ill patients. Ann Intern Med 126:97–106, 1997.

12. Bernabei R, Gambassi G, Lapane K, et al. Management of pain in elderly patients with cancer. JAMA 279:1877–82, 1998.

13. Wolfe J, Grier HE, Klar N, et al. Symptoms and suffering at the end of life in children with cancer. N Engl J Med 342:326–33, 2000.

14. Redford GD. The final answers. Modern Maturity September-October: 43:66–8, 2000.

15. Cleeland CS. Barriers to the management of cancer pain. Oncology (Supplement) April: 9–26, 1987.

16. Ward SE, Goldberg N, Miller-McCauley V, et al. Patient-related barriers to management of cancer pain. Pain 52:319–24, 1993.

17. Von Roenn JH, Cleeland CS, Gonin R, et al. Physician attitudes and practice in cancer pain management: a survey of the Eastern Cooperative Oncology Group. Ann Int Med 119:121–6, 1993.

18. Pargeon KL, Hailey BJ. Barriers to effective cancer pain management: a review of the literature. J Pain Symptom Manage 18:358–68, 1999.

19. Hill CS Jr. Pain management in a drug-oriented society. Cancer. 63(11 Suppl):2383–6, 1989.

20. Hill CS Jr. The barriers to adequate pain management with opioid analgesics. Semin Oncol 20 (Suppl 1):1–5, 1993.

21. Field MR, Cassel CK, eds. Approaching death: improving care at the end of life. Washington, DC: National Academy Press, 1997:188–206.

22. Joranson DE, Gilson AM. Regulatory barriers to pain management. Semin Oncol Nurs 14:158–63, 1998.

23. WHO Expert Committee. Cancer pain relief and palliative care. Geneva: World Health Organization, 1990.
24. Joranson DE, Colleau SM. Medical needs for opioids far from being met. Cancer Pain Release 9:2–3, 1996.
25. Portenoy RK, Kanner RM. Patterns of analgesic prescription and consumption in a university-affiliated community hospital. Arch Intern Med 145:439–41, 1985.
26. Kanner RM, Portenoy RK. Unavailability of narcotic analgesics for ambulatory cancer patients in New York City. J Pain Symptom Manage 1:87–9, 1986.
27. Morrison RS, Wallestein S, Natale DK, et al. "We don't carry that"–failure of pharmacies in predominantly nonwhite neighborhoods to stock opioid analgesics. N Engl J Med 342:1023–6, 2000.
28. Fohr SA. The double effect of pain medication: separating myth from reality. J Palliat Med 1:315–27, 1998.
29. Wall PD. The generation of yet another myth on the use of narcotics. Pain 73:121–2, 1997.
30. Musto DF. The American disease. Origins of narcotic control, 3rd ed. New York: Oxford University Press, 1999.
31. Brecher EM and the Editors of Consumer Reports. Licit and illicit drugs: the Consumers Union Report on narcotics stimulants, depressants, inhalants, hallucinogens and marijuana–including caffeine, nicotine and alcohol. Boston: Little Brown and Company, 1972.
32. Morgan JP. American opiophobia: customary underutilization of opioid analgesics. In: Hill Jr CS, Fields WS, eds. Advances in pain research and therapy. Drug treatment of cancer pain in a drug-oriented society, vol. 11. New York: Raven Press, 1989:181–9.
33. Weissman DE, Joranson DE, Hopwood MB. Wisconsin physicians' knowledge and attitudes about opioid analgesic regulations. Wis Med J 90:671–5, 1991.
34. Wilson P, Kozberg JC, Barnett CL. Summit on effective pain management: removing impediments to appropriate prescribing. Summit Report. State of California, July 29, 1994.
35. Florida Pain Management Commission. Pain Management. A report to the Florida legislature, the Agency for Health Care Administration and the residents of the State of Florida, January 1996.
36. Michigan Official Prescription Program. Evaluation report. Michigan Department of Consumer & Industry Services, Bureau of Health Services and Michigan Controlled Substances Advisory Commission, September 1997.
37. New York State Public Health Council. Breaking down the barriers to effective pain management. Recommendations to improve the assessment and treatment of pain in New York State. Report to the Commissioner of Health, January 1998.
38. Dr. James Winn, Federation of State Medical Boards. Personal communication.
39. US Pharmacist Continuing Education. A review of federal controlled substances laws. ACPE Program No. 430-000-99-029-H03, 2000.
40. United Nations. Single convention on narcotic drugs, 1961. New York: United Nations, 1972.
41. Coyne PG. International efforts in cancer pain relief. Semin Oncol Nurs 13:57–62, 1997.
42. International Narcotics Control Board. Demand for and supply of opiates for medical and scientific needs. Report of the International Narcotics Control Board for 1995. New York: United Nations, 1996.
43. Pain and Policy Studies Group http://www.medsch.wisc.edu/painpolicy.
44. World Health Organization. Achieving balance in national opioids control policy: guidelines for assessment. Geneva: World Health Organization, 2000.
45. Melzack R. The tragedy of needless pain. Sci Am 262:28–33, 1990.
46. Public Law No. 223, 63rd Cong, approved December 17, 1914.
47. Webb et al. v. U.S., 249 U.S. 96.
48. Controlled Substances Act of 1970. Publ No 91-513, 84 Stat 1242, 1970.
49. Joranson DE. Federal and state regulation of opioids. J Pain Symptom Manage 5:S12–23, 1990.
50. US Department of Justice, Drug Enforcement Administration. Prescription Accountability Resource Guide, 1998.
51. Pain & Policy Studies Group. A guide to evaluation. Achieving balance in federal and state pain policy. Madison, WI: University of Wisconsin-Madison, 2000.
52. Code of Federal Regulations, Title 21; Part 1306.07 (C).
53. Pearson L. Fourteenth Annual Legislative update: how each state stands on legislative issues affecting advanced nursing practice. Nurse Pract 27:10–52, 2002.
54. Sigler KA, Guernsey BG, Ingrim NB, et al. Texas effects of a triplicate prescription law on prescribing of Schedule II drugs. Am J Hosp Pharm 41:108–11, 1984.
55. Zullich SG, Grasela TH Jr , Fiedler-Kelly, JB, Gengo FM. Impact of triplicate prescription program on psychotropic prescribing patterns in long-term care facilities. Ann Pharmacother 26:539–46, 1992.
56. Berina LF, Guernsey BG, Hokanson JA, et al. Physician perception of a triplicate prescription law. Am J Hosp Pharm 42:857–9, 1995.
57. Wastila LT, Bishop C. The influence of multiple copy prescription programs on analgesic utilization. J Pharm Care Pain Symptom Control 4:3–19, 1996.
58. Joranson DE, Carrow GM, Ryan KM, et al. Pain management and prescription monitoring. J Pain Symptom Manage 23:231–8, 2002.
59. Joranson DE. Single-copy serialized prescriptions: old regulation in new clothing. APS Bull 2:14–15, 1992.
60. Joranson DE, Gilson AM. State intractable pain policy: current status. APS Bull 7:7–9, 1997.
61. Joranson DE. State pain commission: new vehicles for progress? APS Bulletin 6(1):7–9, 1996.
62. California Board of Registered Nursing. Pain management policy. In: Summit on effective pain management: removing impediments to appropriate prescribing. Sacramento, CA: Department of Consumer Affairs, 1994:42.
63. Joranson DE, Gilson AM, Dahl JL, et al. Pain management, controlled substances and state medical board policy: a decade of change. J Pain Symptom Manage 23:138–47, 2002.

64. Michigan Medical Practice Act. MSA 14.15(16204a). See reference 51, page 220.

65. The Kentucky Board of Medical Licensure, KMA Ad Hoc Committee to Study Guidelines for Prescribing Controlled Substances: Guidelines for Prescribing Controlled Substances, June 20, 1996.

66. Federation of Medical Boards of the United States: Model guidelines for the use of controlled substances for the treatment of pain, May 1998. Available at http://www.medsch.wisc.edu/painpolicy.

67. Joranson DE, Cleeland CS, Weissman DE, Gilson AM. Opioids for chronic cancer and non-cancer pain: a survey of state medical board members. Fed Bull 4:15–49, 1992.

68. Hyman CS. Pain management and disciplinary action: how medical boards can remove barriers to effective treatment. J Law Med Ethics 24:338–43, 1996.

69. Gilson AM, Joranson DE. Controlled substances and state medical board policy: a decade of change. J Pain Symptom Manage 23:138–47, 2001.

70. Burns Ind. Code Ann § 35-42-1-2.5. See reference 51, page 152.

71. K.S.A. § 60-4403 (a). See reference 51, page 169.

72. Shapiro RS. Health care providers' liability exposure for inappropriate pain management. J Law Med Ethics 24:360–4, 1996.

73. Angarola R. Inappropriate pain management results in high jury award. J Pain Symptom Manage 6:407, 1991.

74. The Associated Press, Lexis Nexis Data Base. Oregon disciplines doctor for undertreating pain, Sept 2, 1999.

75. Oregon Board of Medical Examiners: Statement of philosophy. Appropriate prescribing of controlled substances. Adopted May 20, 1999.

76. A Joint Statement from 21 Health Organizations and the US Drug Enforcement Administration. Washington, DC. Promoting Pain Relief and Preventing Abuse of Pain Medications: A Critical Balancing Act. Available at http://www.lastacts.org:80/briefingoct01/consensus.pdf.

77. American Pain Society, American Academy of Pain Medicine: Consensus statement on the use of opioids in chronic pain, 1996. Available at www.ampainsoc.org – under "advocacy."

78. American Pain Society, American Academy of Pain Medicine, American Society of Addiction Medicine. Consensus Statement. Definitions related to the use of opioids in the treatment of pain, 2001. Available at www.ampainsoc.org – under "advocacy."

79. Joranson DE, Ryan KM, Gilson AM, Dahl JL. Trends in medical use and abuse of opioid analgesics. N Engl J Med 283:1710–14, 2000.

80. Dahl JL. New JCAHO standards focus on pain control. Oncol Issues 14:27–8, 1999.

81. Joint Commission on Accreditation of Healthcare Organizations. (2000). Comprehensive accreditation manual for hospitals (CAMH). Oakbrook Terrace, IL.

28 Role of family caregivers in cancer pain management

MYRA GLAJCHEN
Albert Einstein College of Medicine

Introduction

Family caregivers play a vital role in meeting the physical and psychosocial needs of patients with serious illness. The past 5 years have seen accelerating trends toward early hospital discharge, increasingly complex home-based treatment protocols, and the transformation of caregivers' role from promoting convalescence to participating actively in the accomplishment of treatment goals. In spite of the shift in care from the inpatient setting to the home, and the concomitant rise in the expectations of caregivers, the health care system has been slow to recognize the psychosocial and financial burden associated with caregiving.

It is estimated that more than 15 million adults currently provide care to relatives in the United States (1). Of these, most tend to be middle-aged children or older spouses, and predominantly female (2). Until recently, few studies had examined the role of family caregivers in pain management and palliative care, but this trend has changed within the past 5 years. Findings from recent landmark studies convey a picture of rising expectations and unmet needs for caregivers carrying out a variety of medical tasks at home (1–3). For example, Emanuel and colleagues (3) interviewed terminally ill adults and their caregivers to determine how their needs for assistance were being met. Unmet needs were reported by 87% of patients, who required help with transportation (62%), homemaking services (55%), nursing care (29%), and personal care (26%). Most patients relied completely on family and friends to provide this assistance; only 15% relied on paid assistance. For caregivers of cancer patients, such care may translate into 20 or more hours of care a week, the equivalent of a part-time (unpaid) job (2). In another study, caregivers' quality of life was found to be influenced by the cancer patient's stage of illness

and goals of care (4). One prospective, population-based cohort study found that caregiver strain increased mortality risk by 63% within 5 years (1). Caregiver strain is, therefore, a factor of importance to the treating physician. Conclusions from such studies provide valuable points of reference for analysis of the caregivers' role in cancer pain management.

Family caregivers become active members of the health care team with little or no preparation in disease management, sometimes under sudden and extreme circumstances. Specific caregiving responsibilities may change along the disease trajectory and among different care settings. Involvement of family caregivers is essential for optimal treatment of the cancer pain patient, in ensuring treatment compliance, continuity of care, and social support (5,6). Yet the health care system has undervalued caregiving, there is no reimbursement for caregiver education or instruction, and the system has not kept pace with caregivers' needs for education, information, and support.

This chapter discusses the role of the family caregiver in cancer pain management, the impact of caregiving on quality of life, caregivers' adaptational tasks at different points in the disease trajectory, caregivers' coping strategies, and professional strategies for intervention. Selected caregiver resources are listed in the Appendix.

Caregiving roles and responsibilities in cancer pain management

The role of family caregivers in cancer pain management has been documented in recent years. Common responsibilities include assessment and reporting of pain, dispensing medications, refilling prescriptions, providing non-pharmacological therapies, and engaging in decision making that affects treatment planning (Table 28.1).

Table 28.1. *Roles and responsibilities*

Assessing and reporting pain
Managing high-tech treatments
Filling and refilling prescriptions
Administering pain medications
Providing non-drug interventions
Assisting with treatment decision making

Caregivers are expected to assess and report the patient's pain, side effects, and new symptoms. This implies that caregivers must often function as nurses, attempting to determine the source, nature, and amount of pain (7). This can be problematic, given that patients may under-report pain symptoms while caregivers tend to overestimate their loved one's pain (8,9). Caregivers also play an important role in identifying and reporting treatment side effects, most often constipation and drowsiness. As these side effects can cause patients to abandon the pain treatment protocol, educating caregivers about anticipated side effects and strategies for their amelioration is essential.

With the advent of high-tech home care and pain management, family caregivers may be expected to help manage patient-controlled analgesia pumps, epidural catheters, and home infusions (10–12). The technical aspects of these interventions can be terrifying for even the most sophisticated of caregivers. Education of the patient and caregiver unit, followed by a visit or call from a pain nurse, can do much to alleviate such fears.

It generally falls to the caregiver of a patient with cancer to fill and refill pain prescriptions. This presupposes such skills as time management, proficiency with insurance reimbursement, competence in following medical instructions, and mathematical acuity to anticipate the need for refills ahead of time. Developing a long-standing relationship with a neighborhood pharmacy is also helpful to the caregiver at home. Although none of these skills can be presumed, it is generally beneficial to designate one member of the team to pay attention to these aspects of pain management.

The role of family caregivers in fostering or hindering treatment compliance should not be underestimated. Family caregivers frequently dispense pain medication or remind the patient to take a scheduled dose. Administration of pain medication involves deciding which type of medication to give, when, and in what dosage (13). Caregivers can encourage the patient to take medication as prescribed, to take a lesser dose than prescribed, or to "wait until the pain really gets bad." In such cases, a simplified treatment plan involving long- rather than short-acting opioids may

be optimal, and medications should be ordered around the clock, rather than prn (as needed).

Caregivers' knowledge and attitudes about pain management may influence the patient. If caregivers harbor fears of addiction, overdosing, or indirectly causing discomfort through side effects, they may guard the pain medication supply, limit its use, and undermedicate the patient (13). If caregivers stigmatize the use of opioids in general, or specific drugs such as methadone and meperidine, they will most likely project these fears onto the patient with pain.

Caregivers may play a role in providing non-drug pain management such as massage, use of lotions and ointment, heat and cold compresses, distraction, and relaxation (13). These techniques have been shown to be helpful as an adjunct to pain medication. In addition, through trial and error, caregivers may use positioning with pillows, mobilizing the patient, and assistance with ambulation in an effort to promote pain relief. Finally, caregivers provide patients with companionship and emotional support, conversation, and other forms of distraction.

Of more concern to the pain practitioner may be alternative health practices that can exacerbate cancer pain. Toxic side effects such as irreversible neuropathy, bleeding, electrolyte imbalance, and others can result from alternative medical approaches to cancer treatment (14). Desperate families may make erroneous decisions based on biased information in the media and on the Internet. Because patients and caregivers are reluctant to disclose their use of alternative therapies to the physician, it may be helpful to designate this oversight to another team member, such as the nurse or social worker.

Last, caregivers face an overwhelming array of decision making during the course of cancer diagnosis and treatment. Decisions about treatment options, role changes, and finances are generally made by the patient–family unit (6,15). Even in the context of a strong doctor–patient relationship, caregivers may be more open to information from other sources, both informal (family, friends) and formal (the Internet, Cancer Information Service, support groups). Therefore, enlisting the cooperation of family caregivers and including them as the unit of care from the outset are critical ingredients to effective cancer pain management.

Impact of family caregiving on quality of life

Caregivers of cancer patients have described the experience as affecting many domains of life. In general, caregiving is associated with high levels of chronic stress and emotional strain, especially in the context of an illness such as cancer. Ferrell and colleagues (16) developed a conceptual model for studying the impact of pain on quality of life in four distinct dimensions: physical, psychological, social, and spiritual well-being (Table 28.2). This model is applicable to both patients and their caregivers.

The *physical* demands of caregiving are closely related to medical variables, such as disease stage, level of symptomatology, functional ability, fatigue level, and side effect profile. Cancer patients will require varying levels of practical assistance during the course of the illness. If caregivers are on duty 24 hours a day, or just at night, cumulative sleep disruption and fatigue are common.

In the context of advanced disease and pain, it often falls to the family caregiver to manage disease symptoms and treatment side effects in the home setting. The literature has shown that the more time the caregiver spends doing tasks for the patient, the more disrupted will be the caregivers' schedule and emotional well-being. In addition, caregivers of patients in palliative care are shown to have significantly lower quality of life and physical health scores than caregivers of patients in active, curative treatment (4).

From a physical and practical point of view, caregiving has been described as relentless, marked by constant monitoring of the ill person's health status, provision of personal and nursing care, and assuming the duties of the ill family member. Although such physical impact is often obvious to the health care team, the emotional toll of caregiving can be overlooked. In this realm, caregivers describe stress and strain that parallel or surpass that of the patient. Because family members are at increased risk for stress-related problems, and we expect them to continue pain management in the home setting, it is essential to monitor them for emotional distress (6).

Psychological well-being is linked to anxiety, distress, and depression in the patient and caregiver. Family members confronting serious illness have been found to experience as much, if not more, distress as the person with cancer. This distress arises from the caregiver role itself as well as witnessing the patient's suffering (16). In addition, related personality characteristics such as optimism and

pessimism affect the psychological impact of caregiving. Family caregivers burdened by recent loss, stressful life events, or prior illness experiences unrelated to the patient's cancer may enter the new caregiving role already overwhelmed and depleted. Although the psychological needs of the caregiver may be beyond the scope of the pain management team, they are significant, in that they affect the quality of caregiving, as well as the likelihood of premature and unnecessary hospital admissions (15).

Researchers in the field have identified several factors that increase burden in oncology outpatients' caregivers. These include increasing patient dependency, impaired functioning, length of illness, and younger patient age. The impact of pain on caregiver burden has only recently been studied. Early findings suggest first, that patient suffering leads to family suffering, and second, that family caregivers tend to overestimate their family members' pain (15).

Miaskowski and colleagues (5,8) studied the impact of pain on caregivers' mood, health status, and strain among caregivers of oncology outpatients. They found that pain adversely affected the mood states of family caregivers, especially depression and anxiety levels. They found little impairment in health status and moderate caregiver strain among the caregivers of patients with pain. However, the family caregivers were caring for patients with high Karnofsky Performance Status scores who were still in active cancer treatment. These findings, therefore, are not generalizable to the experience of caregivers of patients with more advanced cancer.

Social well-being is affected by both the physical and emotional toll of caring for a loved one with cancer and pain over time. Roles and relationships can be affected if the person with cancer has to delegate family responsibilities to the caregiver. The nature and quality of the previous patient–caregiver relationship are also important considerations in assessment and treatment (17). If marital or relationship strain predates the onset of cancer or pain, the caregiver may approach caregiving grudgingly. Spouses may be elderly and infirm, in need of their own assistance, when caregiving responsibilities are thrust upon them. For adult caregivers, juggling the multiple demands of work, children, spouses, and caregiving for the cancer patient can be overwhelming. Approximately 70% of caregivers for cancer patients are spouses, 20% are adult daughters or daughters-in-law, and remaining 10% friends or extended family members (18). However, not all relationships are created equal, so the quality of that relationship and caregiving should be assessed on a case-by-case basis.

Table 28.2. *Impact on quality of life*

Physical impact
Psychological impact
Social impact
Spiritual impact

The financial impact and hidden costs of cancer pain management may also affect caregiver burden. For people with limited or no insurance, coverage for adequate pain relief may be sparse. More surprising is the financial burden incurred by families who have insurance, from deductibles, co-payments, uncovered services, such as transportation and home care, lost salaries and work, over-the-counter medications, household modifications, and alternative treatments such as herbs and vitamins (11). Limited numbers of prescriptions allowed by some insurers, as well as per month and refill limits, only add to caregiver burden in the context of pain management.

The social impact of cancer and pain can be ameliorated by social support, financial security, and stability at work. Given the chronicity of cancer in recent years, caregivers may find that support in all these areas erodes over time. Encouraging caregivers to network with other families and linking them with formal resources can help to augment informal sources of social support.

Spiritual well-being is increasingly recognized as a factor in pain management for both patients and their caregivers. This refers to the family's degree of religiosity, the meaning of pain to the family, and their existential perspective on hope and suffering (18). Degree of religiosity can be both a hindrance and a help in the pain management equation. To the extent that religion provides comfort, a belief system, and source of social support, it can be helpful to caregivers. To the extent that families believe in stoicism and suffering as the road to salvation, agreeing to administer pain medication can become problematic. Finally, the meaning of pain to the patient and caregiver can profoundly affect treatment outcomes in this area (19). In the setting of a cancer diagnosis, pain is generally emotionally laden in that it signifies advancing disease and eventual death. Because of such fears, patients and their family caregivers may under-report pain and other symptoms.

Adaptational tasks at different points in the disease trajectory

Given that most pain management, much end-of-life care, and even death take place at home, it is increasingly important to understand caregivers' roles at different points along the disease trajectory (20,21) (Table 28.3).

A family's response to cancer will vary according to the family's developmental needs, the demands placed on the family system, the role changes necessitated by the illness, and the repertoire of available coping skills (21). Functional families can act as a buffer for patients deal-

Table 28.3. *Disease trajectory adaptational tasks*

Tasks at diagnosis
Tasks during treatment
Tasks during recurrence
Tasks during terminal illness and dying

ing with cancer pain through four types of support: informational, emotional, instrumental, and affiliational. Advice and information can lessen the burden of decision making for the patient, love and encouragement can reduce isolation and distress, tangible support can meet the patient's concrete needs, and affiliational support can meet socialization needs (21). On the other hand, family problems can undermine the patient's ability to use medical care effectively, impair compliance with pain protocols, and complicate discharge planning (22). Such caregiver behaviors as making excessive demands on staff time, interfering directly with treatment, being unsupportive to the patient, and refusing to comply with medical unit guidelines are challenging clinical issues that require a comprehensive interdisciplinary treatment approach (23).

During the phase of diagnosis and treatment, caregivers experience a complex array of powerful emotions that can equal or surpass those of the person with cancer (24). The caregiver is expected to integrate medical information and play an active role in treatment decision making. This may involve unfamiliar terminology, new treatment settings, and frightening procedures or medications related to pain management (24). During active treatment for cancer, caregivers must juggle competing demands by trying to provide emotional and tangible support for the patient while also meeting ongoing obligations of home, work, and family. The demands of transportation, hospital visits, home care, and insurance can be physically and emotionally exhausting.

In the context of recurrent illness, terminal illness, or the dying process, the caregiver has to meet a new set of challenges in dealing with increasing functional limitations, increasing dependence of the patient, and greater symptom burden (25). If treatment is prolonged, the capacity of caregivers to meet the daily needs of patients is severely strained. In fact, the physical and emotional demands of caregiving reach their peak as the disease progresses to the terminal phase (24–26). In addition to assuming many of the patients' prior domestic responsibilities, family caregivers may be increasingly called on to function as nurses' aides. They may have to forego social activities and work duties that result in isolation and job insecurity. Weitzner and colleagues (4) found that family caregivers of palliative care patients had lower quality-of-life scores and worse overall physical health than caregivers of patients receiving curative treatment. As the cancer patient deteriorates, caregiver quality of life worsens. This is probably related to increased physical demands plus alterations in role functioning as caregivers take on additional responsibilities (27,28).

Coping strategies

Caregivers of cancer patients can acquire and develop coping strategies to help cope with their loved one's pain (Table 28.4).

Obtaining information about pain etiology, medical treatment options, and non-drug interventions can reduce helplessness and promote an active role in pain management. Such information can be found in various formats, including books, resource centers, and web sites, some of which are listed at the end of this chapter. Learning about available resources and knowing where and when to obtain professional help can help caregivers negotiate the health care system and decrease the sense of being overwhelmed.

Second, emotional, social, and peer support can do much to alleviate caregivers' sense of isolation. Caregivers should be encouraged to keep busy, maintain balance, take time away from caregiving, and pursue their own interests and social contacts. Visits from family and friends can serve to change the home environment and should be encouraged (29). Last, support groups with other caregivers can serve a dual purpose in providing both support and socialization.

Third, cognitive reappraisal (i.e., changing the meaning of the situation) has been shown to reduce caregivers' emotional distress. Many caregivers report both positive and negative aspects of caregiving. The positive aspects include an improved relationship with the patient, a sense of satisfaction and mastery over caregiving tasks, and feeling appreciated by the patient (2). Caregivers can be helped to reframe their appraisal of the situation through

individual or group counseling, and through empathic listening by the health care team.

Fourth, caregivers can be taught simple problem-solving techniques, such as taking things one step at a time and selecting what merits attention. Structured educational programs for caregivers have been found to reduce helplessness and improve coping. Such programs can be carried out in a formal setting (30–32) or in the home (11). In-person instruction, reinforced with printed materials, videotapes or audiotapes, promote development of new caregiving skills and offer caregivers an active role in disease and pain management.

Strategies for intervention

Health care professionals are encouraged to include family members in treatment planning and decision making. This is more likely to promote investment on the part of caregivers in the treatment protocol. However, they should not presume similarity nor treat the patient–family as a single unit of care (33). Instead, decisions regarding treatment, a care plan for pain management, and home care referrals should include careful assessment of the caregivers' physical and psychosocial status, as well as the home environment (34,35) (Table 28.5).

Emanuel and colleagues (36) found that caregiver burden was significantly reduced by physicians who practiced active listening. In their study, caregivers experienced less burden and distress if they believed that the treating physician listened to their needs and opinions. In this way, caregivers feel validated in their role, and they receive recognition and support for their caregiving activities.

In addition to listening, health care professionals are encouraged to provide information about pain management, so that common misconceptions about pain etiology, side effects, and opioid tolerance can be addressed (11). Common misconceptions are that pain medicine is addictive, treatment involves painful injections, the use of opioids for pain management signifies a terminal

Table 28.4. *Coping strategies*

Obtaining information
Obtaining emotional and social support
Cognitive reappraisal of the situation
Using problem-solving techniques

Table 28.5. *Professional intervention strategies*

Active listening
Providing information
Providing instruction in the use of pharmacological
    interventions
Providing instruction in the use of non-pharmacological
    interventions
Providing resource information
Considering finances
Providing support for the emotional aspects of caregiving

prognosis, and side effects of pain treatment can be debilitating. If members of the health care team take the time to address them, these misconceptions can be corrected. In the absence of accurate information, patients and caregivers are more susceptible to misinformation from informal sources. Accurate information helps to reduce uncertainty and empowers caregivers by giving them a sense of control. In addition, caregivers derive emotional support from time with the pain professional. In general, caregivers report needing information about their loved one's cancer, symptom etiology, what to expect in the future, treatment side effects, and management of medical emergencies (13).

The health care professional can offer caregivers instruction in the use of pharmacological and non-drug pain interventions to promote an active role in the care plan. Education for caregivers about pain etiology, rationale for selecting a treatment approach, around-the-clock dosing, anticipated side effects, and treatment of those side effects should become a routine part of medical practice. In addition, most caregivers report that they discover non-pharmacological pain management techniques informally, or by trial and error. A brief instructional session, reinforced with materials in print or electronic form, can serve as a catalyst for these techniques and provide guidance for the proper use of heat, cold, massage, positioning, imagery, distraction, and other techniques. This can be supplemented with referrals to support groups and educational programs in person, on-line, or by teleconference.

Recently, programs have been developed to teach caregivers intervention skills in the physical and psychological aspects of patient care (37,38). Conceptualizing caregiver skill, rather than impact or burden, allows for measurement, outcome assessment, and proactive teaching. This represents a fruitful line of inquiry for future research.

The health care professional can provide caregivers with resources for physical care, home health aides, respite programs, counseling, support groups, financial assistance programs, and others (15). They can provide guidance in negotiating the health care system, which can become unmanageable for overburdened and fatigued caregivers.

The Internet provides an important educational tool for patients and caregivers. However, a list of web sites is no substitute for professional communication; many sites presuppose a high reading level, and finding the correct information requires skill in negotiating search engines (39).

When developing a pain management care plan, members of the team should take financial realities into account, as cost can become a major factor in noncompliance (11). Costs associated with cancer pain management

include co-payments, deductibles, over-the-counter drugs, as well as hidden costs from transportation, tolls, parking, non-drug materials, environmental modifications, dietary needs, and lost wages.

Conclusion

Helping family caregivers cope increases their effectiveness as caregivers and improves their own quality of life (6). In addition to the practical assistance described previously, caregivers benefit from support and guidance for the emotional aspects of caregiving. Open communication about the patient's mood swings; the caregivers' shift from partner, parent, or child to caregiver; and the concomitant suffering or resentment can be therapeutic. Medical personnel should discuss the emotional aspects of relieving pain, such as fears of hurting the patient, fears of giving an overdose, and fears of creating intolerable side effects (13). Encouragement can be provided about the management of anger, depression, and hopelessness. Other opportunities for emotional expression and social support should be identified and maximized. If caregivers are helped to maintain hope and a positive attitude, they will be more likely to continue caregiving. Early recognition of psychological vulnerability among families is essential to develop specific interventions to promote coping, alleviate anxiety, and encourage problem solving (25,40).

References

1. Schulz R, Beach SR. Caregiving as a risk factor for mortality: The Caregiver Health Effects Study. JAMA 282:2215–19, 1999.
2. United Hospital Fund. A survey of family caregivers in New York City: findings and implications for the health care system. New York: United Hospital Fund, 2000.
3. Emanuel EJ, Fairclough DL, Slutsman J, Emanuel LL. Understanding economic and other burdens of terminal illness: the experience of patients and their caregivers. Ann Intern Med 132:451–9, 2000.
4. Weitzner MA, McMillan S, Jacobsen PB. Family caregiver quality of life: differences between curative and palliative cancer treatment settings. J Pain Symptom Manage 17:418–28, 1999.
5. Miaskowski C, Kragness L, Dibble S, Wallhagen M. Differences in mood states, health status and caregiver strain between family caregivers of oncology patients with and without cancer-related pain. J Pain Symptom Manage 13:138–47, 1997.
6. Warner JE. Involvement of families in pain control of terminally ill patients. Hospice J 8(1–2):155–70, 1992.

7. Taylor EJ, Ferrell BR, Grant M, Cheyney L. Managing cancer pain at home: the decisions and ethical conflicts of patients, family caregivers and homecare nurses. Oncol Nurs Forum 20:919–27, 1993.

8. Miaskowski C, Zimmer EF, Barrett KM, et al. Difference in patients and family caregivers' perceptions of the pain experience influence patient and caregiver outcomes. Pain 72:217–26, 1997.

9. Kornblith AB, Herr HW, Ofman US, et al. Quality of life of patients with prostate cancer and their spouses: the value of a database in clinical care. Cancer 73:2791–802, 1994.

10. Ferrell BR, Taylor EJ, Grant M, Corbisiero RM. Pain management at home: struggle, comfort and mission. Cancer Nurs 16(3):169–78, 1993.

11. Ferrell BR, Dean G. Ethical issues in pain management at home. J Palliat Care 10(3):67–72, 1994.

12. Coyle N, Cherny NI, Portenoy RK. Subcutaneous opioid infusions at home. Oncology 8(4):21–7, 1994.

13. Juarez G, Ferrell BR. Family and caregiver involvement in pain management. Clin Geriatr Med 12(3):531–47, 1996.

14. Montbriand MJ. An overview of alternate therapies chosen by patients with cancer. Oncol Nurs Forum 21:1547–54, 1994.

15. Vachon MLS. Psychosocial needs of patients and families. J Palliat Care 14(3):49–56, 1998.

16. Ferrell BR, Rhiner M, Cohen MZ, Grant M. Pain as a metaphor for illness. Part I. Impact of cancer pain on family caregivers. Oncol Nurs Forum 18:1303–9, 1991.

17. Hinton J. Can home care maintain an acceptable quality of life for patients with terminal cancer and their relatives? Palliat Med 8(3):183–96, 1994.

18. Ferrell BR. The family. In: Doyle D, Hanks GWC, MacDonald N, eds. Oxford textbook of palliative medicine. Oxford: Oxford University Press, 1998:909–17.

19. Yeager KA, Miaskowski C, Dibble SL, Wallhagen M. Differences in pain knowledge and perception of the pain experience between outpatients with cancer and their family caregivers. Oncol Nurs Forum 22(8):1235–41, 1995.

20. Glajchen M. Psychosocial issues in cancer care. In: Miaskowski C, Buchsel P, eds. Oncology nursing: assessment and clinical care. St. Louis: Mosby, 1999:305–18.

21. Kristjanson LJ, Ashcroft T. The family's cancer journey: a literature review. Cancer Nurs 17:1–17, 1994.

22. Blanchard CG, Albrecht TL, Ruckdeschel JD, et al. The role of social support in adaptation to cancer and survival. J Psychosoc Oncol 13:75–95, 1995.

23. Zabora JR, Smith ED, Baker F, et al. The family: the other side of bone marrow transplantation. J Psychosoc Oncol 10:35–46, 1992.

24. Sales E. Psychosocial impact of the phase of cancer on the family: an updated review. J Psychosoc Oncol 9:1–18, 1991.

25. Anderson JL. The nurses role on cancer rehabilitation: a review of the literature. Cancer Nurs 12:85–94, 1989.

26. Rose K. How informal carers cope with terminal cancer. Nurs Stand 11(30):39–42, 1997.

27. Hansom LC, Danis M, Garrett J. What is wrong with end-of-life care? Opinions of bereaved family members. J Am Geriatr Soc 45:1339–44, 1997.

28. Cherny NI, Coyle N, Foley K. Guidelines in the care of the dying cancer patient. Hematol Oncol Clin North Am 10(1):261–86, 1996.

29. Steele RG, Fitch MI. Coping strategies of family caregivers of home hospice patients with cancer. Oncol Nurs Forum 23(6):955–60, 1996.

30. Bucher JA, Houts PS, Nezu CM, Nezu AM. Improving problem-solving skills of family caregivers through group education. J Psychosoc Oncol 16(3/4):73–84, 1999.

31. Glajchen M, Moul JW. Teleconferencing as a method of educating men about managing advanced prostate cancer and pain. J Psychosoc Oncol 14:73–87, 1996.

32. Robinson KD, Angeletti KK, Barg FK, et al. J Cancer Educ 13:116–21, 1998.

33. Ward SE, Berry PE, Misiewicz H. Concerns about analgesics among patients and family caregivers in a hospice setting. Res Nurs Health 19:205–11, 1996.

34. Berry PE, Ward SE. Barriers to pain management in hospice: a study of family caregivers. The Hospice J 10(4):19–33, 1995.

35. Jepson C, McCorkle R, Adler D, et al. Effects of home care on caregivers' psychosocial status. J Nurs Scholarship 31:115–20, 1999.

36. Emanuel EJ, Fairclough DL, Slutsman J, et al. Assistance from family members, friends, paid care givers and volunteers in the care of terminally ill patients. N Engl J Med 341:956–63, 1999.

37. McCorkle R, Pasacreta JV. Enhancing caregiver outcomes in palliative care. Cancer Control 8(1):36–45, 2001.

38. Schumacher KL, Stewart BJ, Archbold PG, et al. Family caregiving skill: development of the concept. Res Nurs Health 23(3):191–203, 2000.

39. Berland GK, Elliott MN, Morales LS, et al. Health information on the Internet: accessibility, quality, and readability in English and Spanish. JAMA 285(20):2612–21, 2001.

40. Ferrell BR, Johnston Taylor E, Grant M, Corbisiero RM. Pain management at home: struggle, comfort and mission. Cancer Nurs 16(3):169–78, 1993.

Appendix: Selected Caregiver Resources

Web Sites

Caregivers.com
www.caregivers.com
Provides information from AgeNet on caregiving for aging relatives. Includes listings of care managers, senior care facilities, housing options, hospice search, lawyer search, and geriatrician search.

Caregiving.com
www.caregiving.com
Publishes a newsletter, handbook, and manual for family caregivers, as well as a monthly advice column and support group.

Familycare America

www.familycareamerica.com

Provides general information about local resources, tools, and products for older or seriously ill people and their caregivers. Also provides support groups and discussion forums.

National Alliance for Caregivers

www.caregiving.org

Provides resources, tips, events, survey results, reports, and products. Provides a network of partners and affiliates.

Well Spouse Foundation

www.wellspouse.org

A member organization for partners of the chronically ill or disabled. Provides support groups in some areas, letter writing campaigns, a bi-monthly newsletter, and an annual conference.

Department of Pain Medicine and Palliative Care, Beth Israel Medical Center

www.StopPain.org

Provides information for caregivers of patients with advanced medical disease, regarding the practical and emotional aspects of caregiving. Also provides access to a user-friendly, free Caregiver Resource Directory.

Cancer Care

www.Cancercare.org

Provides a brief caregiver section on dealing with side effects, tips on caregiving, emotional issues, the workplace, and links to other on-line resources.

Books/guides

American Cancer Society. Caring for the patient with cancer at home: a guide for patients and families. Atlanta: American Cancer Society, 1998.

Beedle J, Dunn L, eds. The carebook: a workbook for caregiver peace of mind. Portland, OR: Lady Bug Press, 1991.

Brammer L, Bingea M. Caring for yourself while caring for others: a caregiver's survival and renewal guide. New York: Vantage Press, 1999.

Brandt A. Caregiver's reprieve: a guide to emotional survival when you're caring for someone you love (the Working Caregiver series). San Luis Obispo, CA: Impact Publishers, 1997.

Cancer Care. A helping hand: the resource guide for people with cancer. New York: Cancer Care, Incorporated, 1996.

Glajchen M, Portenoy RK, Fraidin L, Goelitz, A. The caregiver resource directory: a practical guide for family caregivers, 2nd ed. New York: Beth Israel Medical Center, 2001.

Hereema C. A caregiver's guide to giving medicines. Upper Saddle River: NJ, Prentice Hall, 1999.

Houts P. American College of Physicians home care guide for cancer: for family and friends giving care at home. Philadelphia: American College of Physicians, 1994.

Ilardo J, Rothman C. I'll take care of you: a practical guide for family caregivers. Oakland, CA: New Harbinger, 1999.

Levine C, ed. Always on call: when illness turns families into caregivers. New York: United Hospital Fund, 2000.

Lipsyte R. In the country of illness: comfort and advice for the journey. New York: Alfred A. Knopf, 1998.

McFarlane R, Bashe P. The complete bedside companion: a no-nonsense guide to caring for the seriously ill. New York: Fireside, 1999.

McGonigle C. Surviving your spouse's chronic illness: a compassionate guide. New York: Henry Holt & Company, 1999.

Meyer M, Derr P, Hatfield M. The comfort of home: an illustrated step-by-step guide for caregivers. Portland, OR: Care Trust Publications, 1998.

National Family Caregivers Association. The resourceful caregiver: helping family caregivers help themselves. St. Louis: Mosby, 1996.

Olshevski J, Katz A, Knight B. Stress reduction for caregivers. Philadelphia: Brunner/Mazel, 1999.

Ortho Biotech. Strength for caring: education and support for family cancer caregivers. Raritan, NJ: Ortho Biotech, Inc, 1998.

Schonhoff S, Speaker J. Family caregiver guide: a comprehensive handbook for caring for your loved one at home. Dubuque, IA: Simon & Kolz Publishing, 1998.

Visiting Nurse Associations of America. Caregiver's handbook: a complete guide to home health care. New York: DK Publishing, 1998.

Index